HOSPITALS & HEALTH FACILITIES

LINKS

HOSPITALS & HEALTH FACILITIES

Author: Jacobo Krauel & Carles Broto Comerma
Editorial coordination: Jacobo Krauel
Graphic design & production: Roberto Bottura, architect
Collaborator: Oriol Vallés, graphic designer
Text: Contributed by the architects, edited by Jay Noden

© LINKSBOOKS
Jonqueres, 10, 1-5
08003 Barcelona, Spain
Tel.: +34-93-301-21-99
Fax: +34-93-301-00-21
info@linksbooks.net
www.linksbooks.net

© This is a collective work. In accordance with Intellectual Property Law "collective works" are NOT necessarily those produced by more than one author. They have been created by the initiative and coordination of one person who edits and distributes them under his/her name. A collective work constitutes a collection of contributions from different authors whose personal contributions form part of a creation, without it being possible to separately attribute rights over the work as a whole.

© All rights reserved. No part of this book may be used or reproduced in any manner whatsoever without written permission except in the case of brief quotations embodied in critical articles and reviews.

Printed in China

HOSPITALS & HEALTH FACILITIES

LINKS

INDEX

07 INTRODUCTION

08 JDS Architects
Psychiatric Hospital (PSY)

16 Nickl & Partner
Mother and Child Center

26 Burger Grunstra Architects
Martini Hospital

42 Allford Hall Monaghan Morris
Kentish Town Health Centre

52 C. F. Møller Architects
Akershus University Hospital

68 Carvajal + Casariego / Baquerizo Cruz Petrement
San Pedro Hospital

84 Perkins Eastman
Queens Hospital Center: Ambulatory Care Pavilion

92 Pinearq. S.L
Quirón Hospital

110 Corea, Quijano, Codina. Secretaria Salud Pública Rosario
Clemente Alvarez Emergency Hospital

120 Argola Arquitectos
Tajo Hospital

Carvajal + Casariego/ Baquerizo Cruz Petrement Reina Sofía Hospital	**140**
KMD Architects CHA Women and Children's Hospital	**154**
Corea & Moran Arquitectura Mahón Hospital	**174**
Estudio Lamela Center For Alzheimer Patients	**186**
Tonet Sunyer Arquitecte - LKS Estudio Villablino Hospital	**204**
Estudio Entresitio CEDT Daimiel	**220**
Groupe-6 Arras Hospital	**238**
Stantec Architecture Ltd. Peterborough Regional Health Centre	**244**
Carvajal + Casariego / Baquerizo Cruz Petrement Marqués de Valdecilla Hospital	**254**
CSPE & Anshen + Allen Meyer Children's Hospital	**276**
Anshen + Allen The Bexley Wing, St James's Institute of Oncology	**290**

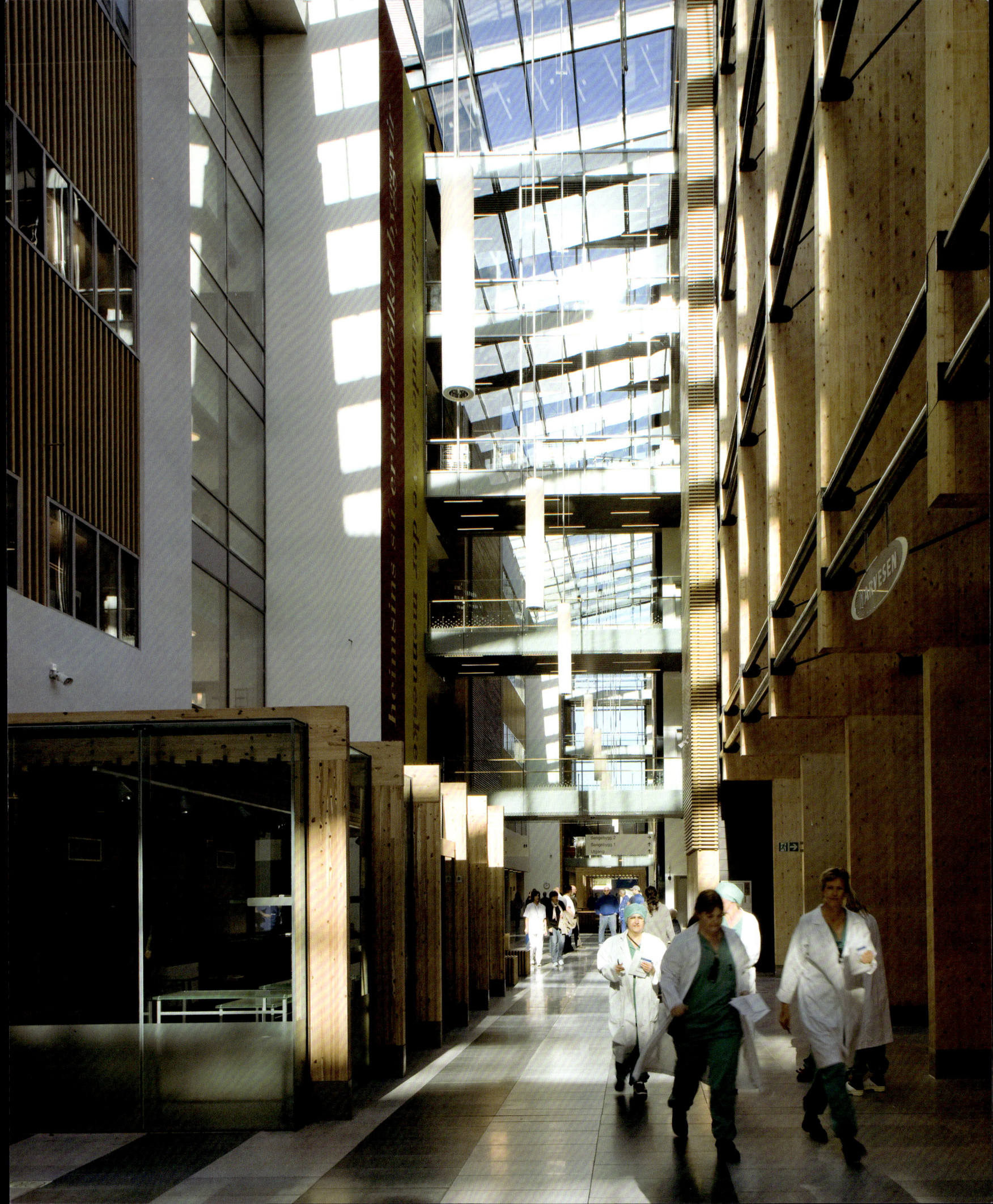

INTRODUCTION

As this new century dawns concerns for healthcare, keeping fit and taking care of our bodies are, without doubt, among the most central concerns of our society.

Now we have understood that life often begins and ends in hospitals, and have seen how healthcare centers themselves along with the professionals who work in them endeavor to make our journey through life as bearable and healthy as possible, a new take on hospital architecture is also beginning to show a human side.

The challenging task of developing the architecture for clinics and hospitals should be seen as an art. These skilful professionals are capable of providing us with a desirable level of well-being, while at the same time avoiding hospital stays being what many people still consider to be excessively uncomfortable.

The projects presented in this book reveal the new trends in architecture for hospitals of the future. This is a formidable undertaking in which the functionality required by all hospitals, which needs to be adaptable to changing computer systems and sophisticated medical equipment, must combine with an aesthetic that is pleasant for patients, visitors and medical staff alike.

This combination is complemented with circulation and access systems that must be comfortable and efficient, since at times a matter of minutes can prove crucial in a building of this type.

Hospitals often function as small towns: people come and go, there are different specialist departments to attend to different needs, people sleep, eat and shop there, and often a stay may be extended unexpectedly. This is why throughout these projects one can appreciate the presence of natural light, which has become a fundamental factor in allowing the different spaces to be transformed into environments that meet the demands these centers make today. Some situations, for example, may call for a simple, quiet shady area, while others require the brightness and clarity of fluorescent lighting.

The selection of projects presented in this book show some of the most modern and innovative projects in the field. Work carried out by architects who are sensitive to these changes in mentality and which is accompanied here by plans and constructive details that help to understand the different channels of expression. This truly representative and up-to-date compilation would suggest that the days when healthcare centers were synonymous with coldness and discomfort are coming to an end. Today's hospitals offer a new class of space; one which upholds the high standards that we as a society are coming to expect.

JDS Architects

Psychiatric Hospital (PSY)

Helsingør, Denmark

Photographs: Nikolaj Møller

As the basis for the development of this design, Danish studio JDS architects interviewed patients, personnel and relatives connected with the psychiatric hospital. Although the exercise did not reveal concrete truths, a series of paradoxes became evident. The PSY needed to combine the efficiency of a central organization with the freedom and autonomy of a decentralized complex. It needed to allow control and protection while maintaining a free and open atmosphere.

In terms of function the PSY is a logistically optimized hospital and in terms of experience it is anything but a hospital. Located in a natural setting, surrounded by grassland, within view of small areas of woodland and on the edge of a small lake, the hospital offers its patients a calming atmosphere, yet one which is full of life. The building itself is a far cry from the traditionally imposing psychiatric blocks of the past. The PSY develops horizontally, across one or in places two levels, and is therefore on a scale that is easy to grasp for patients and visitors alike, and not at all imposing. Homely spaces have been created which are clutter-free, but at the same time warm and friendly. Passageways are wide and both vertical and horizontal surfaces are finished in white and light green with the occasional splash of more intense colors, which help to distinguish different areas. The color scheme has been carefully chosen to be both serene and stimulating.

All façades are glazed affording patients views of their natural surroundings from wherever they are in the building and allowing natural light to flood the interiors. In this way the PSY forms a strong connection with the exterior in an environment where patients can feel at ease and totally safe.

The building consists of a series of modules that reach out from a central communal area. Each module has views of the surroundings as well as at least two other modules. This avoids patients feeling 'lost' inside the building since they always have several reference points close to hand. The arrangement also enables staff to reach all parts of the hospital quickly and helps those unfamiliar with the hospital to find their way around. The landscaped spaces between the modules generate semi-enclosed outdoor areas, which are delineated by the building itself or the natural elements that surround it. These spaces include wooden garden furniture and flowerbeds and can be accessed directly from the building through French windows.

The PSY can be reached directly from the main hospital by way of a long glazed corridor which connects the two buildings. A service road also provides direct access.

Client:
Frederiksborg County Council
Surface area:
6,000 sqm (64,600 sqft)
Finish Date:
2006
Collaborators:
Plot Architects, BIG Architects
Cost:
€ 11 million

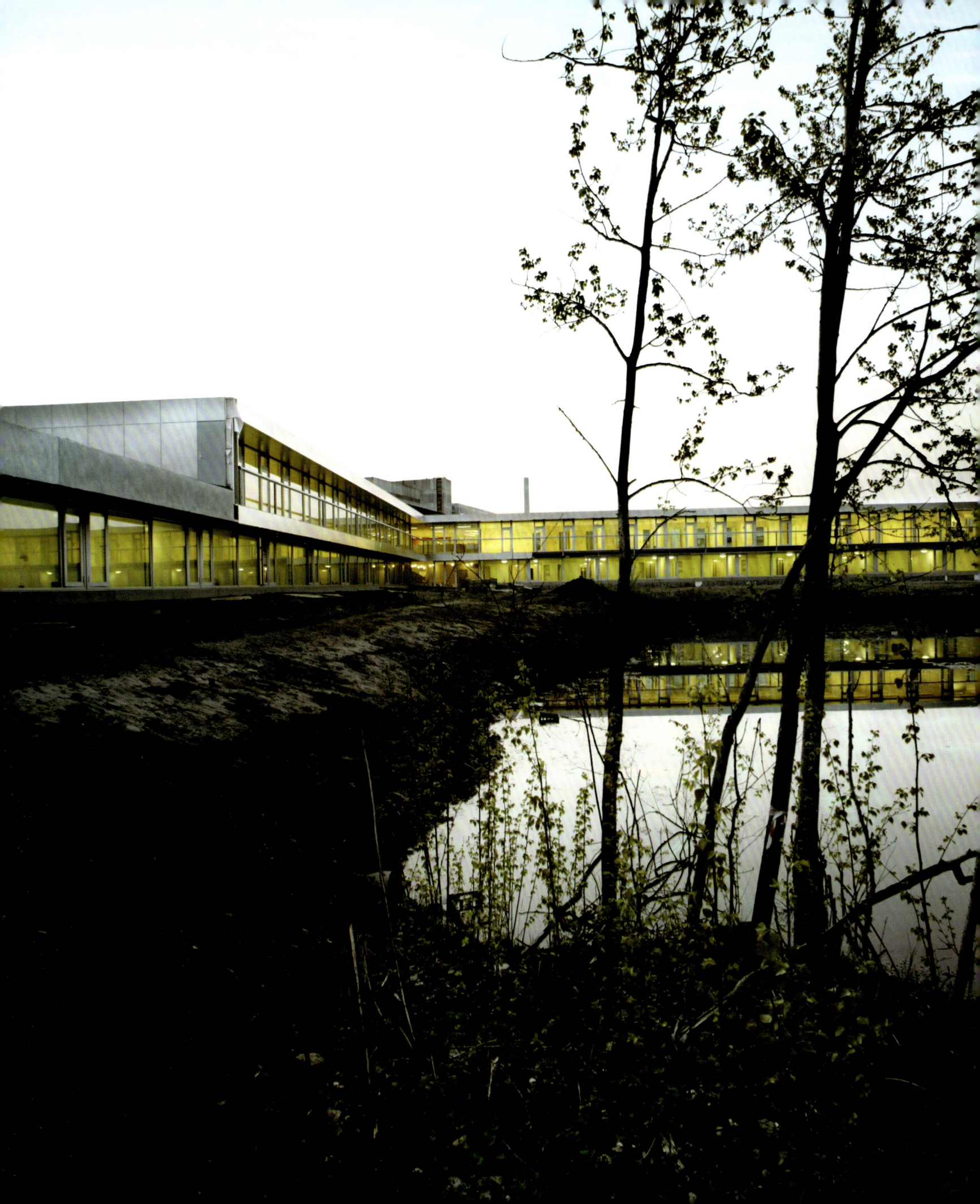

10

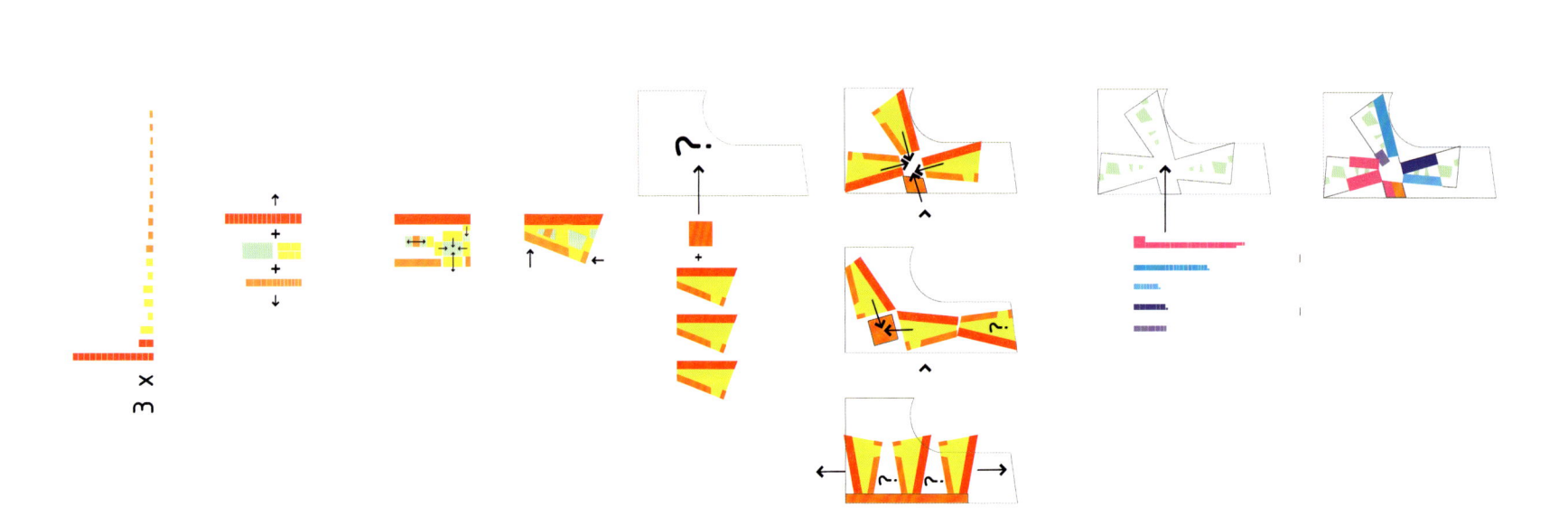

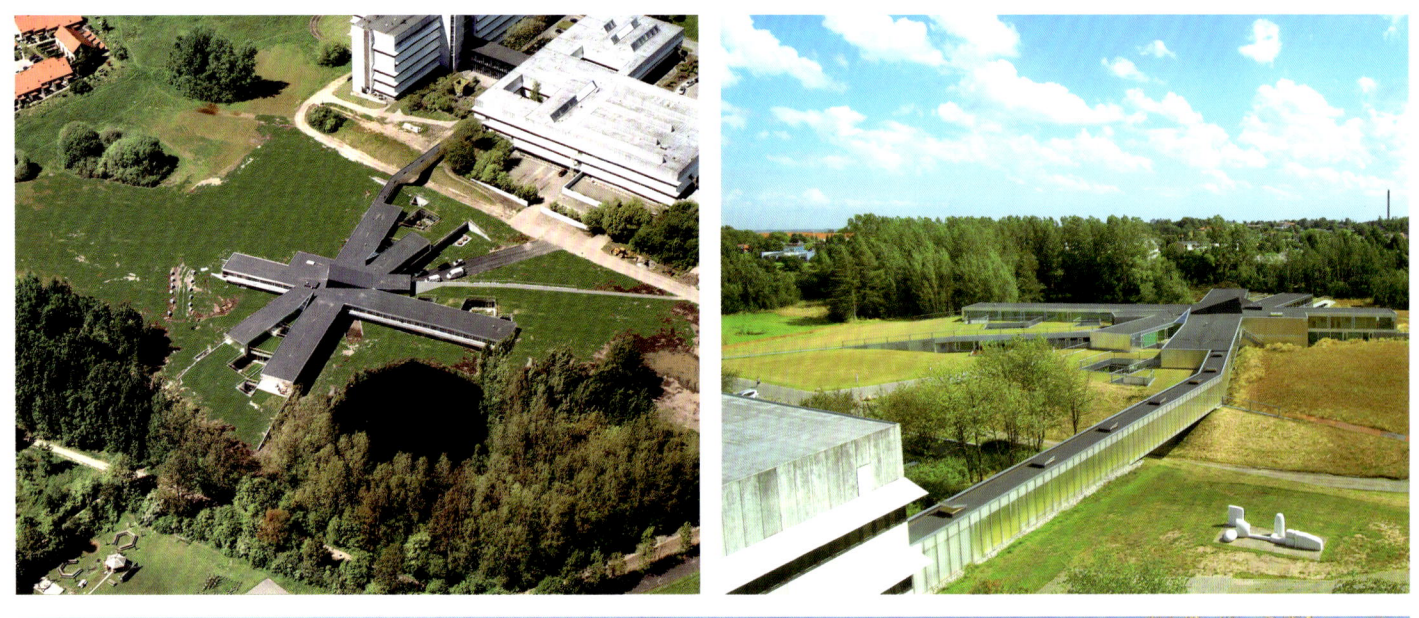

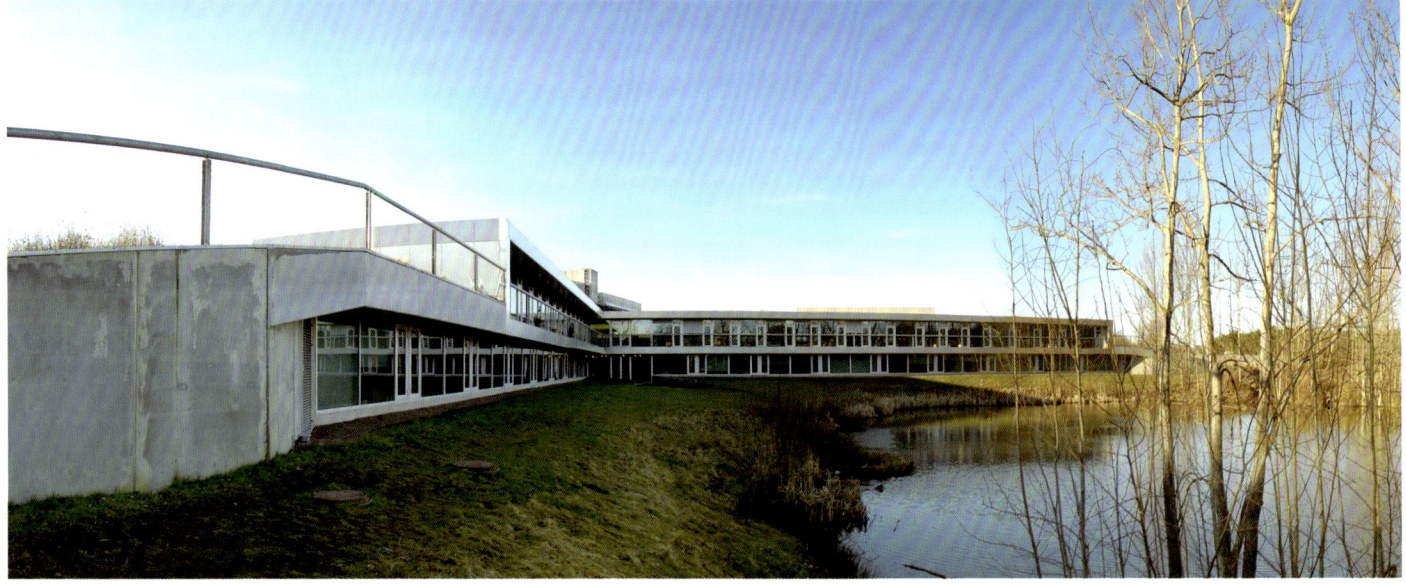

11

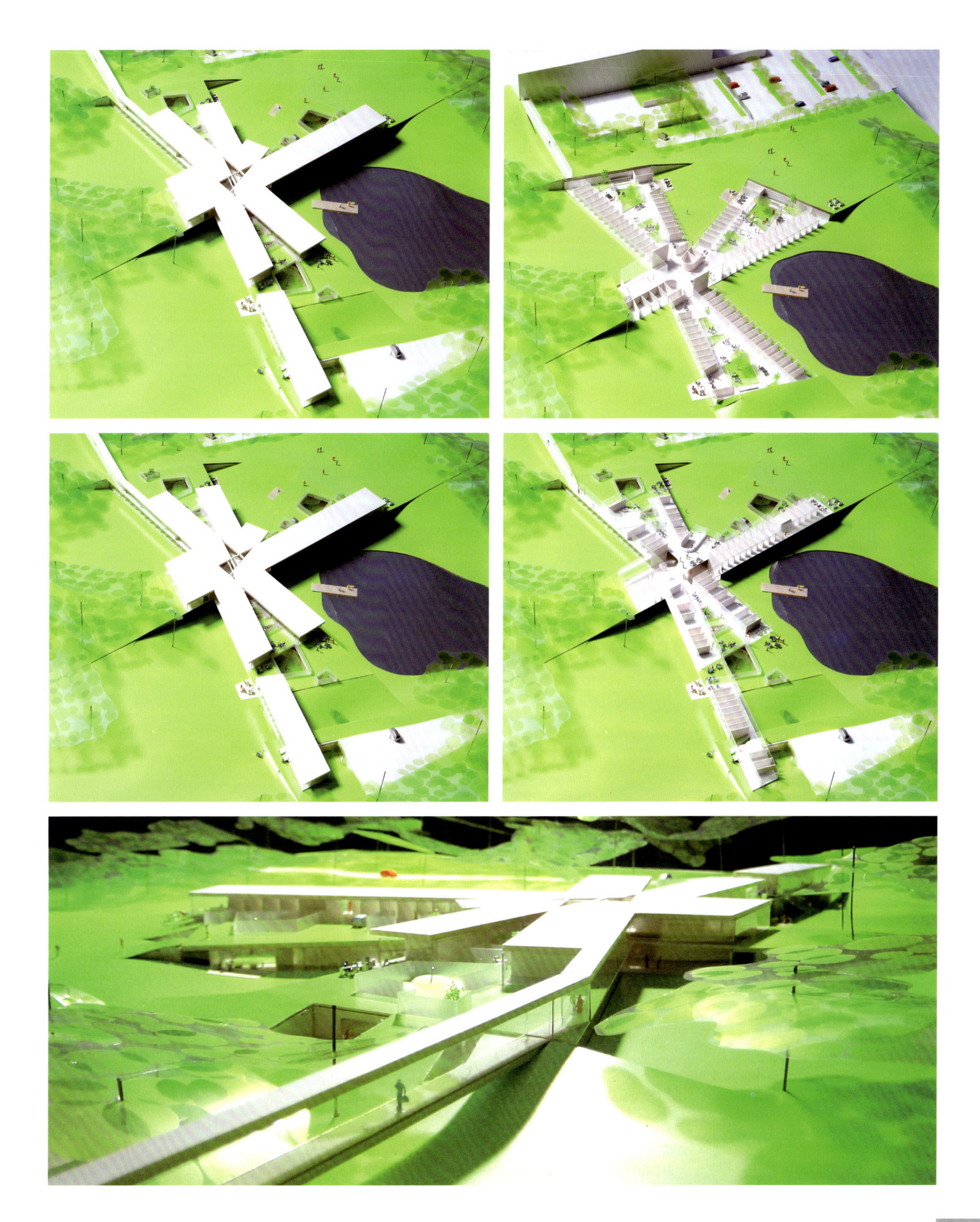

← Konference 2725

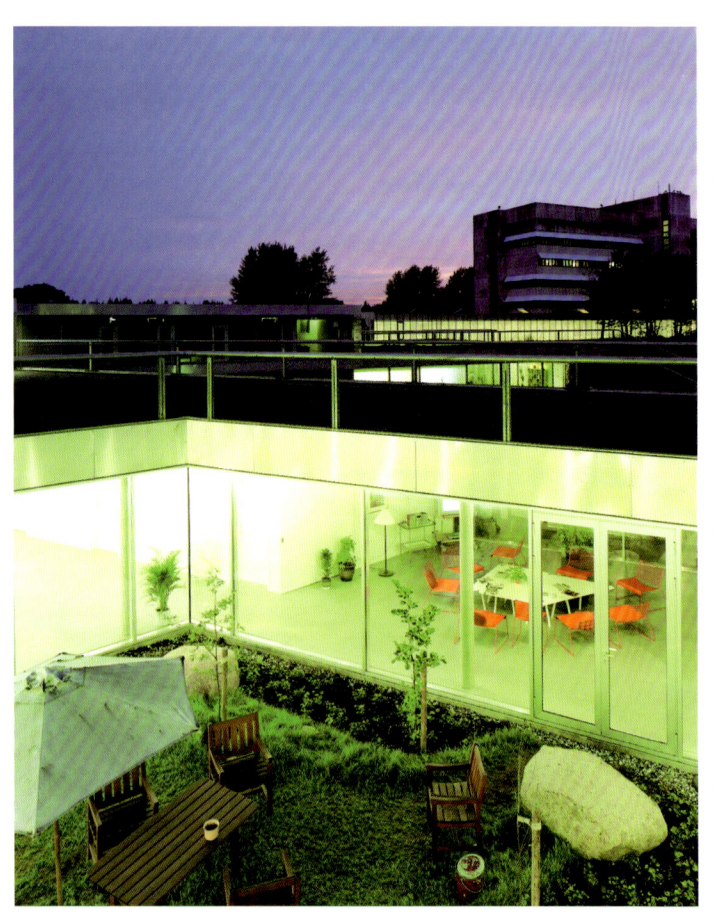

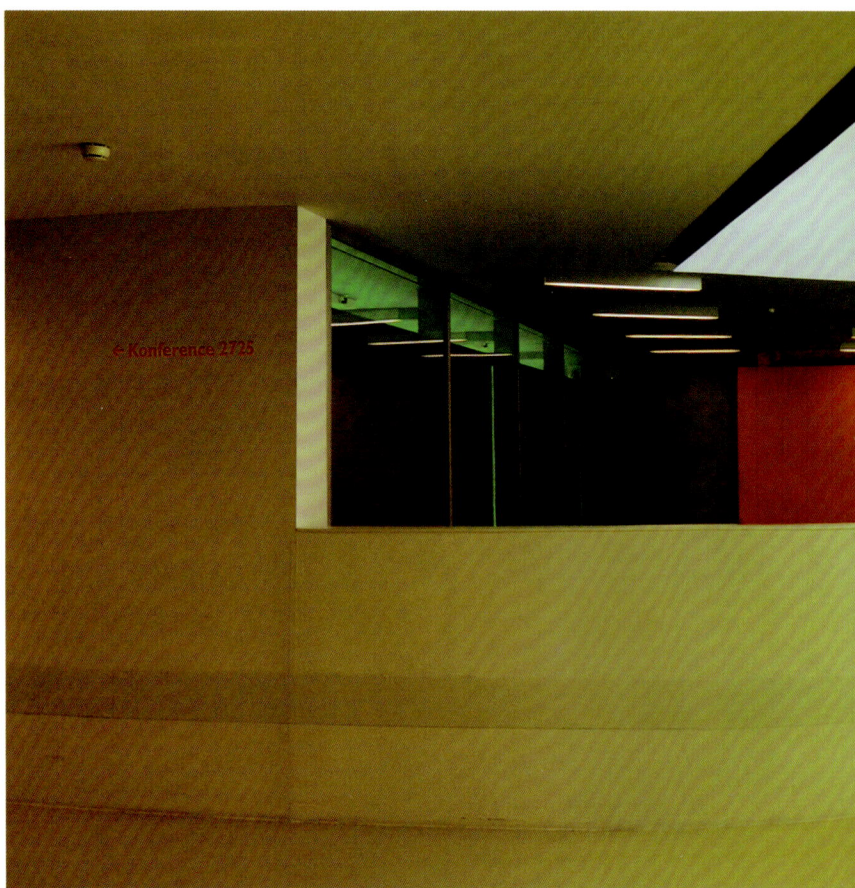

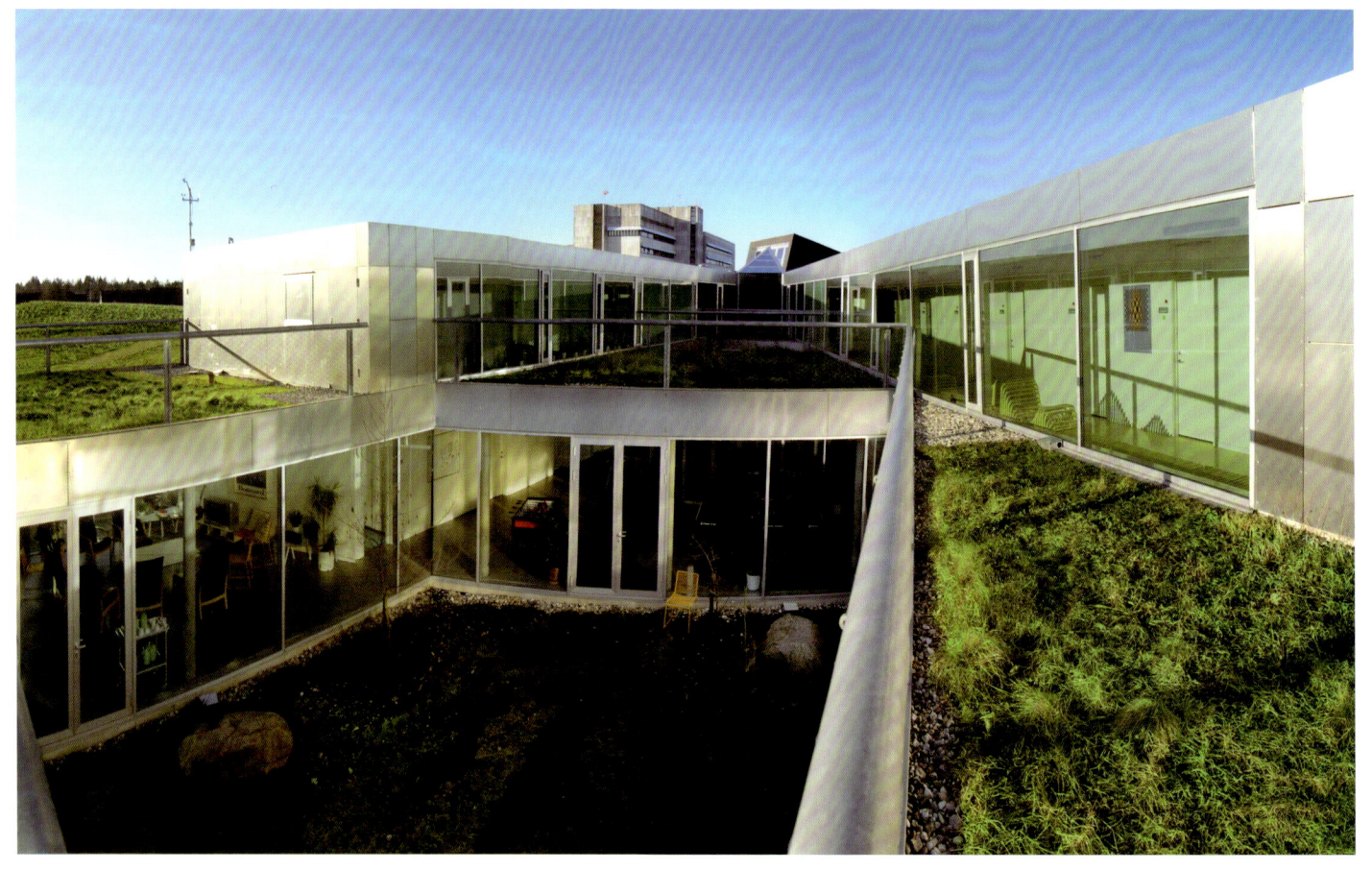

13

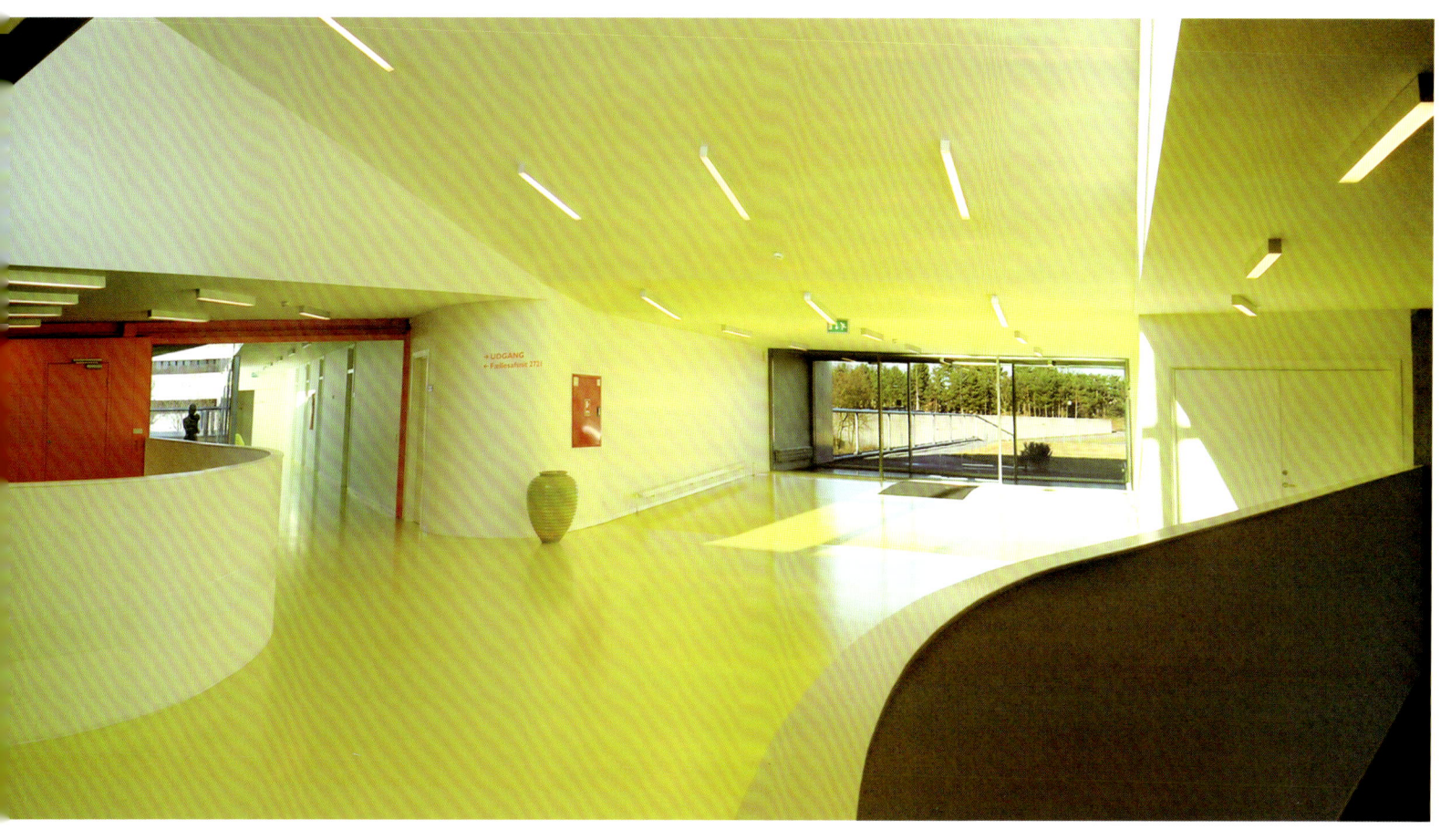

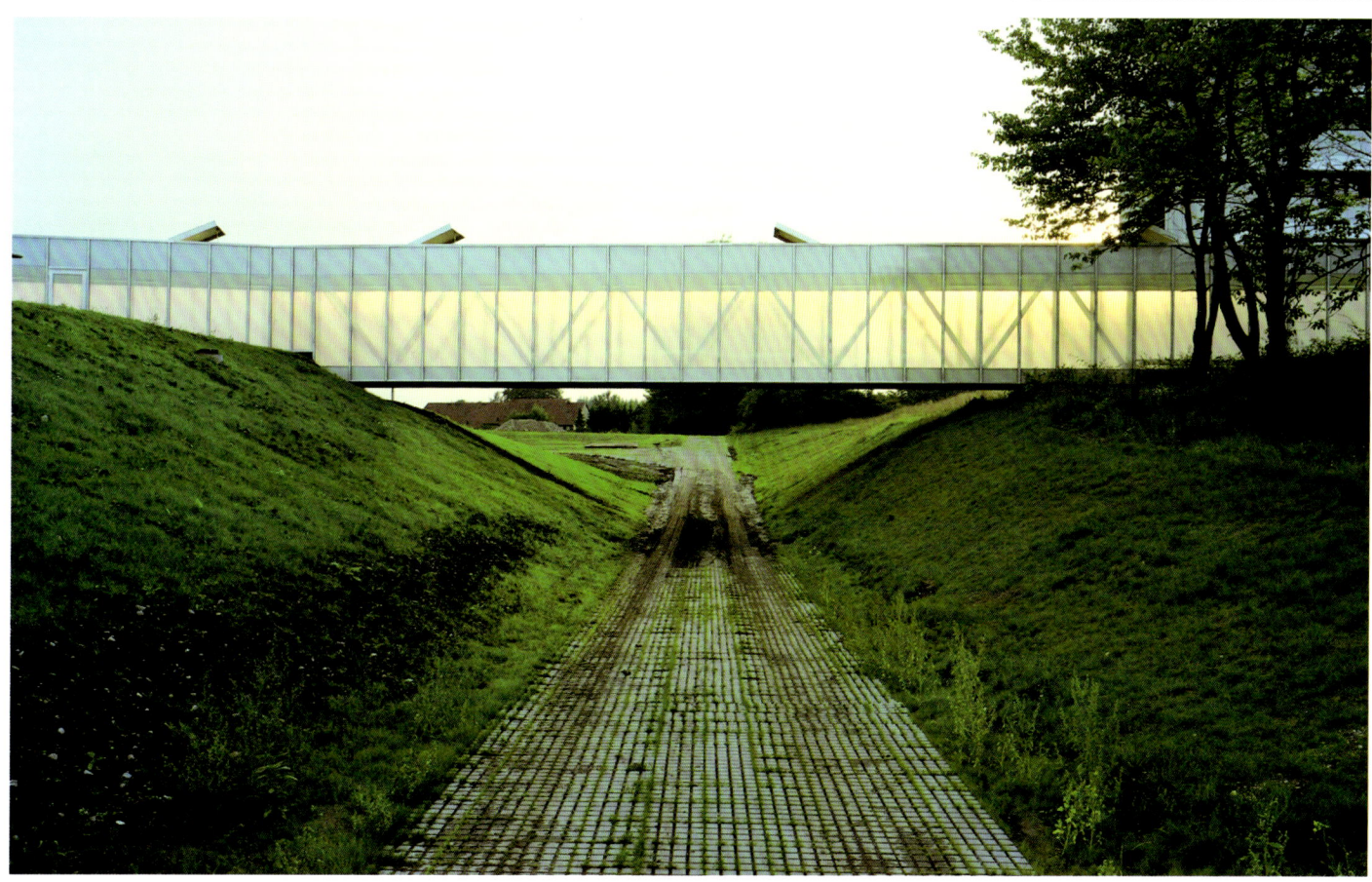

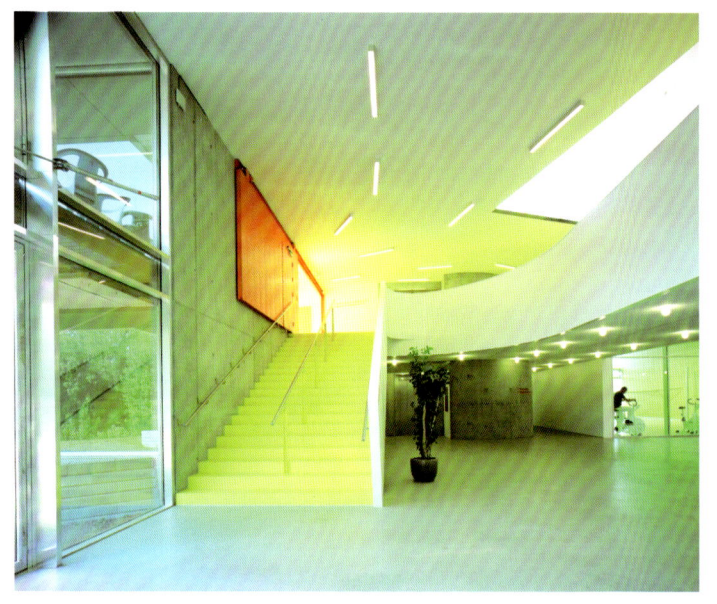

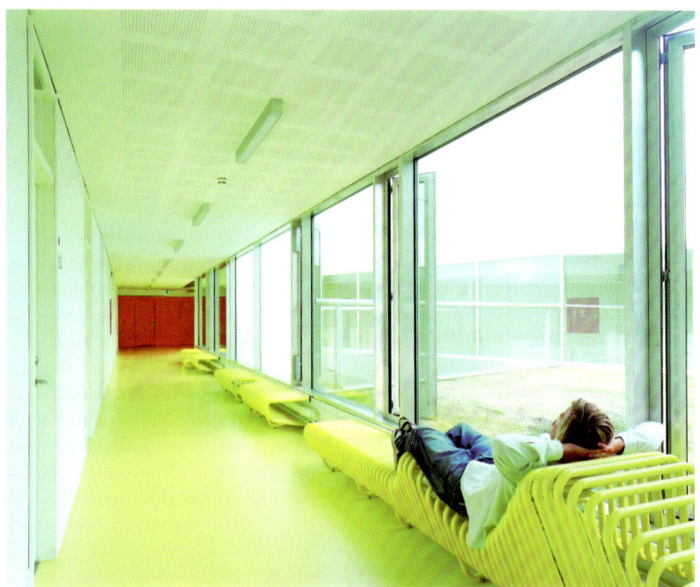

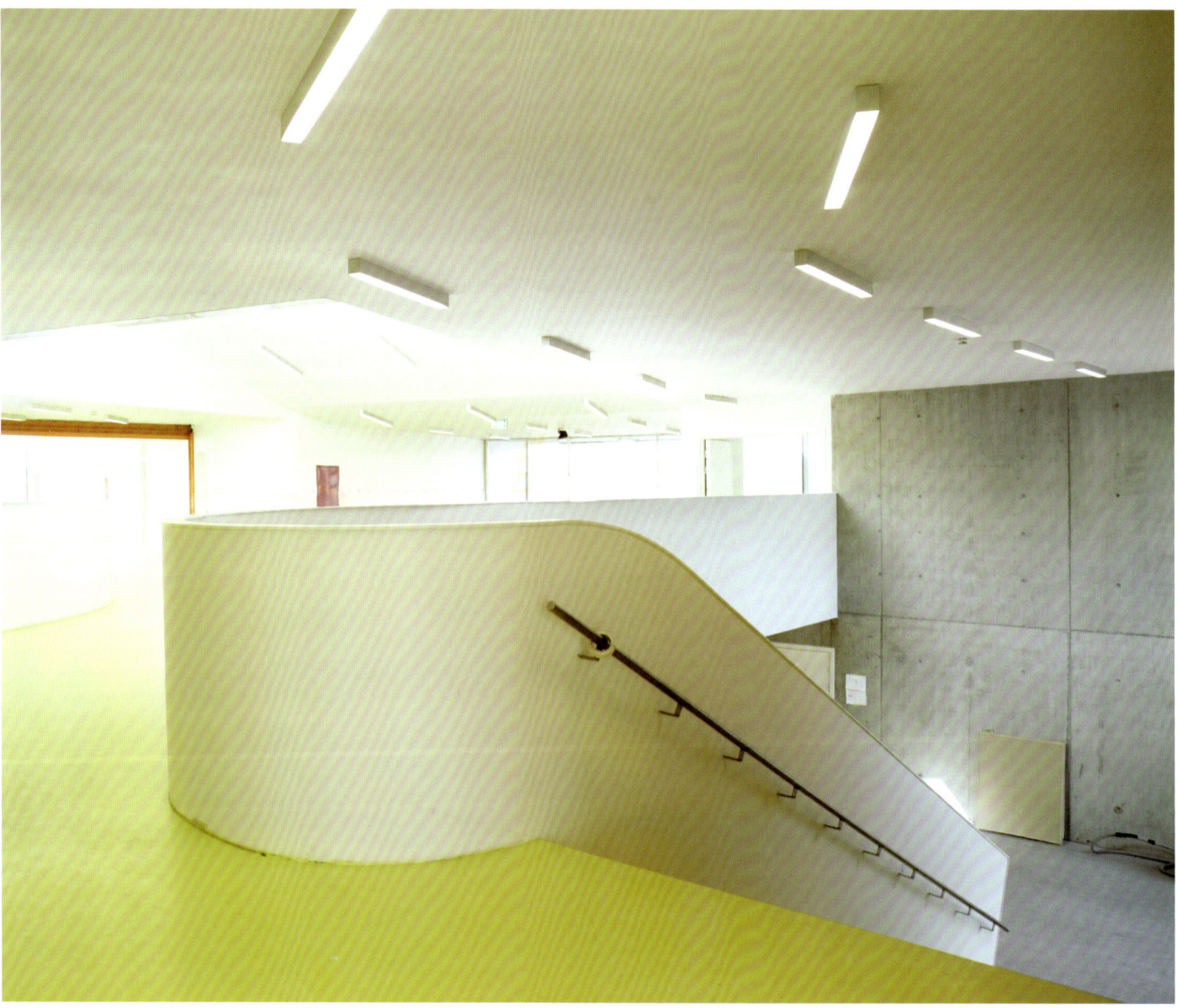

15

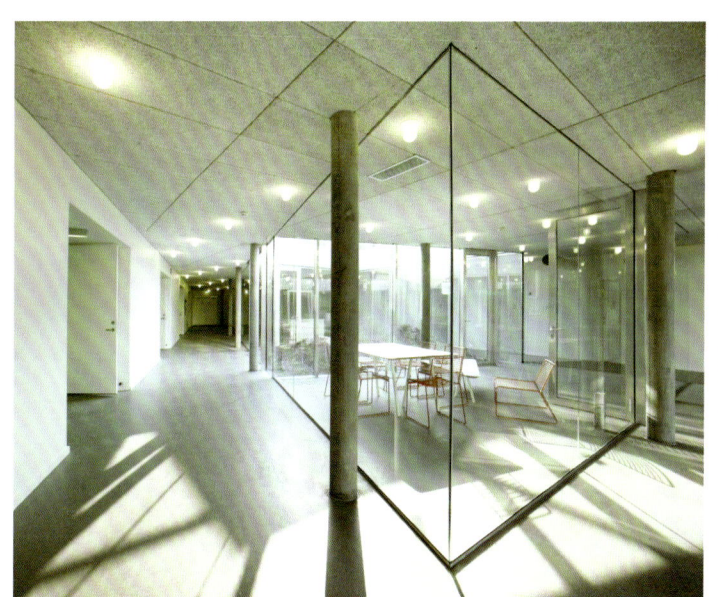

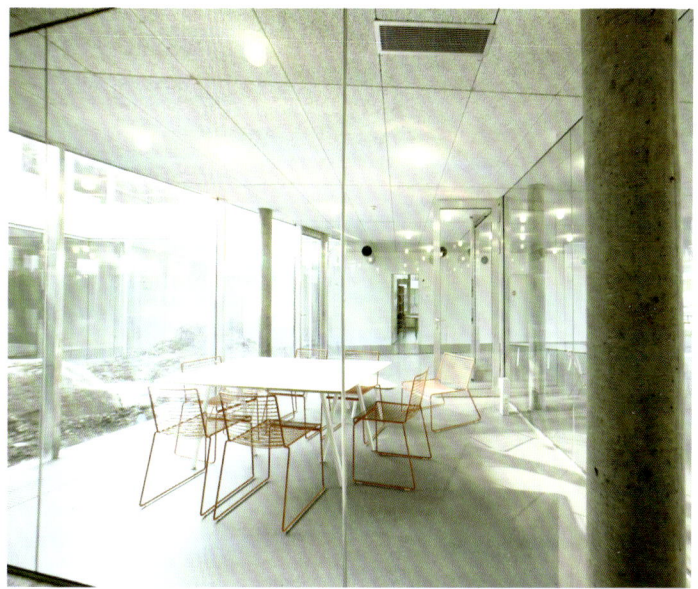

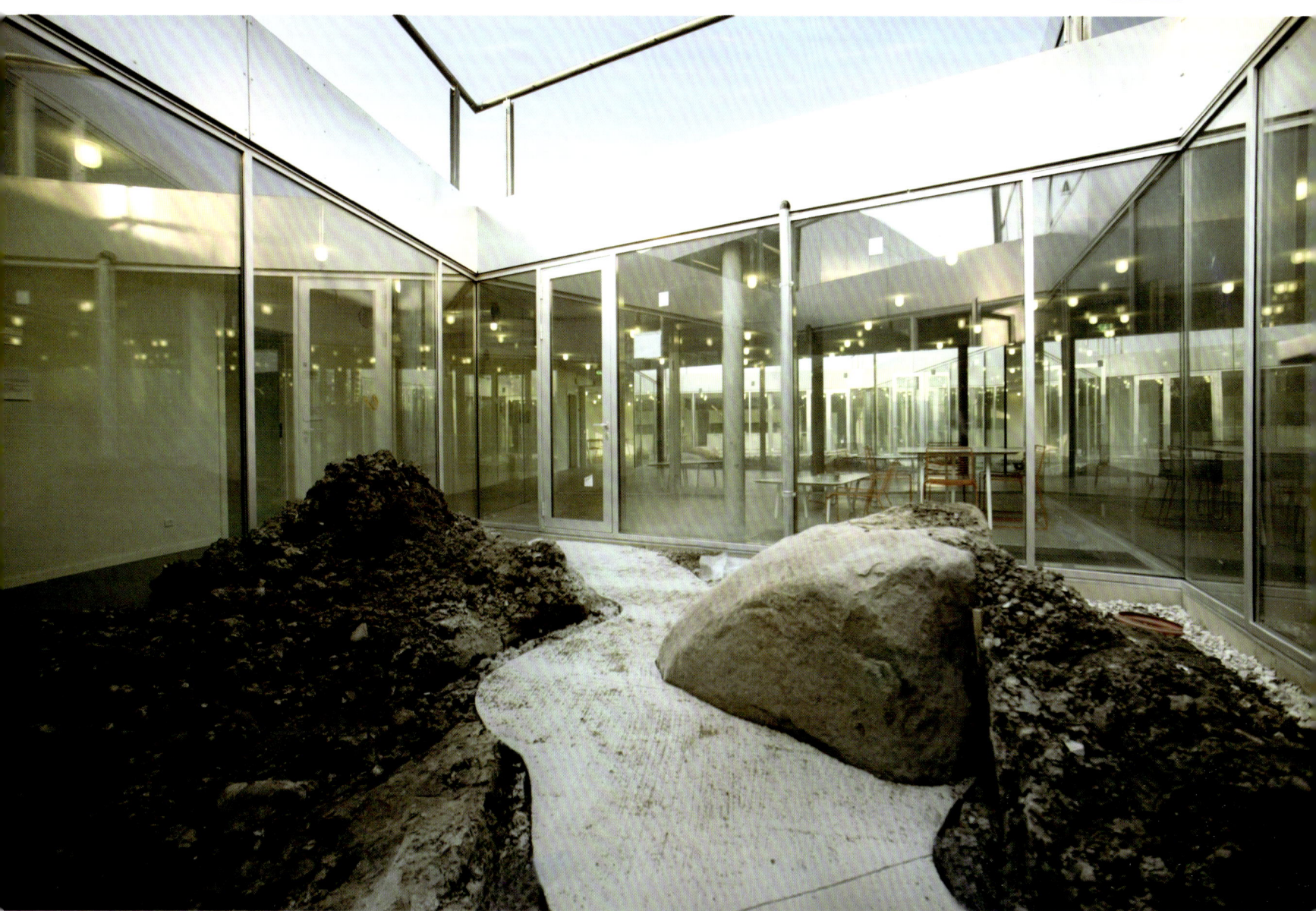

Nickl & Partner

Mother and Child Center

Heidelberg, Germany

Photographs: *Stefan Müller-Naumann*

Due to a lack of space in the original building, the construction of the new pediatric clinic became a matter of urgency. The design was inspired by the famous brightly colored cube puzzle invented by the Hungarian engineer and architect Ernő Rubik in the 1970s: a simple shape that is playful yet capable of clearly ordering highly complex processes and supporting a high level of functionality. The primary colors are a subtle way of orienting patients, their visitors, and staff within the building. In the sunlight, horizontal panes of colored glass along the façade cast bright and ever changing images across the walls of the patients' rooms. Bright colors are also used in the foyer and for the furnishings. The idea of the Rubik's cube has been translated into a workable concept through the division of functions: each principal function is assigned its own building. Patients are treated and cared for in the cube building. The garden level hosts the intensive care units, the first floor the busy outpatient clinic areas, and the three floors above that contain the nursing wards with patients' rooms.

The façade of the three nursing floors is composed of a dual-layer glass skin, with a maintenance ledge giving depth to the façade and at the same time acting as a sunscreen for the rooms. With a façade made of wooden slats and a projecting bay, the area known as the 'Children's Planet' – a care facility for relatives of sick children – has its own distinctive form. Similarly, each of the other corners of the building has been given its own design: the all-glass staircases in the northwest and southeast corners are accentuated by horizontal panes, and the double-flight staircases are suspended from the ceilings of each story, thus giving the space a light and elegant feel.

A deep sense of commitment to the young patients, their families and the staff is conveyed by coherent details and outstanding architectural choices combined with attractive aesthetics. High creative standards are combined with user friendliness in order to make a stay in an unfamiliar functional environment (which often engenders anxiety) as pleasant as possible. Thus the patients' rooms face towards the full-length glass façade and offer beautiful views across the Odenwald forest. Interior courtyards carved from the solid volume of the building ensure plenty of natural light.

The open space is characterized by a forecourt with curved benches and a large play area, which allows ample opportunity for outdoor activity. Climbing plants will ensure that the garden levels and the surrounding parkland grow together in tandem.

Client:
University of Heidelberg
Surface area:
19.900 sqm (202,000 sqft)
Start date:
March 2005
Finish date:
January 2008
Project team:
Prof. Hans Nickl, Prof Christine Nickl-Weller, Gerhard Eckl, Nils Langbein
Cost:
€ 47,500,000

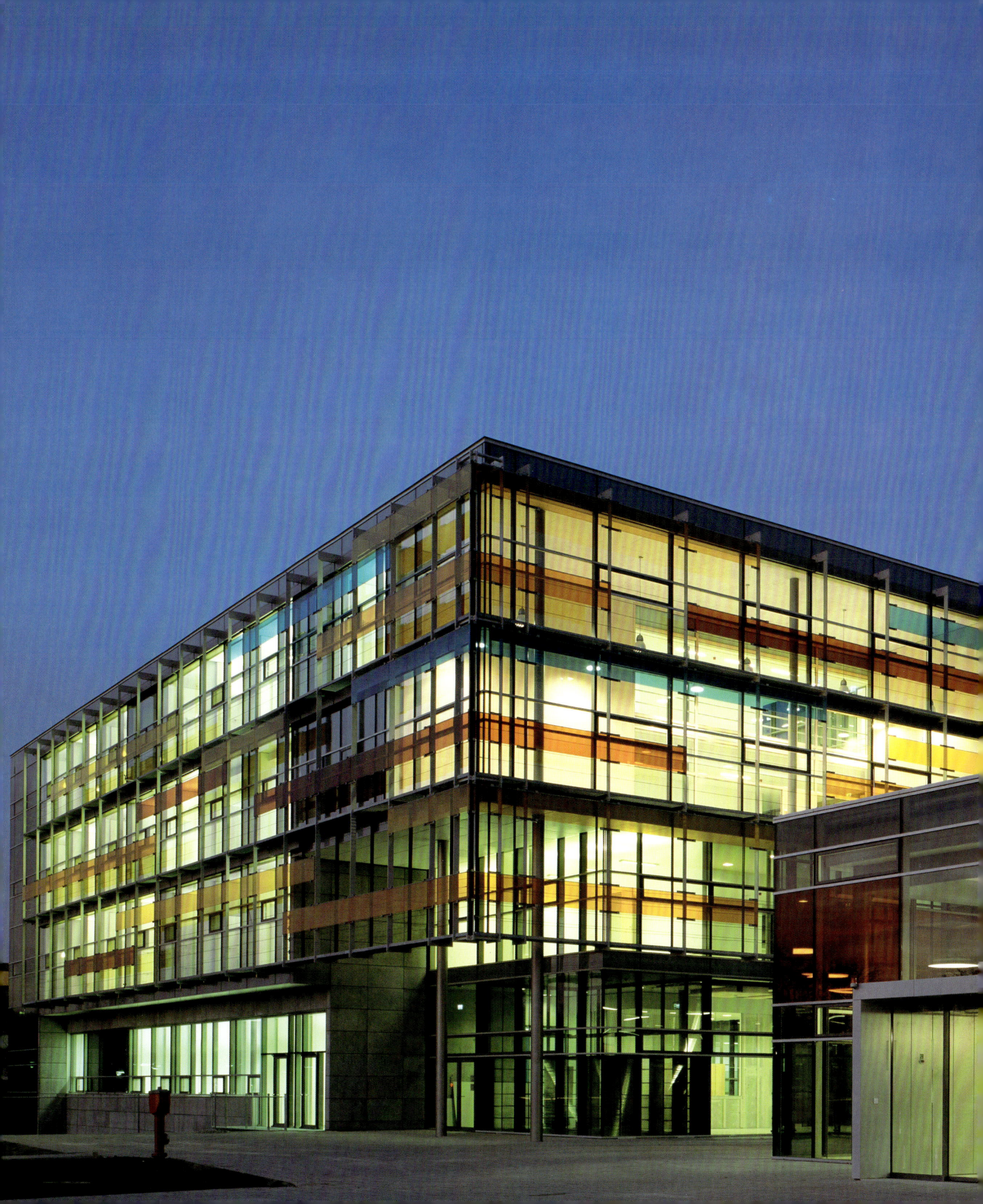

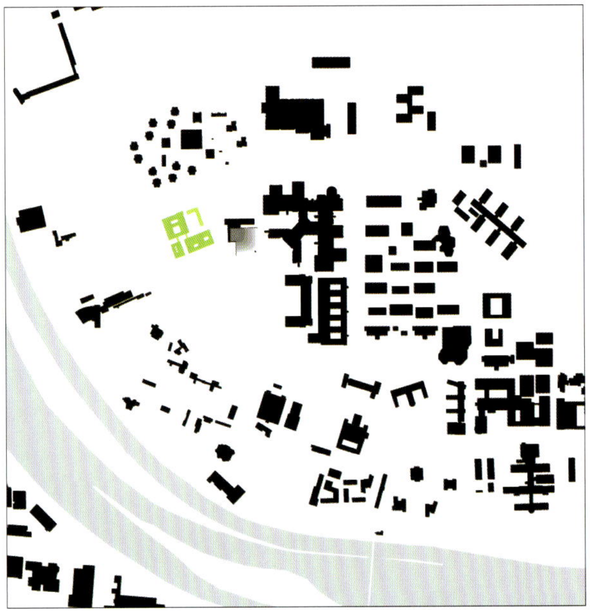

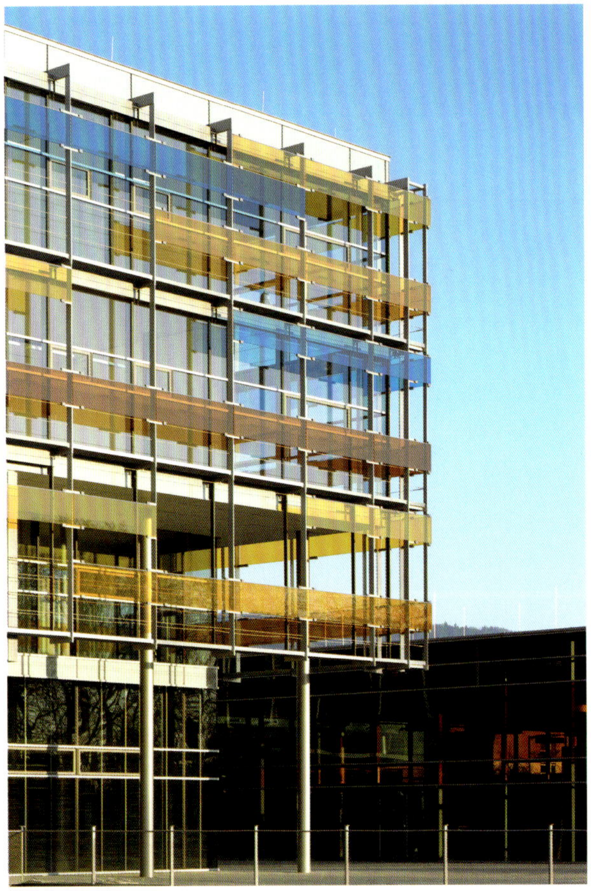

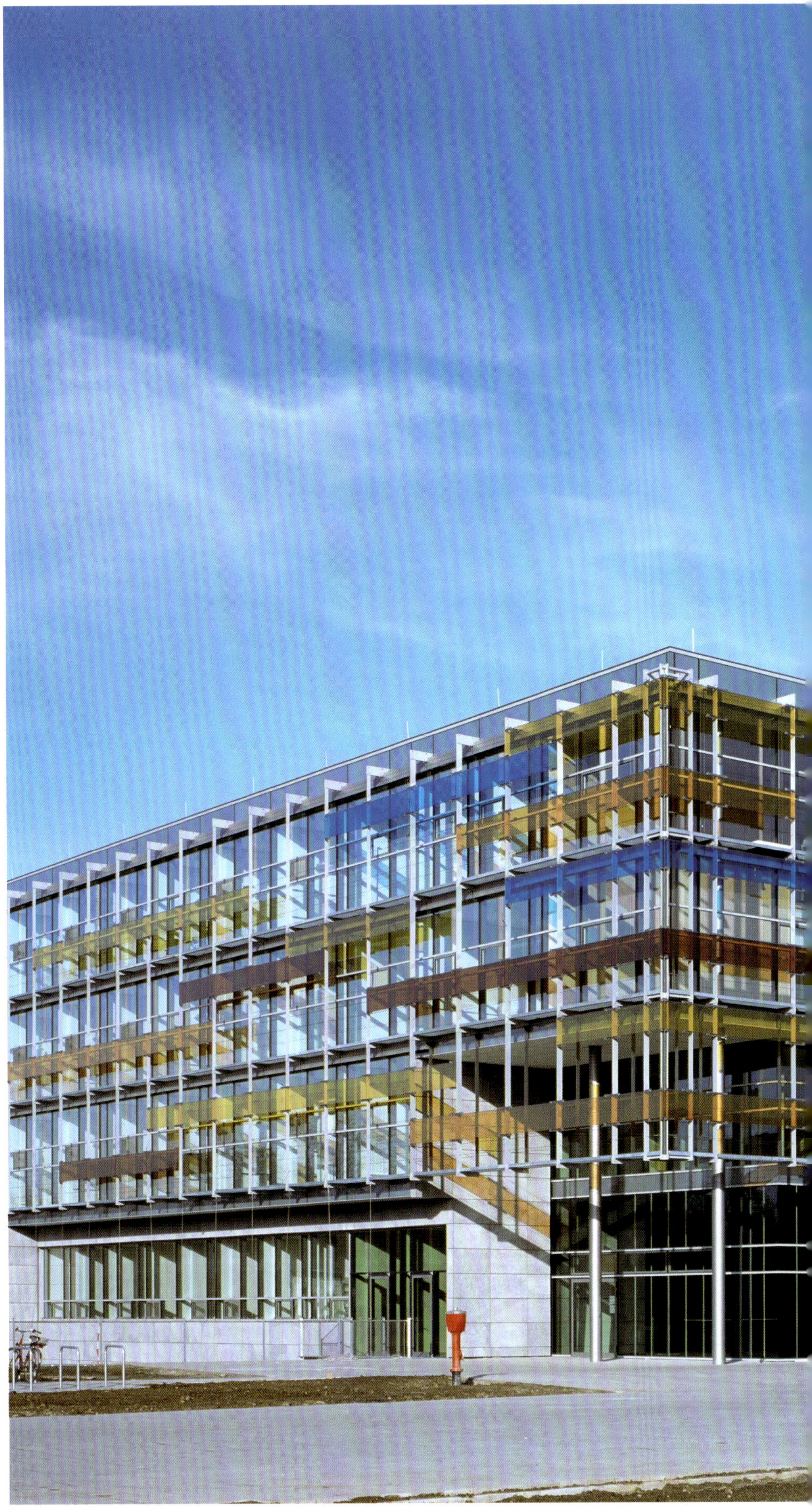

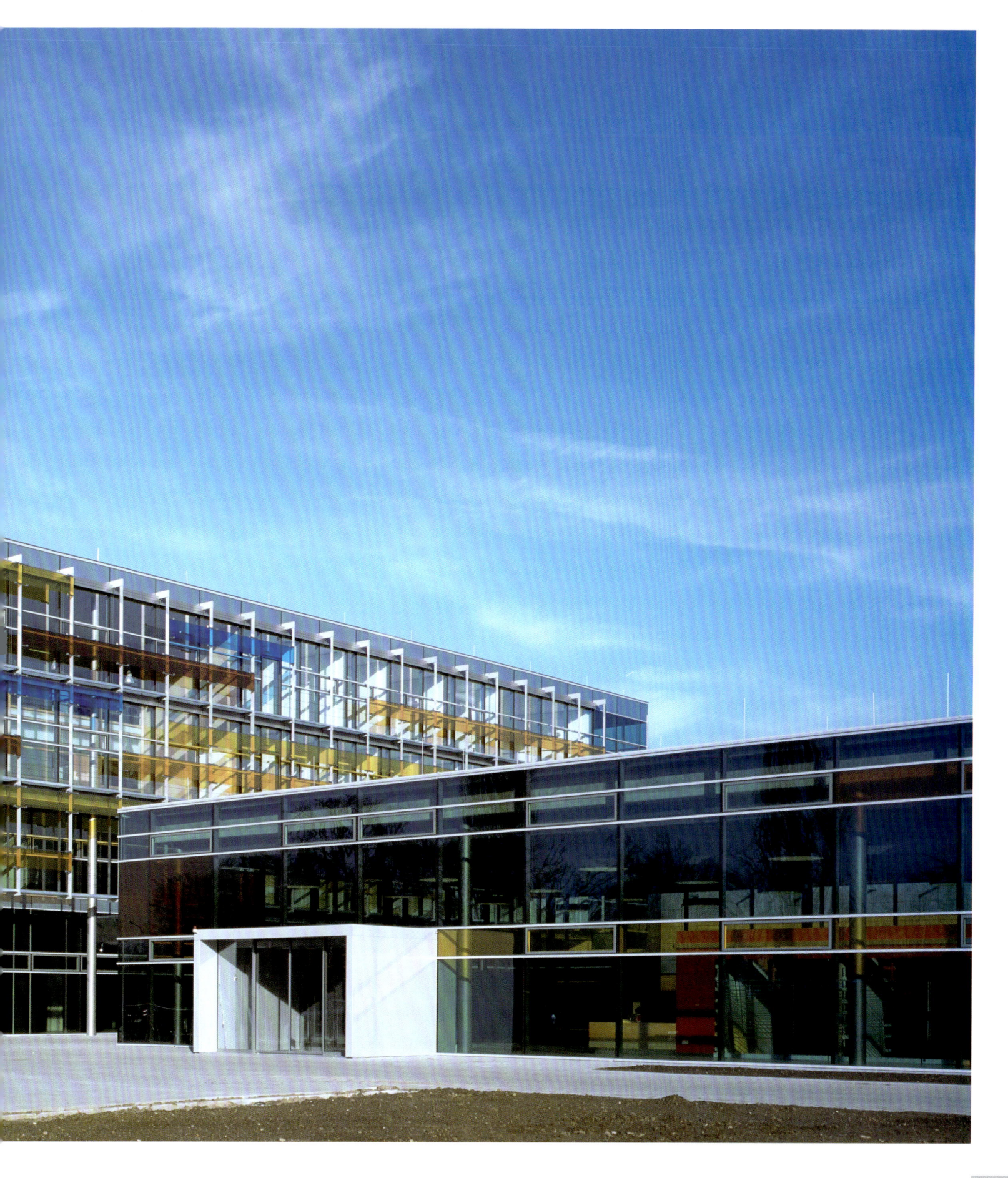

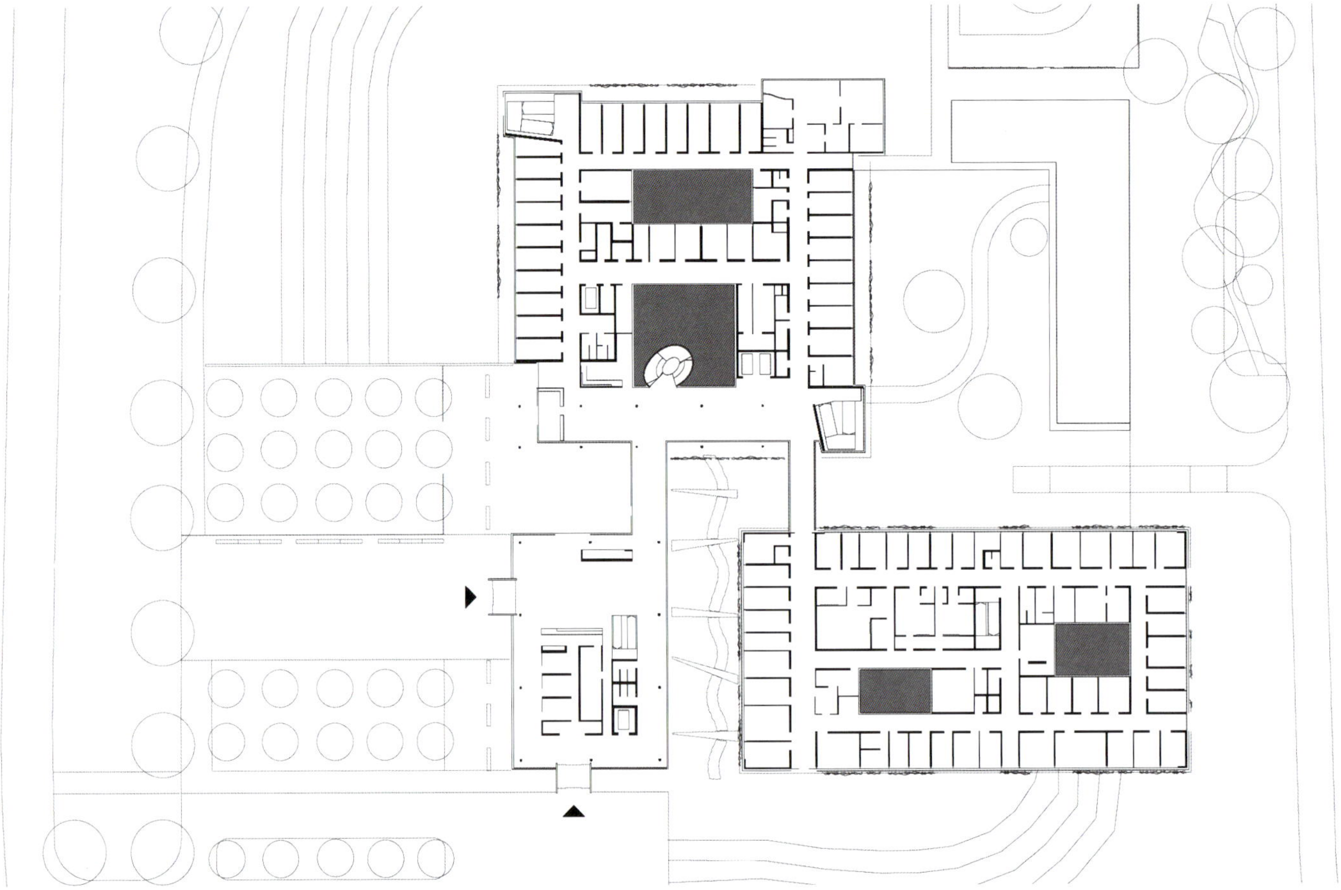

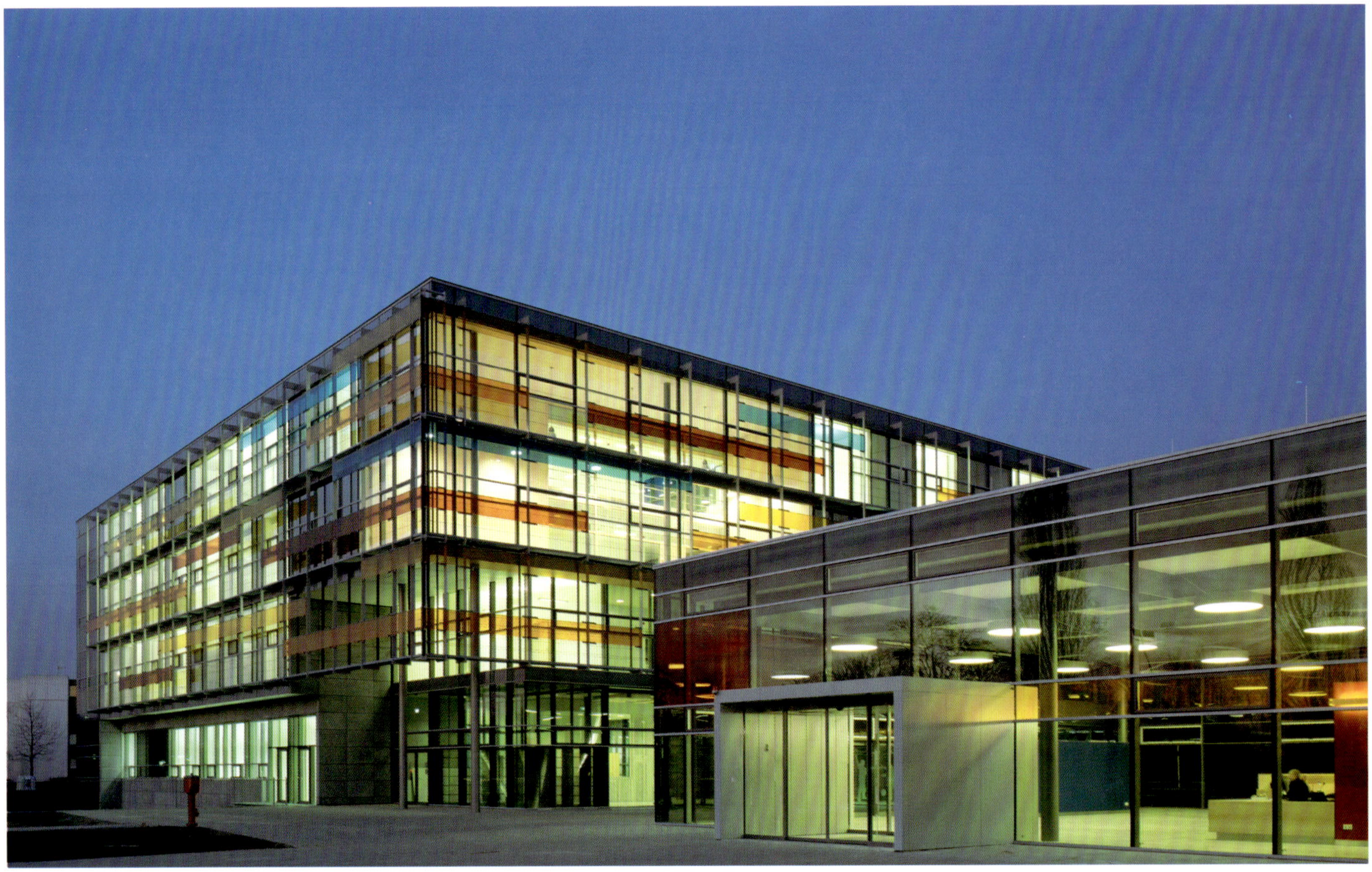

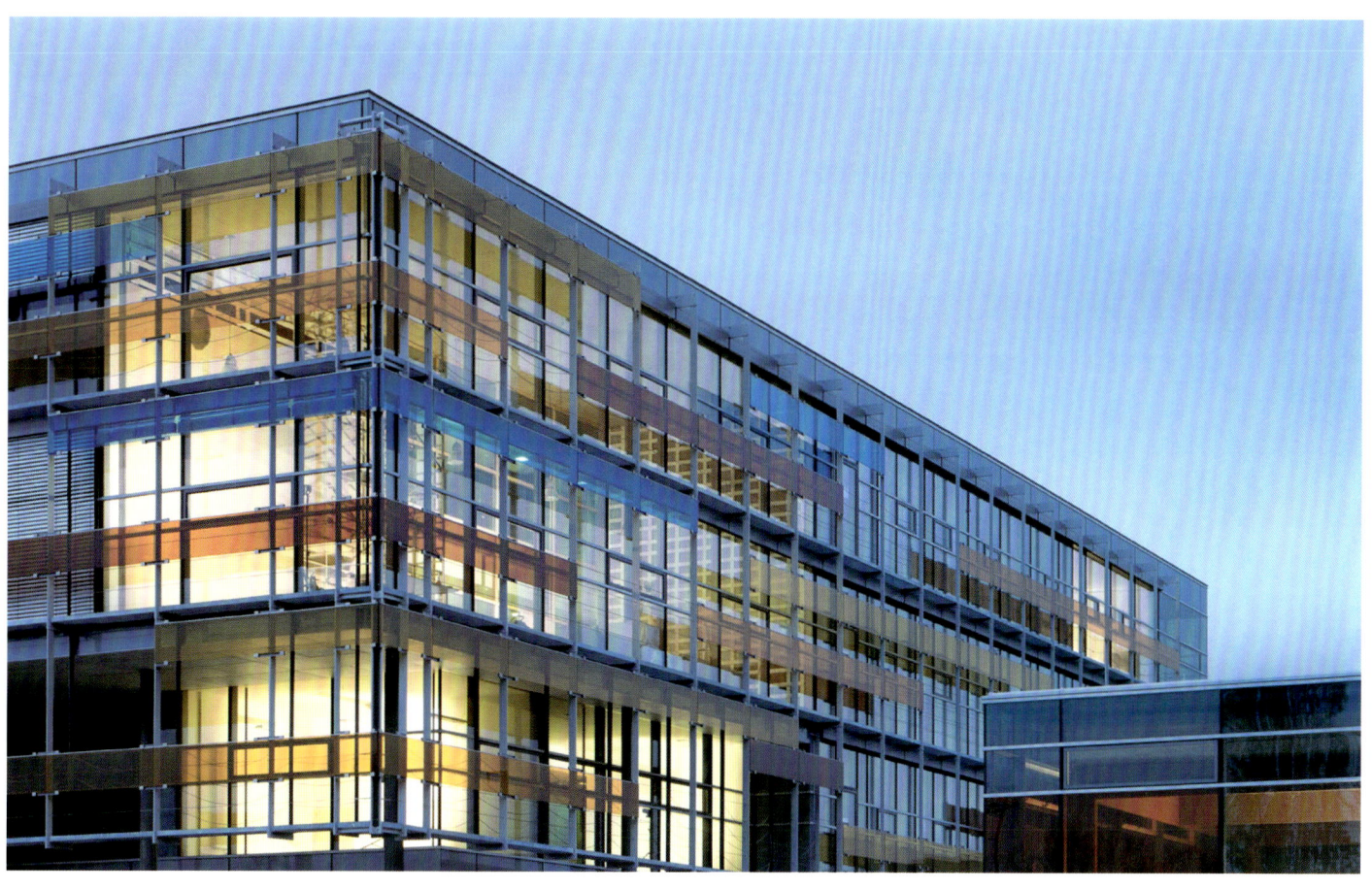

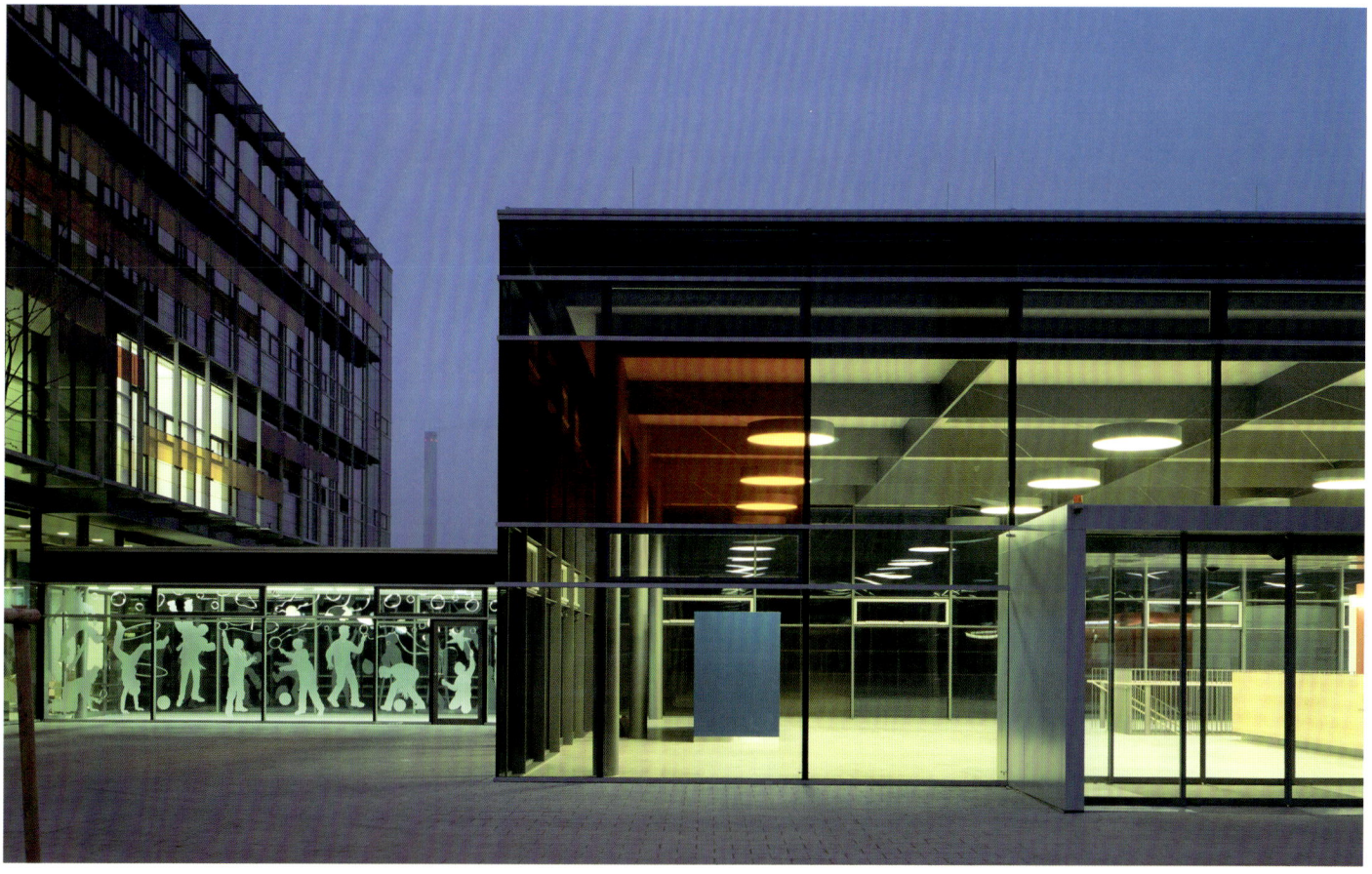

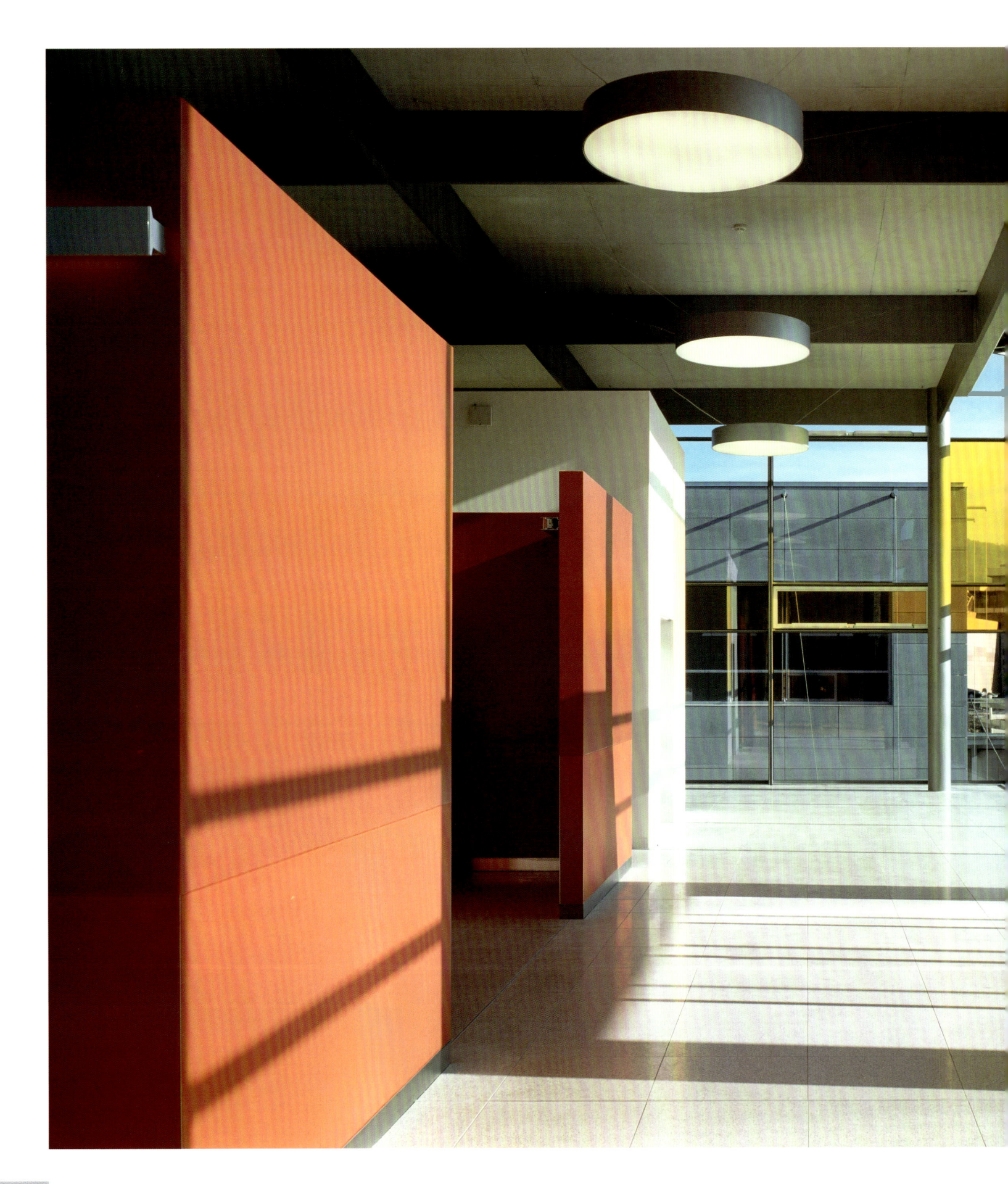

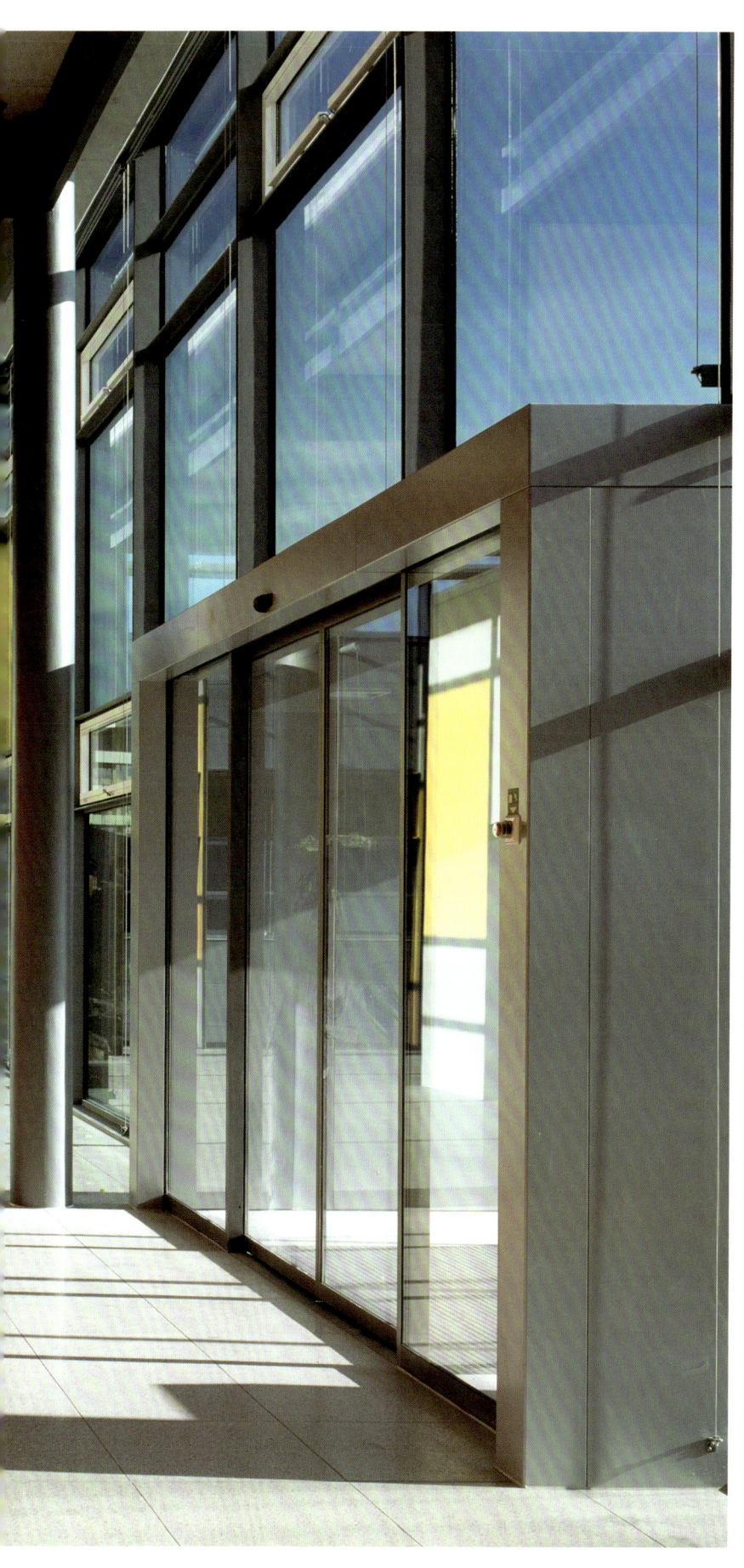

The design was inspired by the famous brightly colored cube puzzle invented by the Hungarian engineer and architect Ernő Rubik in the 1970s: a simple shape that is playful yet capable of clearly ordering highly complex processes and supporting a high level of functionality.

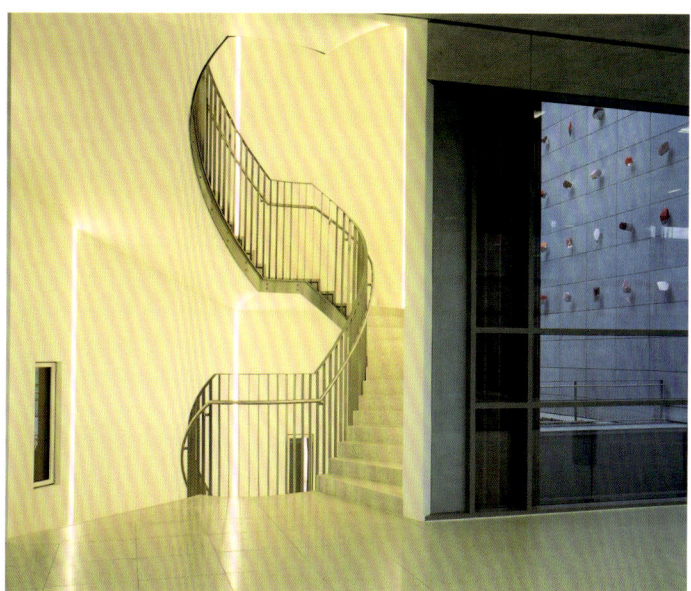

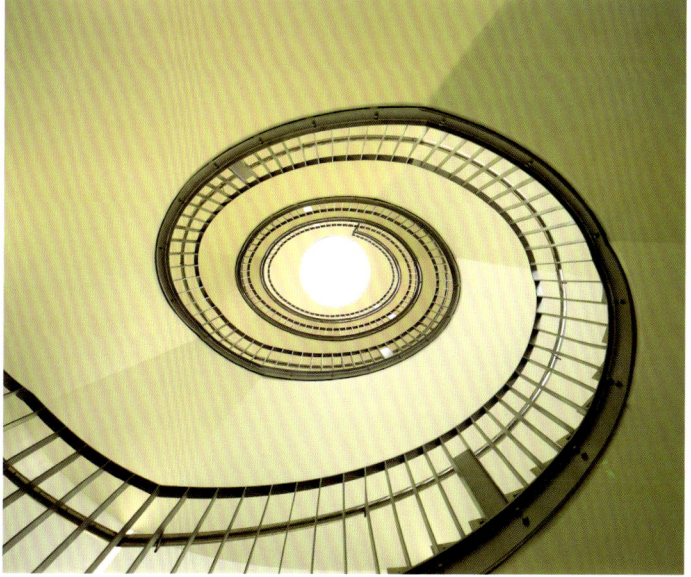

The primary colors are a subtle way of orienting patients, their visitors, and staff within the building. In the sunlight, horizontal panes of colored glass along the façade cast bright and ever changing images across the walls of the patients' rooms.

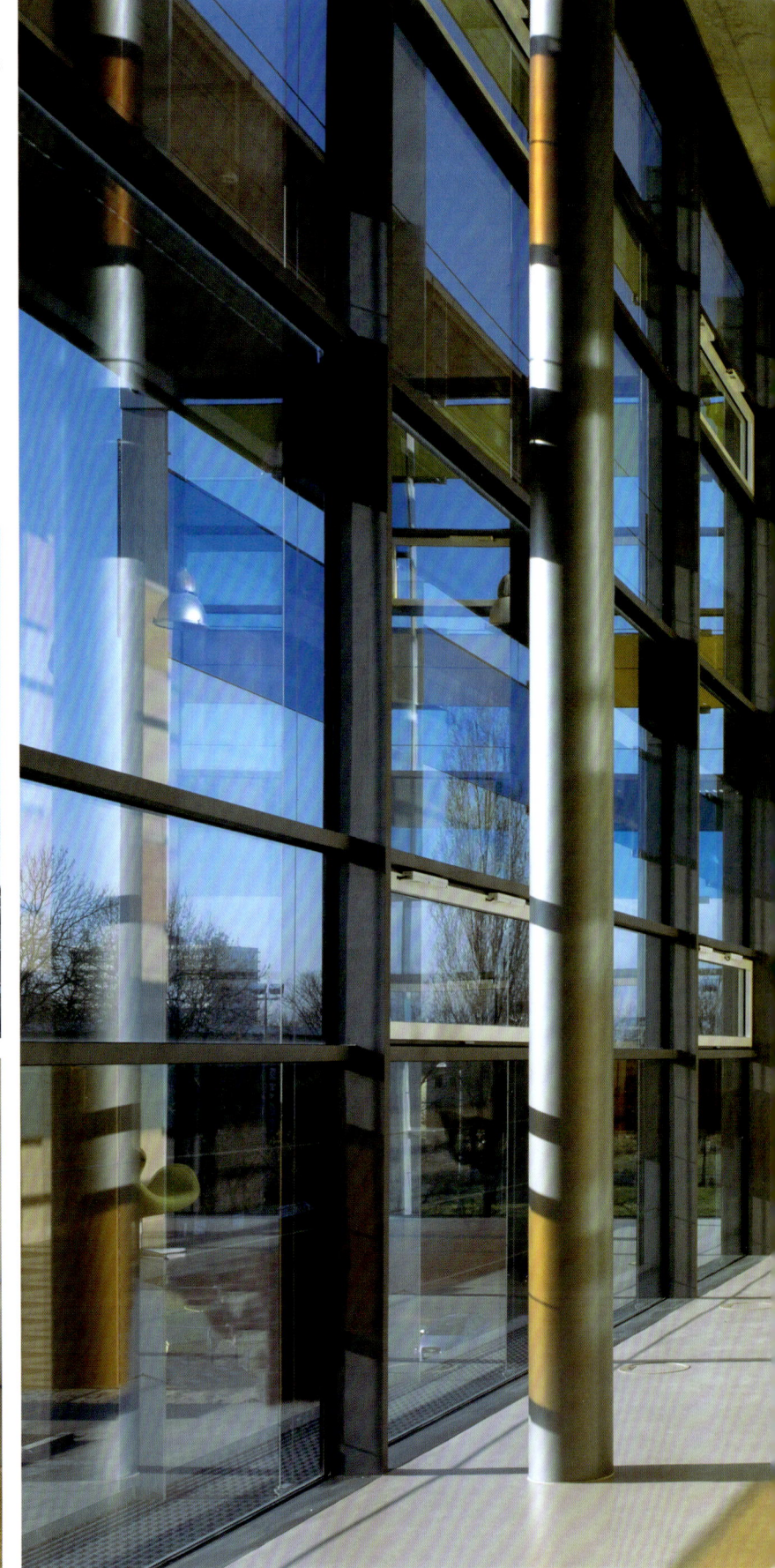

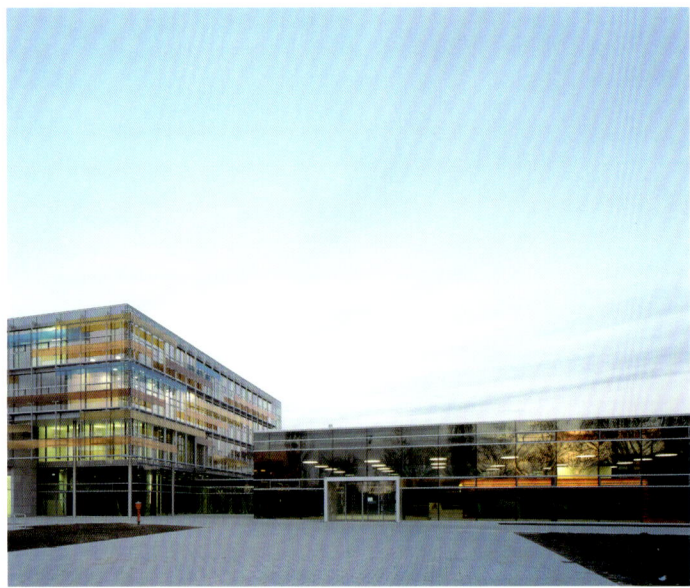

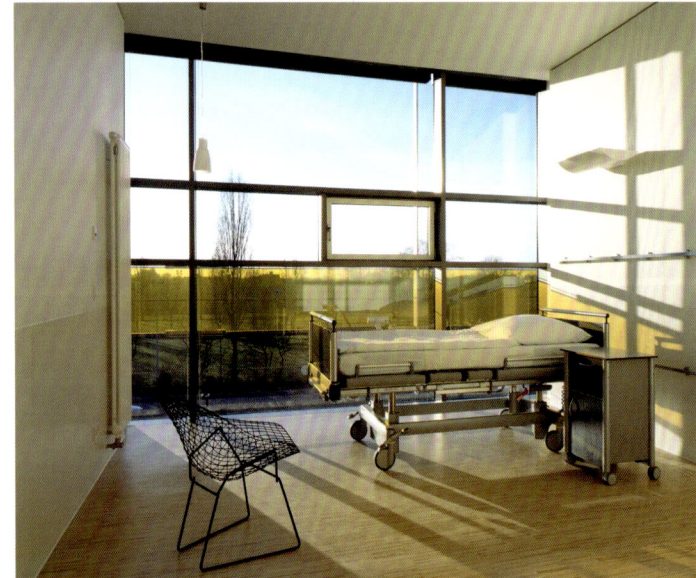

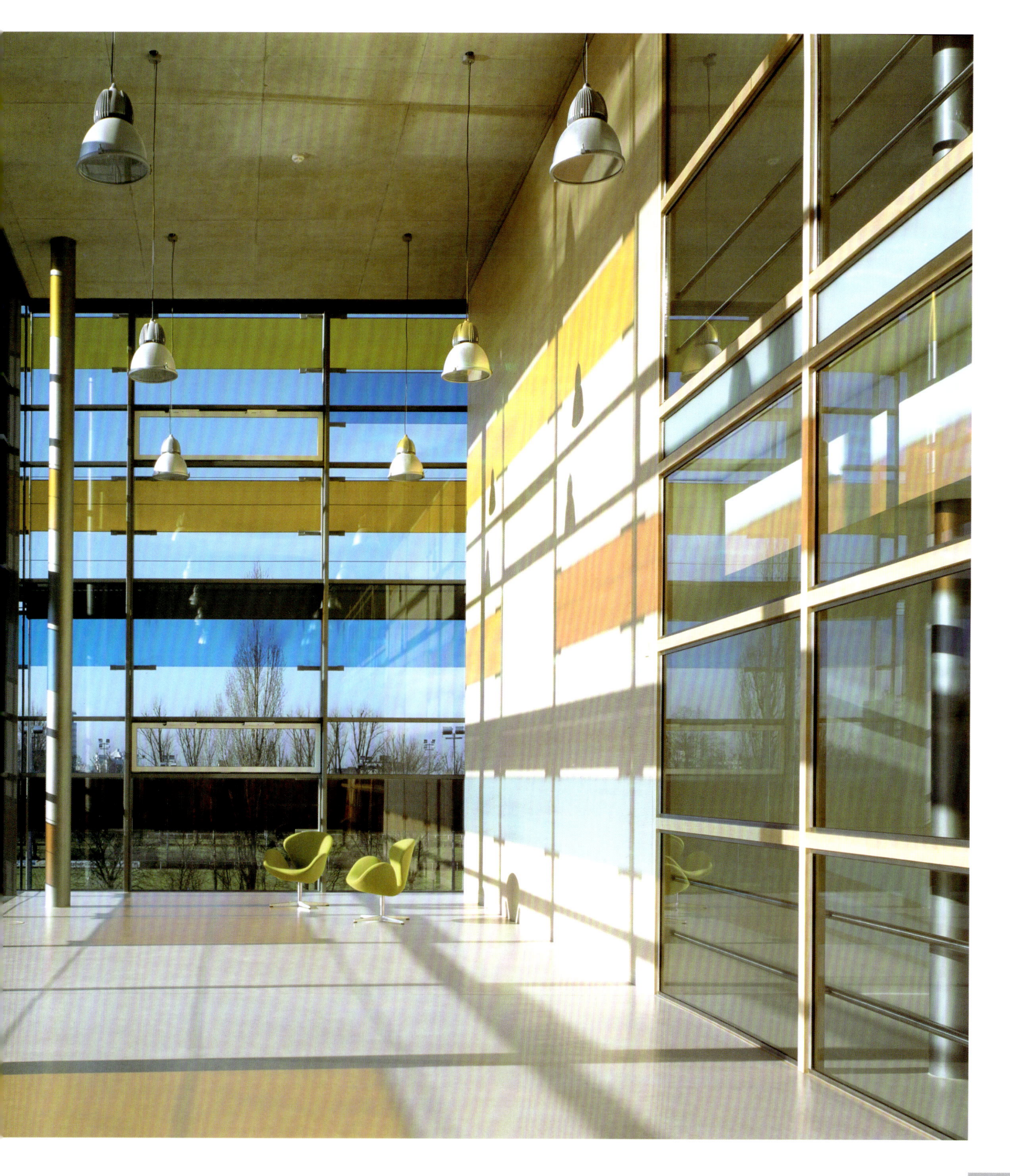

Burger Grunstra Architects

Martini Hospital

Groningen, Netherlands

Photographs: Mr. Rob Hoekstra, Mr. Derk Jan de Vries

Needs and requirements in healthcare facilities are constantly changing due to modifications in technology and medical knowledge. This was the basic concept behind Burger Grunstra's design for the Martini Hospital.

Research led to the design of a uniform building block measuring 60 x 16 m (200 x 52 ft) with a floor surface area of 1,000 sqm (10,800 sqft). These dimensions afforded the unit the ability to undergo complete functional changes both during the design phase as well as afterwards, once in use. The 16 m (52 ft) width is a deviation from the typical dimensions of Dutch Hospitals to allow for an increase in daylight penetration. This also contributes to the building's functional flexibility: it is better to have a light-filled storeroom than a dark work area.

The architects were able to integrate IFD principles (a Dutch initiative that stands for Industrial Flexible Demountable) right down to the detailing. With the help of system partition walling, technical couplings and fixed furniture, changes can be made at room level without disturbing adjacent rooms. Fixture points for electrics, medical gases and water are portable, as are reception desks and cupboards. The F from Flexible has therefore led to the D from Demountable and makes the I from Industrial development possible. The metal system partition walling not only offers a particularly flexible layout but also presents new design possibilities to create a less clinical atmosphere in the hospital rooms.

The 270 sqm (2,900 sqft) double-skin façade, consisting of just four timber frame elements and an outer glazed membrane, protects the building from the noise of the nearby traffic and from Holland's cold and wet winter climate. The four exterior materials: plaster, steel, glass and timber in combination with the colors applied make the building clearly recognizable as a healthcare facility. The boxes in the glass façade and the dynamics of the sunshades and slats give the impression of a moving building, reflecting its adaptability to changes in healthcare.

The interior design of the Martini hospital also aims to be flexible. Dutch artist Peter Struycken was commissioned to produce a color harmonious palette, which finally consisted of 46 different tones. This has been randomly applied throughout the interior, breaking up and enlivening the long corridors. The colors do not correspond to specific functions or departments in order to enhance the hospital's high degree of flexibility.

Client:
Martini Hospital
Surface area:
60,000 sqm (646,000 sqft)
Start Date:
2004
Finish Date:
2007
Color artist:
Peter Struycken
Contractor:
VOF Jorritsma - J.P. van Eesteren
Cost:
€ 155 million

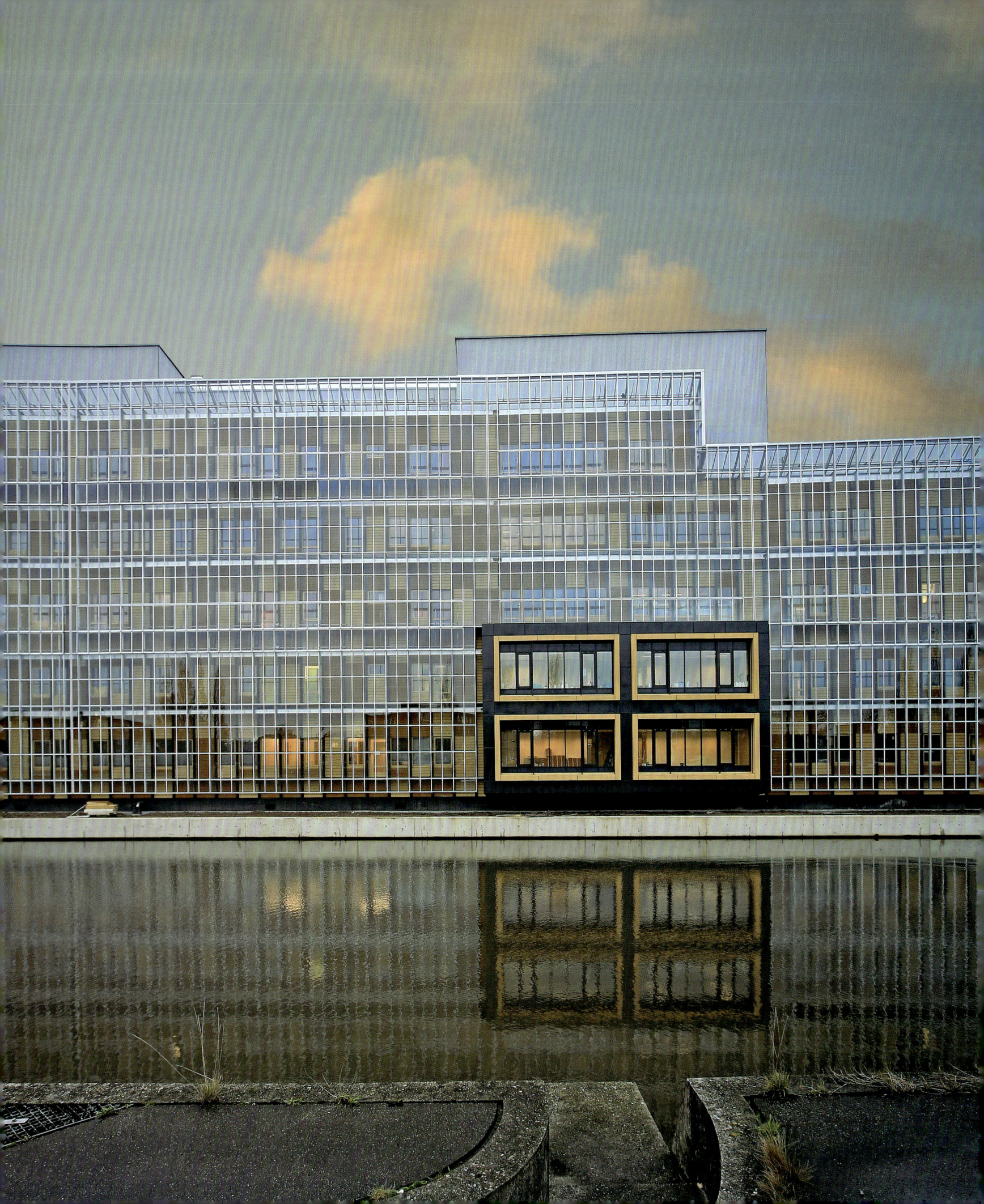

Site plan

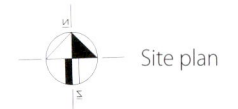

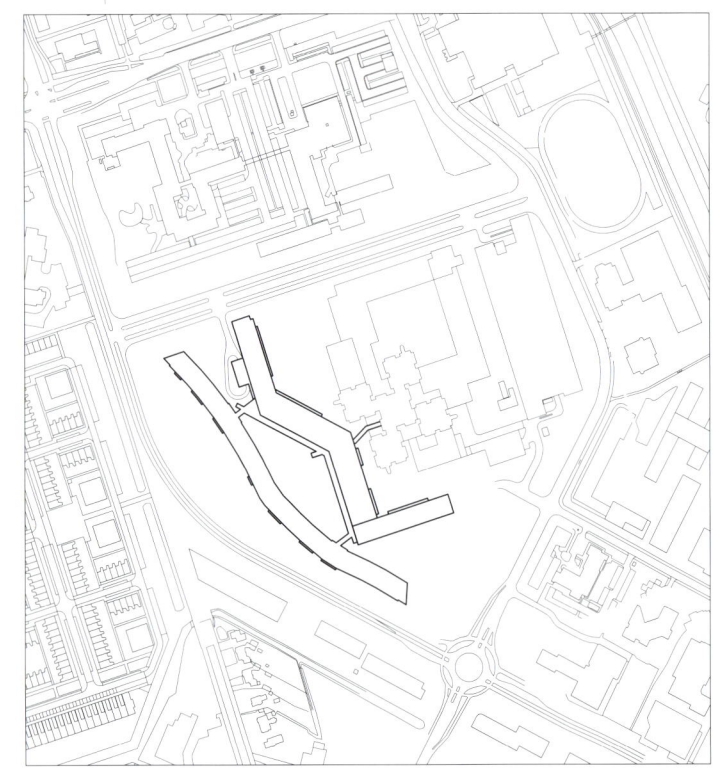

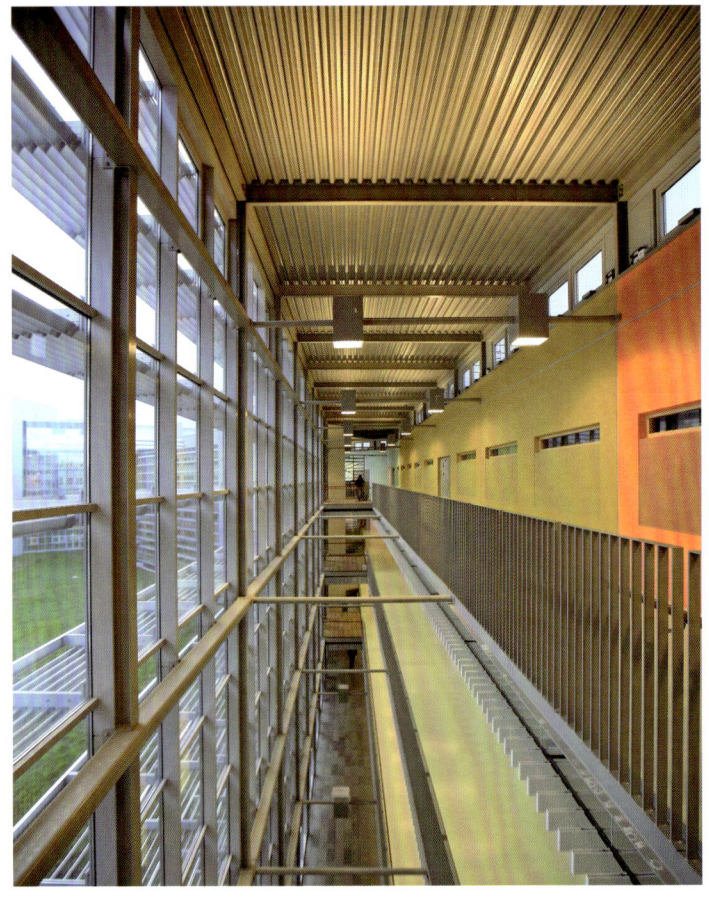

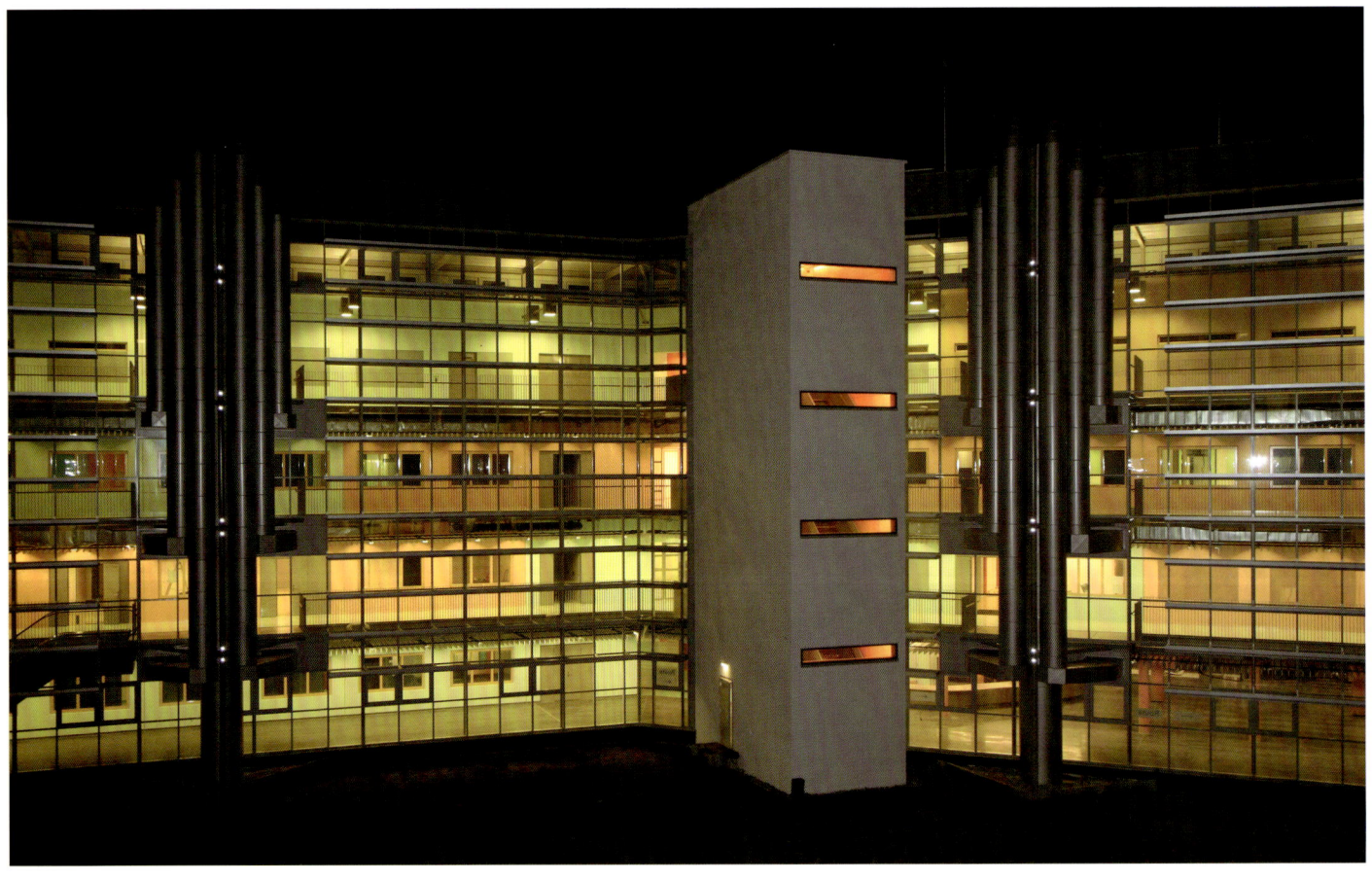

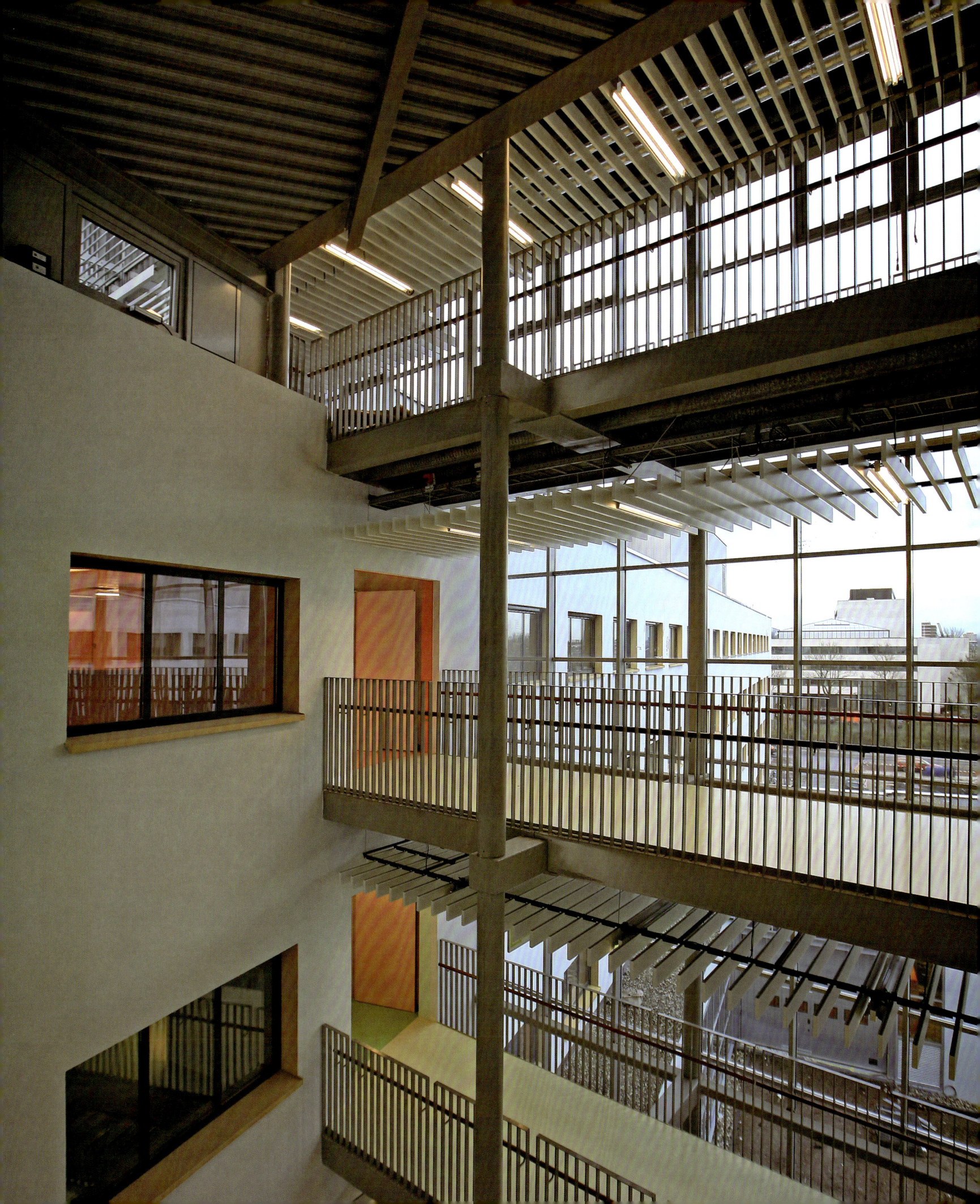

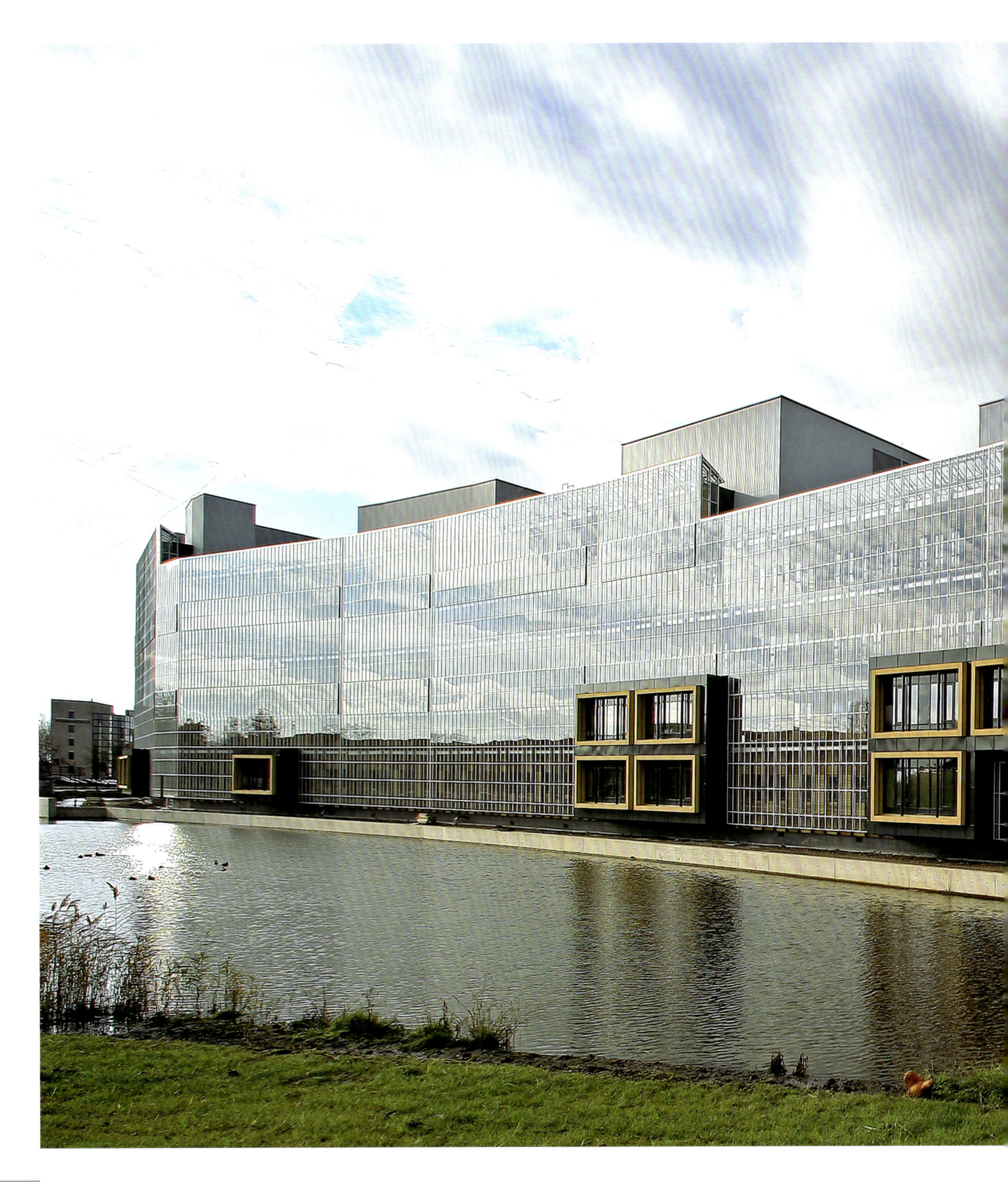

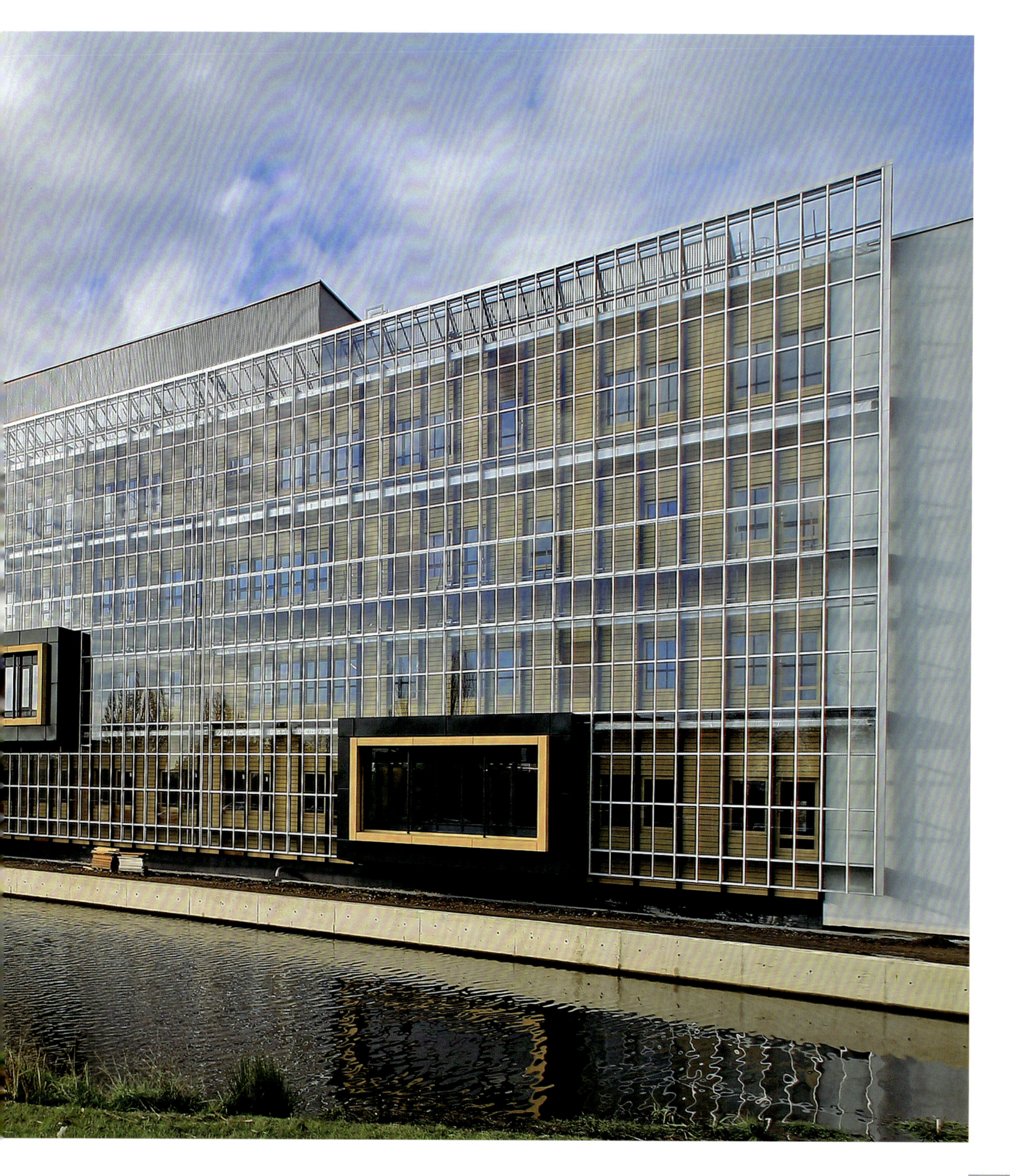

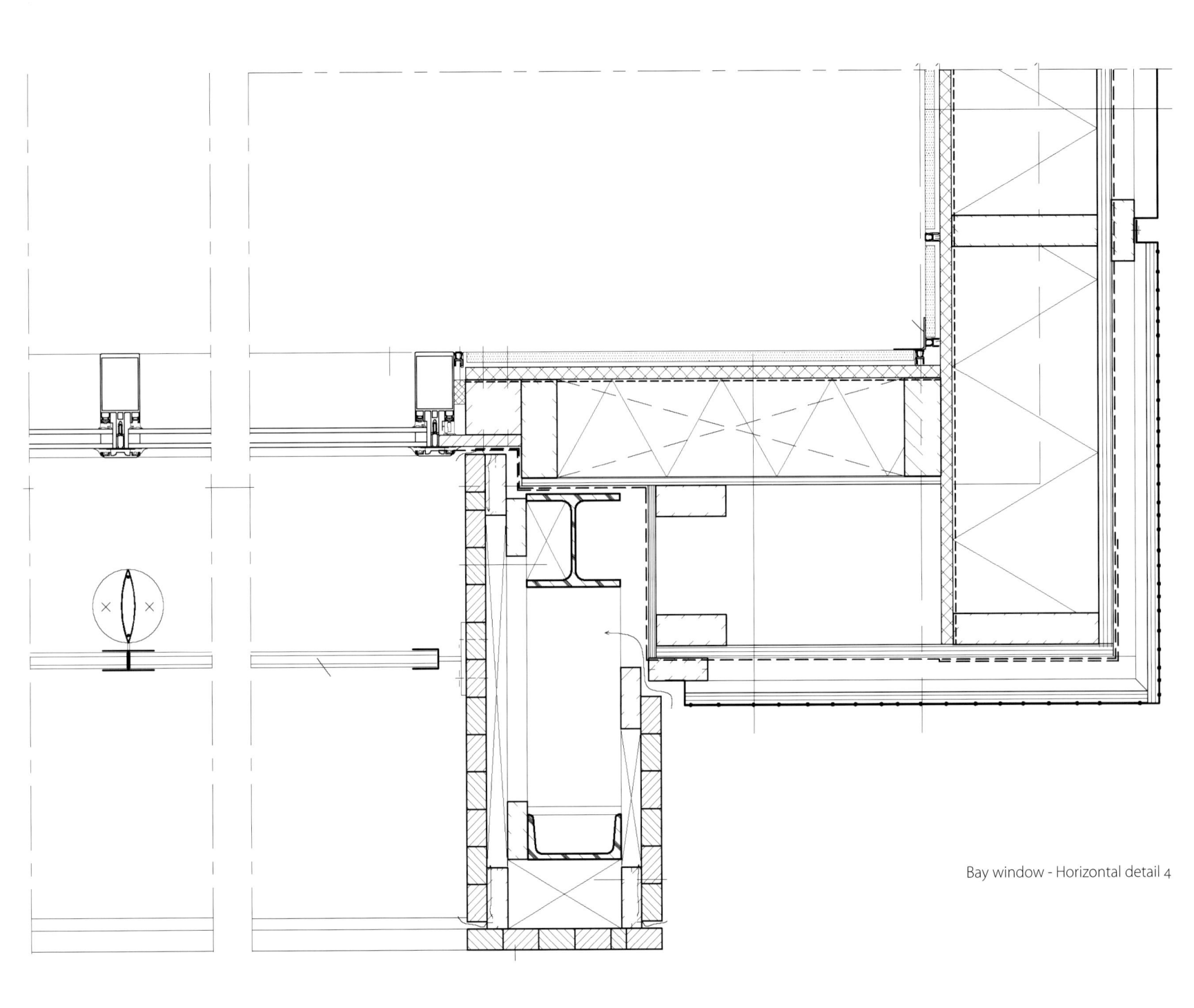

Bay window - Horizontal detail 4

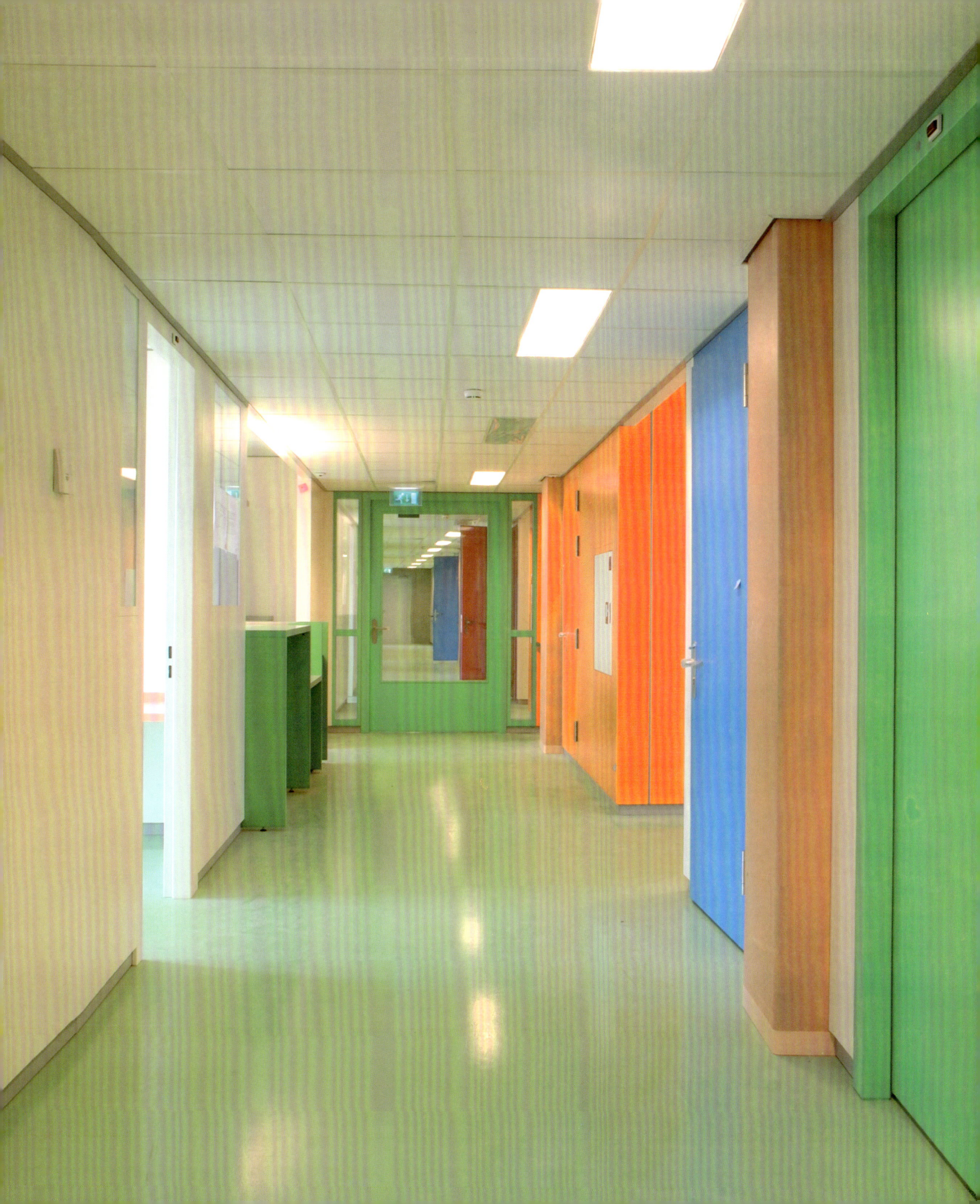

Ground floor plan

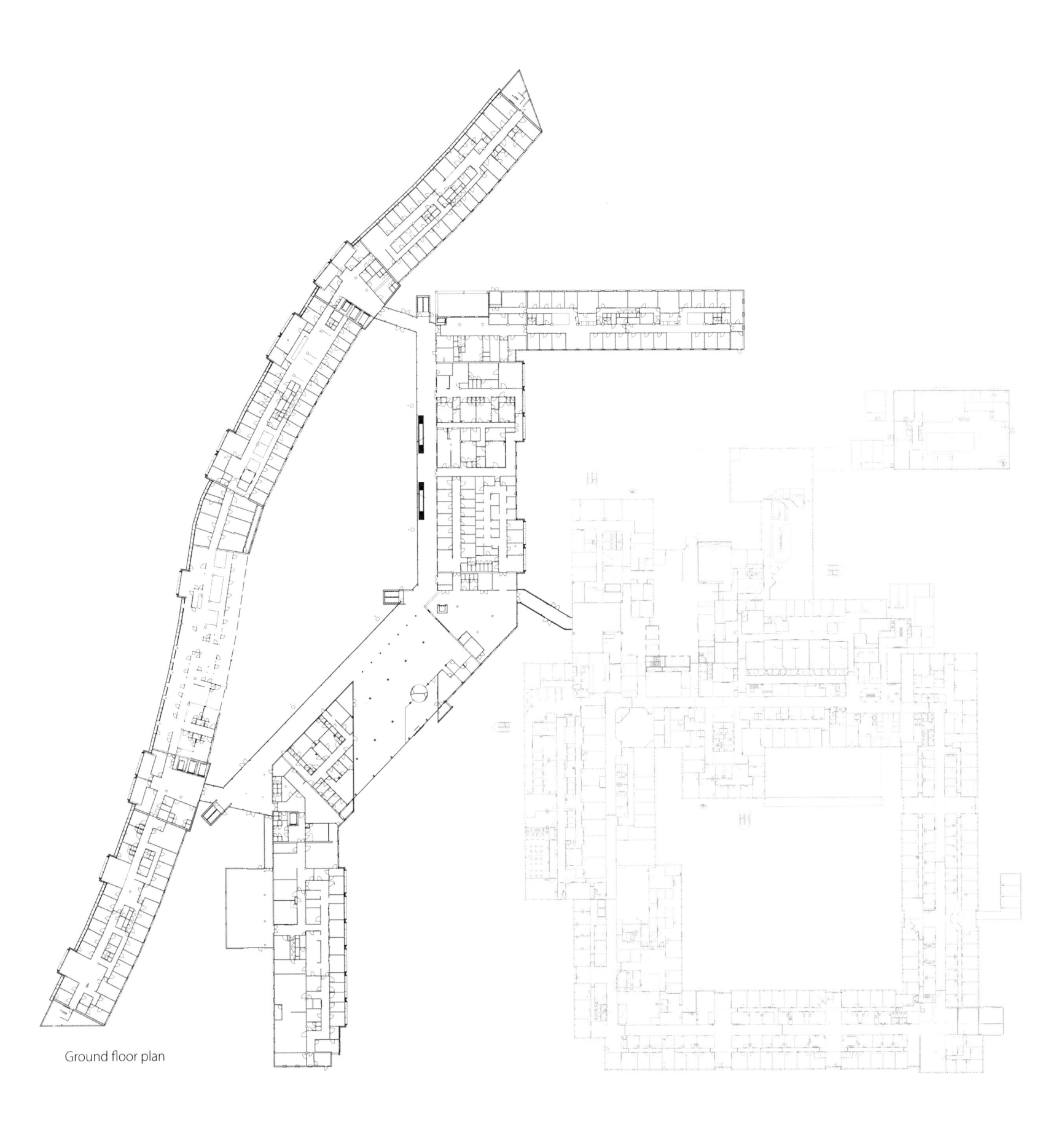

Third floor plan

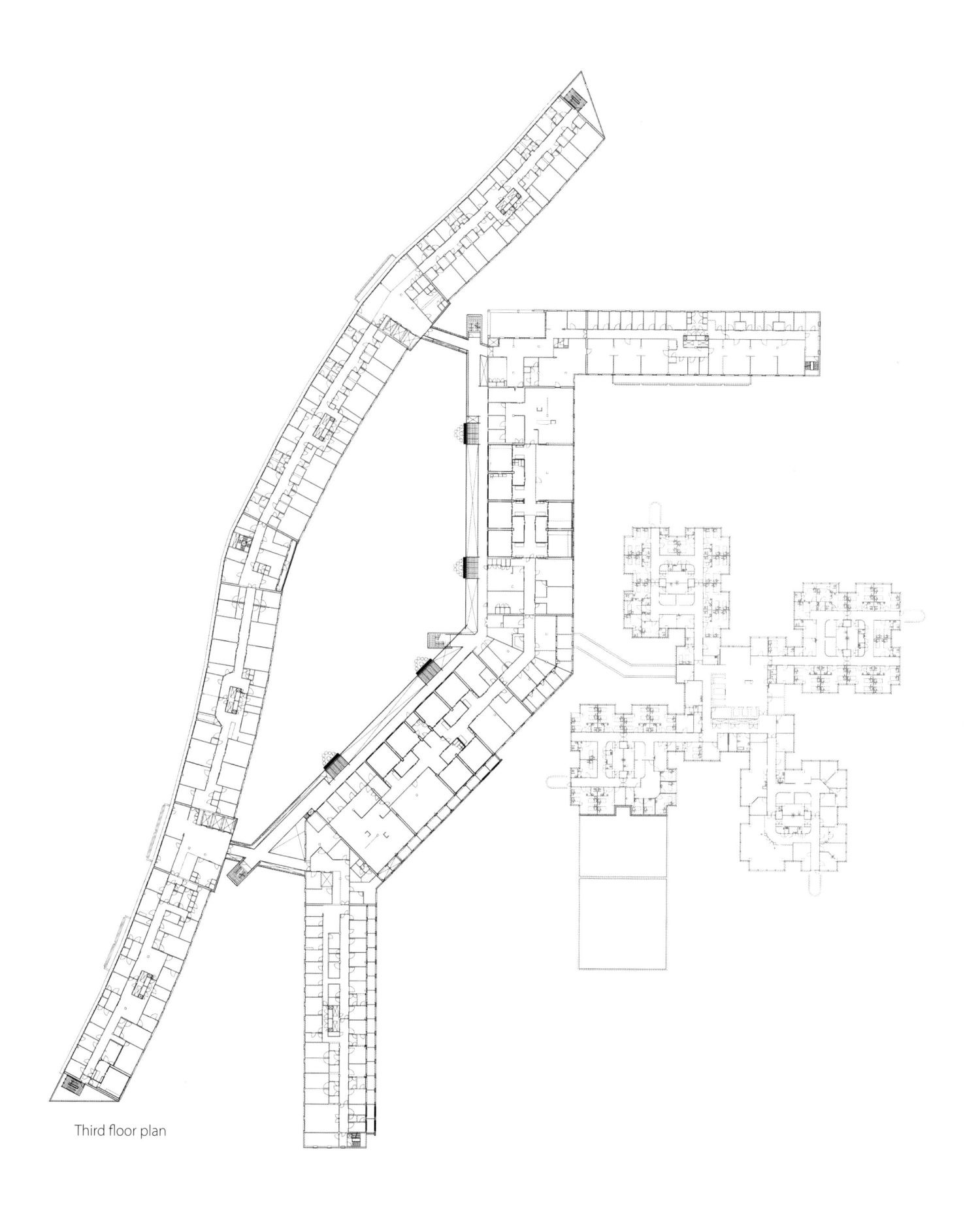

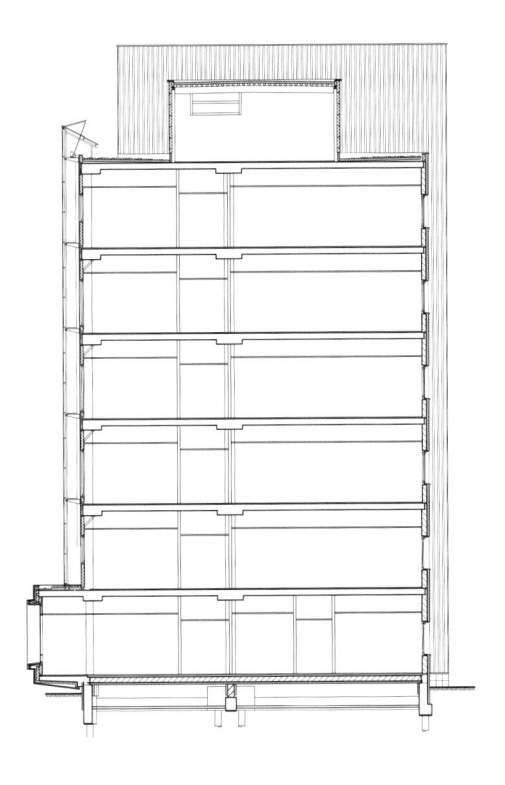

Cross section plan

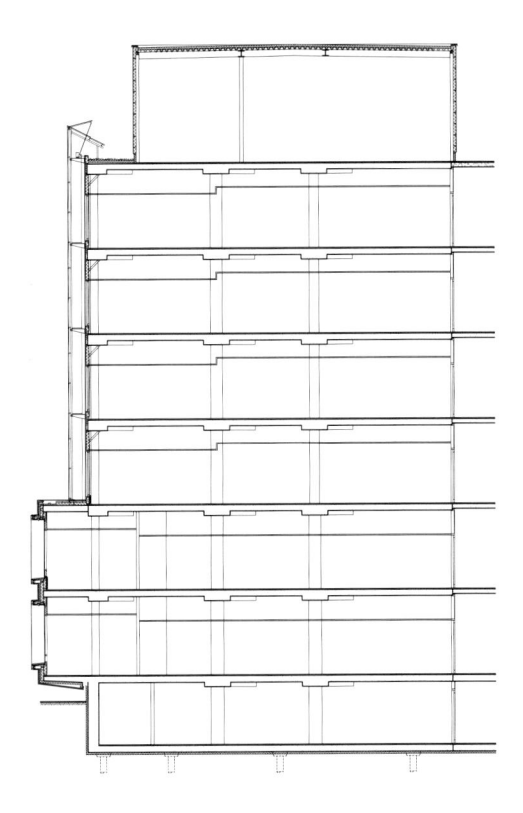

Cross section plan

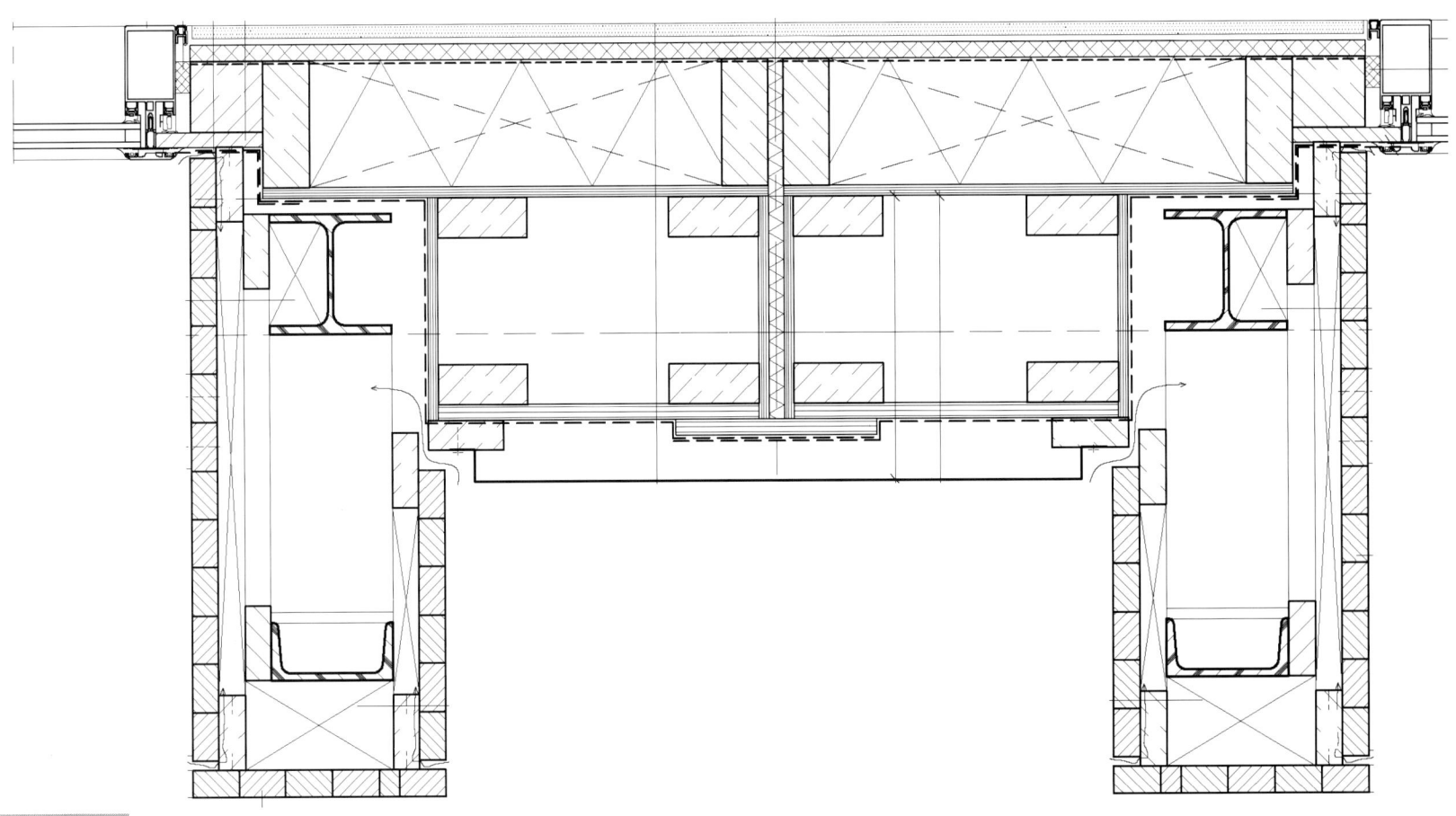

Bay window - Horizontal detail 1

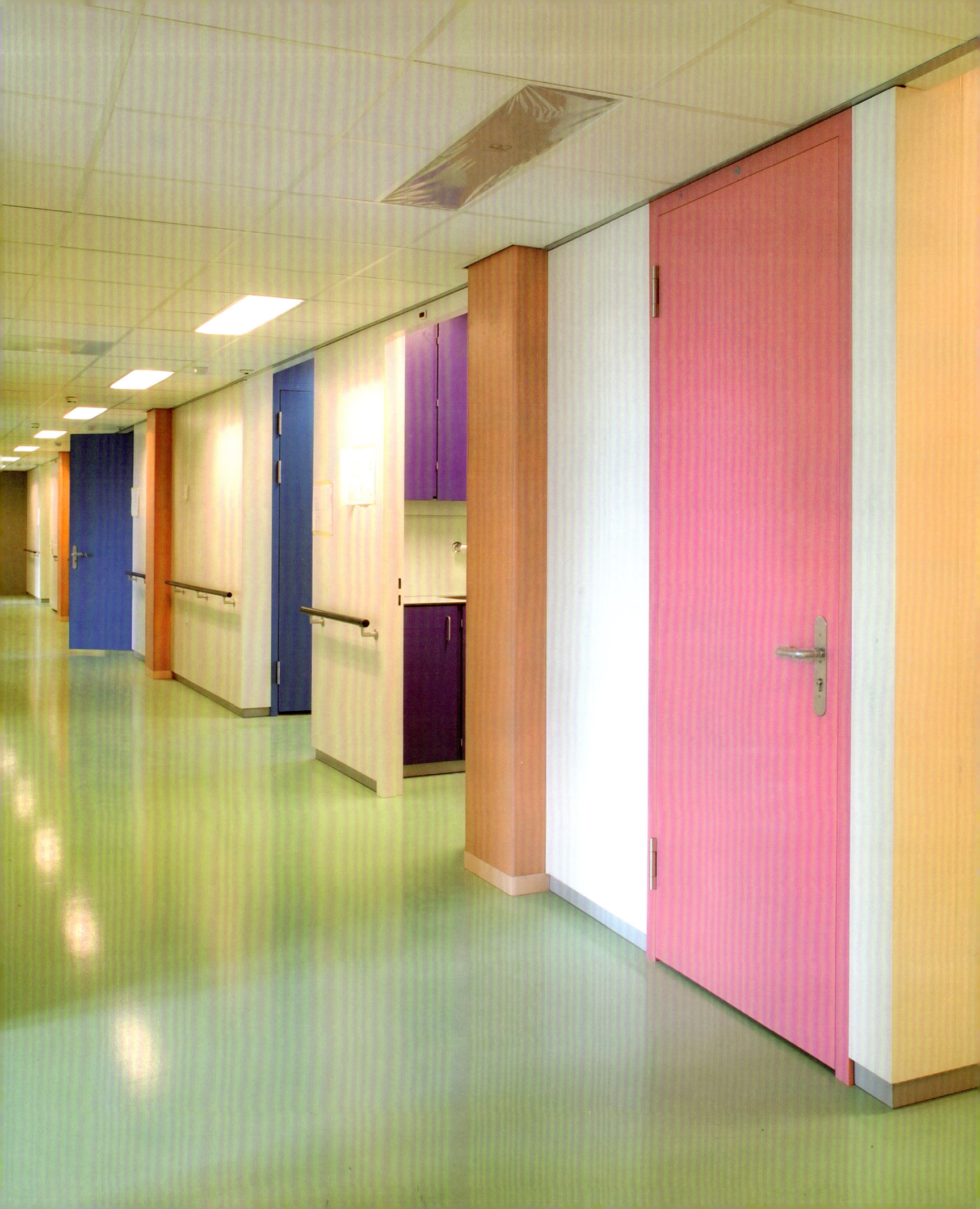

38

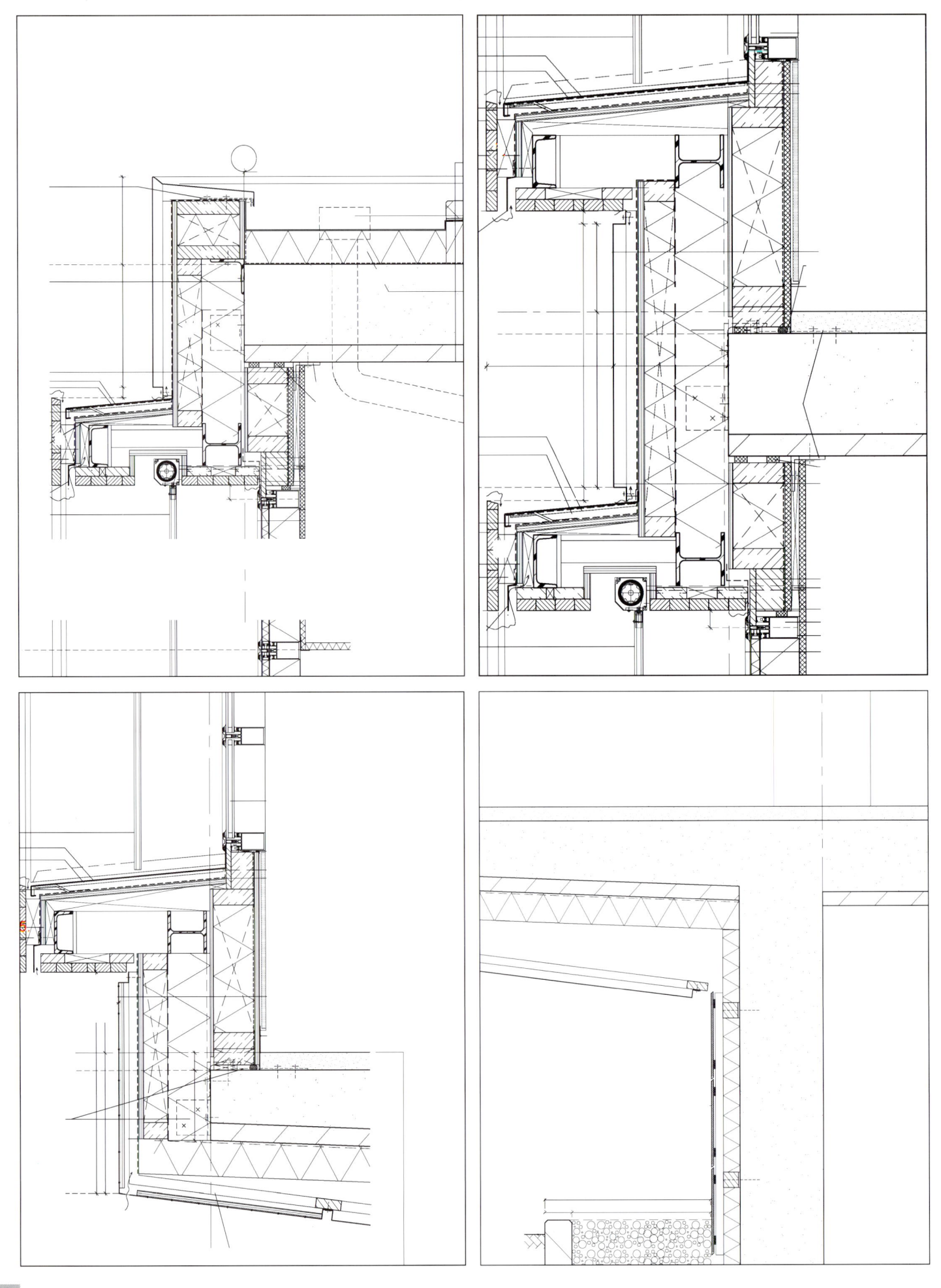

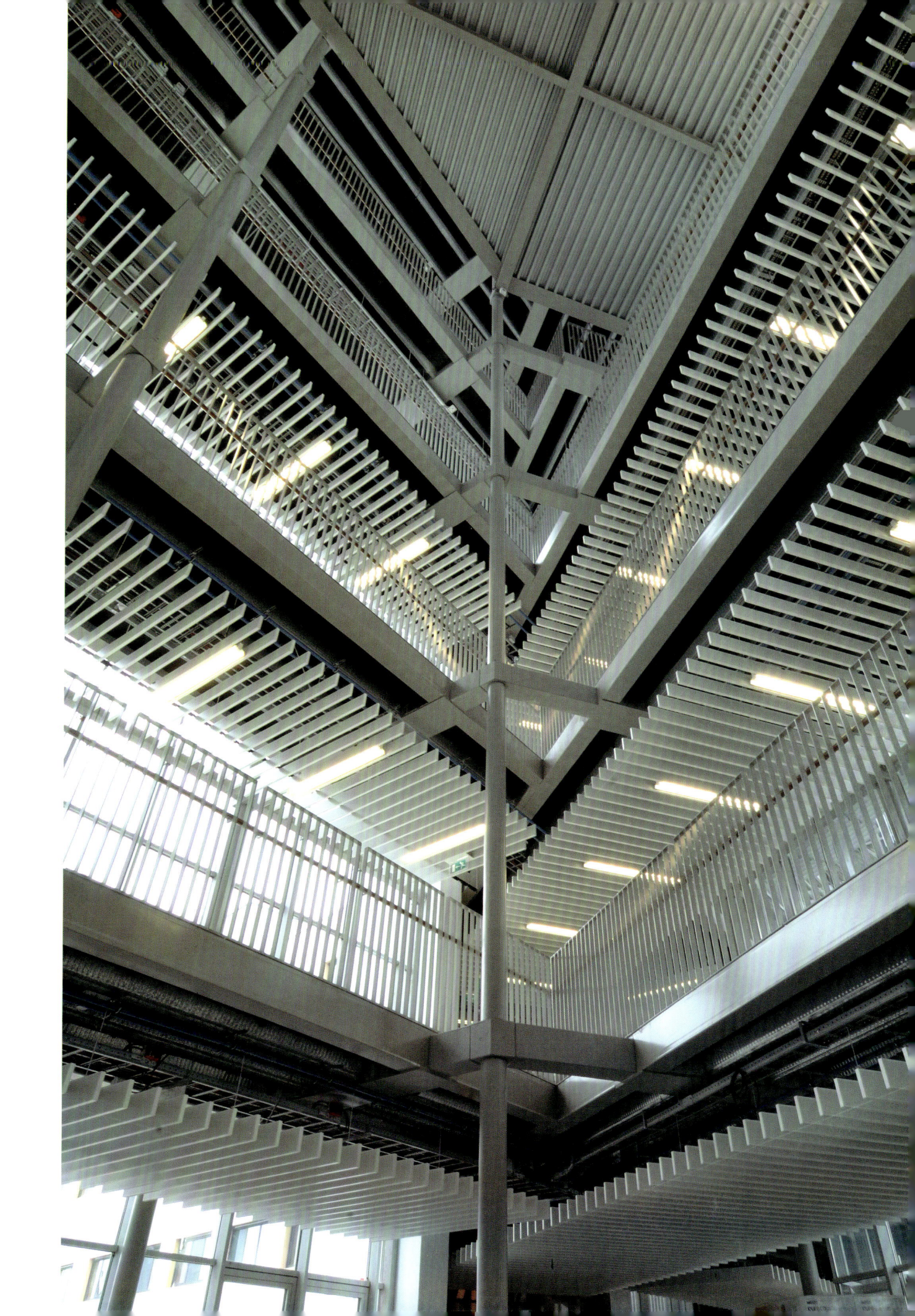

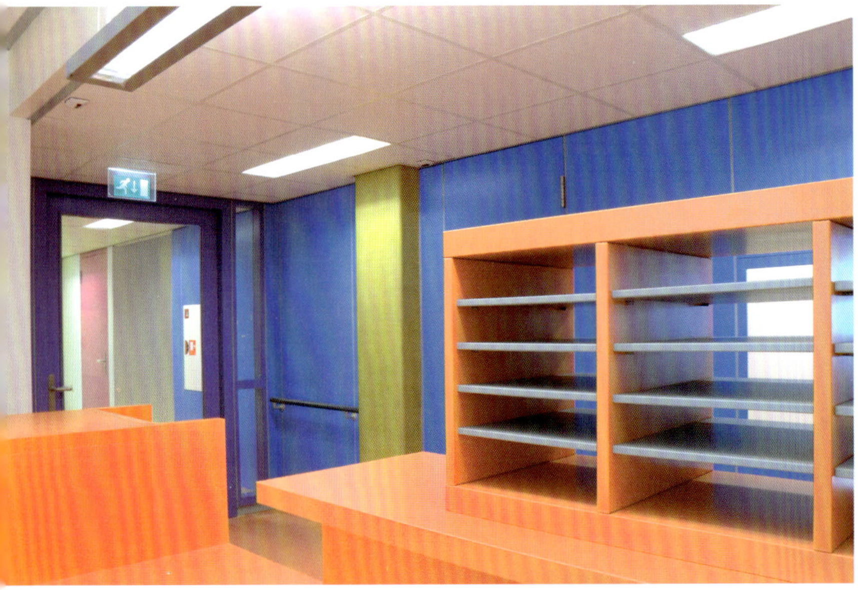
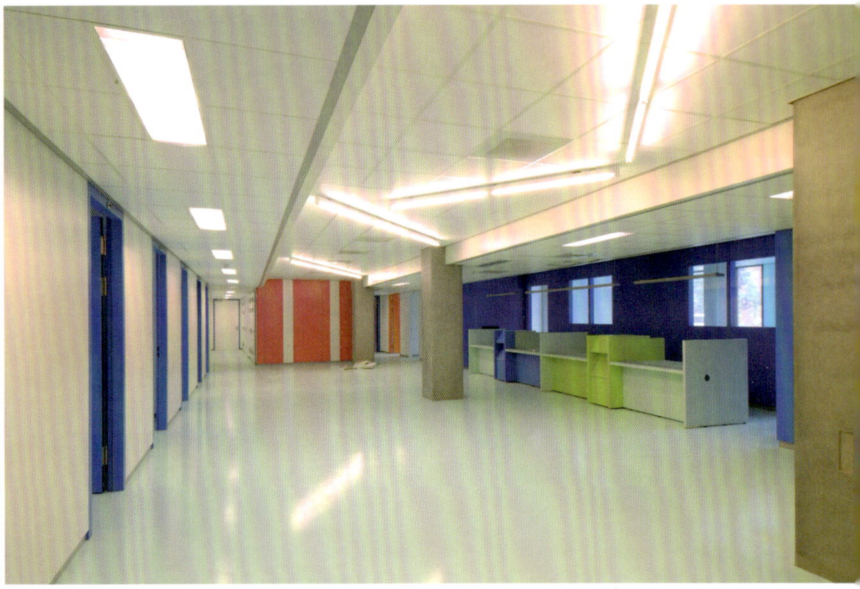
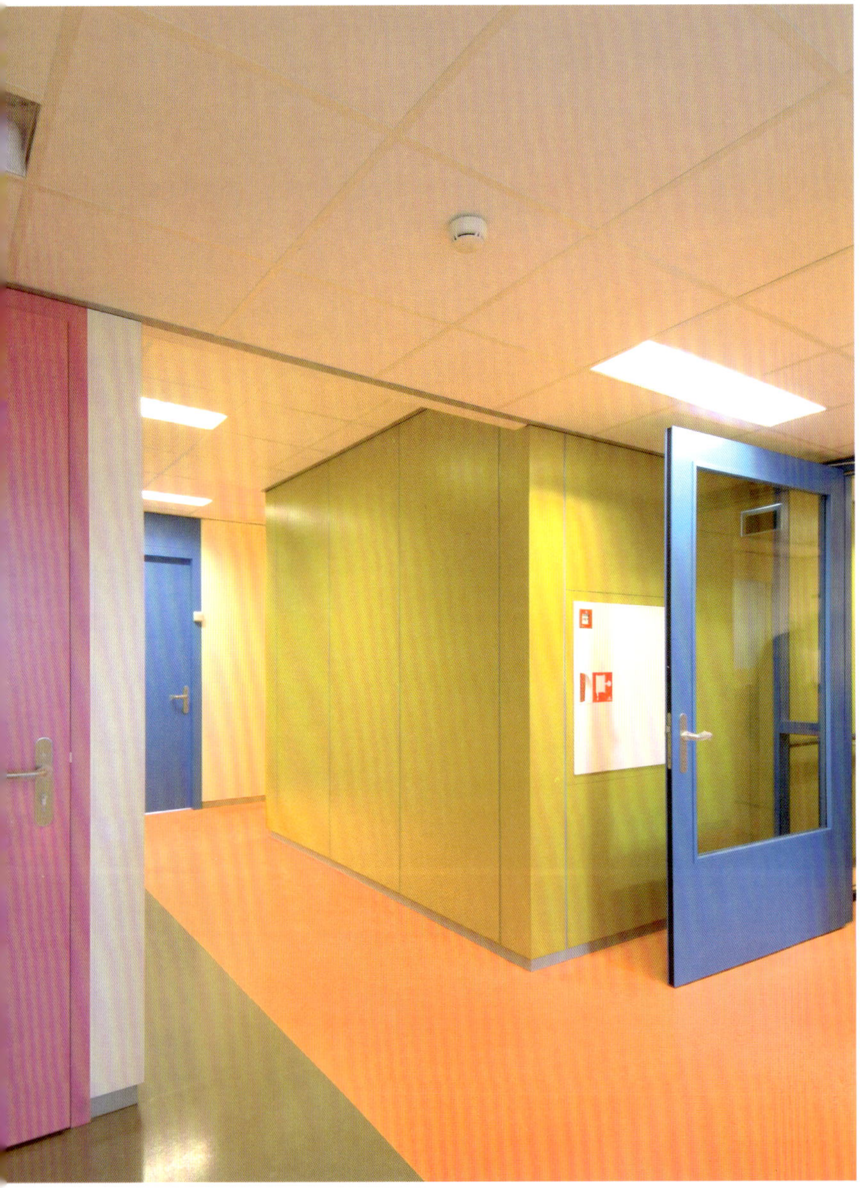
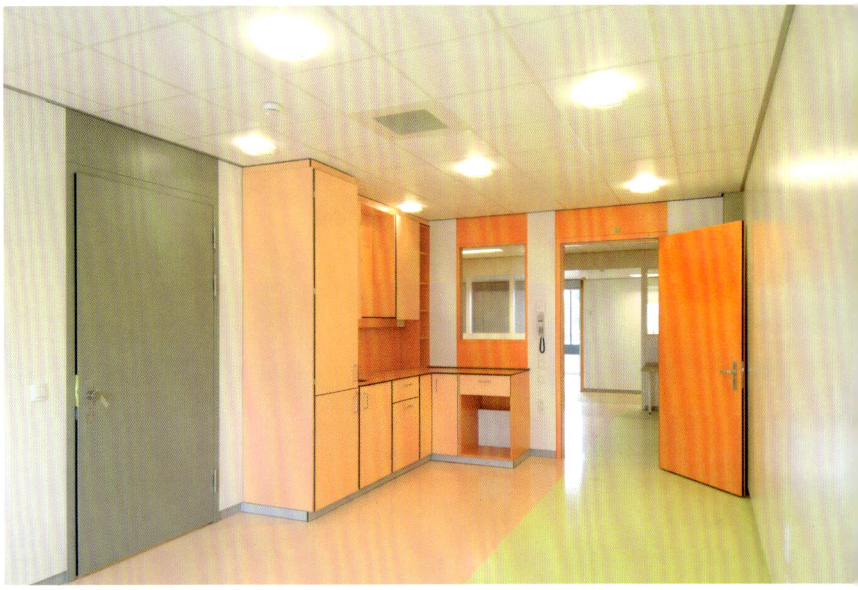
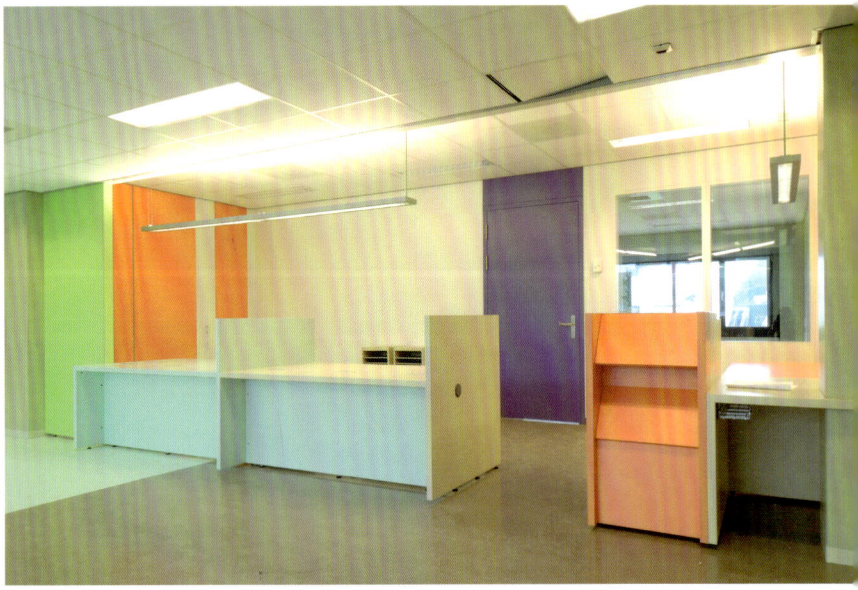

41

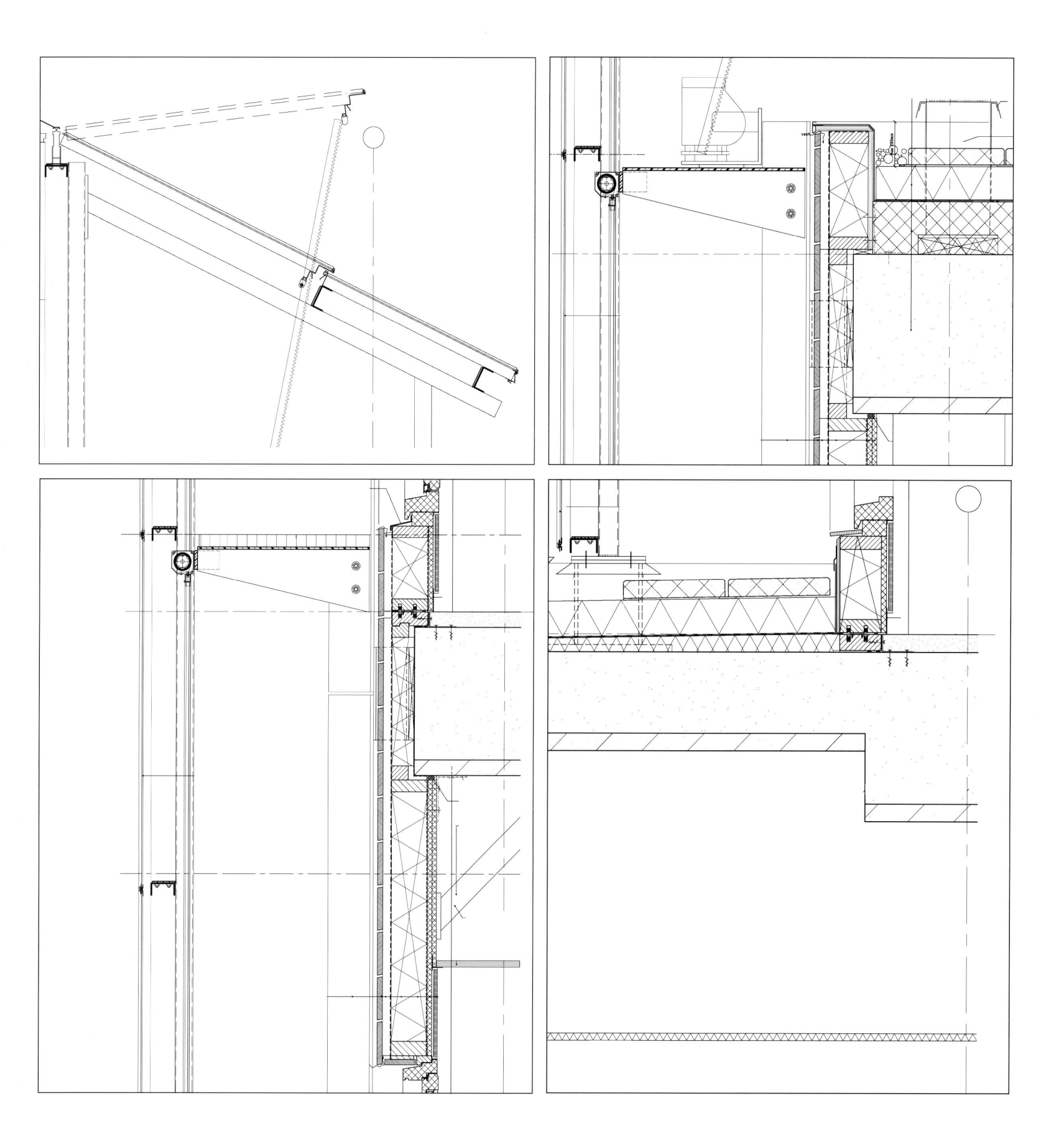

Allford Hall Monaghan Morris

Kentish Town Health Centre

London, UK

Photographs: Rob Parrish, Timothy Soar

Kentish Town Health Centre (KTHC) is a new health building in central London, housing a large GP practice and a wide range of health facilities. The goal of the project was to create a building where not only medicine but also health and art came together for the community. Ideas of transparency and connectivity were embraced by the architects and the whole team worked collaboratively to create a building that expresses the new, holistic approach to healthcare.

KTHC creates a bold civic presence that responds to its environment. Referencing the brick and stucco, architectural repetition, scale and forms of the surrounding housing, the ground floor is articulated as a brick plinth, with the rendered forms of the upper floors floating above. Cantilevered rooms at first and second floor provide substantially larger floor plates at these levels whilst allowing a small ground floor footprint and reducing the overall mass of the building. The building houses a large GP practice, pediatric, dental services, children's services, breast screening and diagnostic imaging, plus supporting office space, staff facilities, library and meeting rooms.

Fully accessible ground and first floors accommodate all public and clinical space, whilst the second floor is a private space for use by staff with teaching rooms. Some areas and rooms on the ground floor have been designed to be used out of clinic hours, and consequently have their own, discrete routes of access and security. Circulation and waiting areas visually connect the different floors and spaces and staff can communicate by talking from bridges and leaning through hatches between consulting floors. Generous staff accommodation, special tea points and break out areas mean that different staff groups can easily meet to discuss and liaise about clients to avoid replication and unnecessary appointments.

Internally, the building has been designed around the concept of a street – a generous public/private space that welcomes users and leads them to the reception at the heart of the building from where all services are accessed. This double or triple-height space running through the building is enlivened by bridges, views, colorful graphics and a bold signage system by Studio Myerscough that creates a stimulating internal streetscape whilst providing ease of use for the diverse needs of the many users. Arts Council funding has been secured to deliver a program of art throughout the building. The materials and fit-out elements of the building have been selected to be both robust and highly flexible. Within communal areas a cost-effective lighting strategy has been designed to reinforce the linearity and volumetric nature of the spaces.

Client:
Camden Primary Care Trust and James Wigg Practice
Surface area:
3,432 sqm (37,000 sqft)
Finish Date:
December 2008
Structural Engineer:
Elliot Wood Partnerships
Graphic Designer:
Studio Myerscough
Landscape Architect:
Jinny Bloom Landscape
Contractor:
Morgan Ashurst Plc
Cost:
£10.1 million

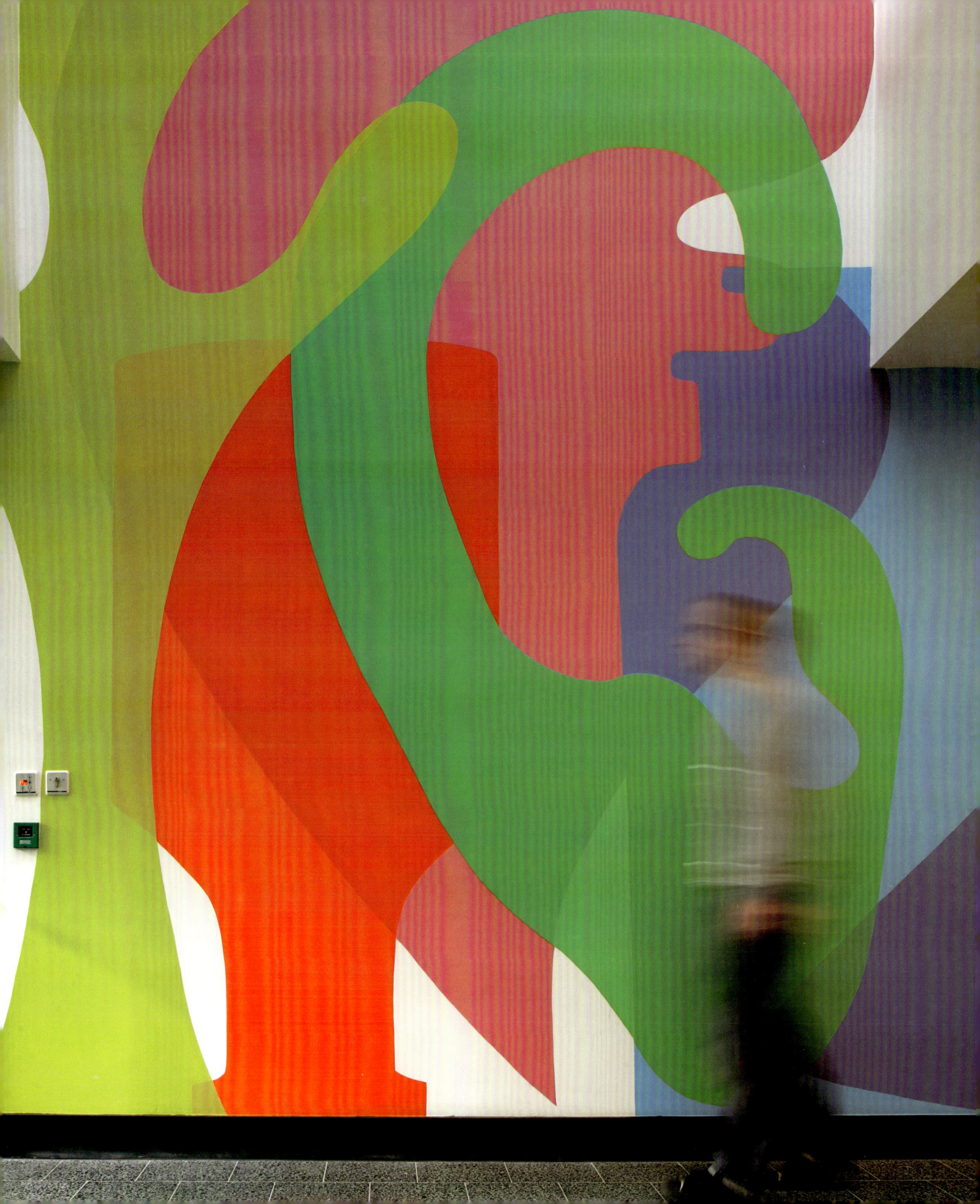

44

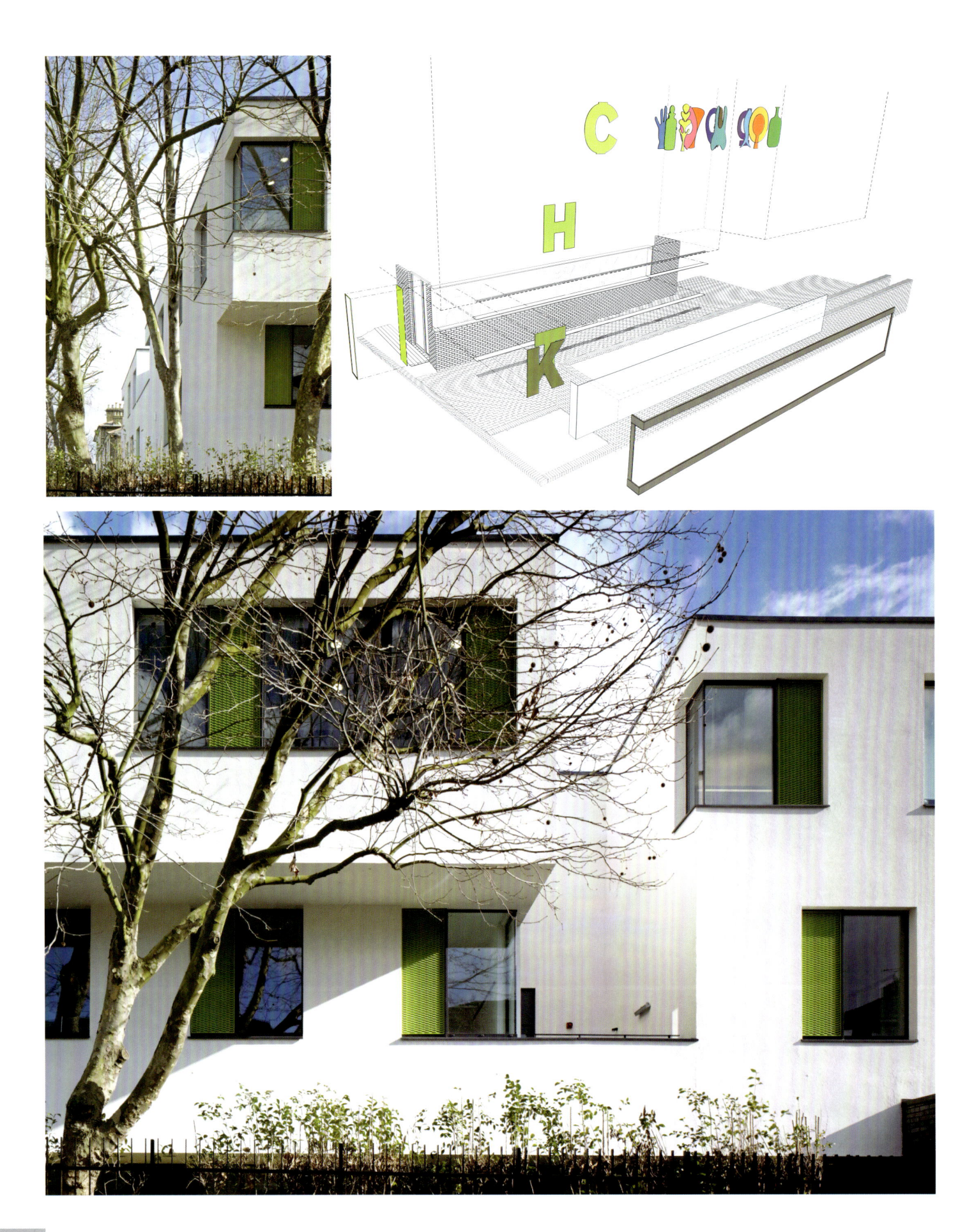

London-based graphic design firm Studio Myerscough designed the colorful graphics and bold signage used throughout the building.

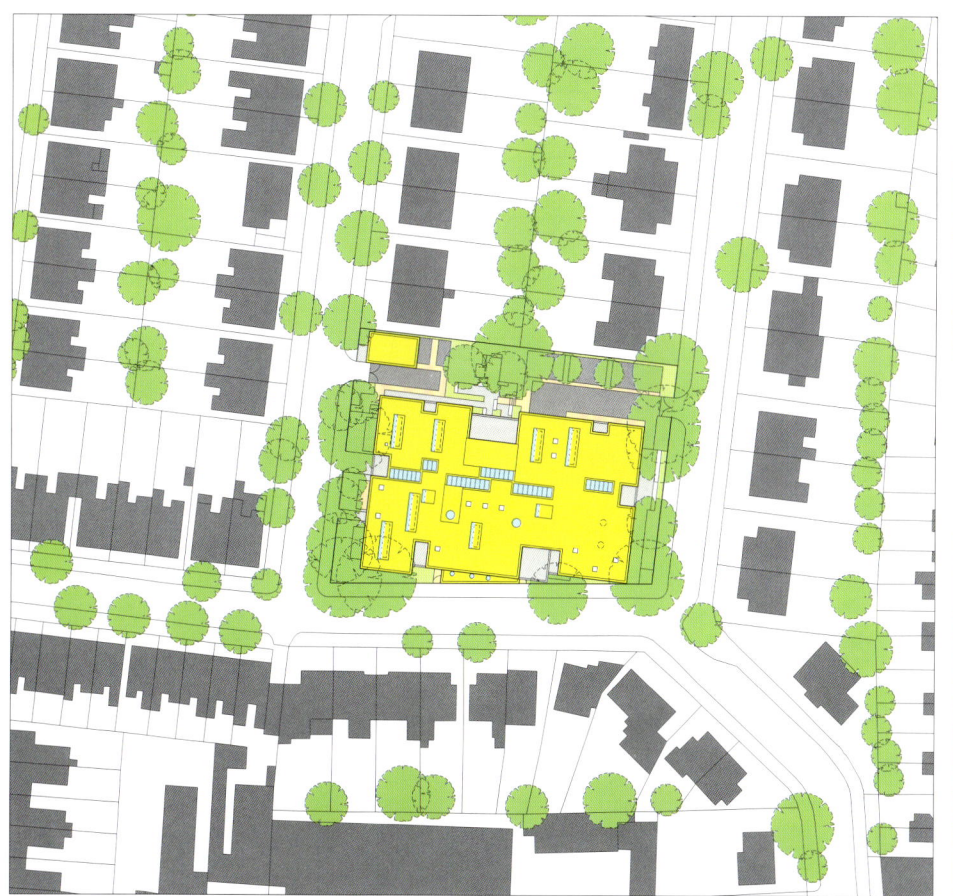

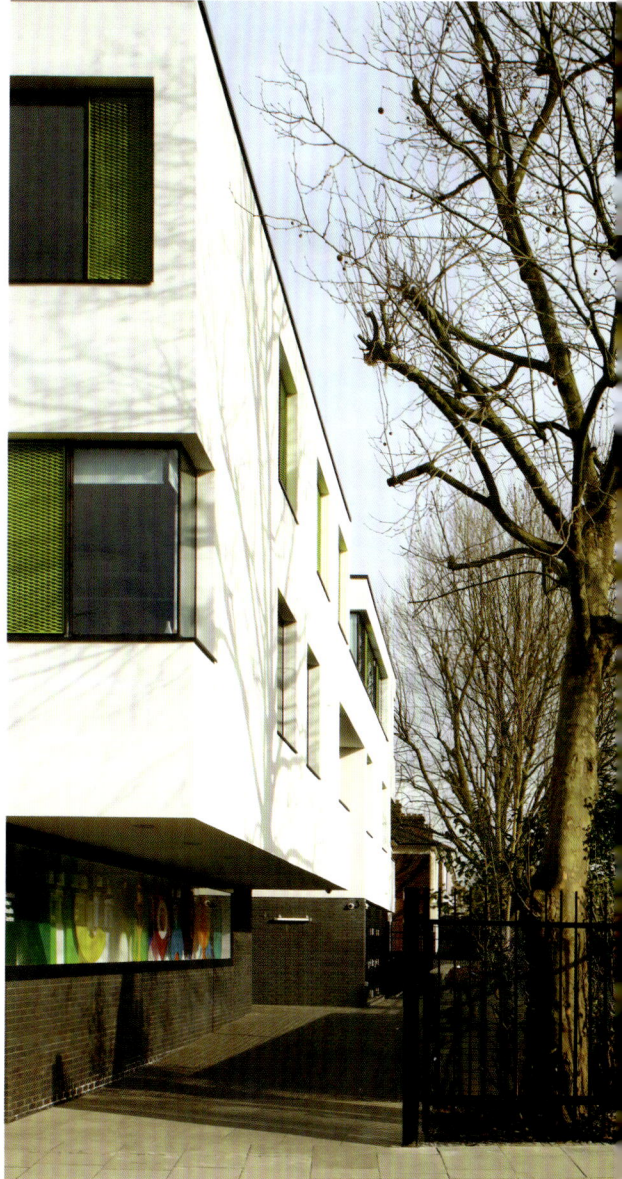

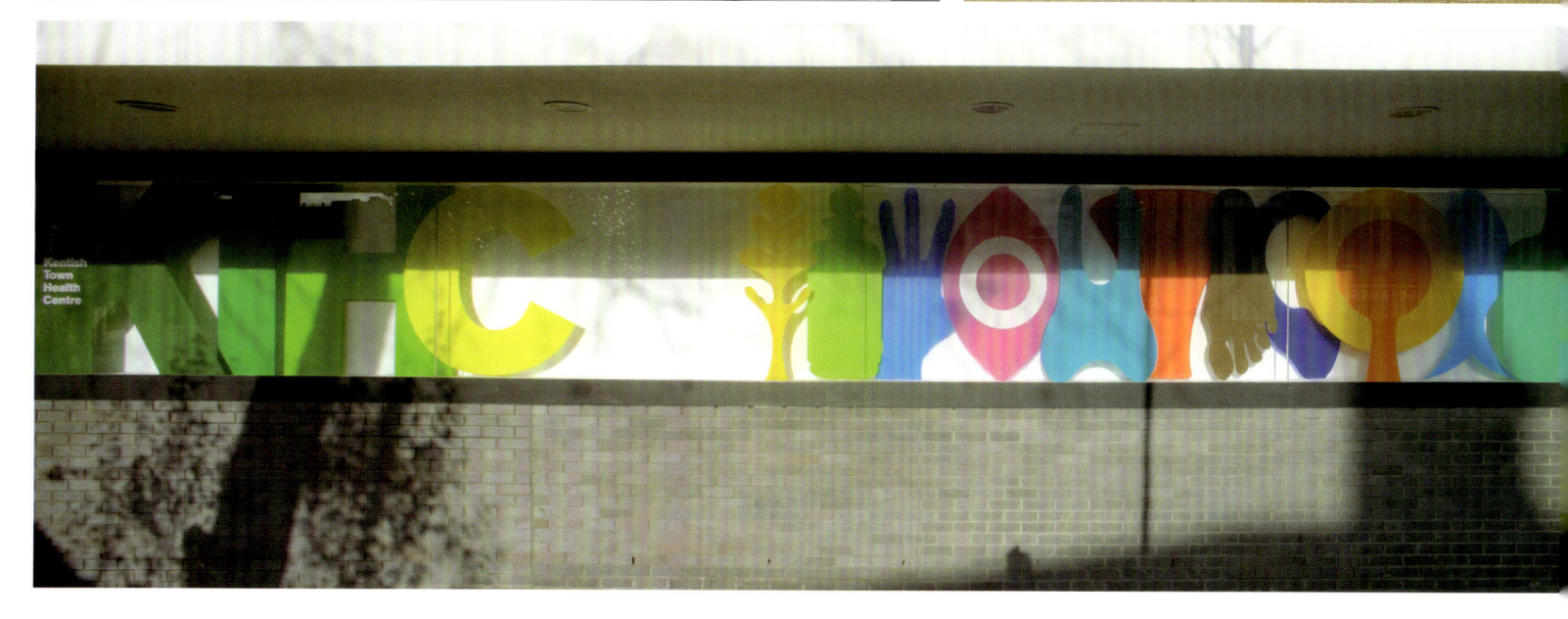

First floor plan

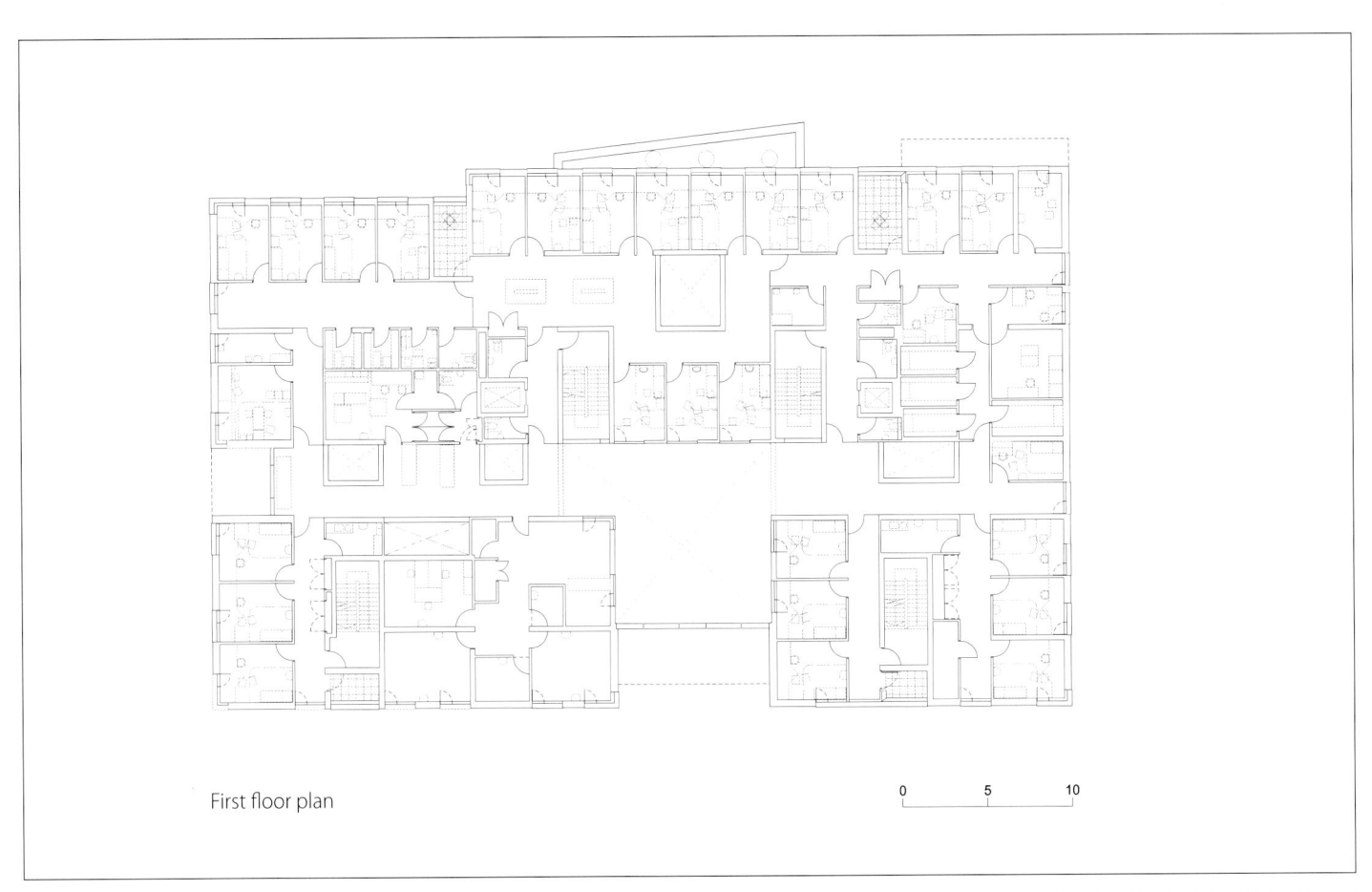

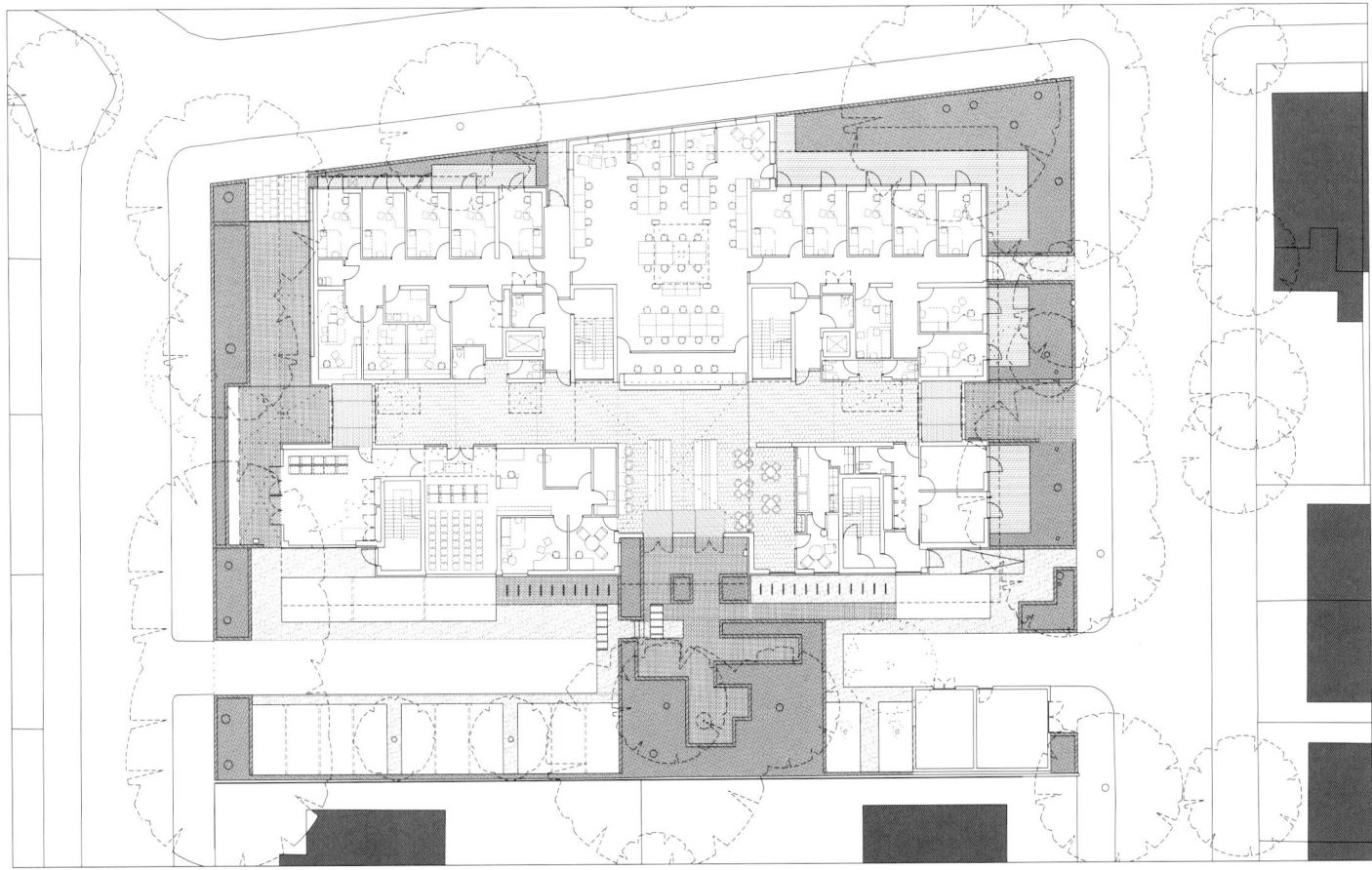

0　5　10

Ground floor plan

Second floor plan

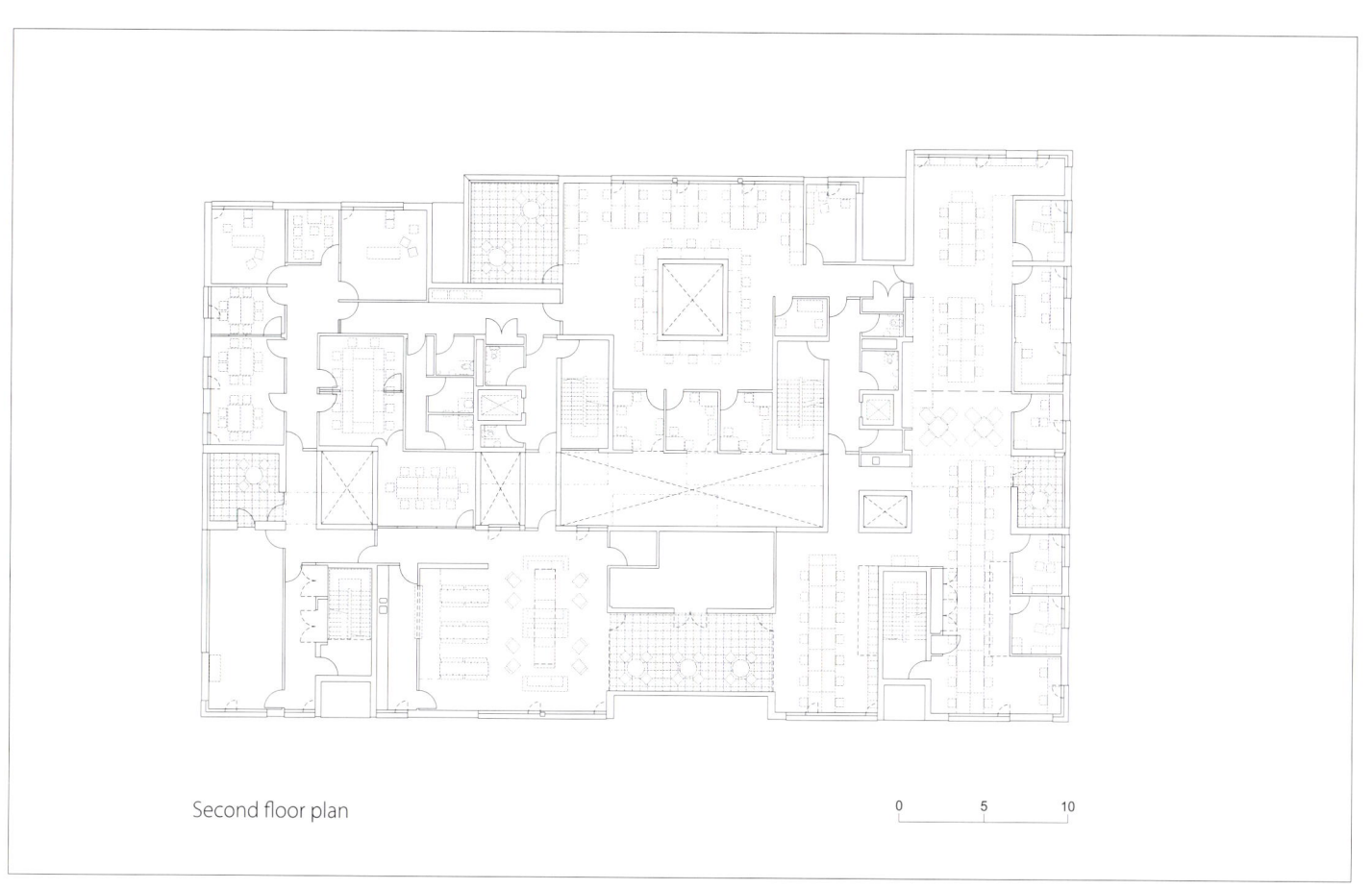

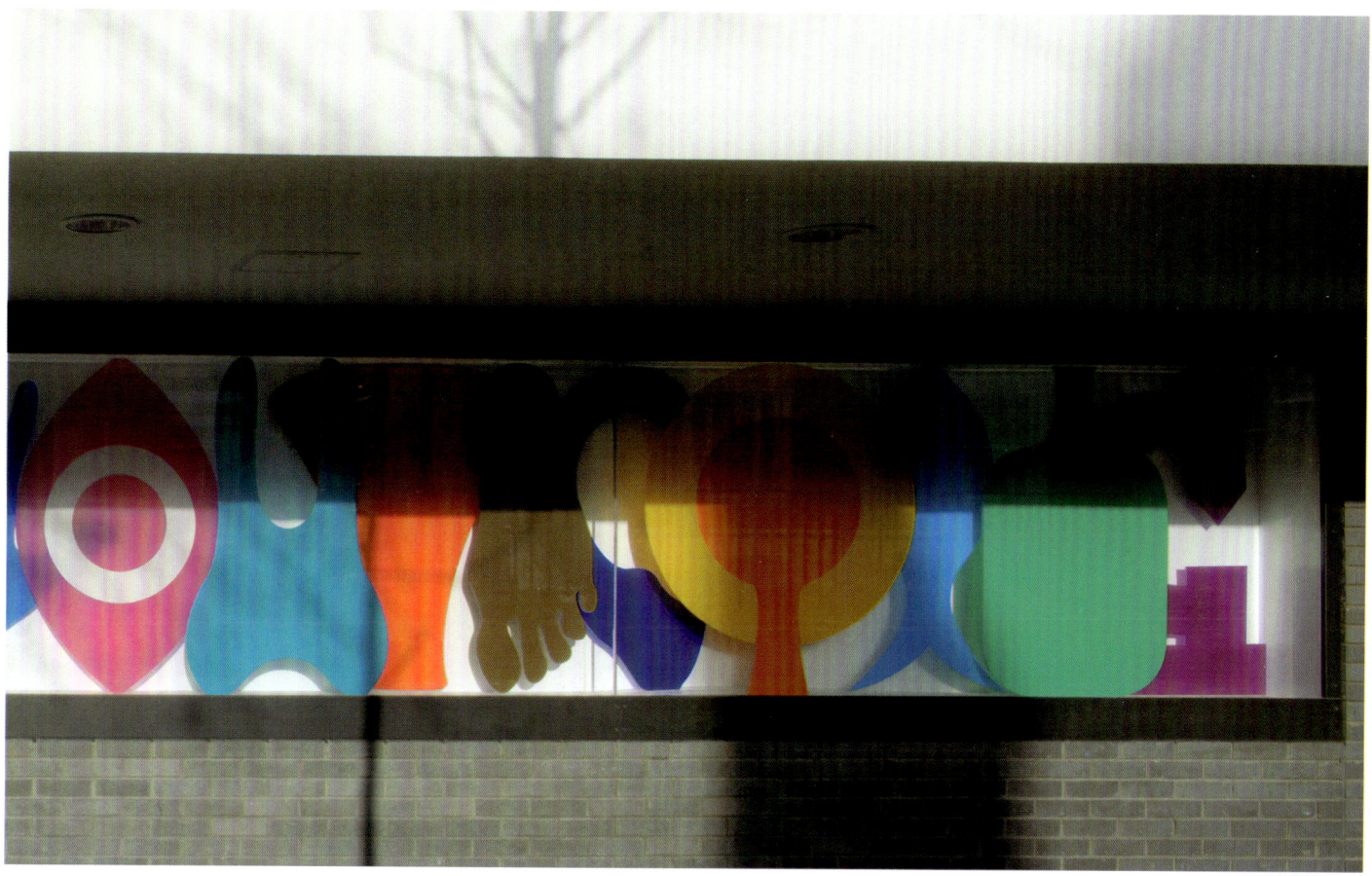

48

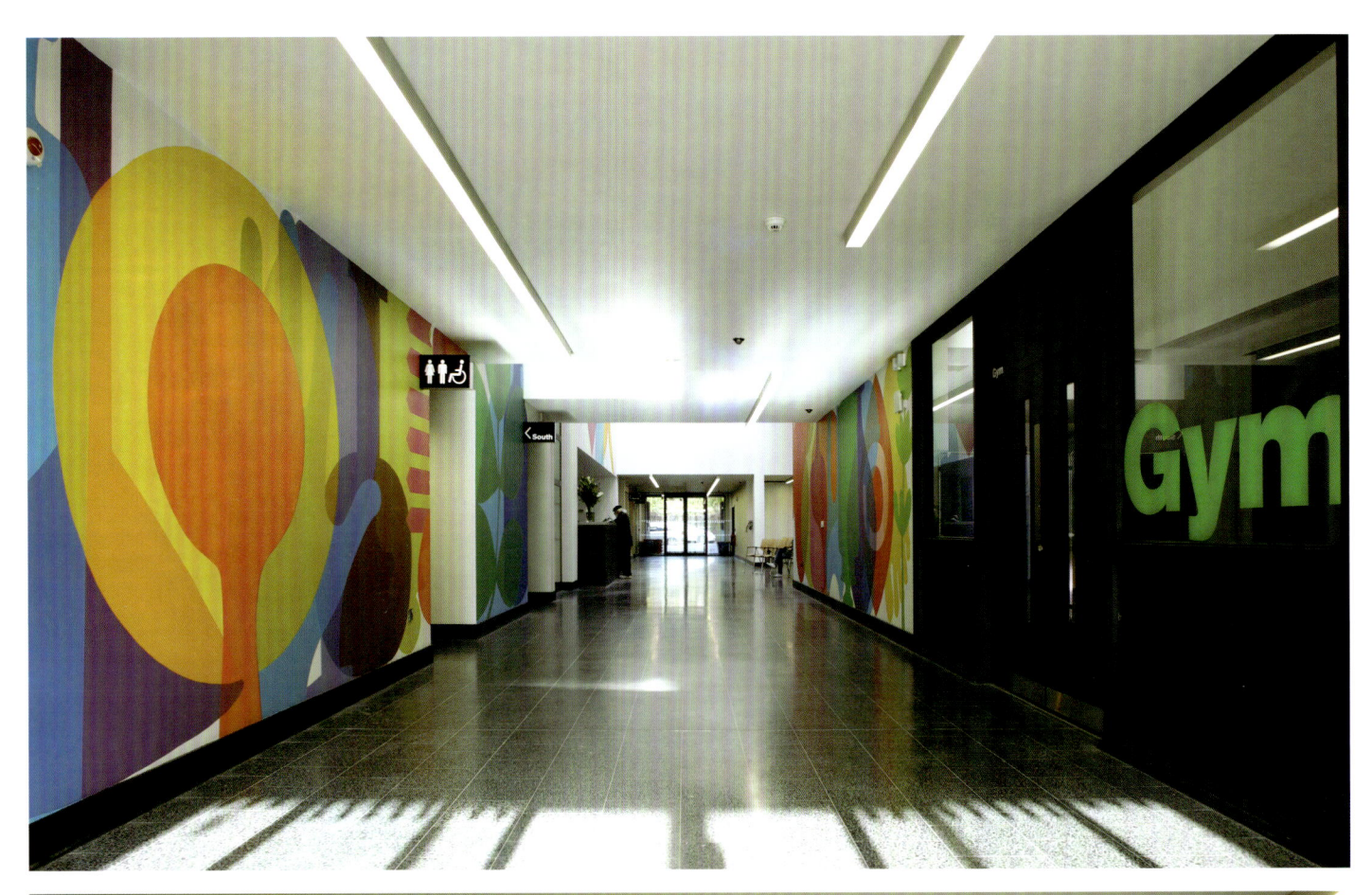

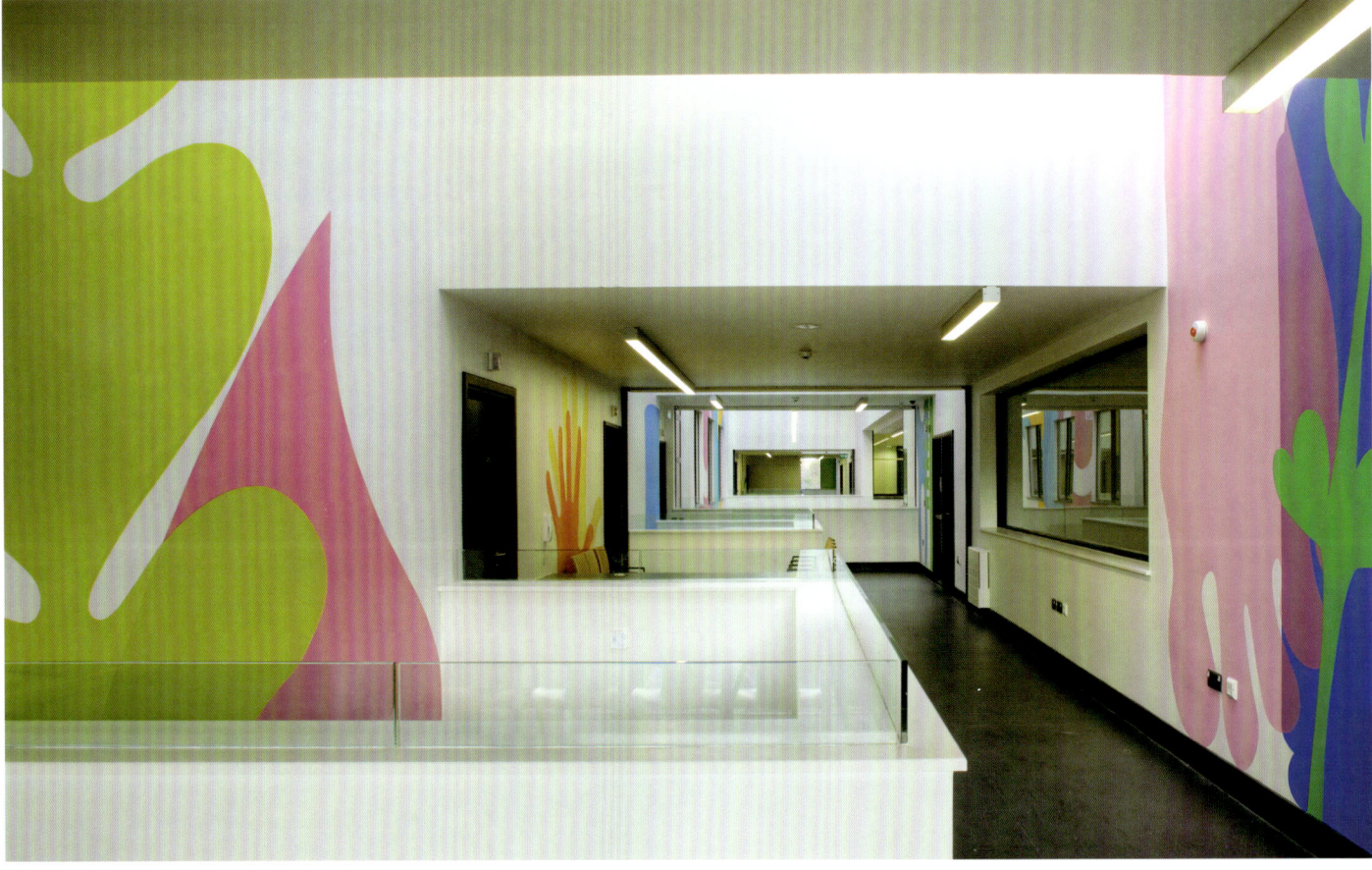

Within all rooms a hanging rail system allows employees to customize their space from a wide selection of fixtures. Interchangeable IPS panels allow the switch from clinical to counseling use with green, black and white selected to provide a calming, neutral environment.

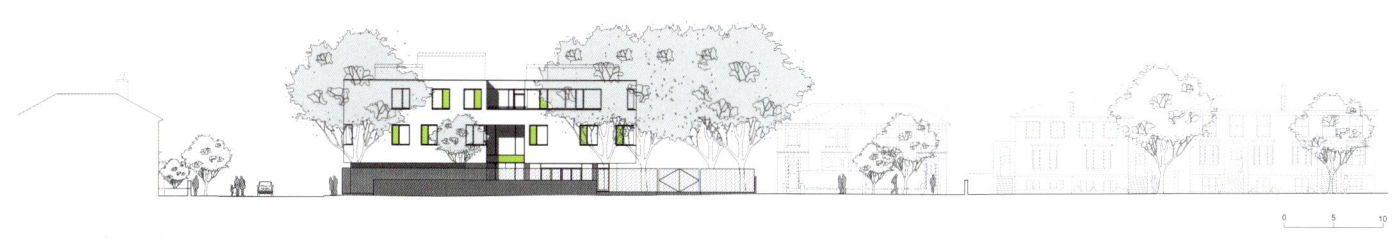

East View

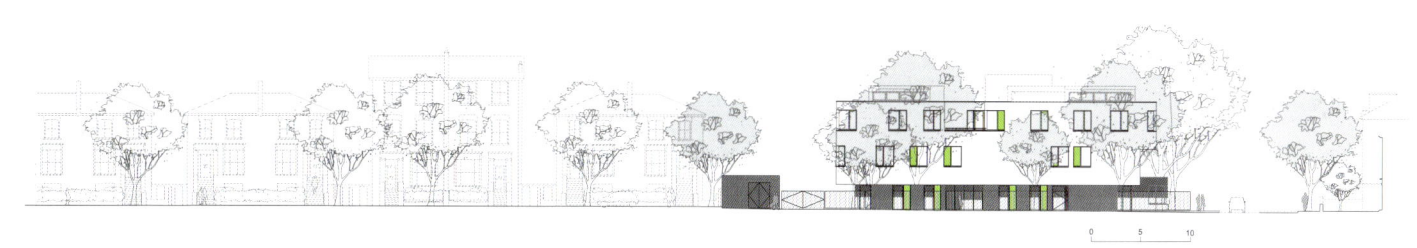

West View

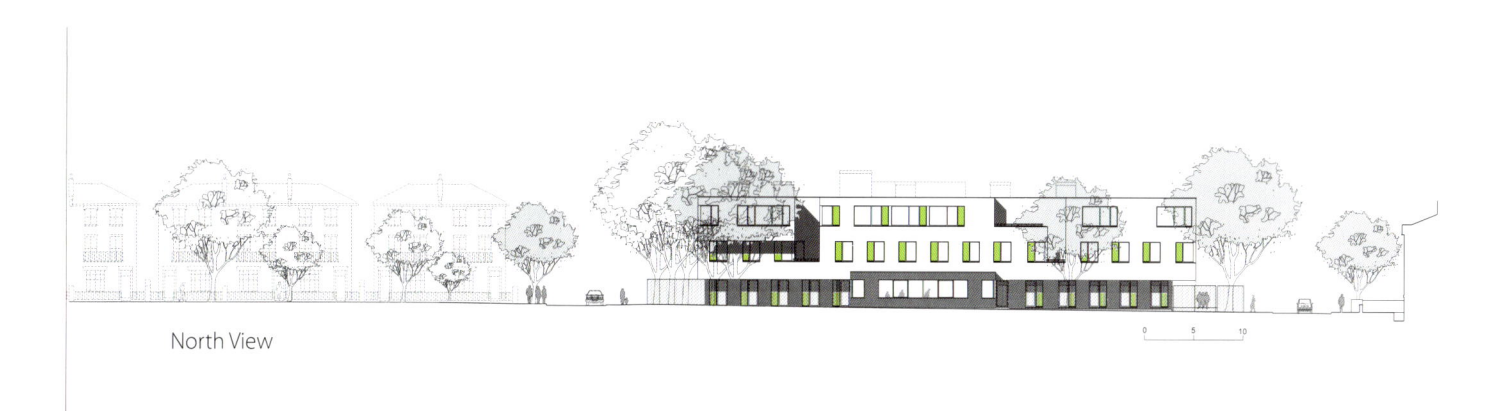

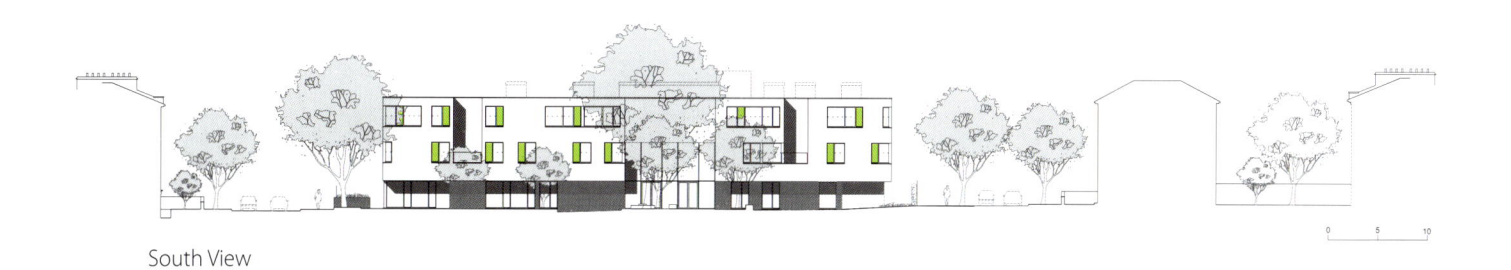

North View

South View

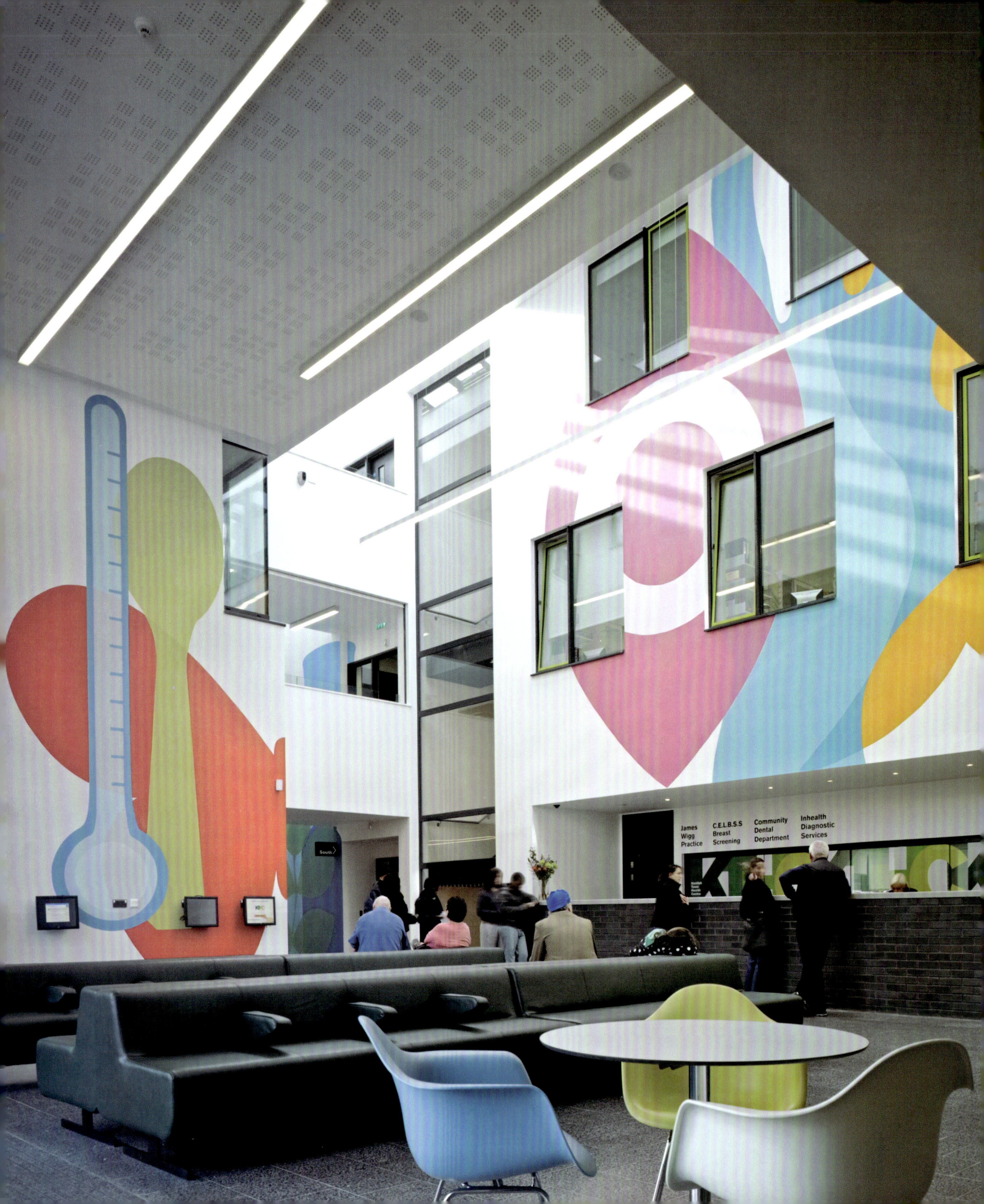

James Wigg Practice
C.E.L.B.S.S Breast Screening
Community Dental Department
Inhealth Diagnostic Services
South

The colorful triple height atrium creates a stack effect within the main street, drawing fresh air throughout the building assisted by wind catchers, and temperature-responsive openers on the roof lights.

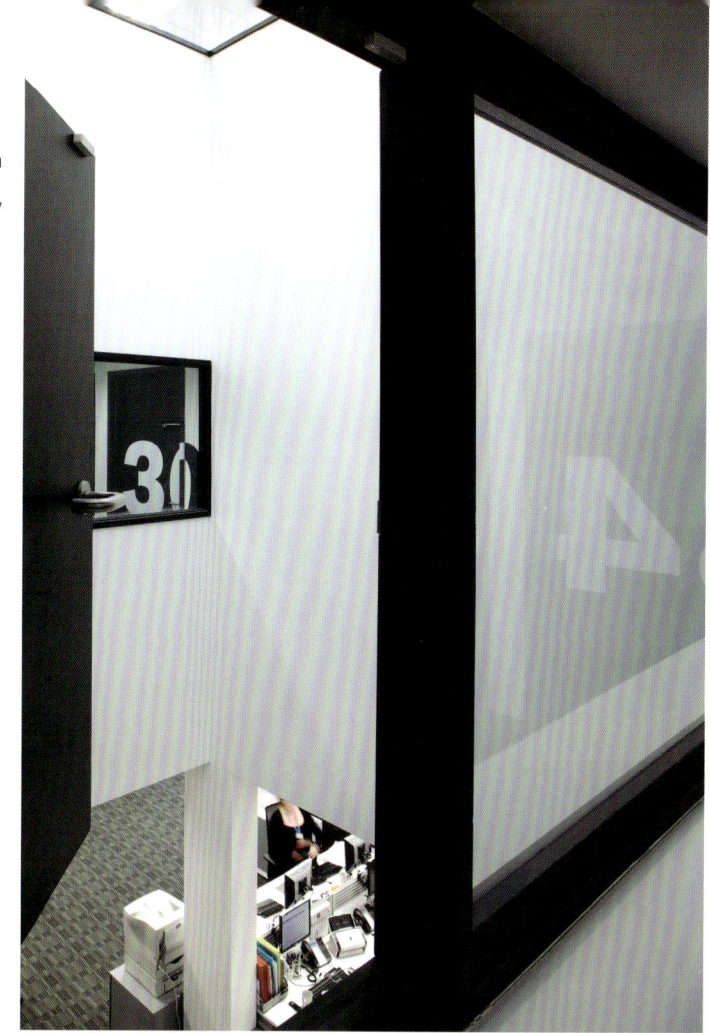

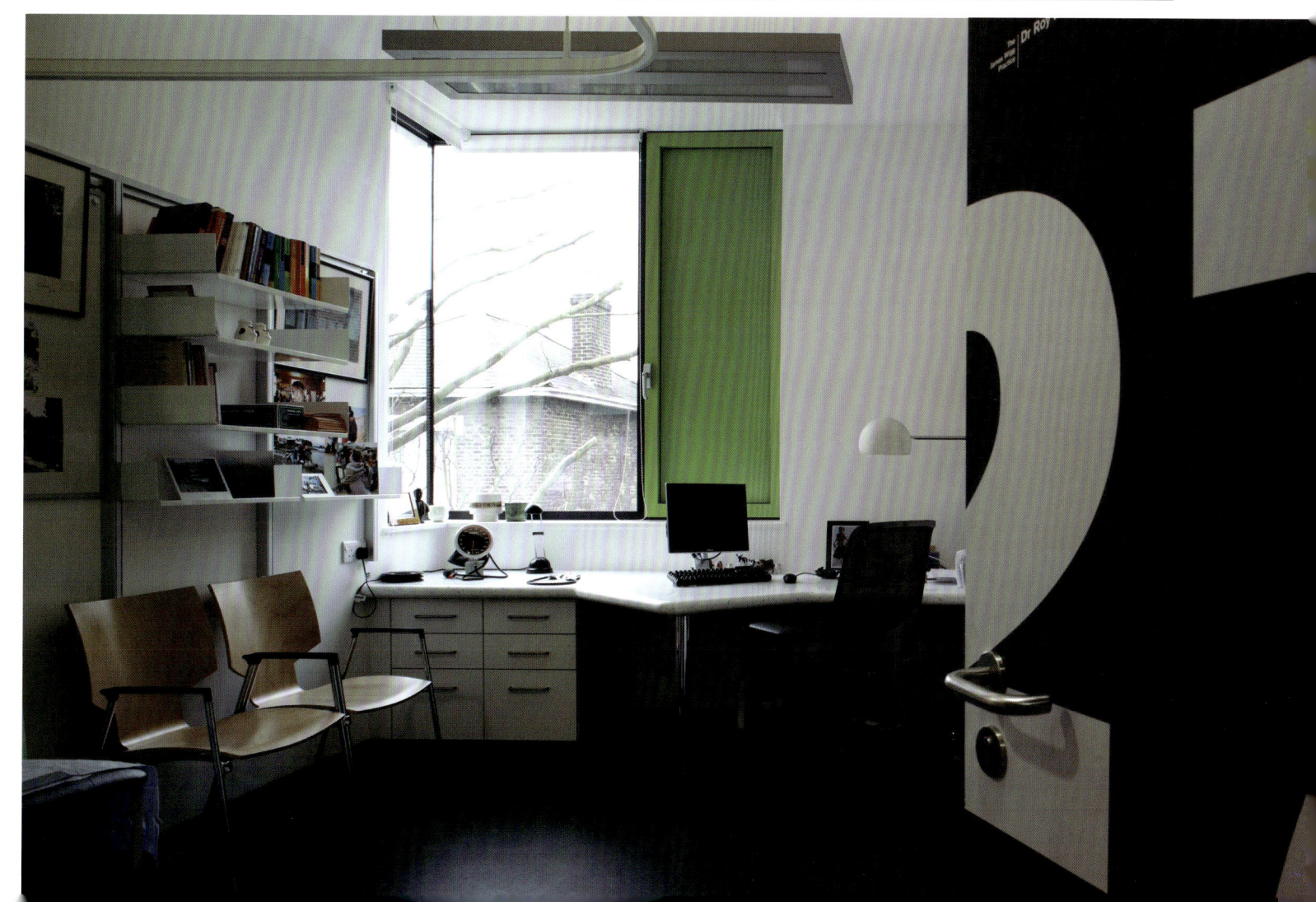

C. F. Møller Architects

Akershus University Hospital

Oslo, Norway

Photographs: *Torben Eskerod, C. F. Møller Architects*

The new university hospital is not a traditional institutional construction; it is a friendly, informal place with open, well-structured surroundings which form a welcoming image for patients and their families. Akershus University Hospital has been designed to emphasize security and clarity in experientially rich surroundings, where everyday functions and familiar materials are integrated into the hospital's structure. Although the individual parts of the development each have their own character and the material expression throughout the development varies, the project is united into a whole by means of a general architectural theme centered on panels and transparency. In this way continuity is created between the individual parts of the complex to aid orientation, while users of the hospital also benefit from a varied visual experience.

A glass-covered main thoroughfare, in which wood is the predominant material, links the various buildings and departments. The "glass street" begins in the foyer at the entrance area, where the main reception desk welcomes visitors, and concludes in the foyer and separate entrance area of the children's department. This central element in the development unites the various materials in an overall composition in which the large colored panels, designed by Icelandic artist Birgir Andrésson, form a natural element and provide a 'palette' for the color scheme of the hospital. The glass street has a town-like structure, with public and semi-public zones defined as squares and open spaces, offering the everyday functions of a town: church, pharmacy, hairdresser, florist, café and kiosk, as well as traffic nodes and other services for the benefit of patients, relatives and staff. In natural continuation of these functions, a number of other services, such as health information, polyclinics and outpatient surgeries, are located near the street level of the thoroughfare.

The hospital's structure helps to ensure that the patient remains the natural focus in the physical design, despite the strict and demanding logistical requirements which underlie all hospital constructions. Just as the overall complex is made up of clear and comprehensible units, so the individual wards are built up from smaller elements. The wards are situated around four courtyards which ensure a well-defined daily life for the patients, with a manageable level of social contact, assisted by a clear staff interface. The wards of the children's department are equipped with generous windows that give the children individual views of both the sky and the surrounding greenery from their beds. The well-equipped facilities for parents secure excellent contact between the children and their families.

Client:
Helse Sør-Øst RHF
Surface area:
137,000 sqm (1,475,000 sqft)
Start date:
2000
Finish date:
2008
Landscape Design:
Bjørbekk & Lindheim AS, Schønherr Landskab A/S
Cost:
€ 1 billion

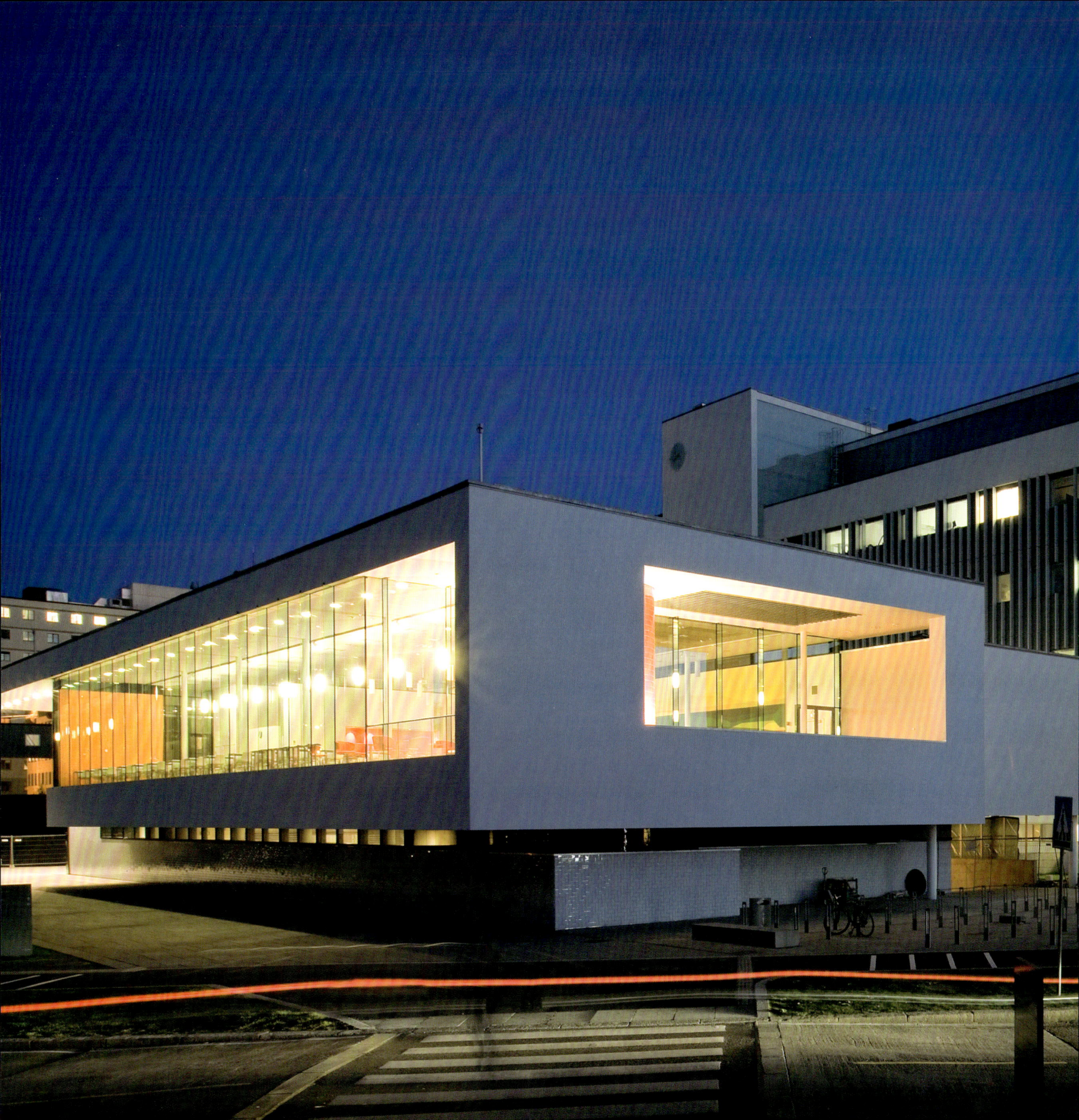

54

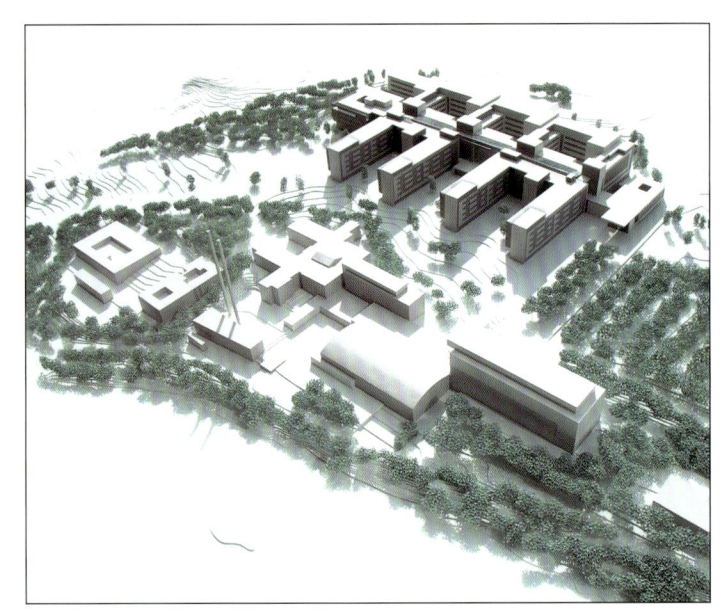

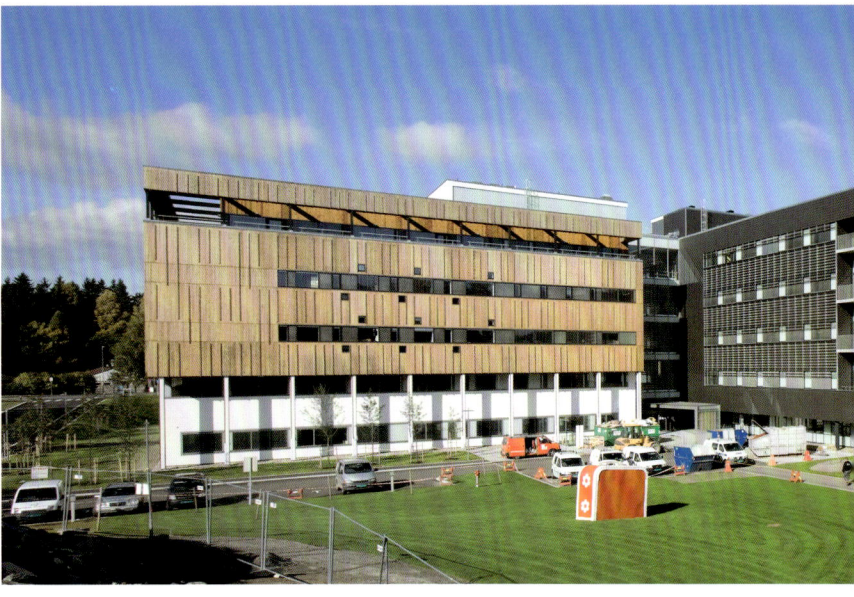

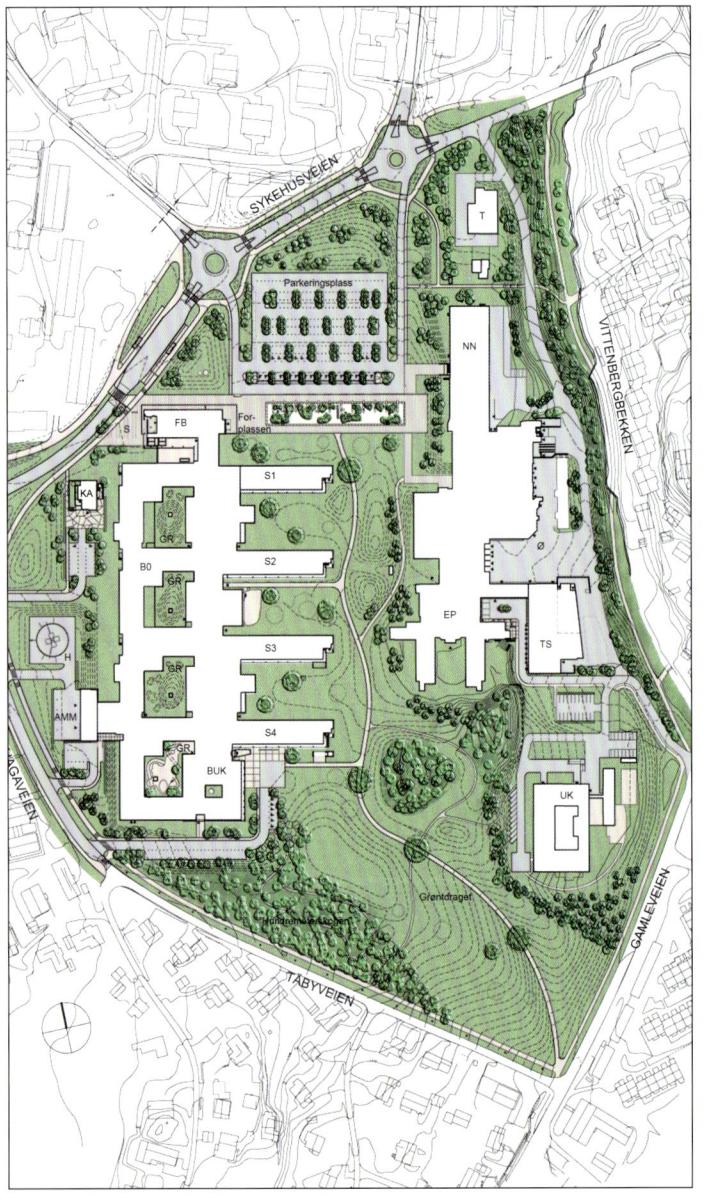

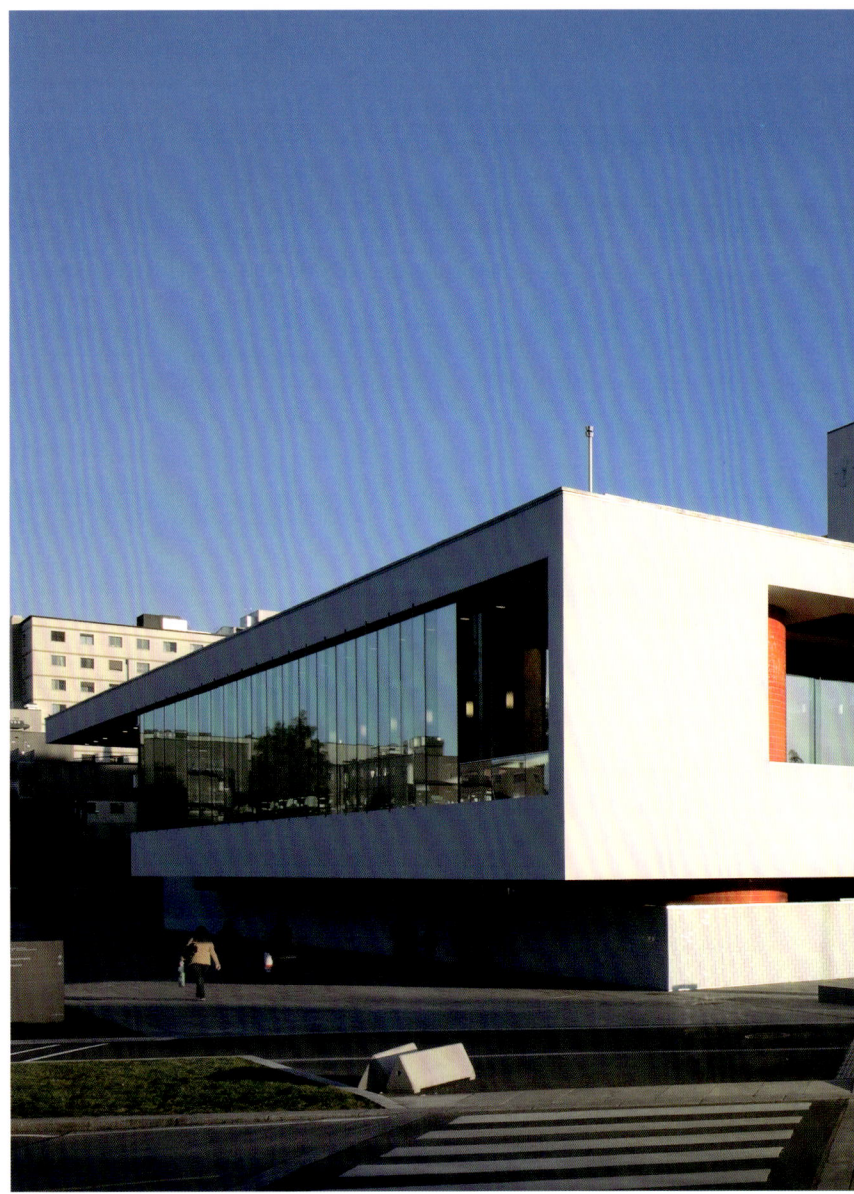

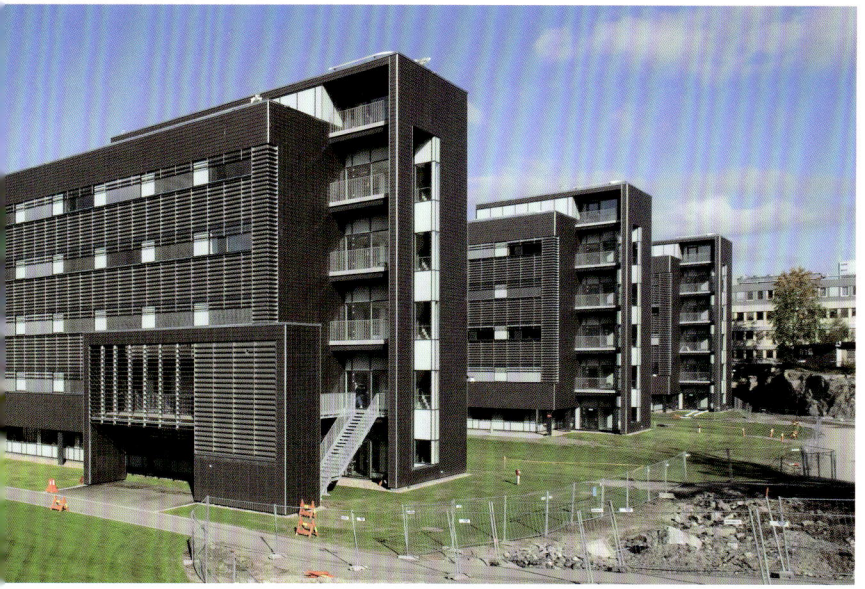

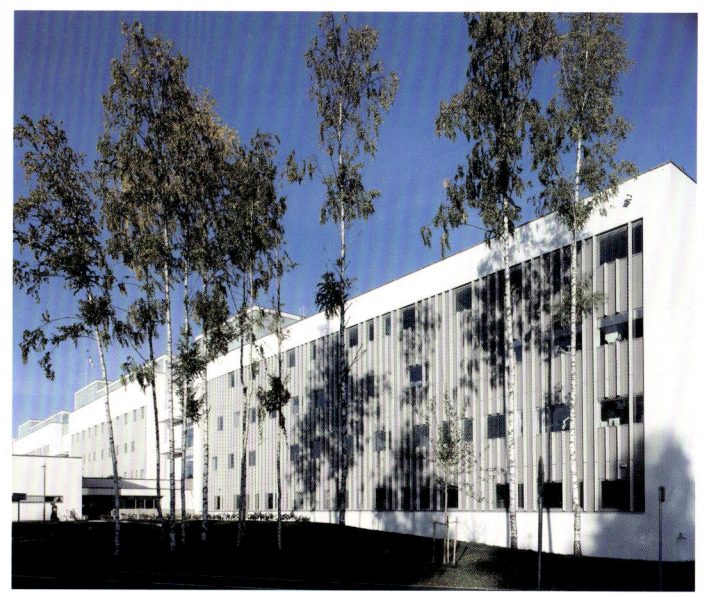

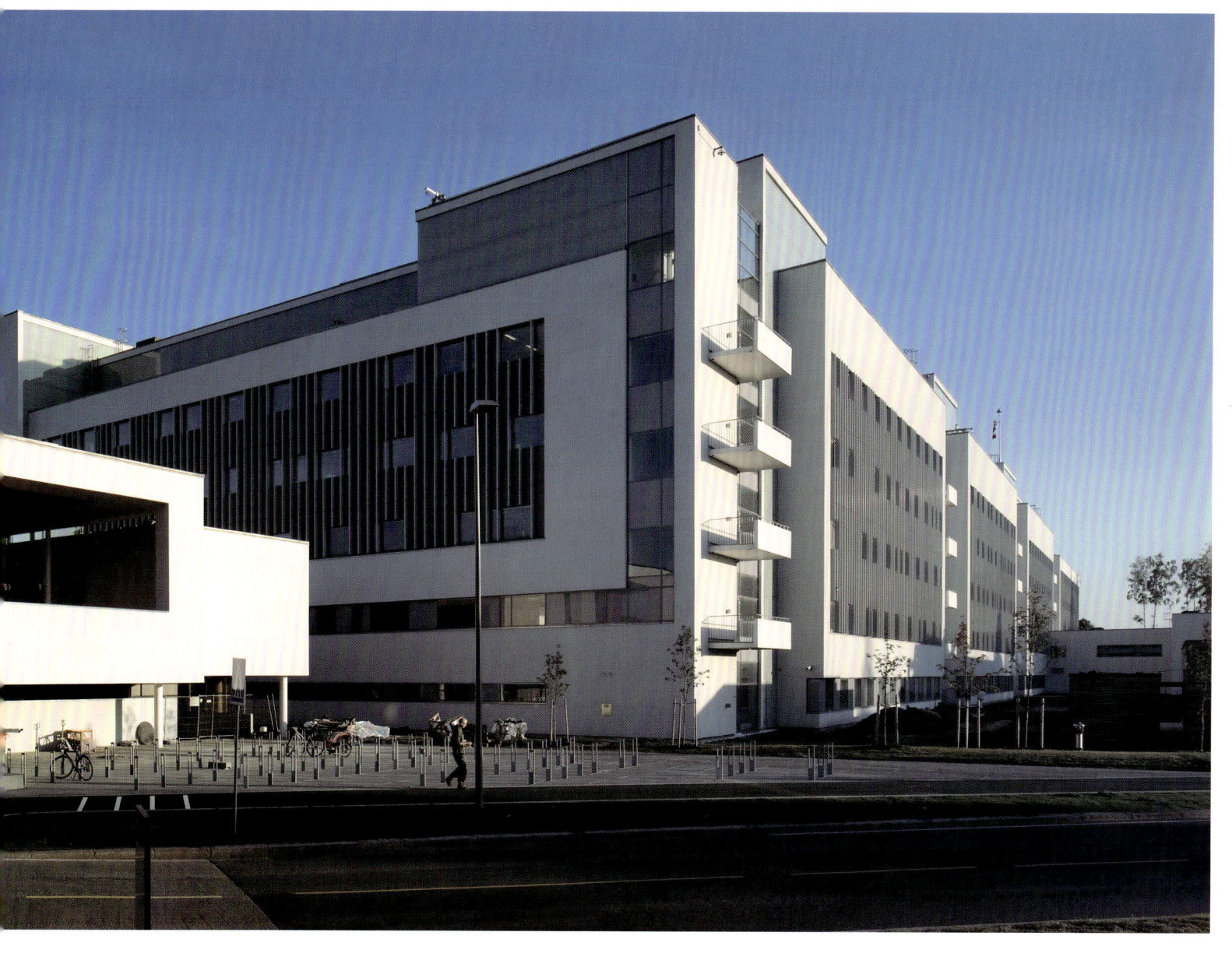

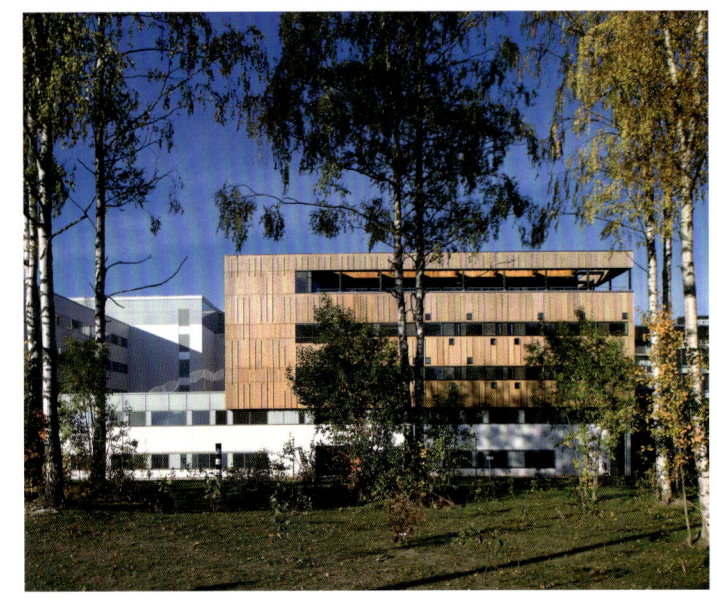

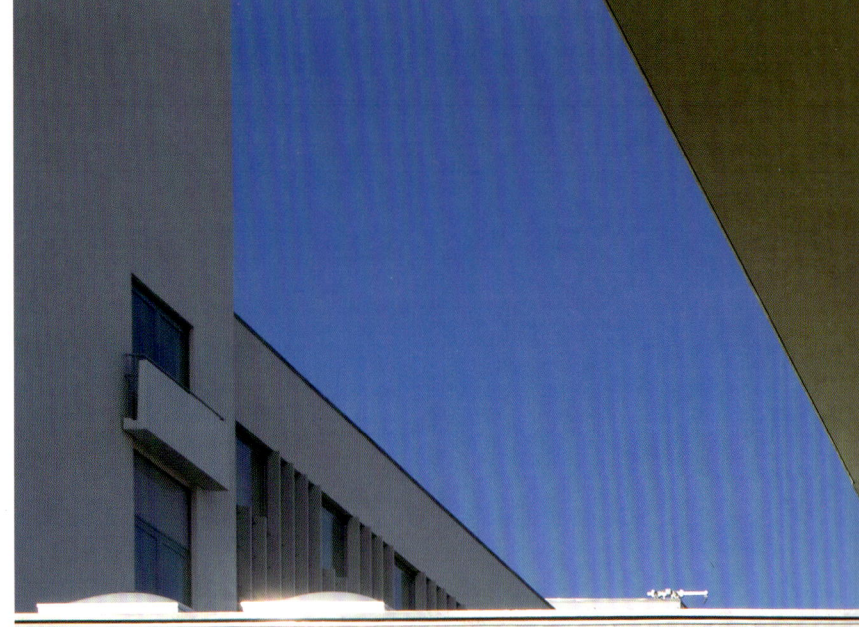

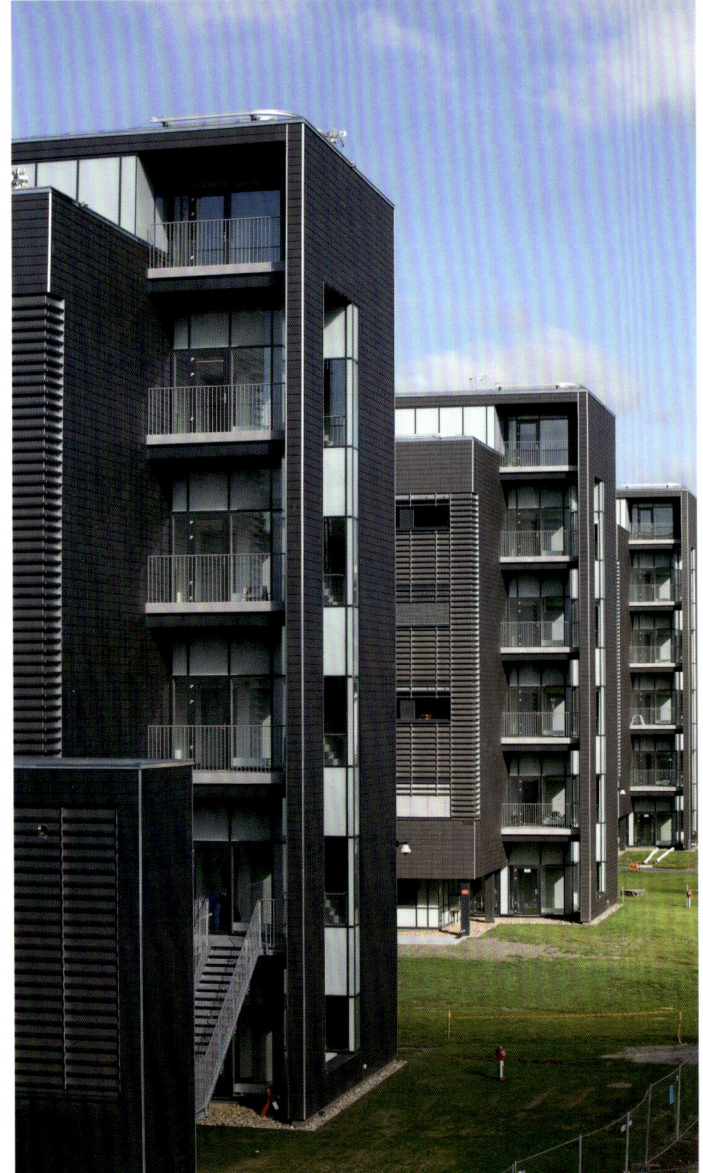

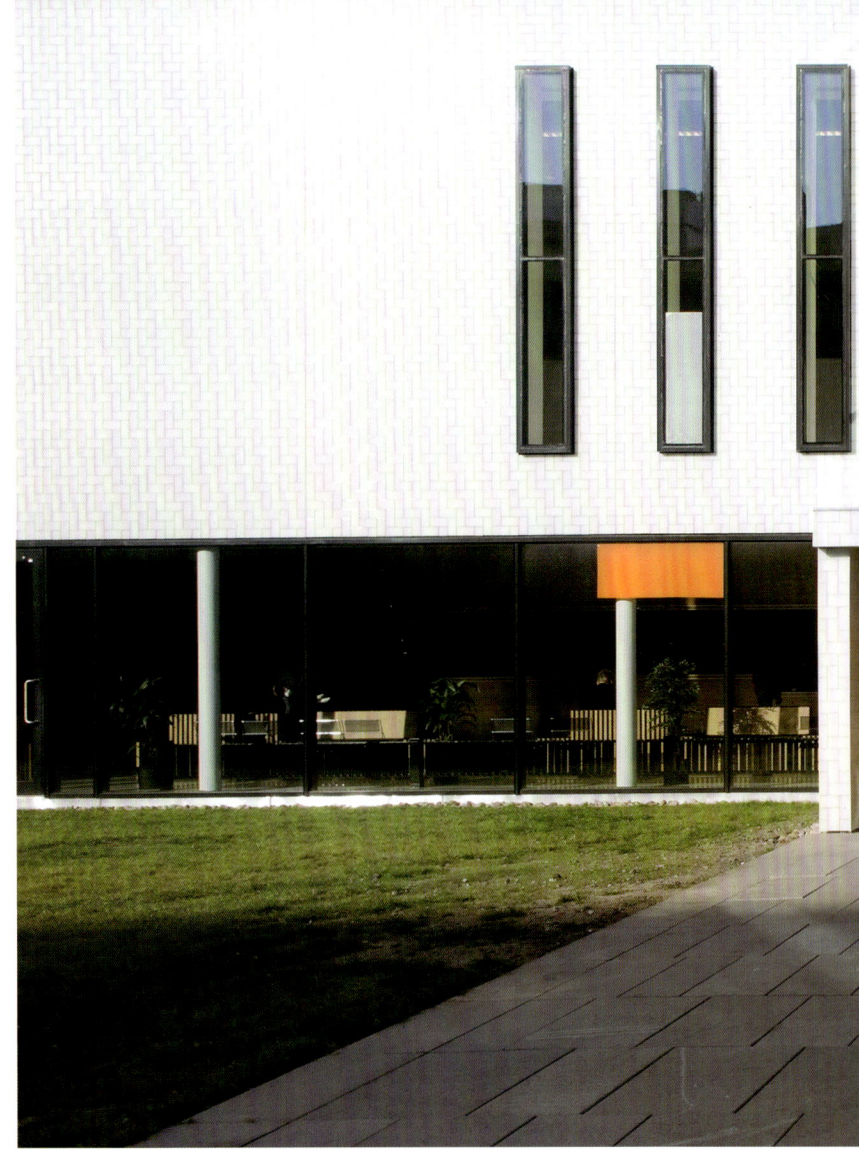

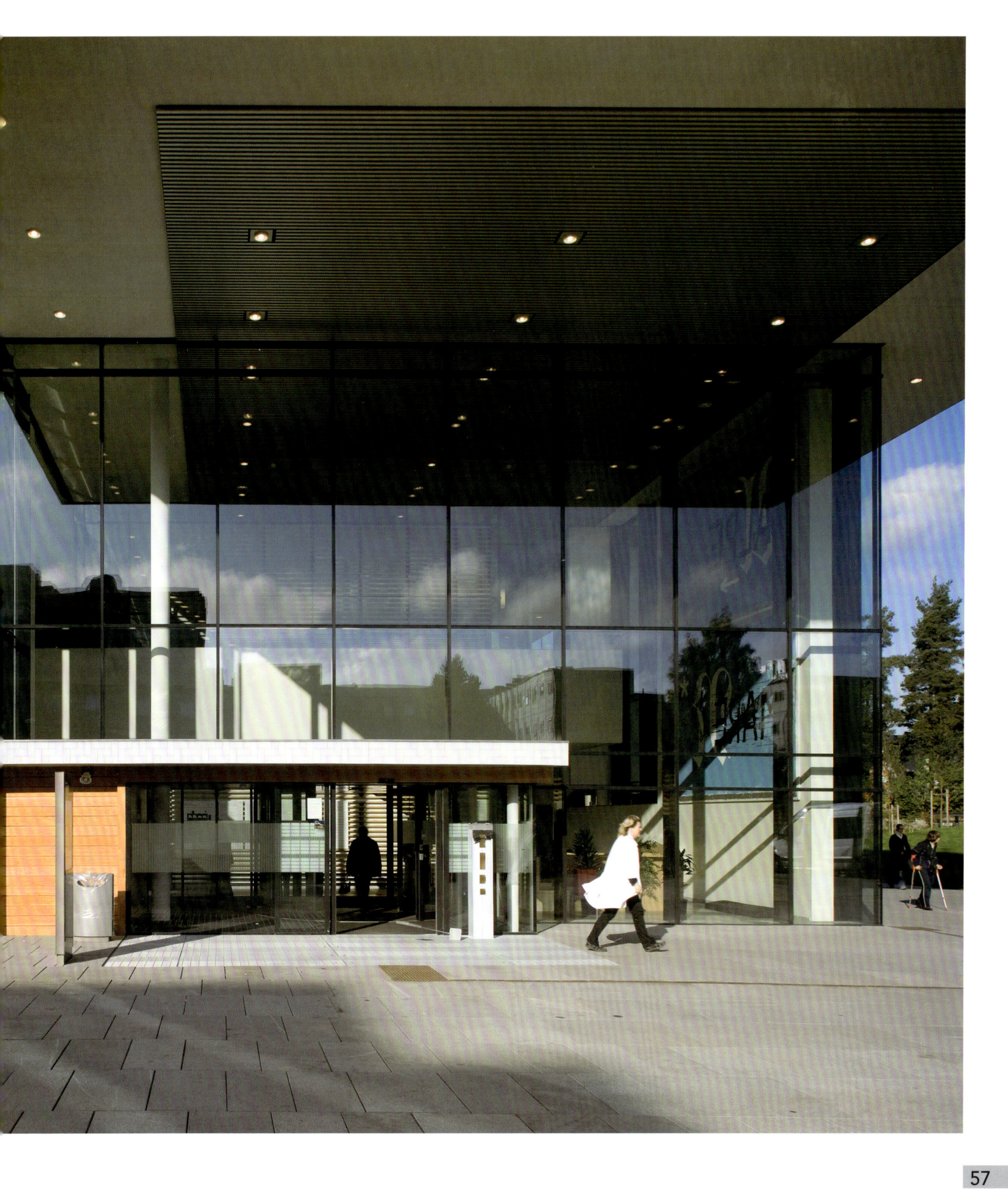

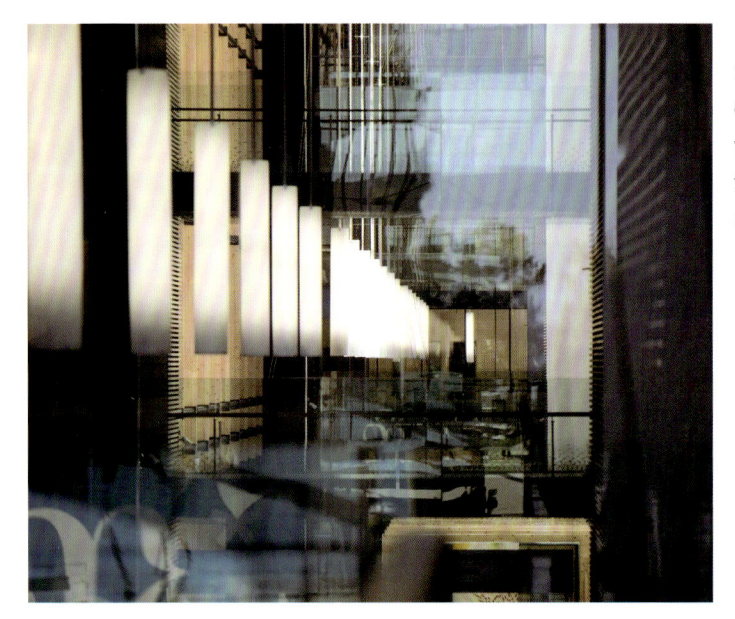

The "glass street" begins in the foyer at the entrance area, where the main reception desk welcomes visitors, and concludes in the foyer and separate entrance area of the children's department. This central element in the development unites the various materials in an overall composition in which the large colored panels, designed by Icelandic artist Birgir Andrésson, form a natural element and provide a 'palette' for the color scheme of the hospital.

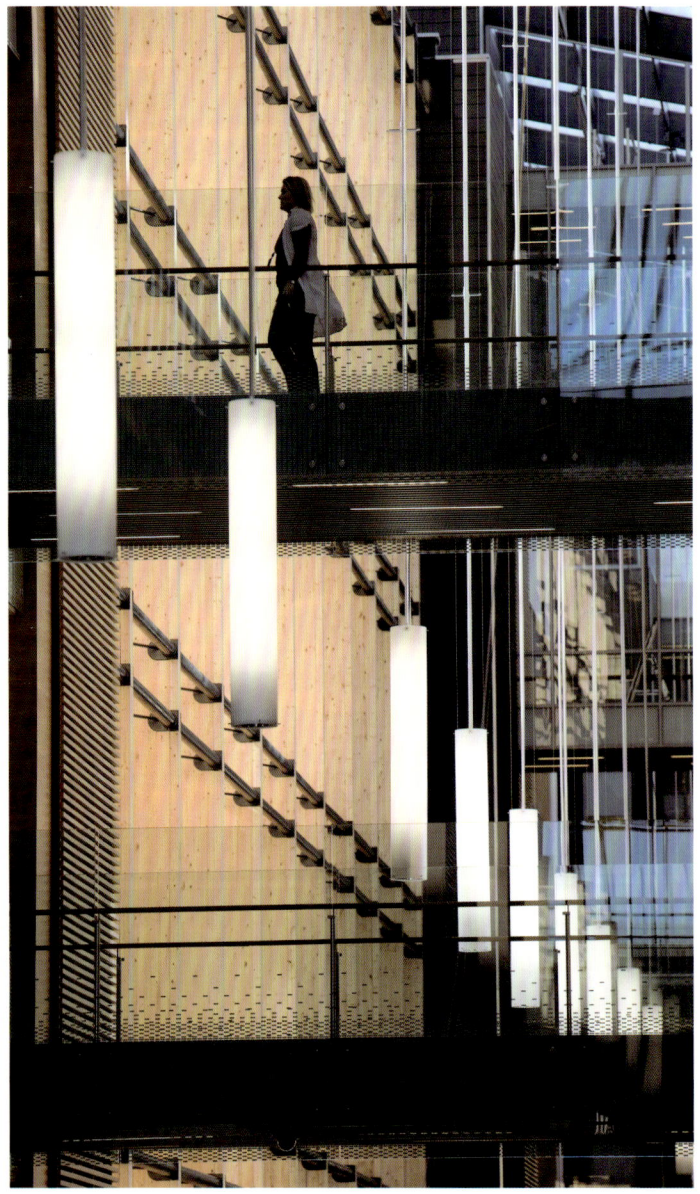

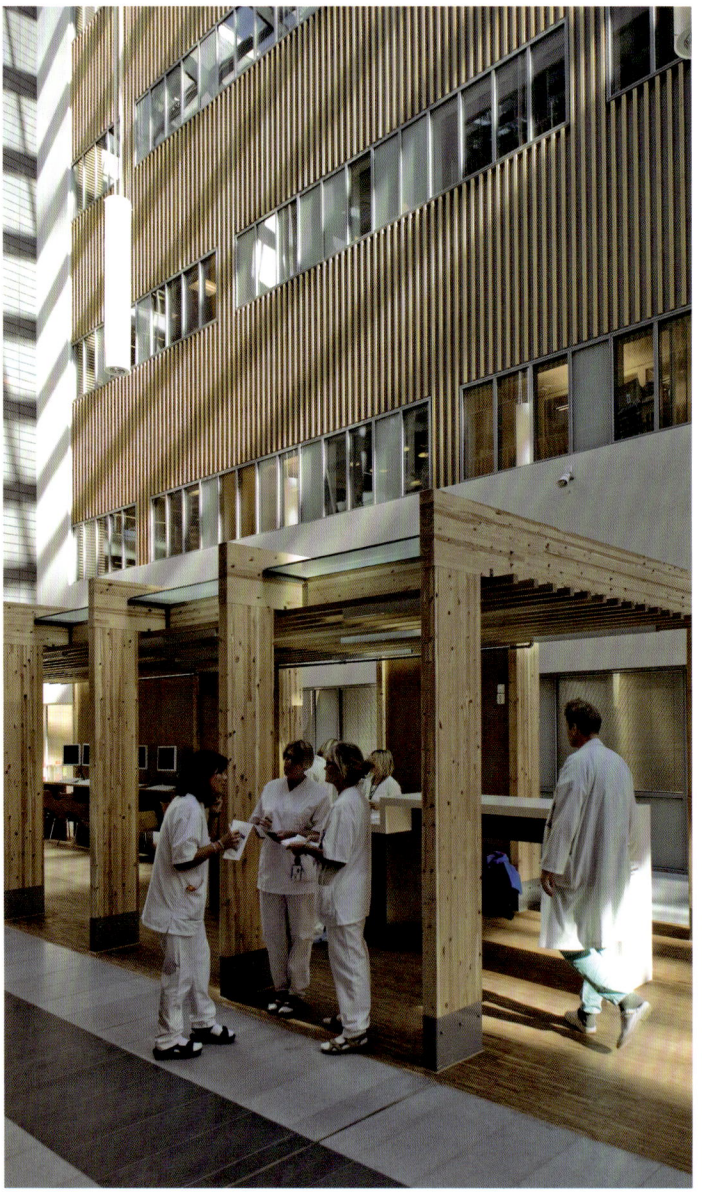

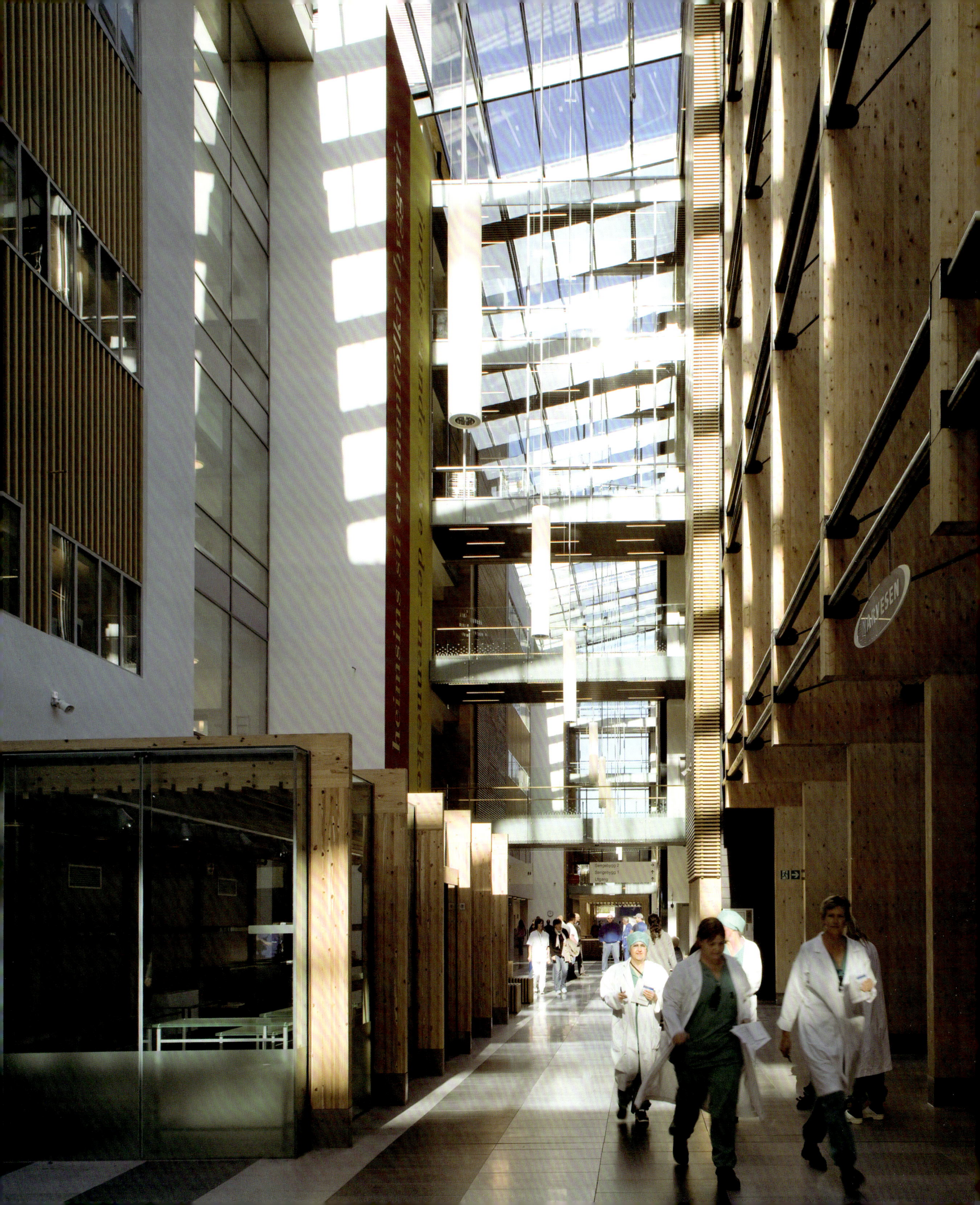

First floor plan

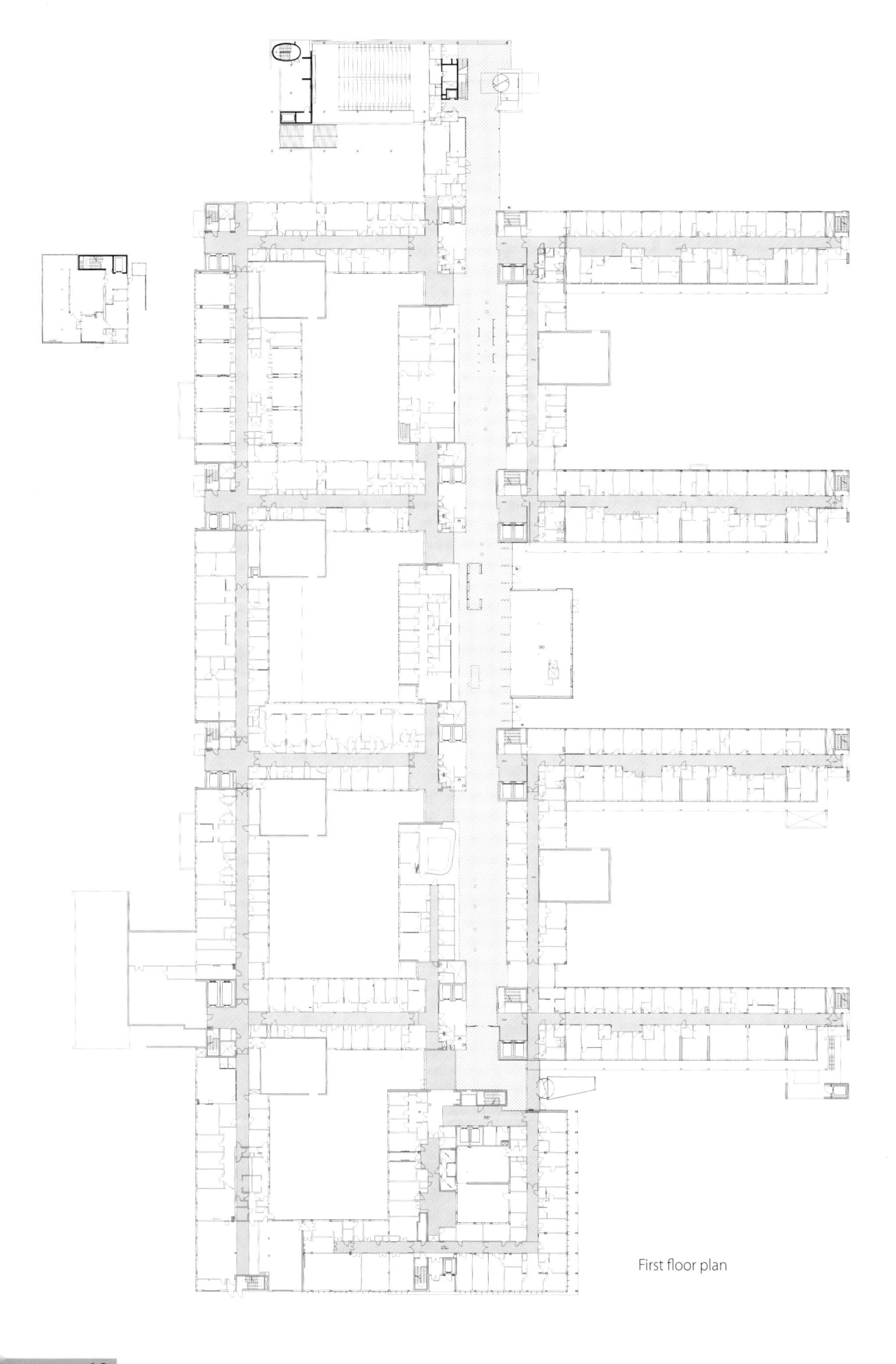

Second floor plan

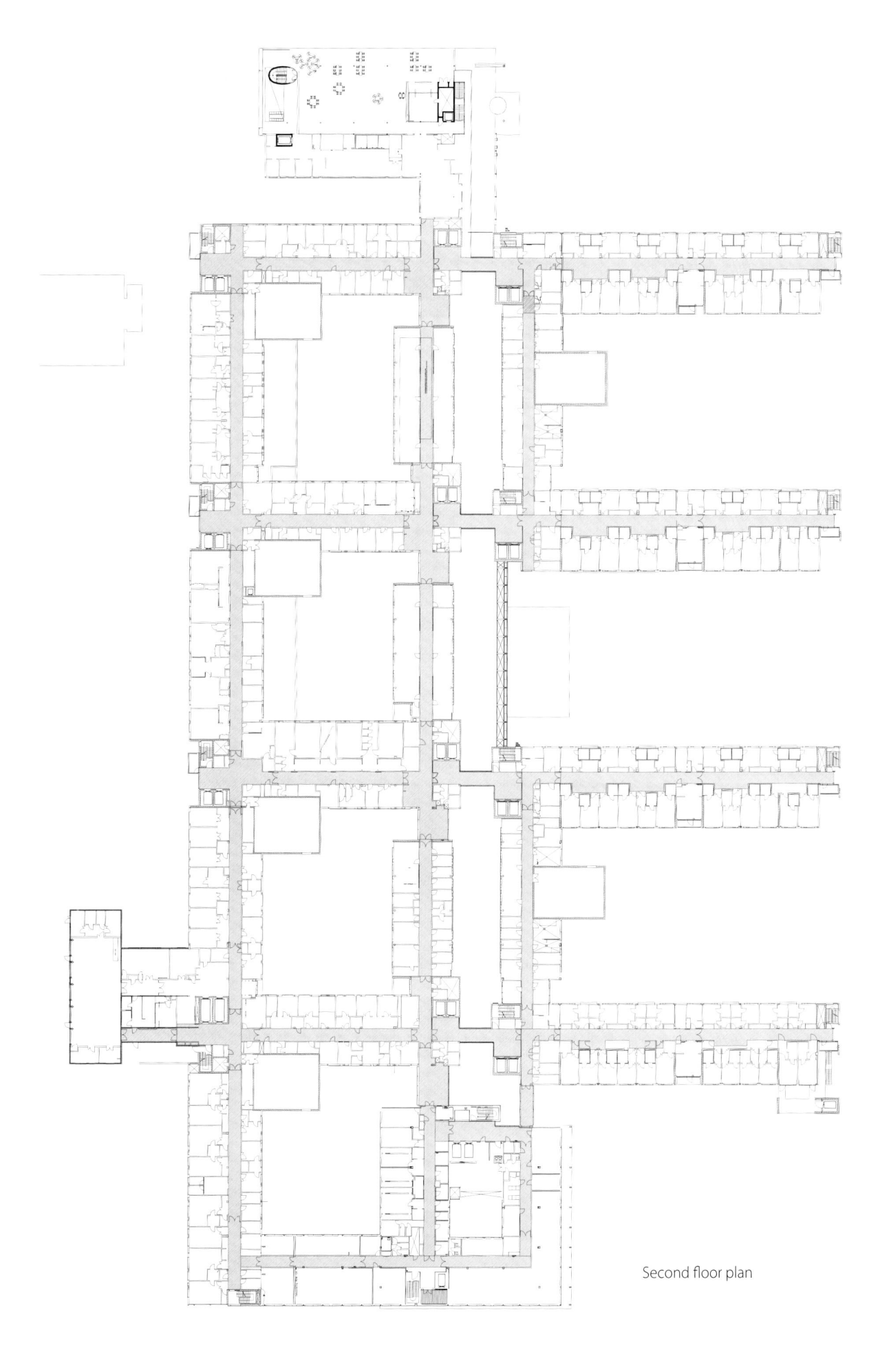

Fifth floor plan

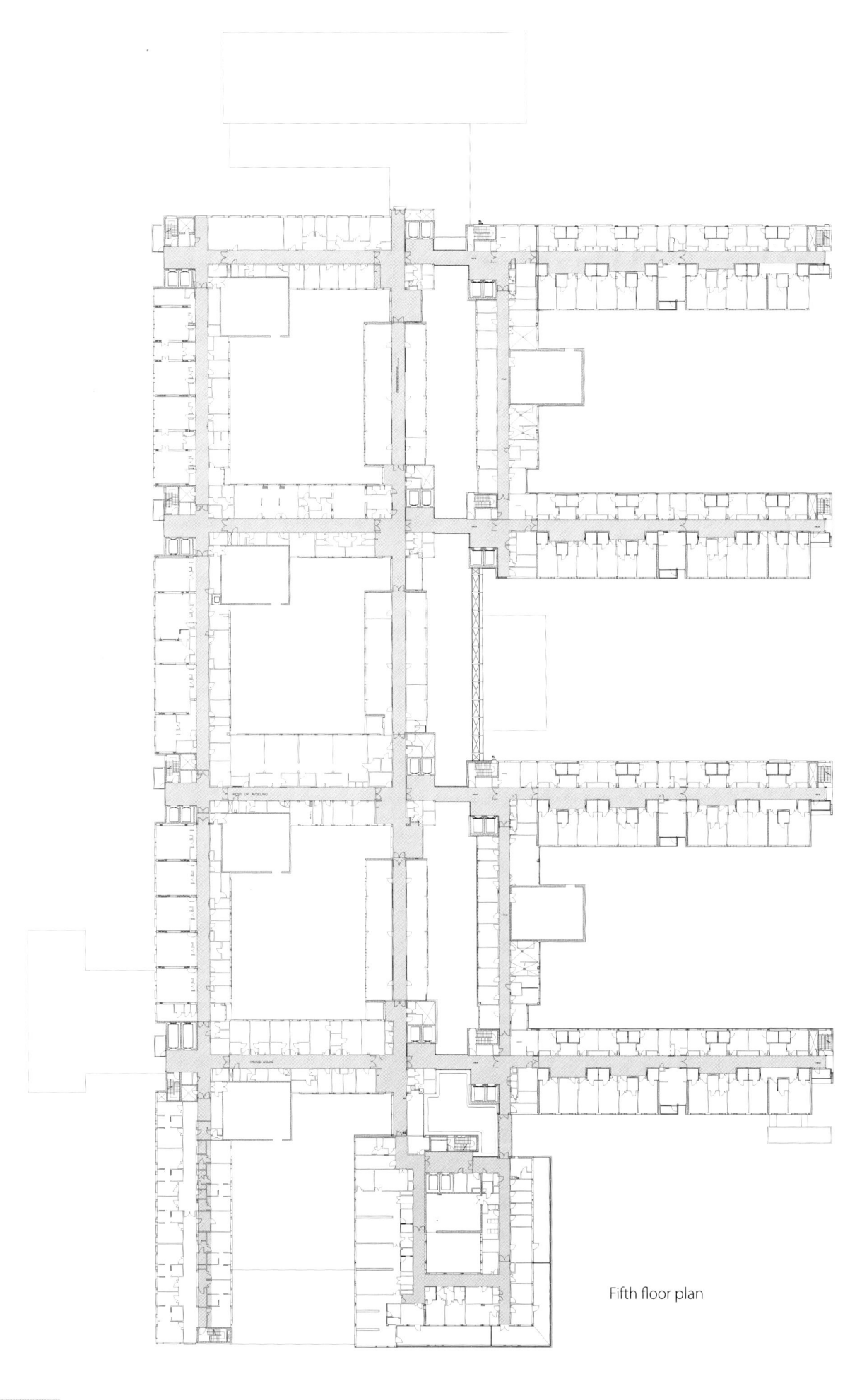

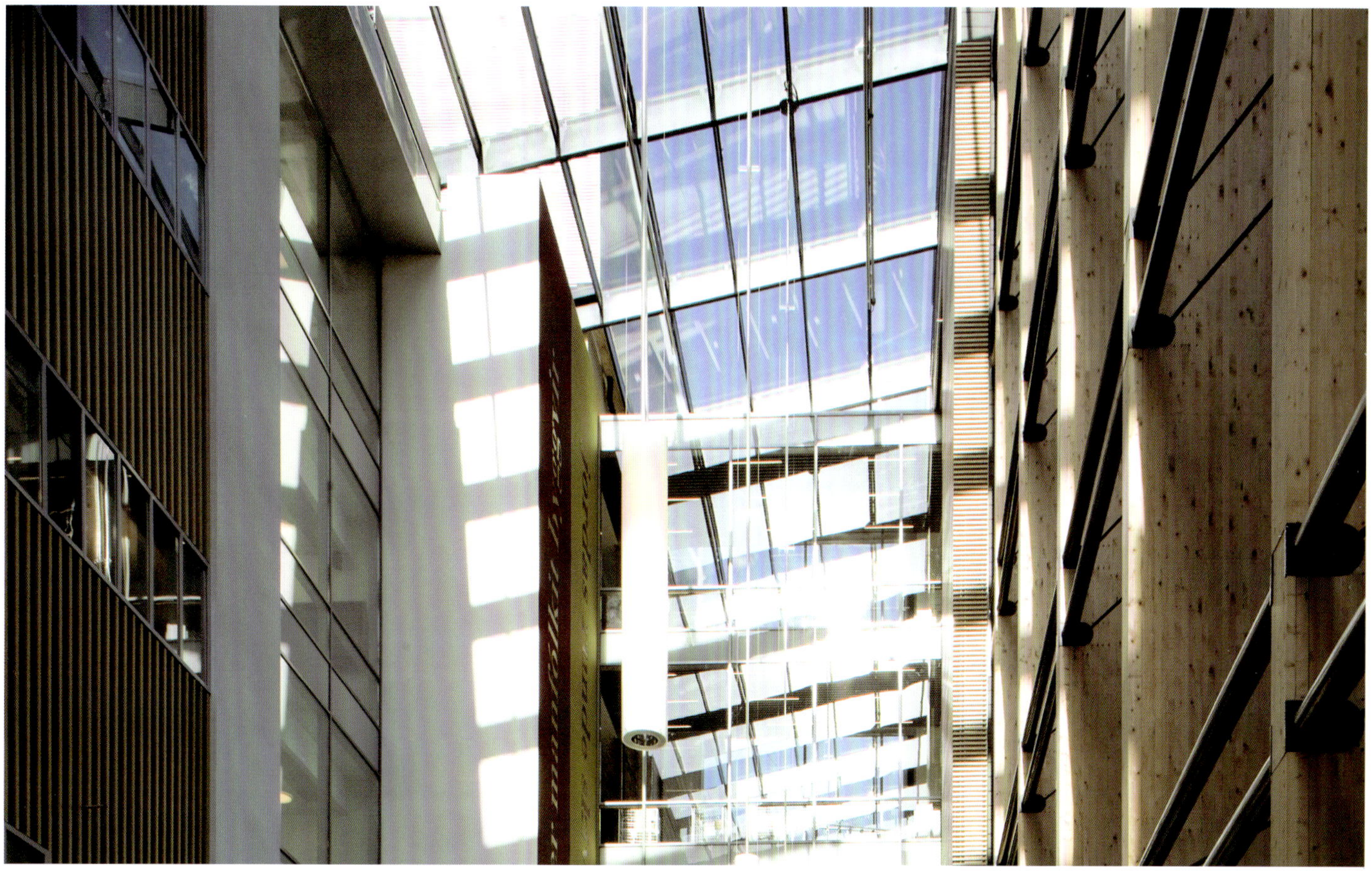

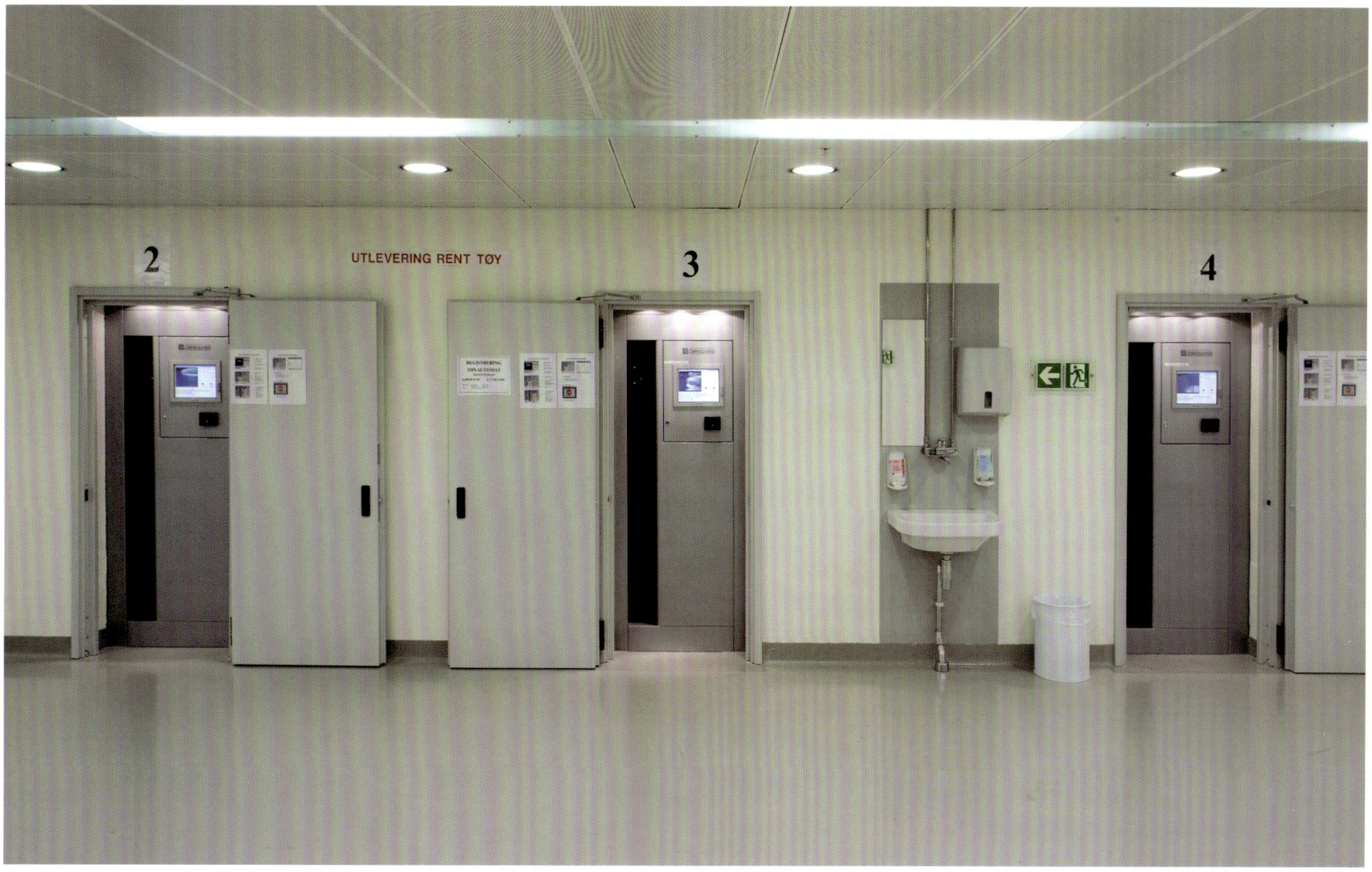
2
UTLEVERING RENT TØY
3
4

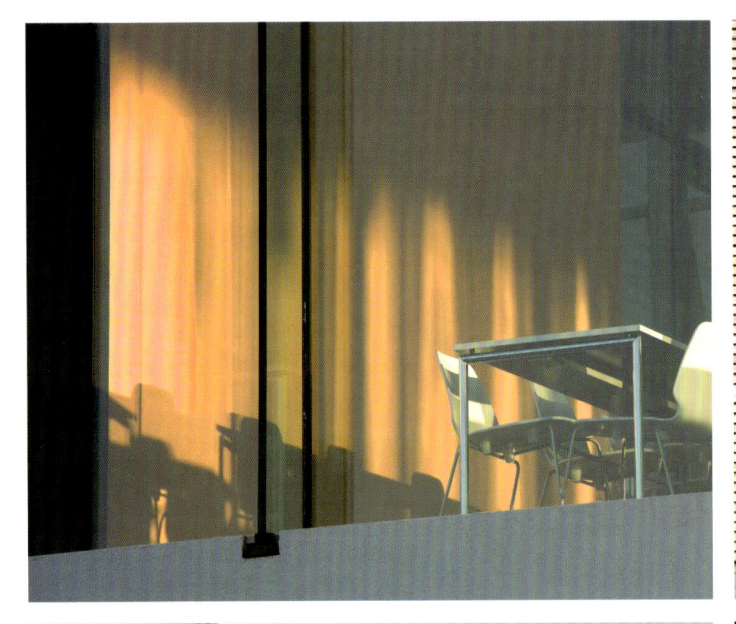

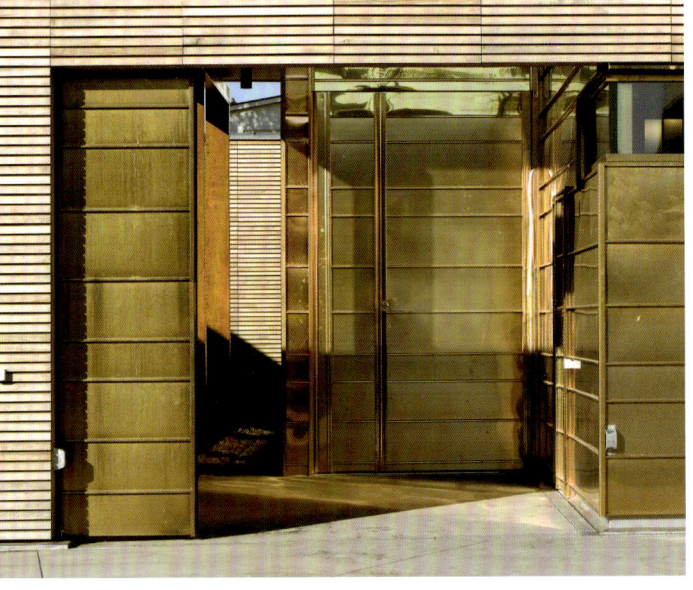

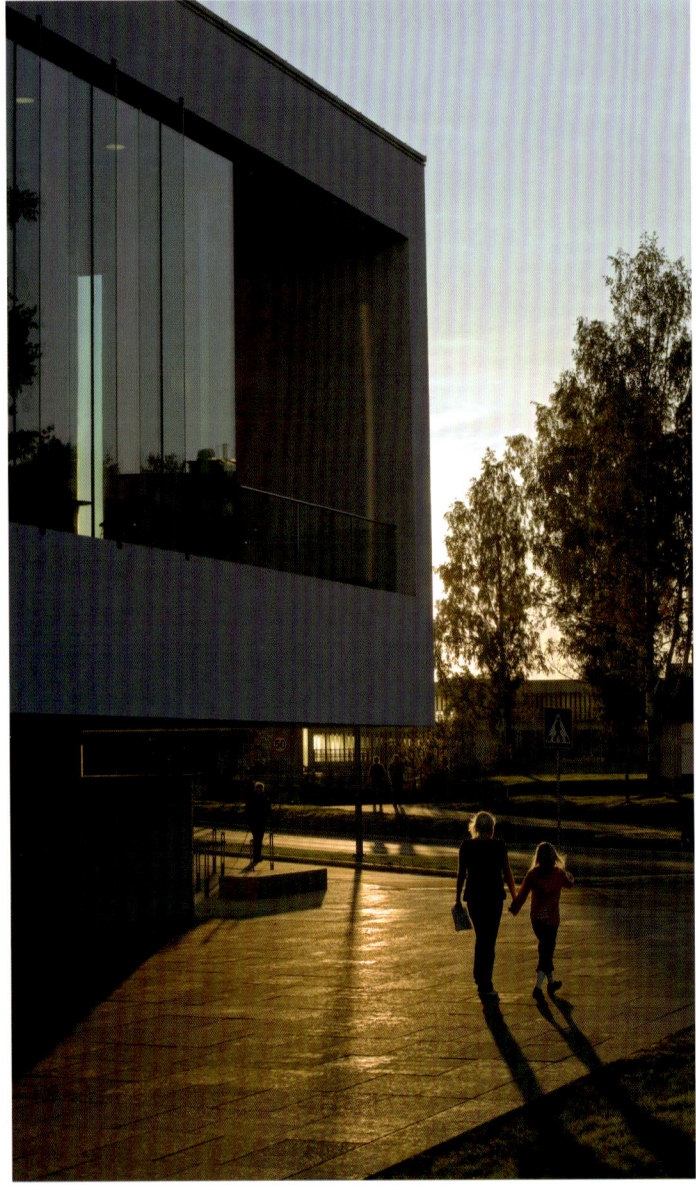

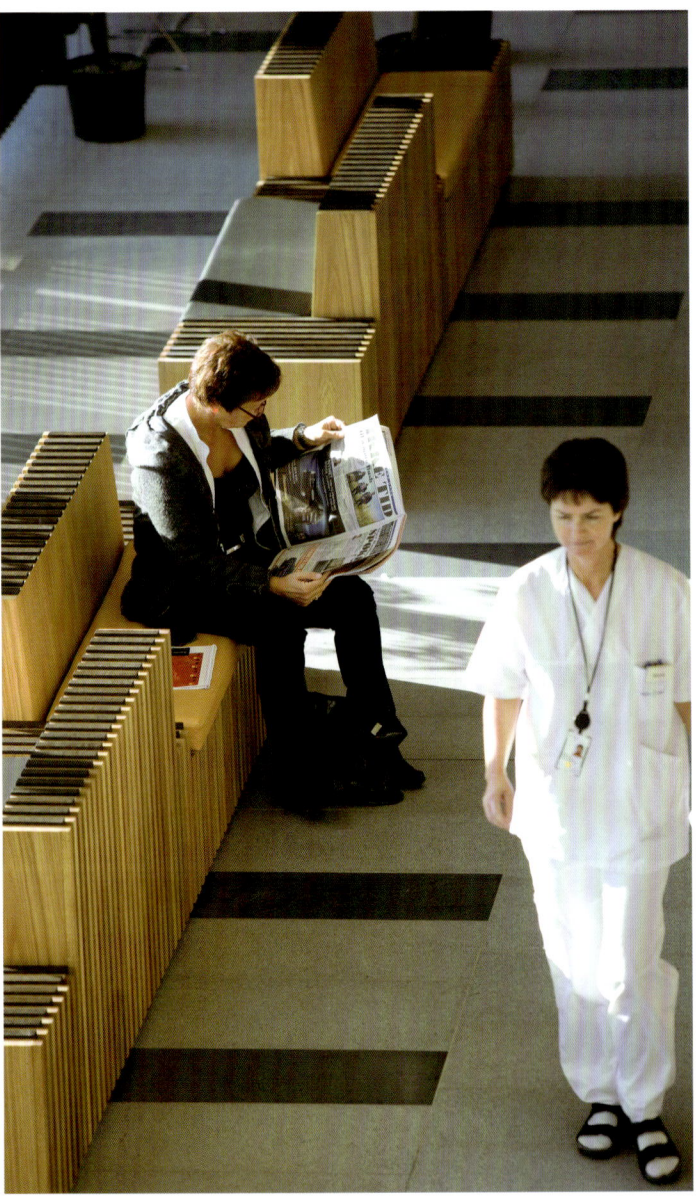

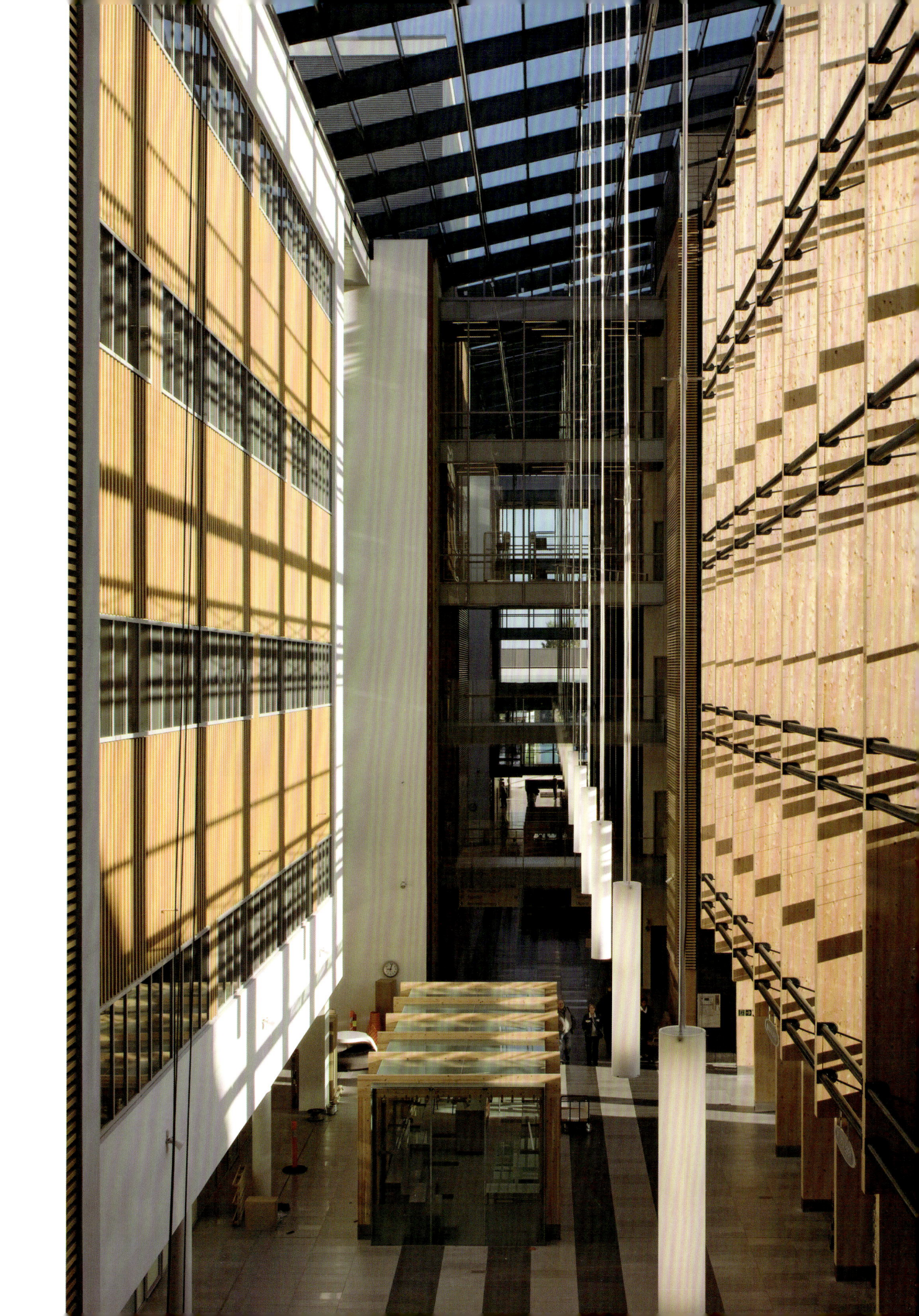

66

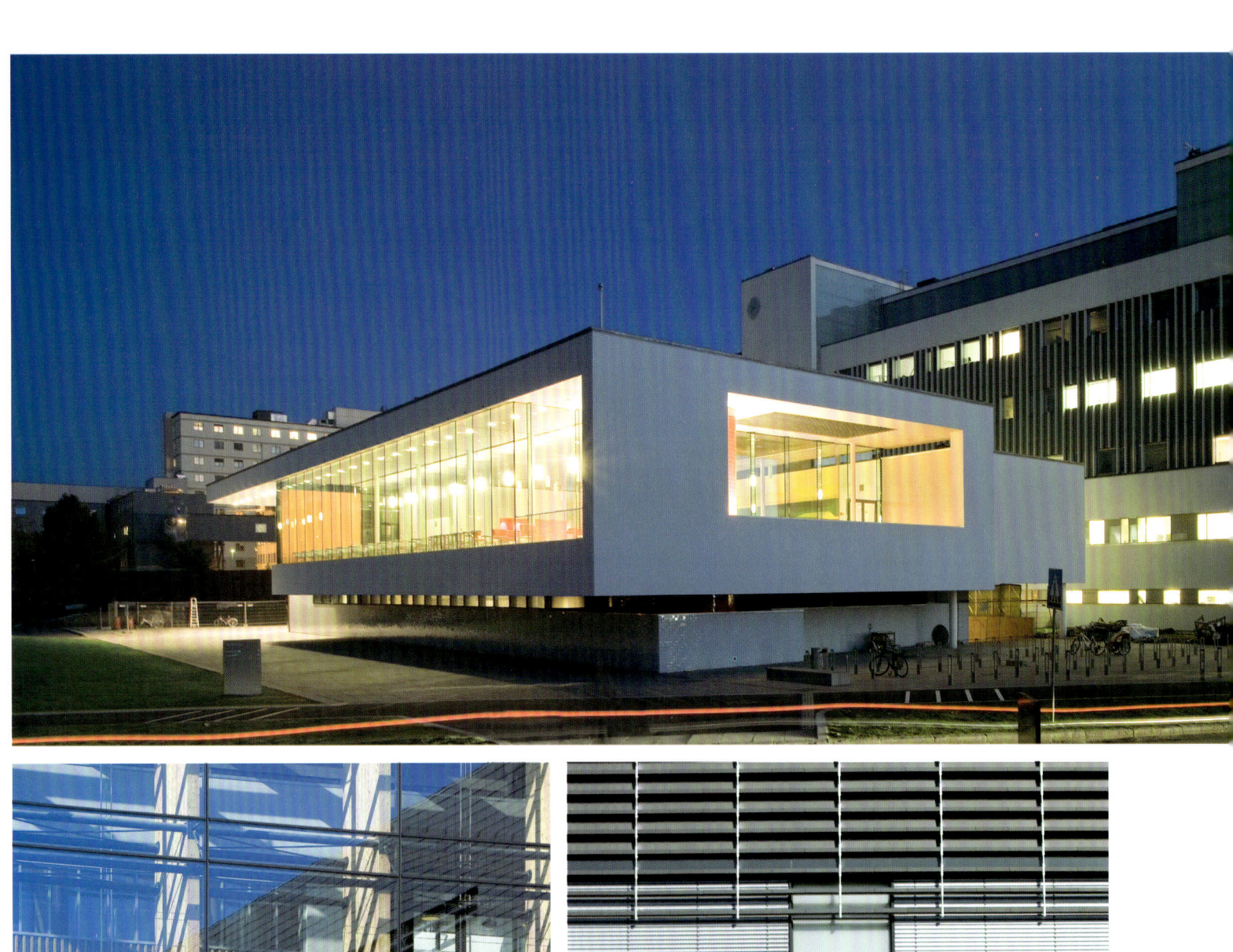

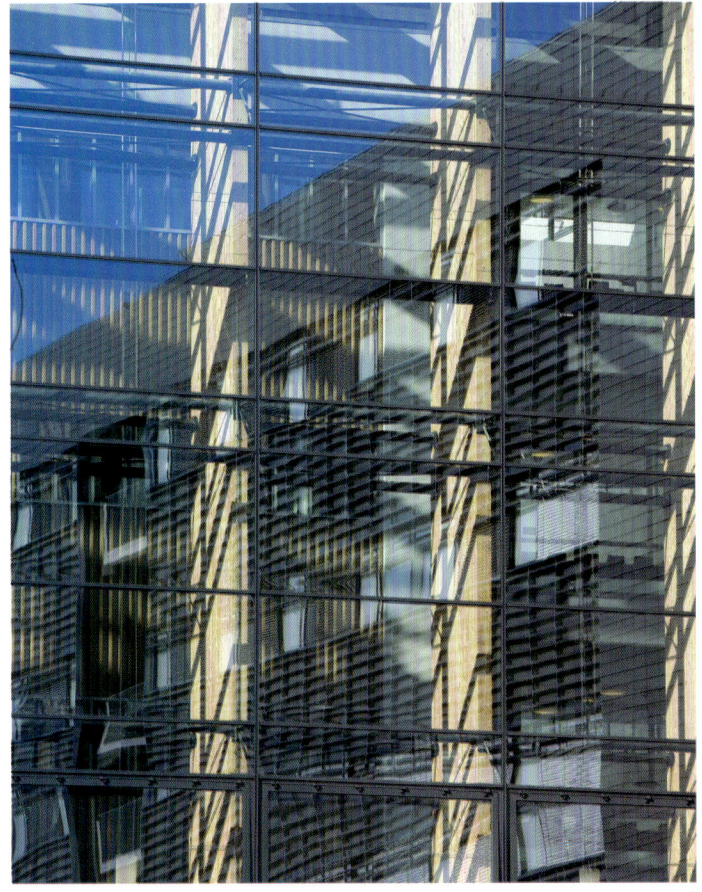

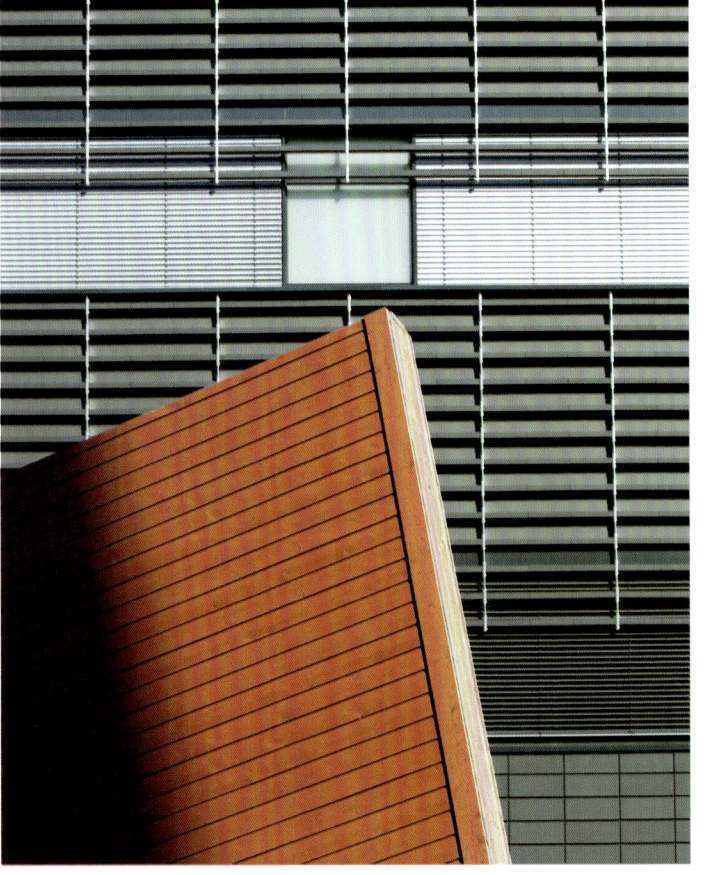

67

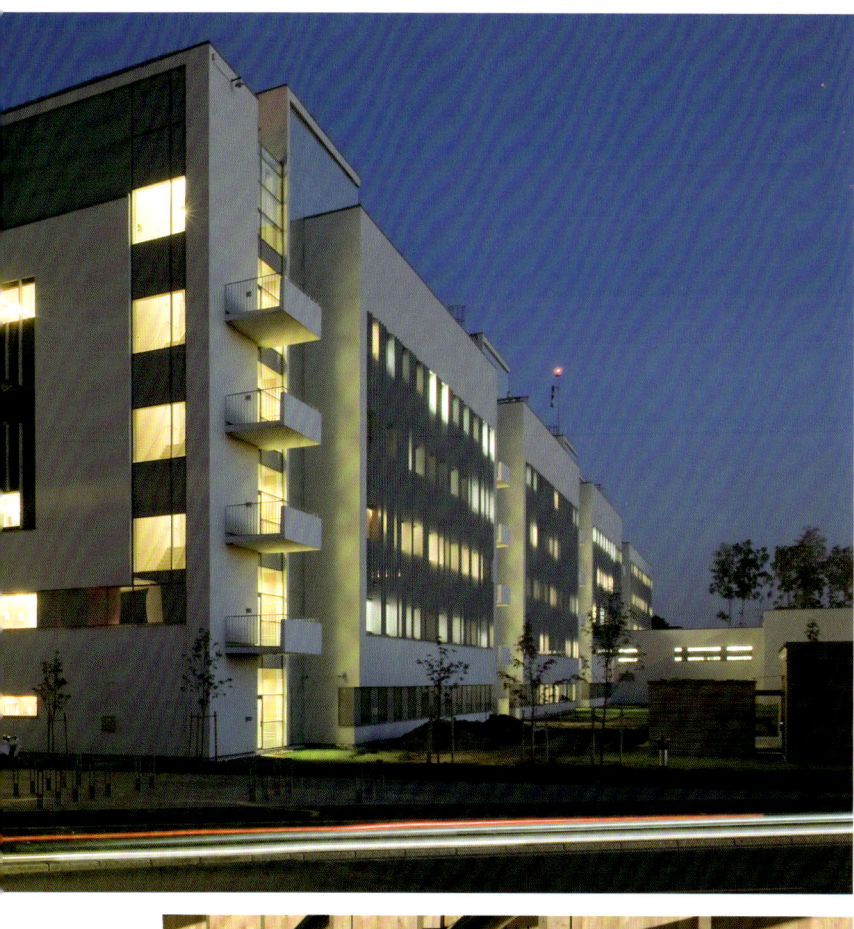

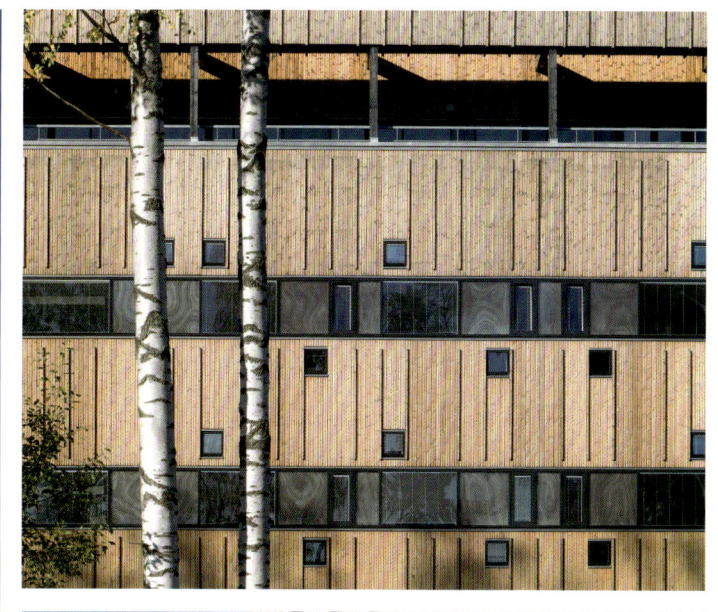

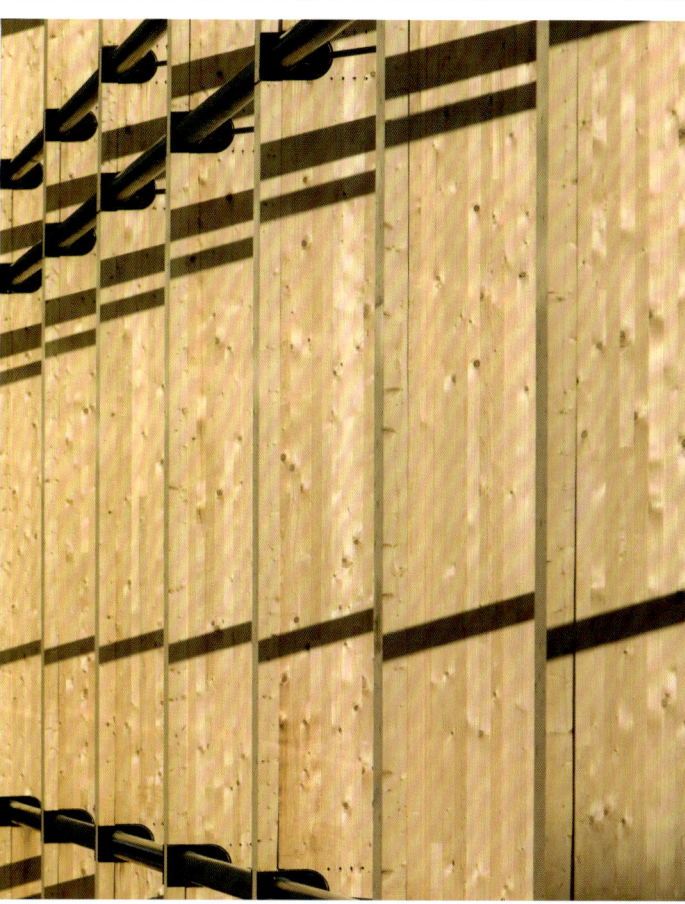

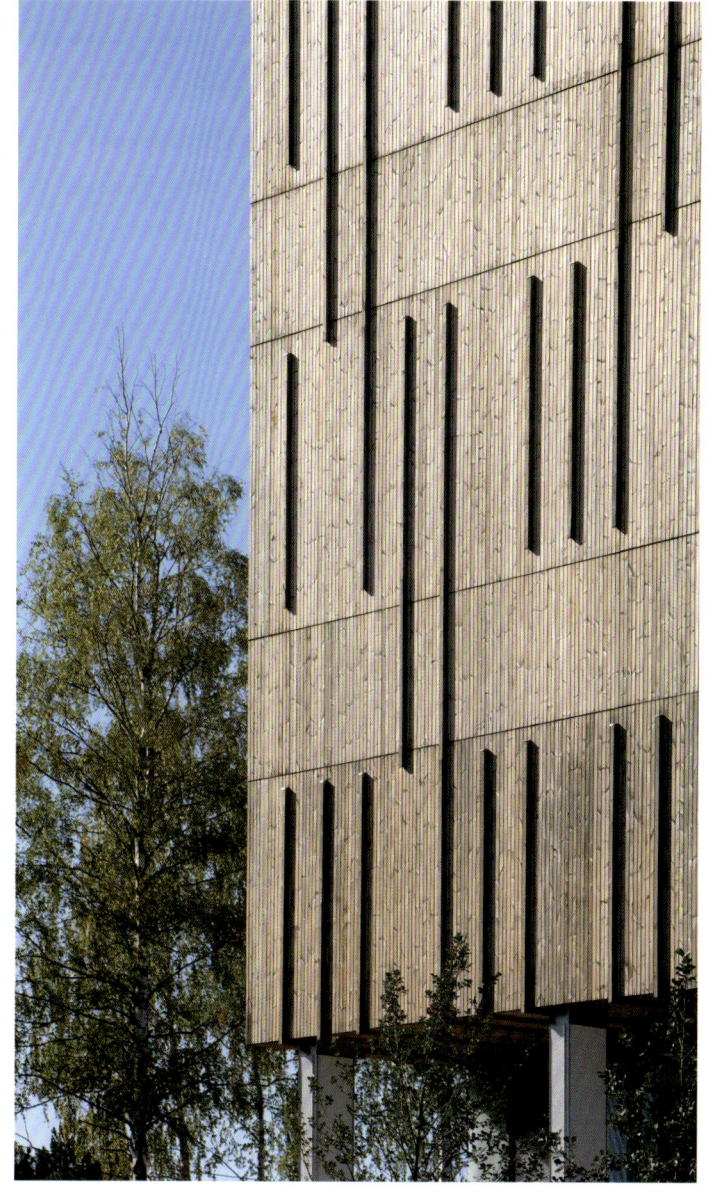

Carvajal + Casariego
Baquerizo Cruz Petrement

San Pedro Hospital

Logroño, Spain

Photographs: *José Manuel Cutillas, Carvajal Casariego*

The old San Pedro Hospital was a six-story building constructed in the 50s for patients suffering from tuberculosis set within a spacious landscaped plot that extends towards the south. Reformed in the 90s, the hospital maintained its original functional program, with bedrooms and terraces overlooking the garden to the south and the service access points to the north. A circular annex building with a changed floor plan designed to accommodate the installations completed the project.

The initial welcoming feel afforded by the original building with its gardens and terraced south façade led the architects to develop a solution based on the preservation, where possible, of these elements. It was decided to extend the hospital northwards, by way of a new façade with large windows and views to the city, thus changing the image of the current façade, which had few expressive qualities. The south façade, on the other hand, was to be respected and formally integrated into the new building. The rest of the building was to be extended with a maximum height of two stories following a grid in which covered and open courtyards, passageways and gardens alternate to form a configuration unlike the traditional vision of an overly compact hospital.

The east façade now accommodates the main entrances for visitors and outpatients, beneath a canopy formed by the management building and the library. The rest of the entrances (supplies and services) are resolved through a perimeter, landscaped walkway. An external and internal circulation network was created with clearly differentiated uses. The passageways are well lit and provide views of the gardened courtyards. Interior circulation has been made as clear as possible through orthogonal passageways which make use of color as an organizational element. This defines the different functional areas and adapts the scale of the building to that of the staff and patients.

The large dimensions of the north façade offer a changing image of the hospital via fragmented reflections on folded stainless steel panels, thus avoiding the appearance of a single, static block. On the east façade the continuity of the curtain wall from the first floor contrasts with the open, dynamic character of the canopy.

The materials used have been chosen especially for the function of the different areas. The floors are stone in the public areas, terrazzo in the general and circulation areas and PVC in areas for patients. For the vertical cladding joins have been avoided where possible and have been protected with skirting boards made from phenolic panels and strips of stainless steel in areas where traffic is more intense. The false ceilings have been studied in great detail to achieve ideal acoustics, lighting and temperature control for patients in beds, staff and other users.

Client:
The Rioja Health Council
Surface area:
126,000 sqm (1,356,252 sqft)
Start date:
1999
Finish date:
2007
Project team:
Pedro Casariego, Genaro Alas,
José Manuel Baquerizo, Fernando Cruz,
Carlos Petrement, Gádor de Carvajal, Juan Casariego
Collaborators:
P.Reznak, F.López, M.Pascual, V.Aguilar-Amat,
A.Navarro, A.Montero, P.Martínez, S.Martínez, J.Asua,
M.Hidalgo, N.Merayo
Contractors:
UTE ACS, Necso, Mabesa

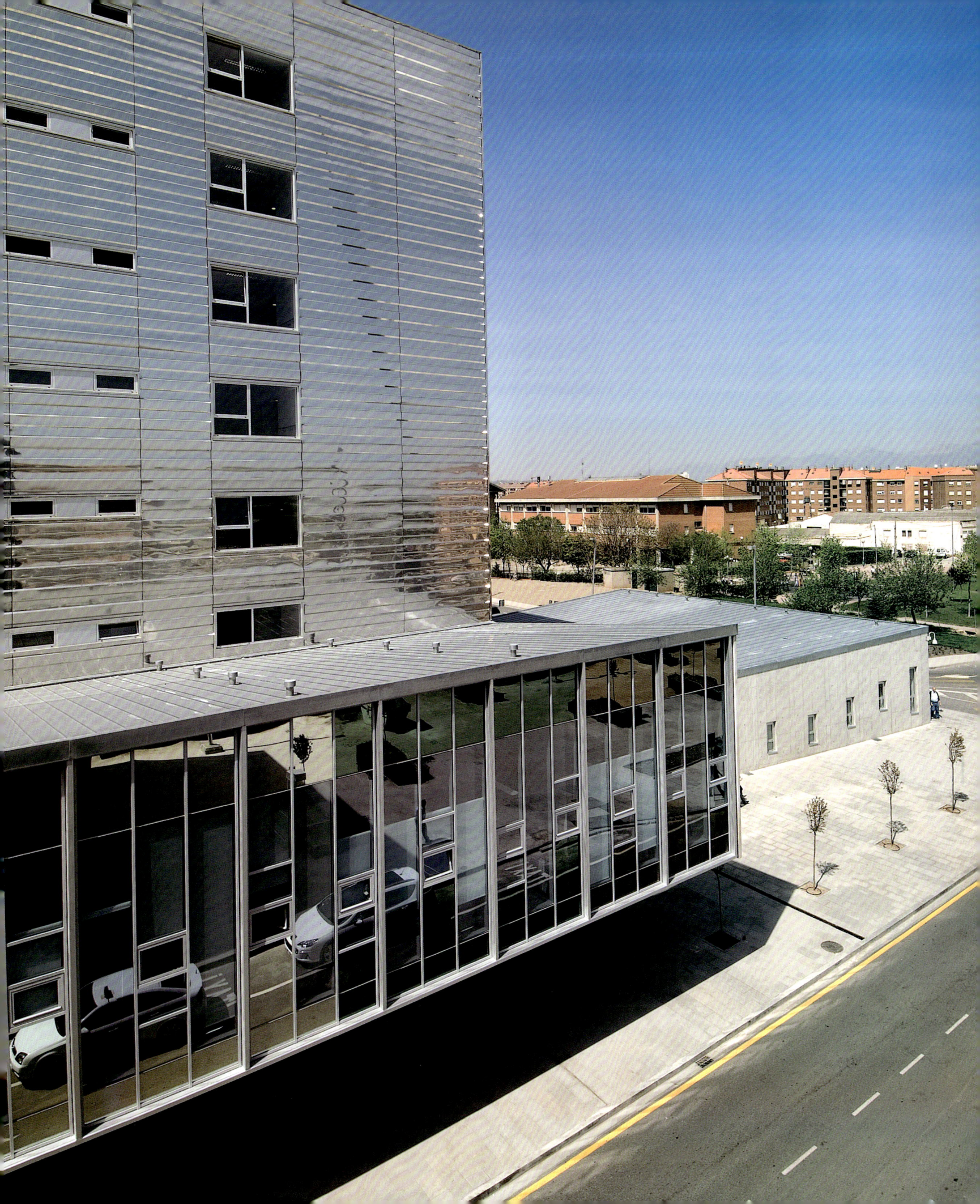

70

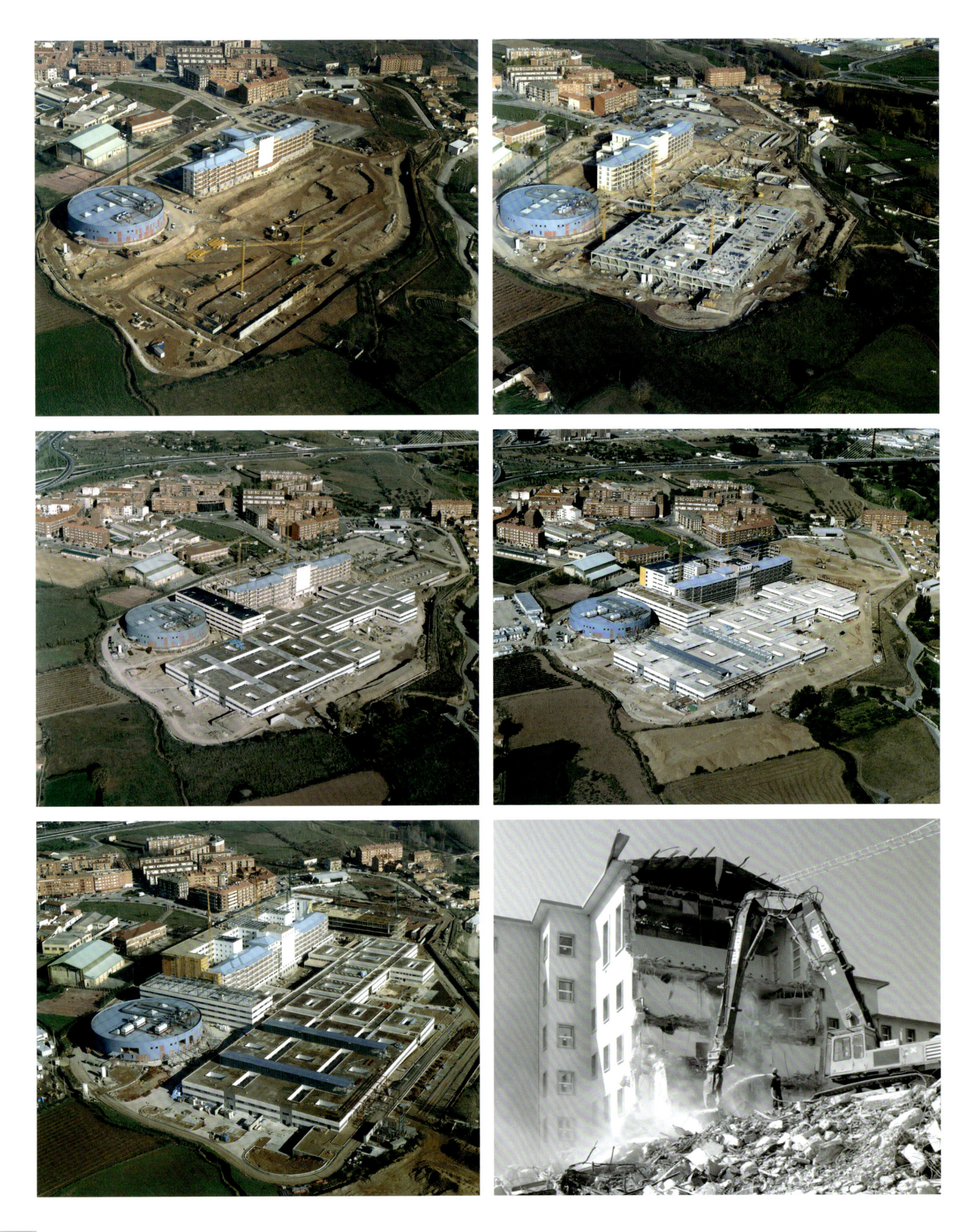

71

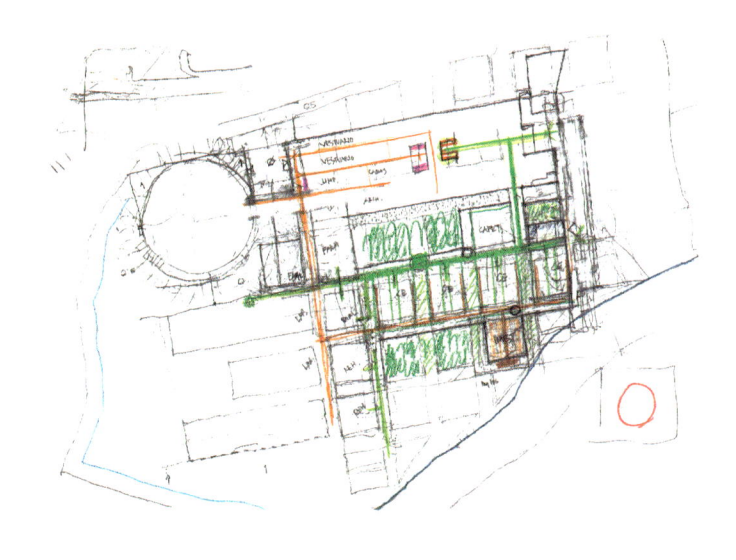

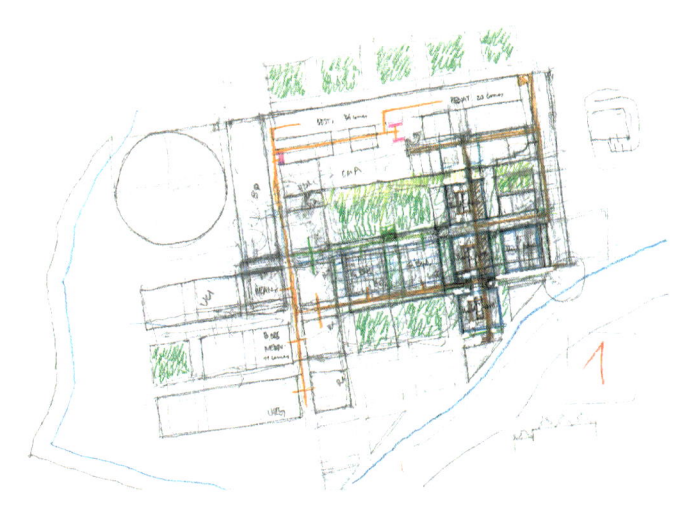

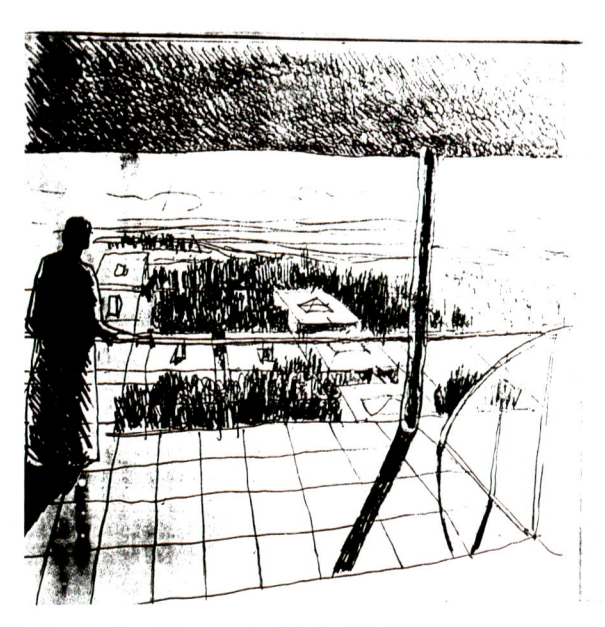

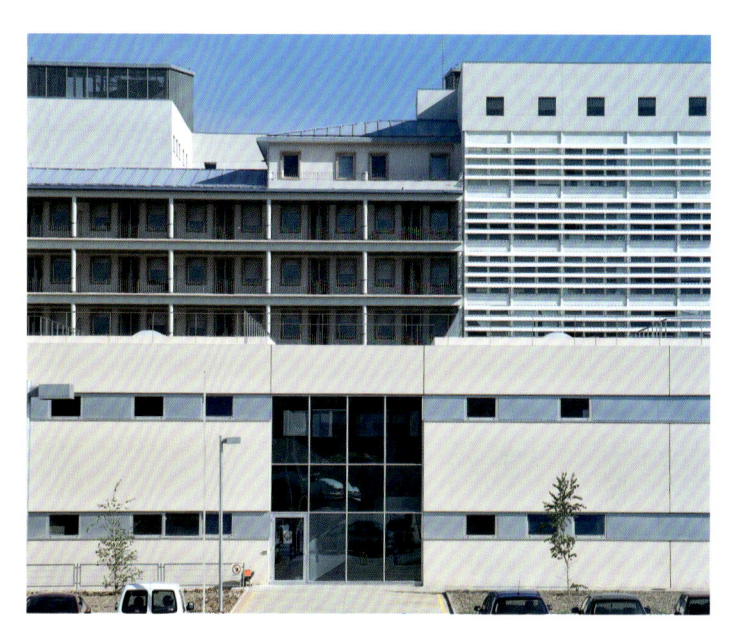

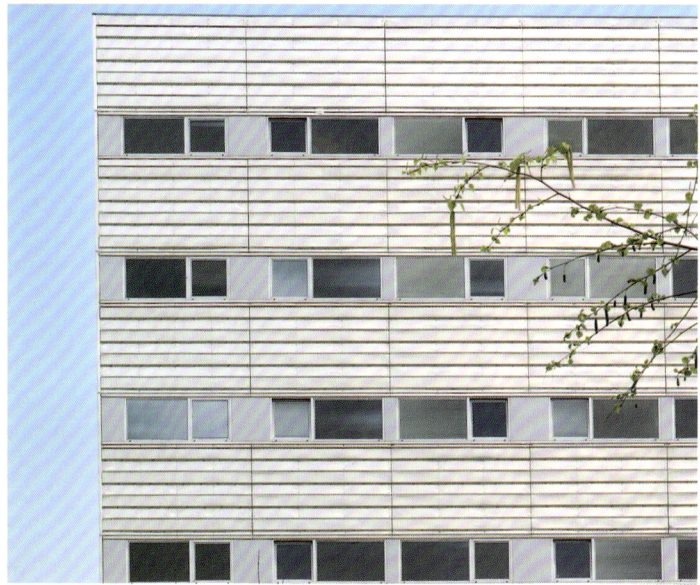

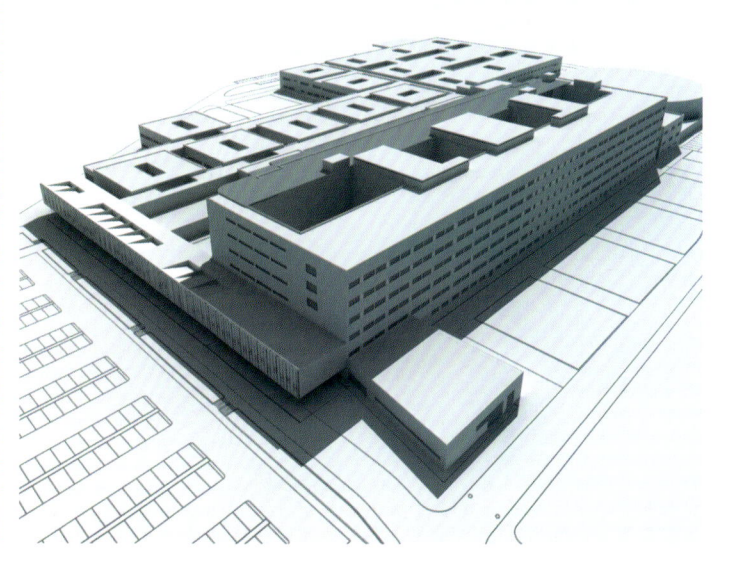

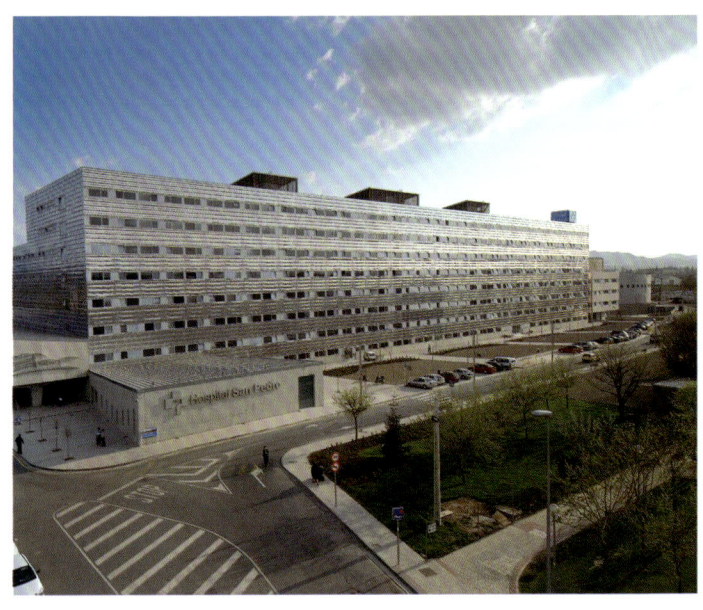

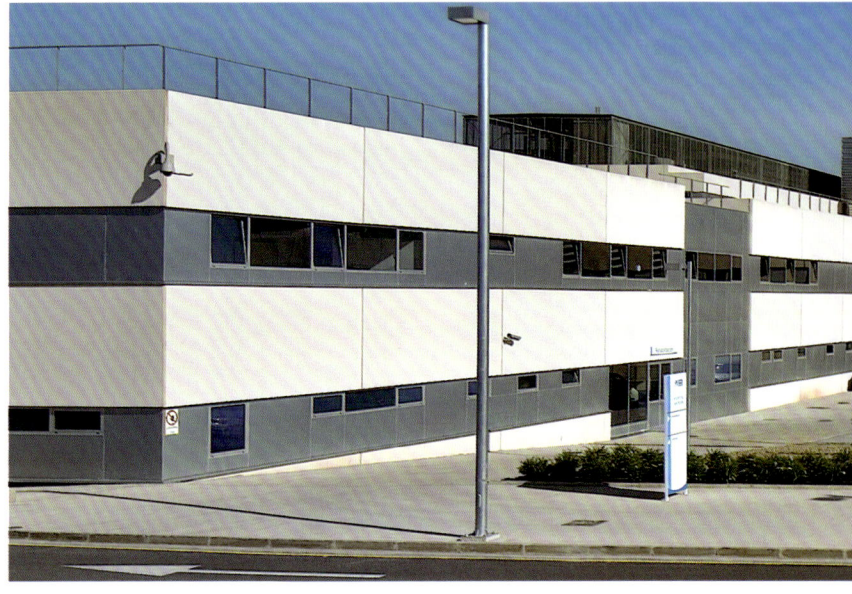

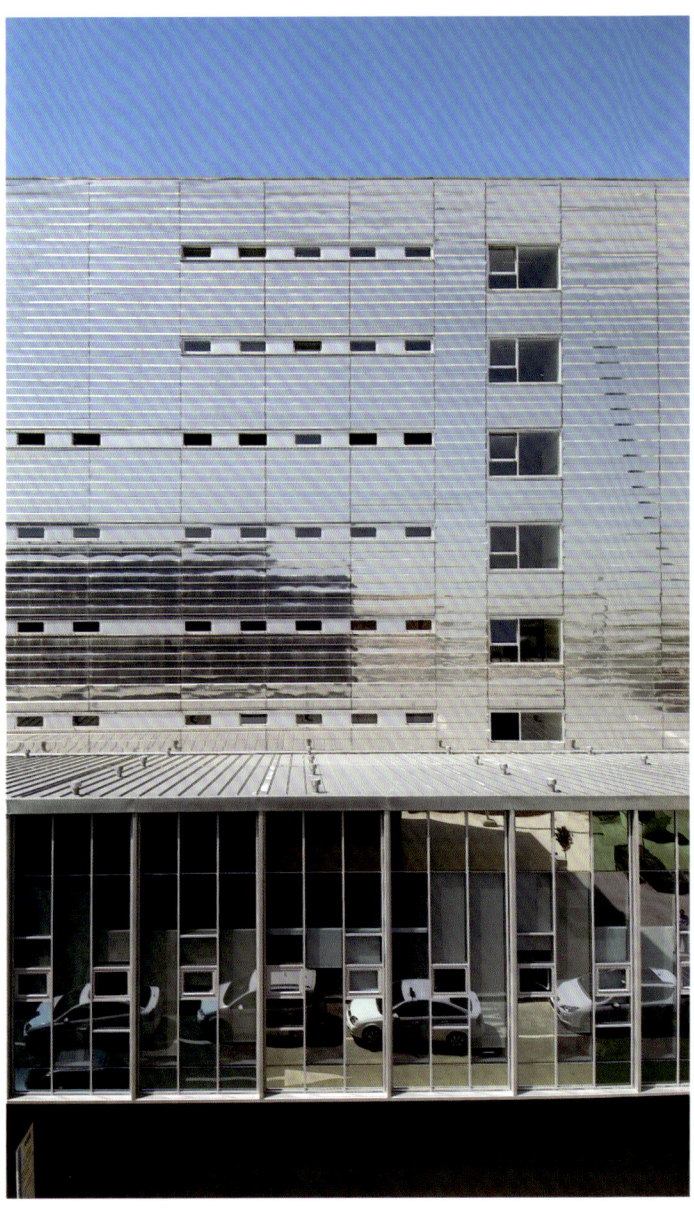

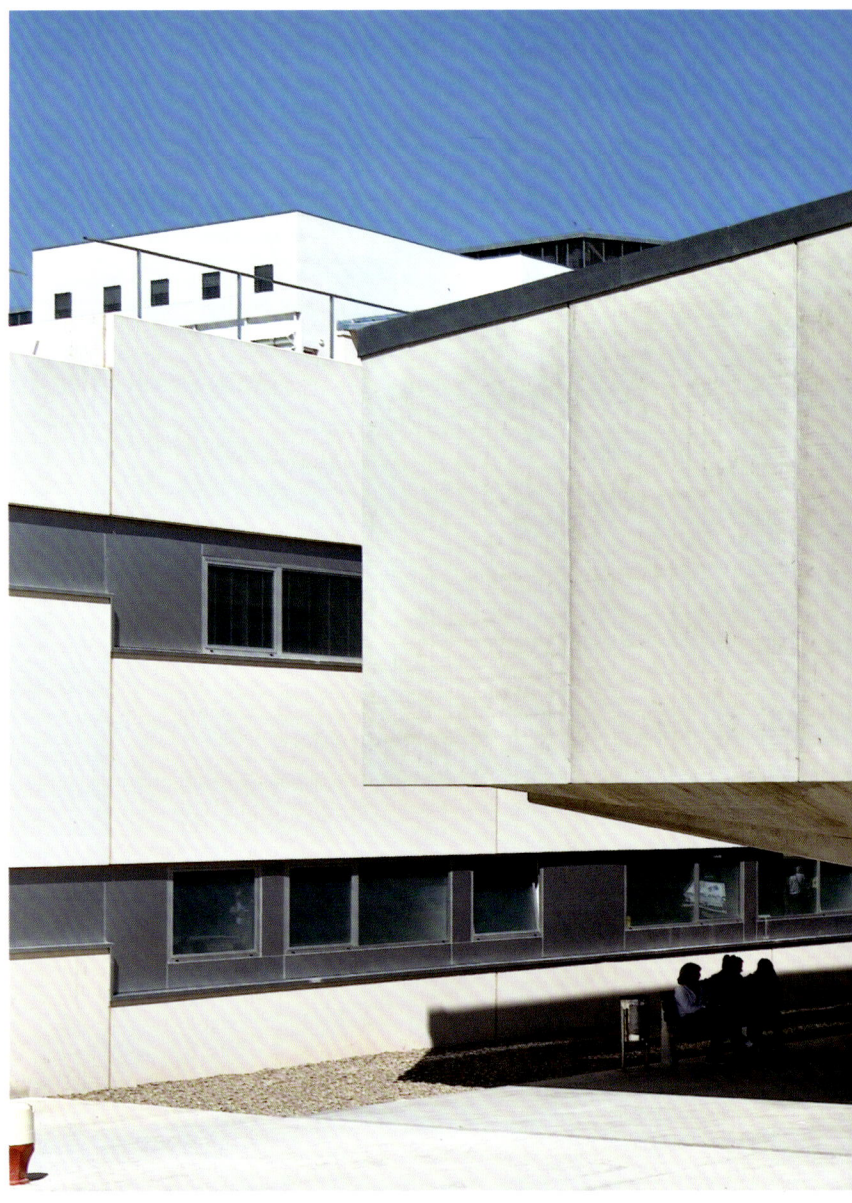

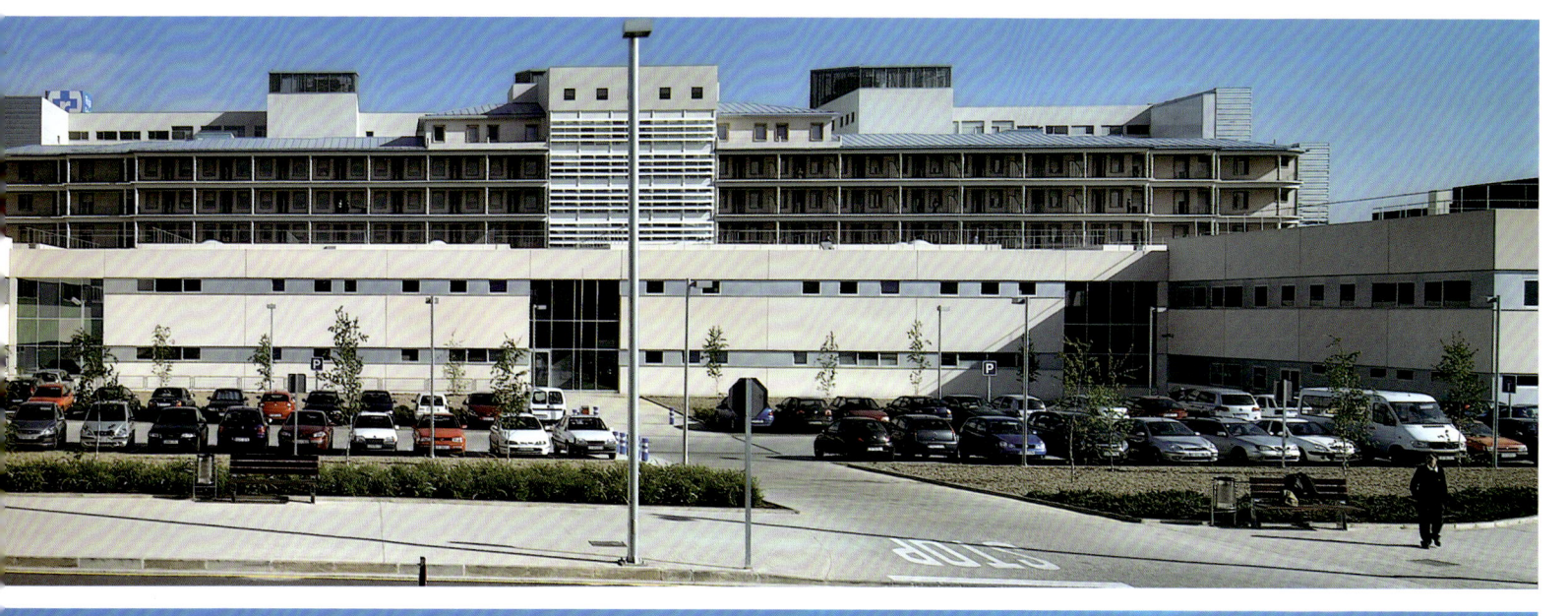

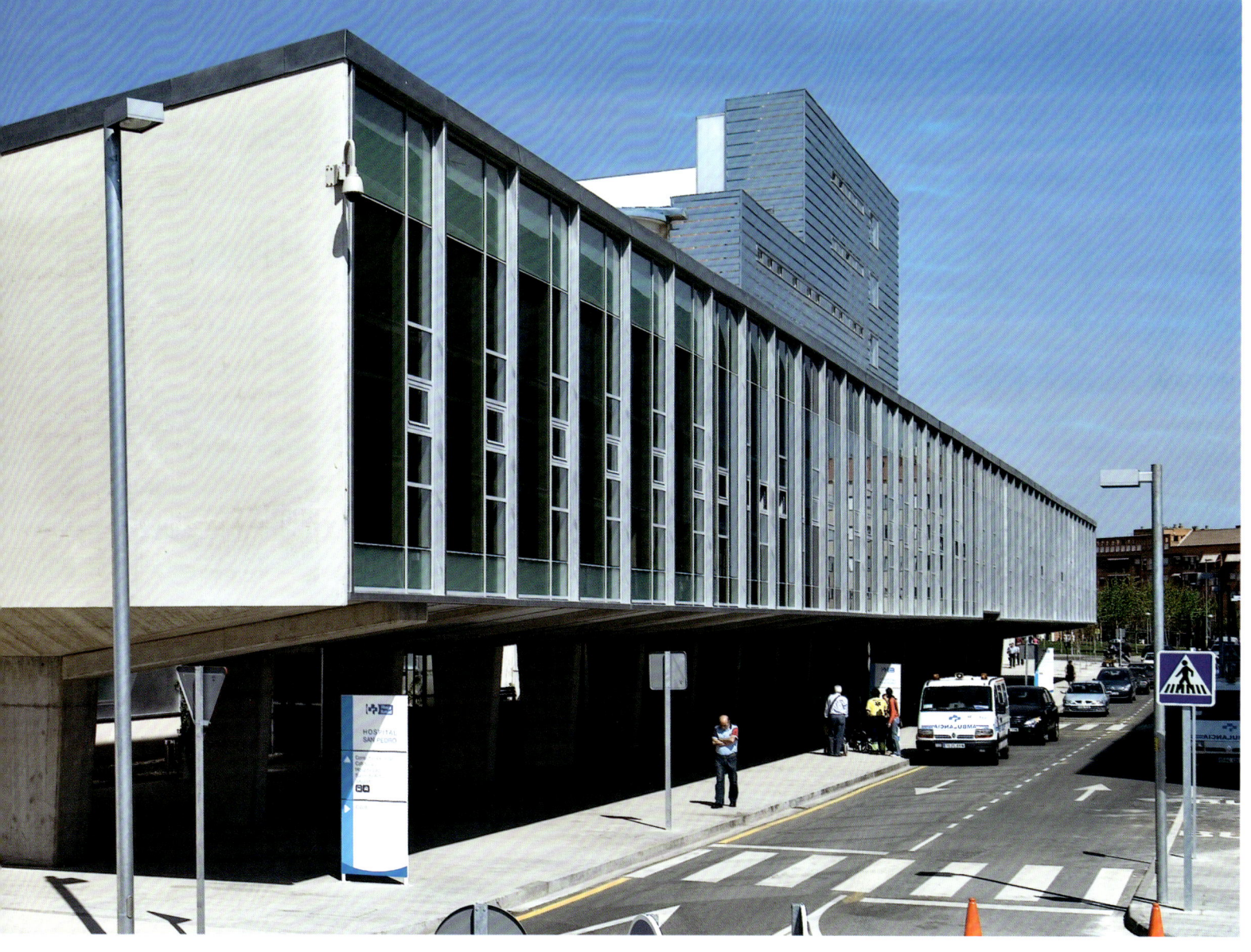

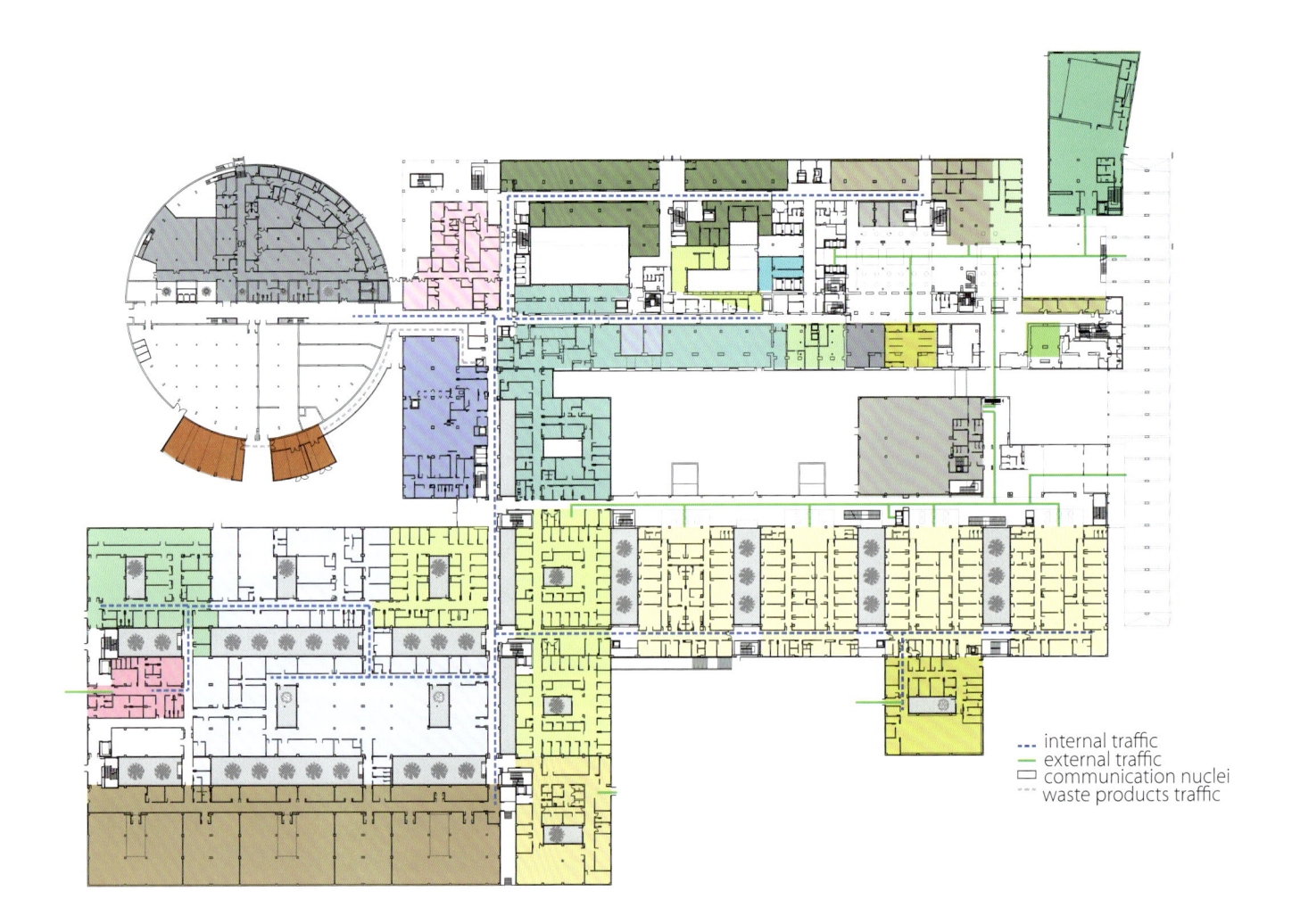

Ground floor plan

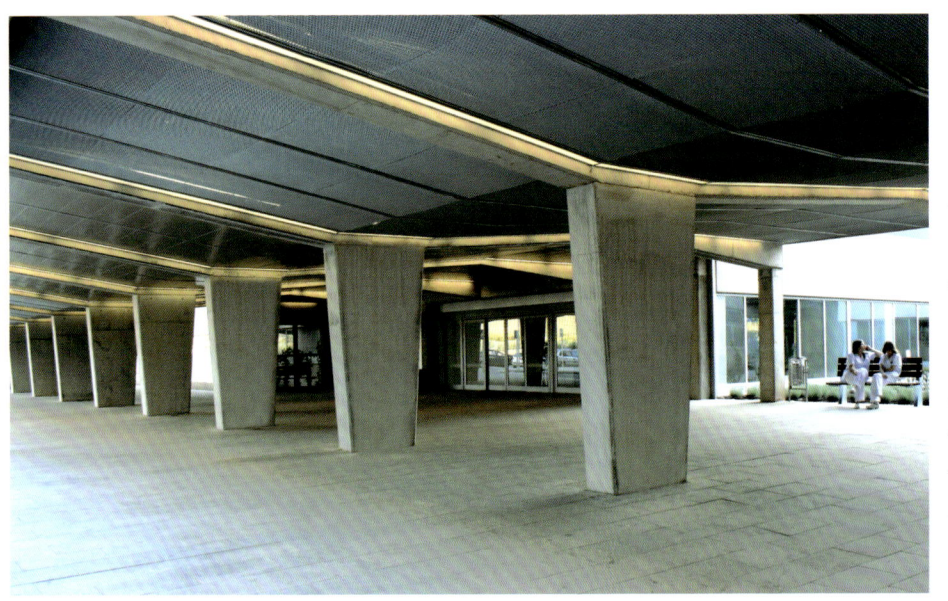

- - - internal traffic
— external traffic
▢ communication nuclei
- - - waste products traffic

The old San Pedro Hospital was a six-story building constructed in the 50s for patients suffering from tuberculosis set within a spacious landscaped plot that extends towards the south. Reformed in the 90s, the hospital maintained its original functional program, with bedrooms and terraces overlooking the garden to the south and the service access points to the north. A circular annex building with a changed floor plan designed to accommodate the installations completed the project.

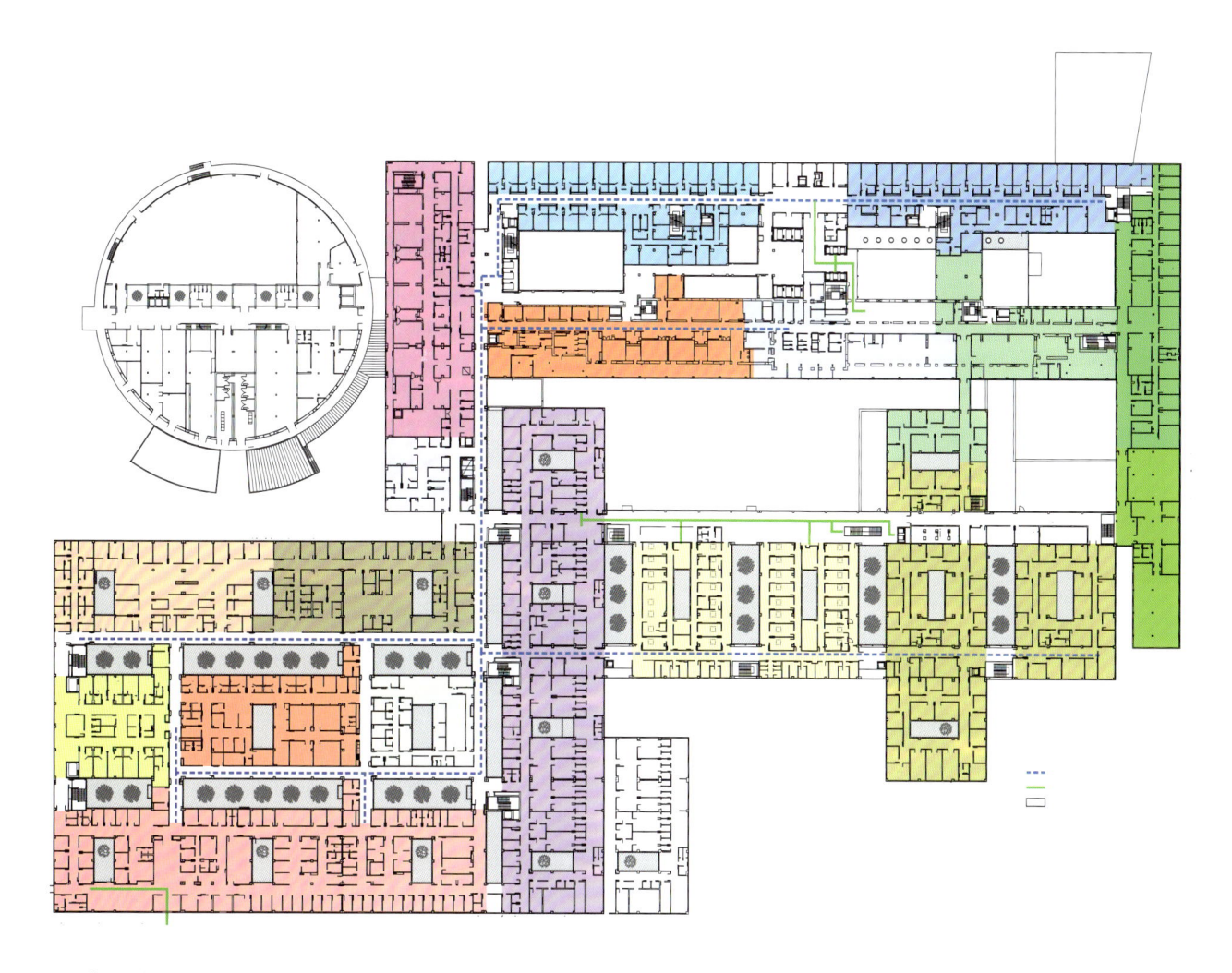

First floor plan

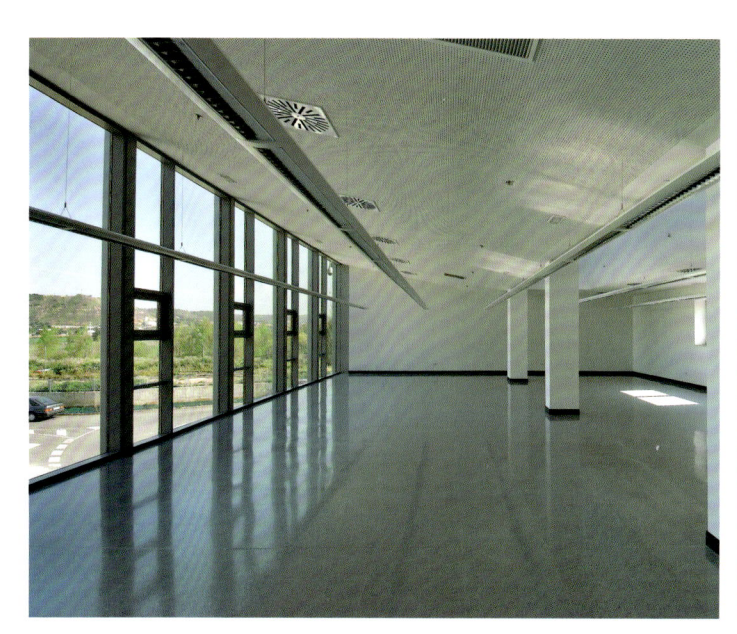

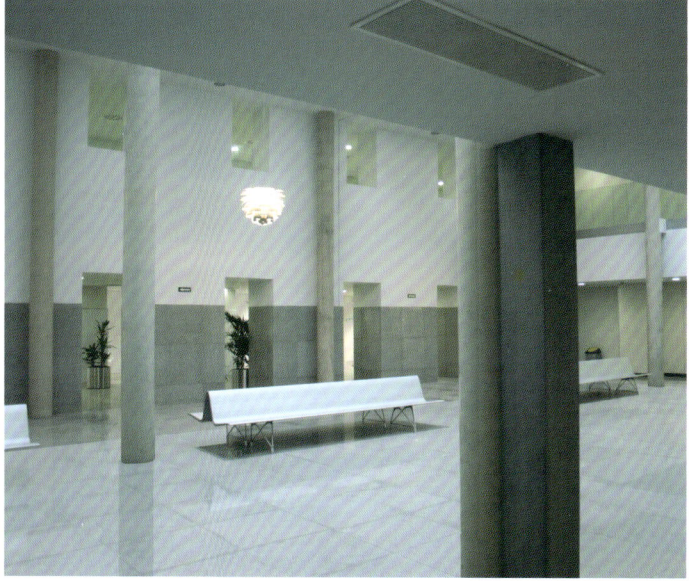

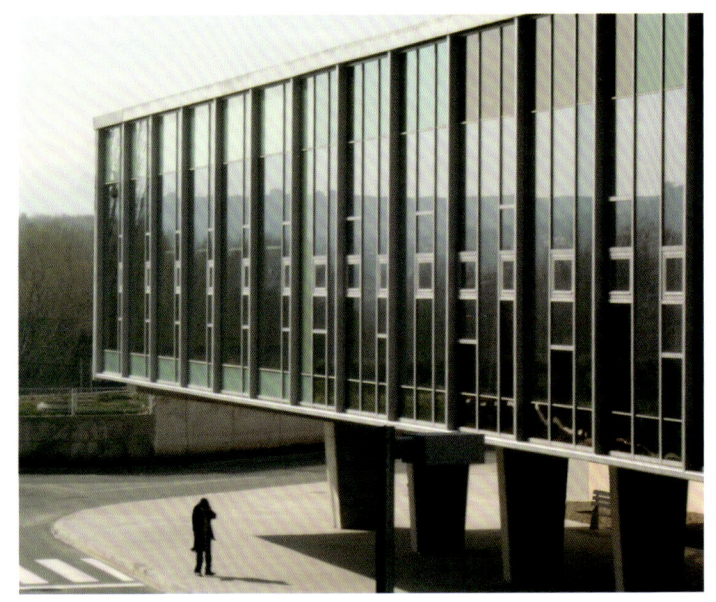

The initial welcoming feel afforded by the original building with its gardens and terraced south façade led the architects to develop a solution based on the preservation, where possible, of these elements. It was decided to extend the hospital northwards, by way of a new façade with large windows and views to the city, thus changing the image of the current façade, which had few expressive qualities.

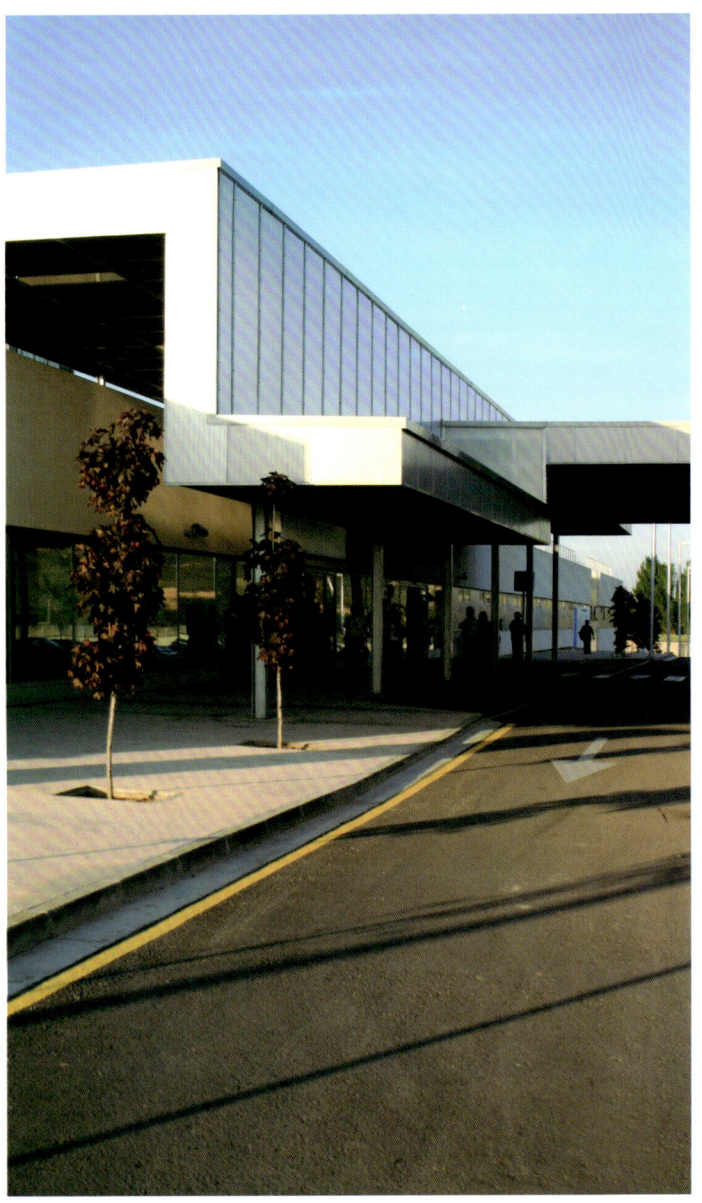

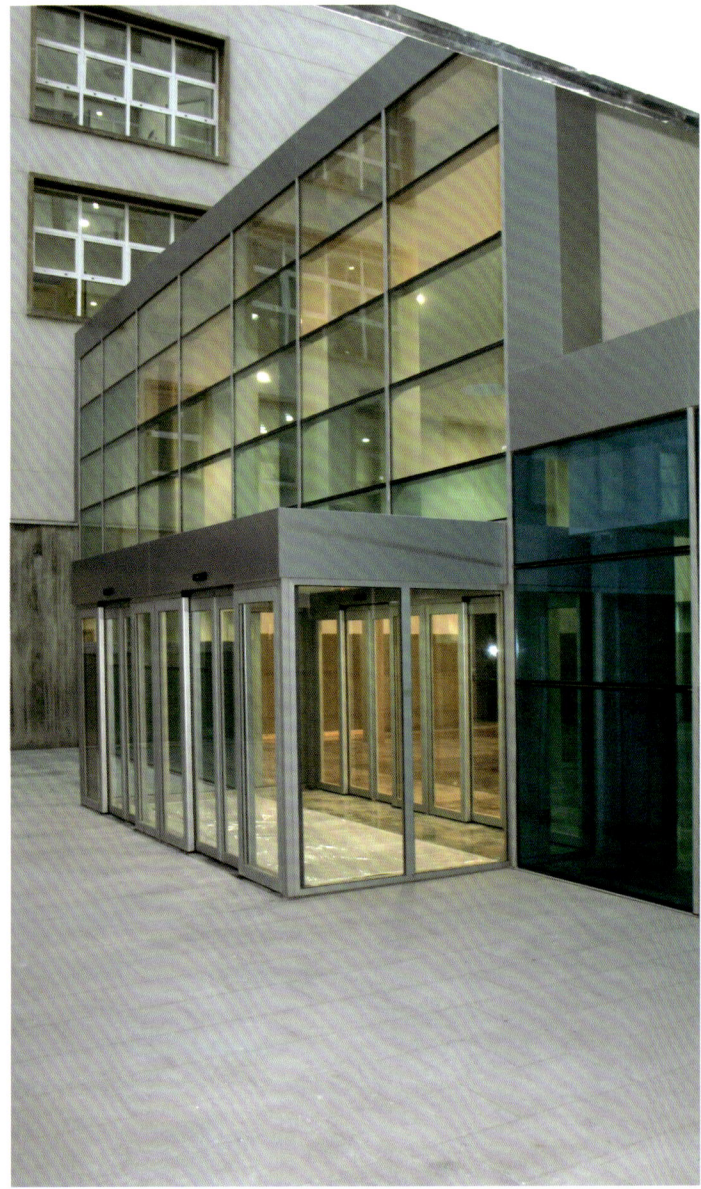

77

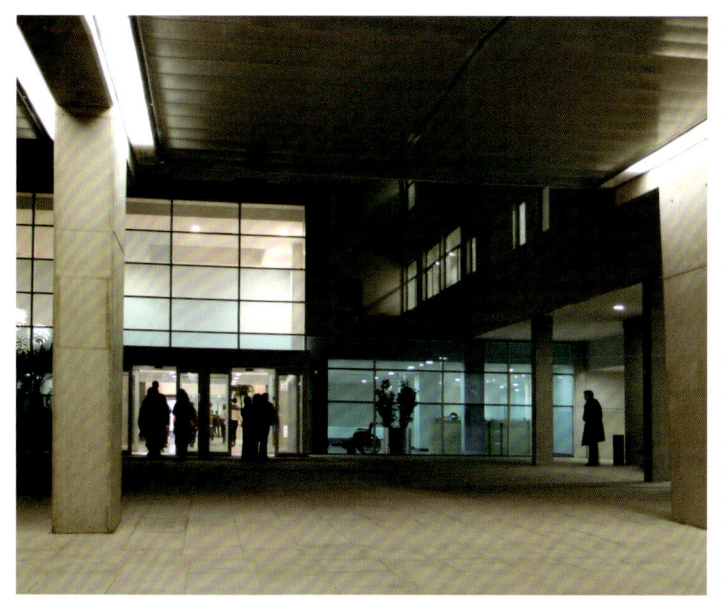

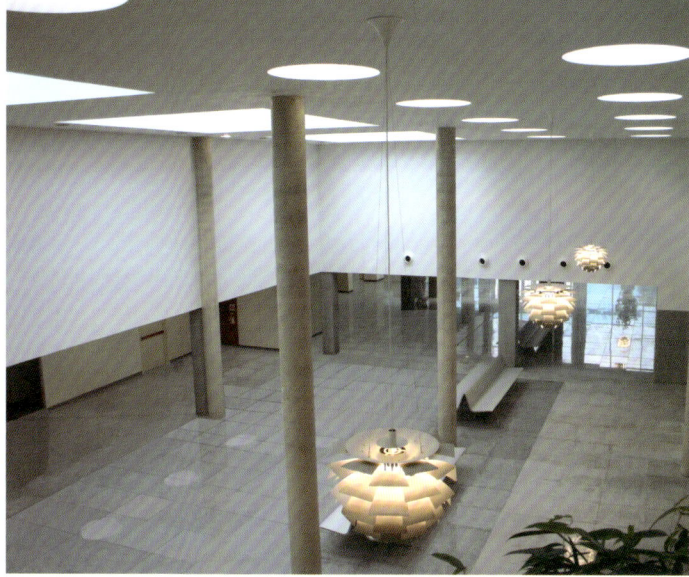

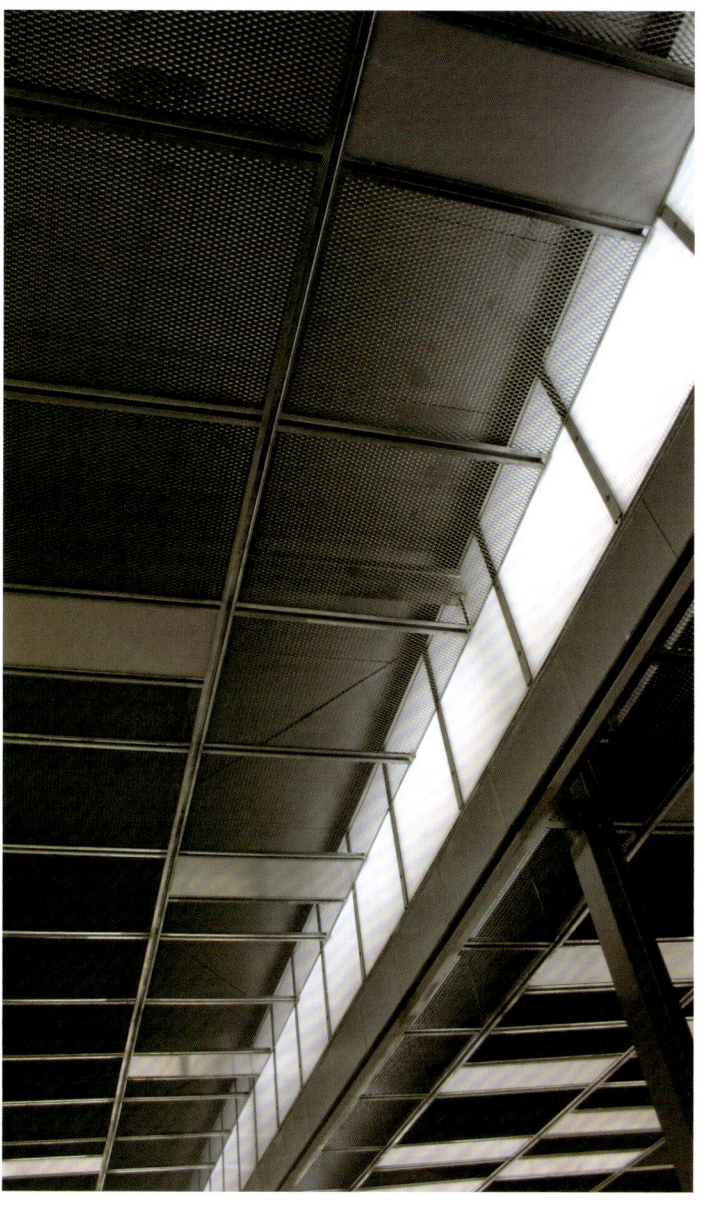

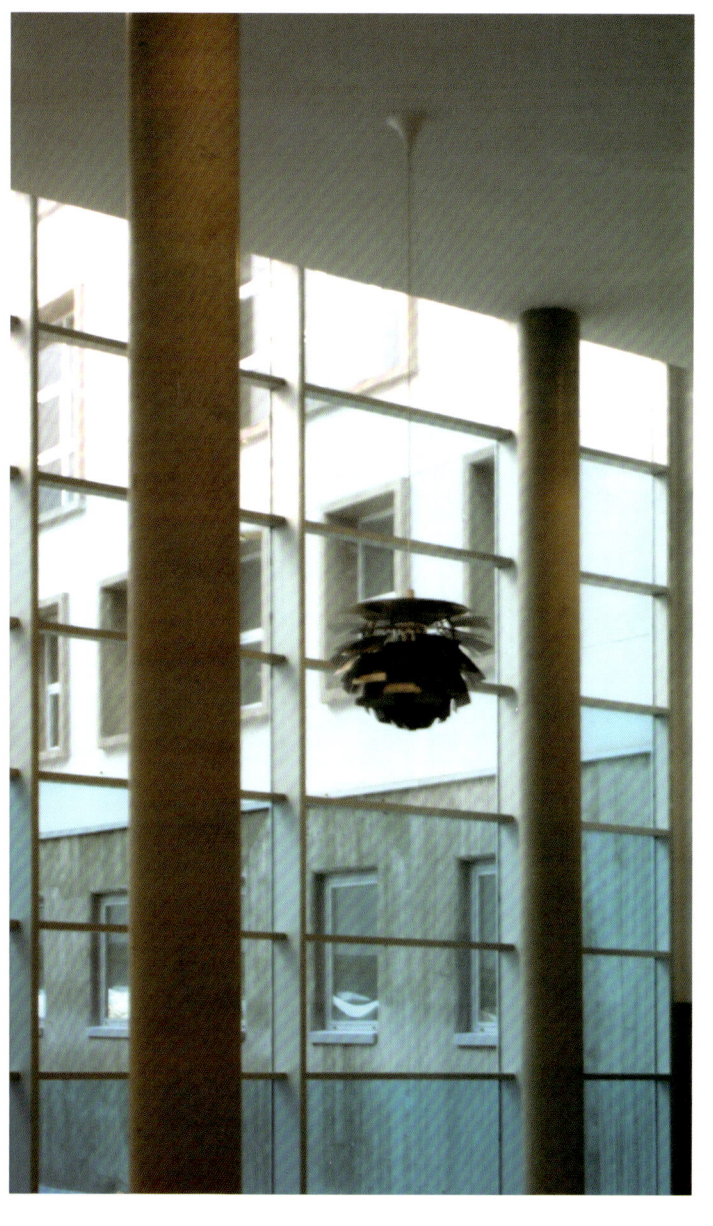

Section AA   North frontal elevation

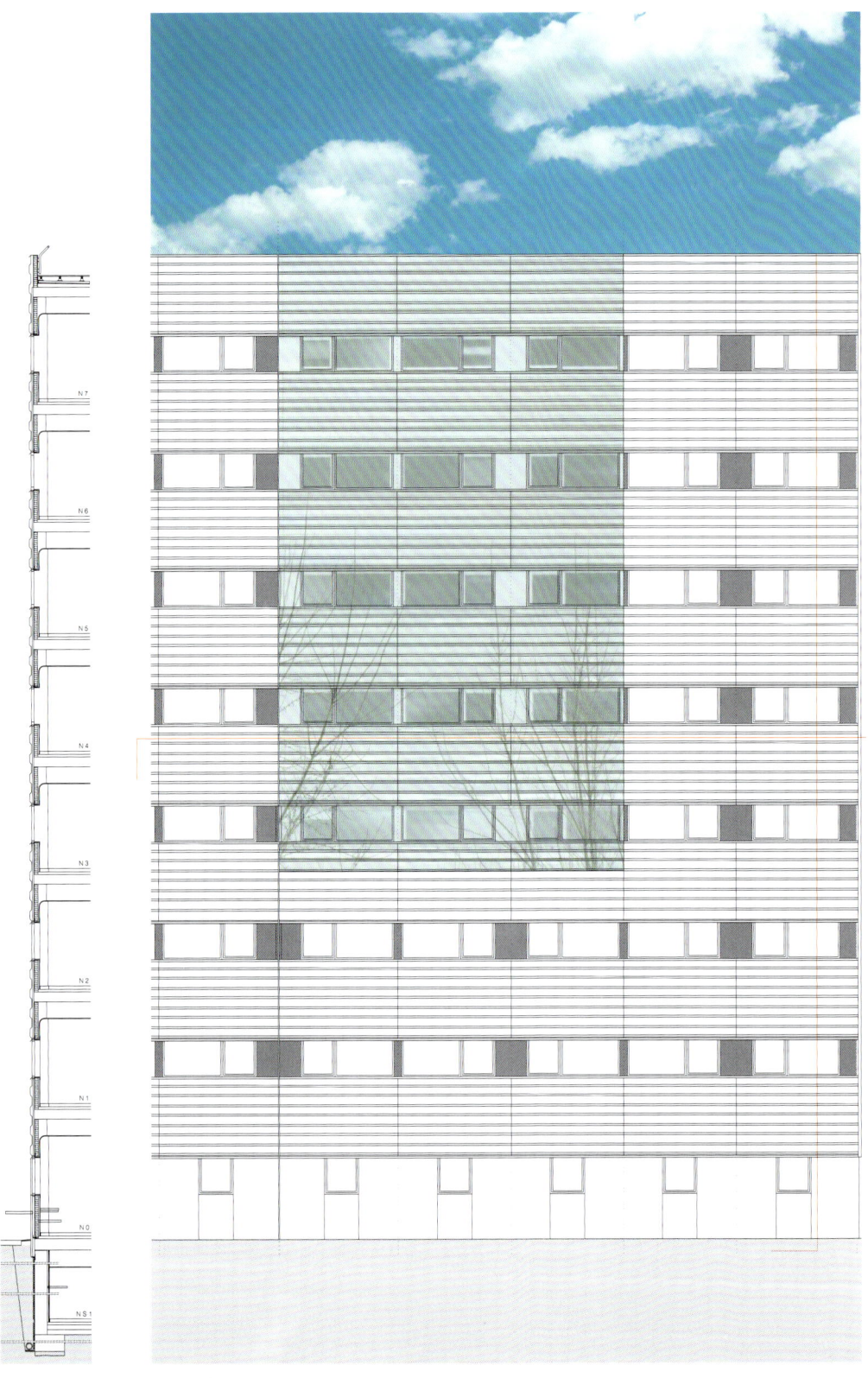

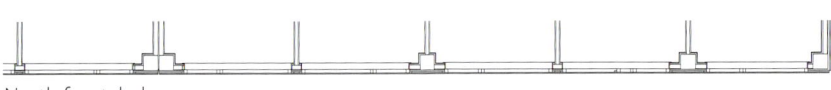

North elevation with detail

North frontal plan

78

Elevation 3

Elevation 2

Elevation 1

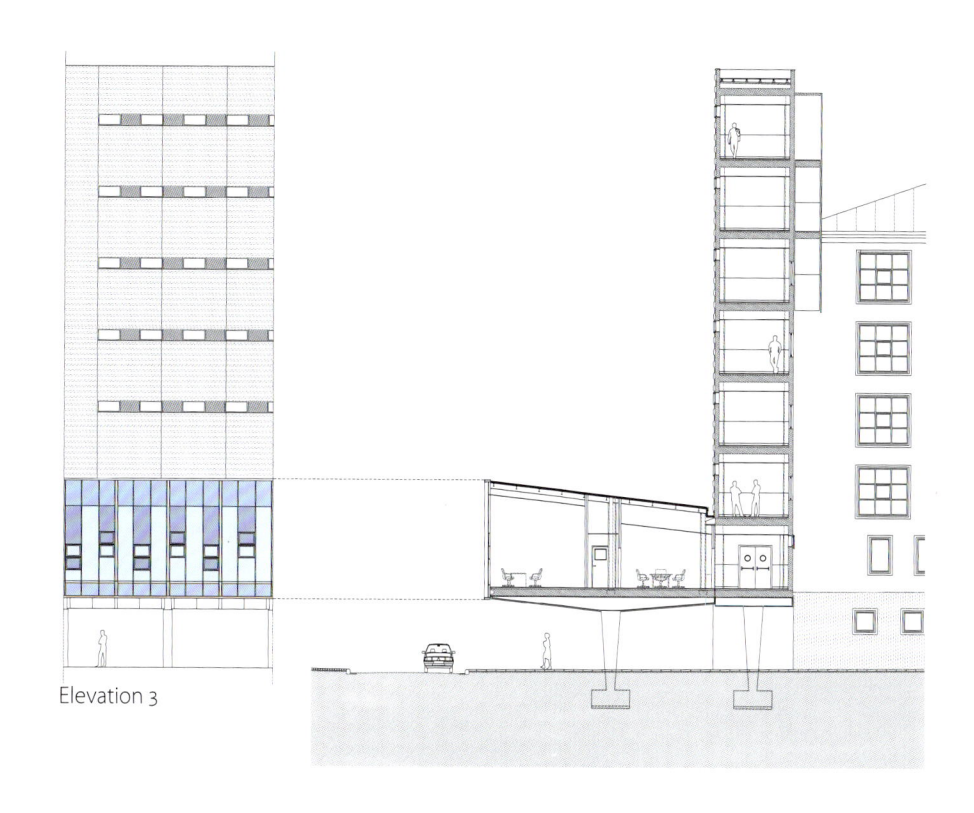

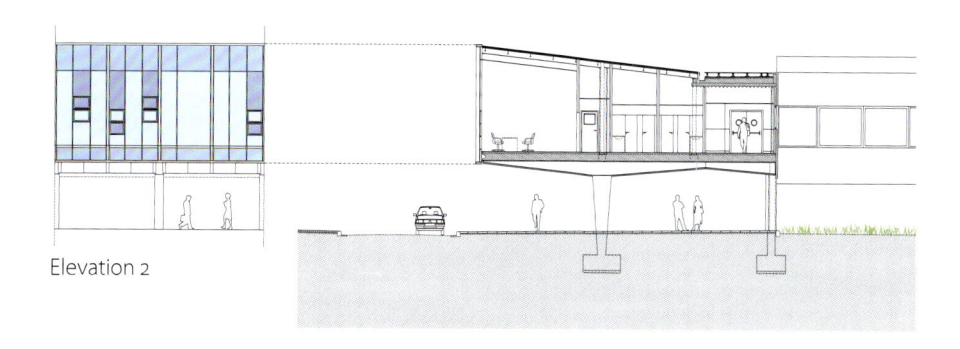

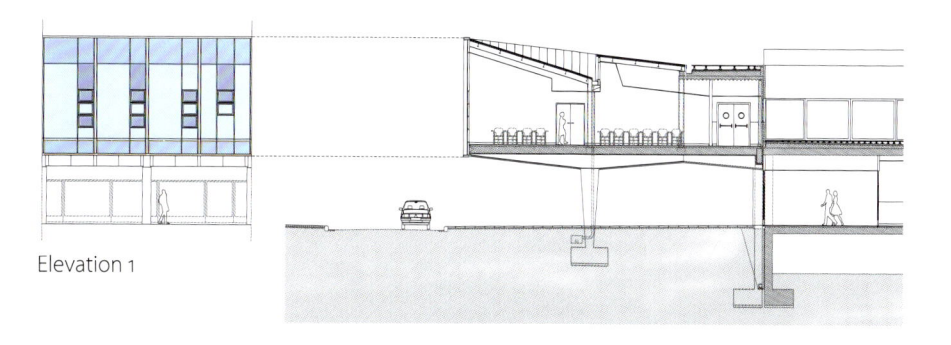

Management pavillion detail

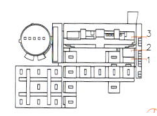

79

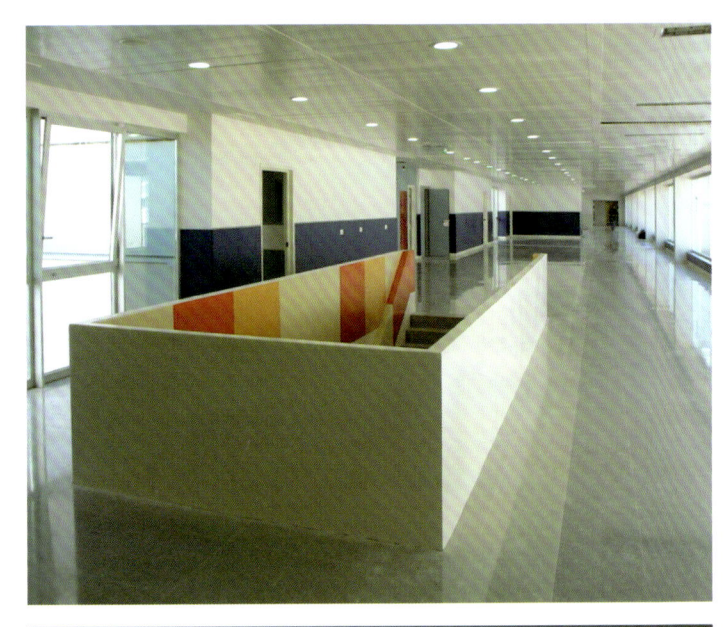

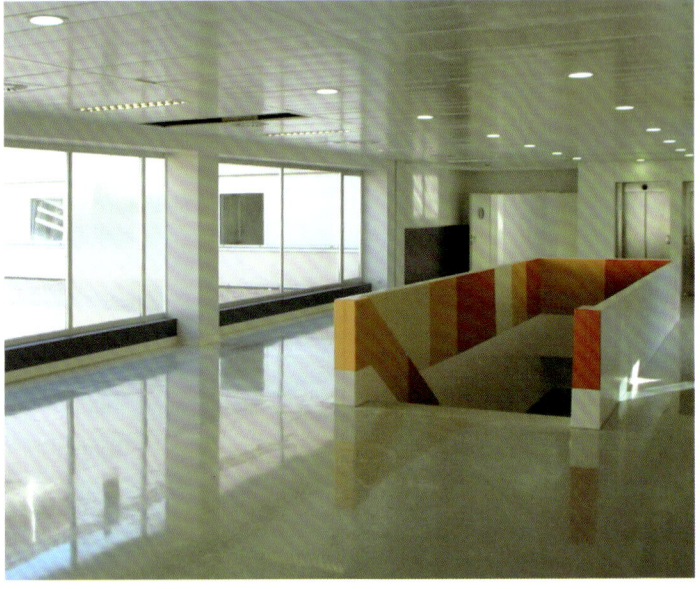

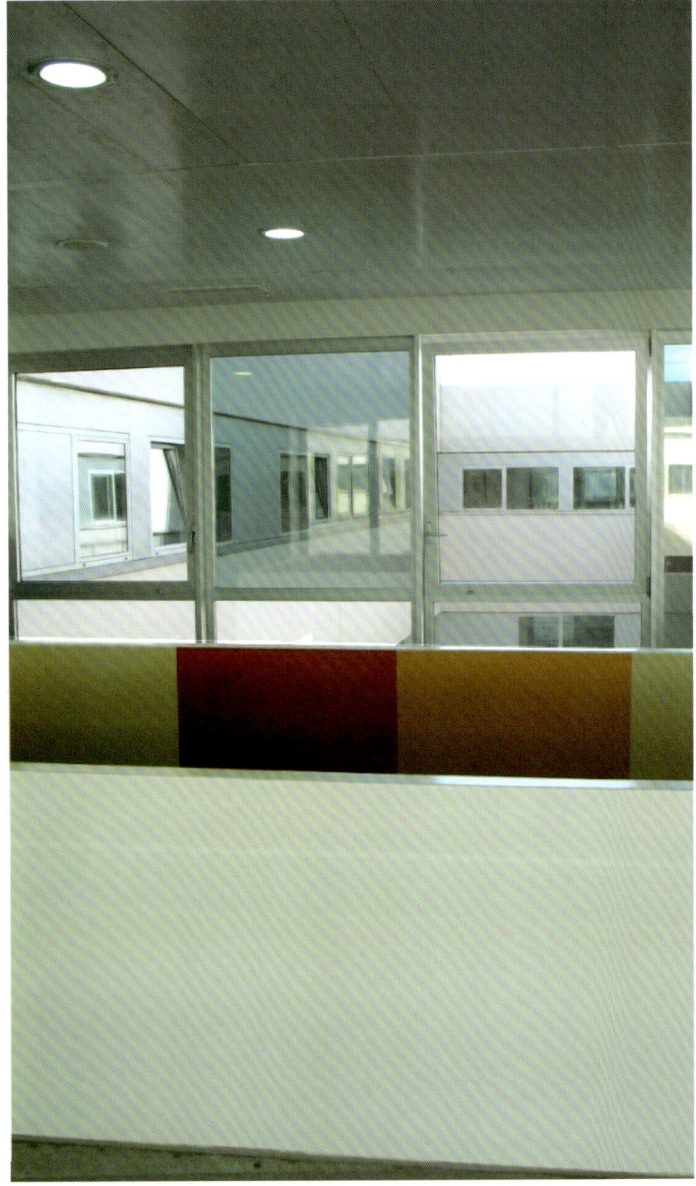

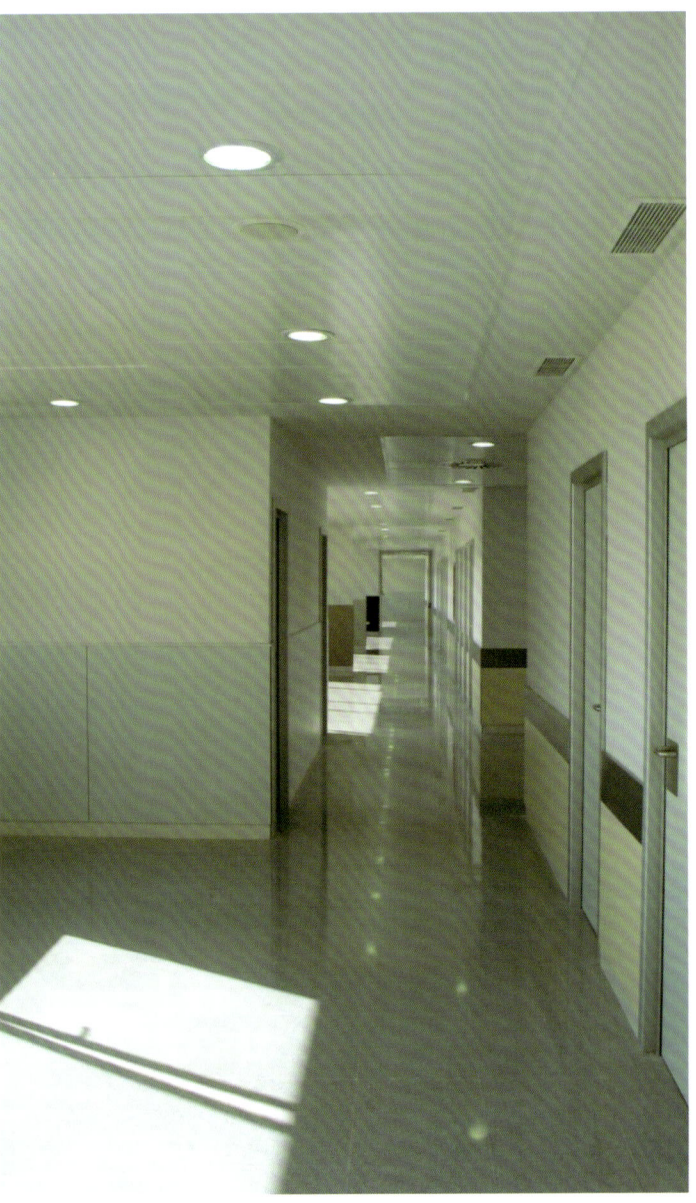

Coffee shop section

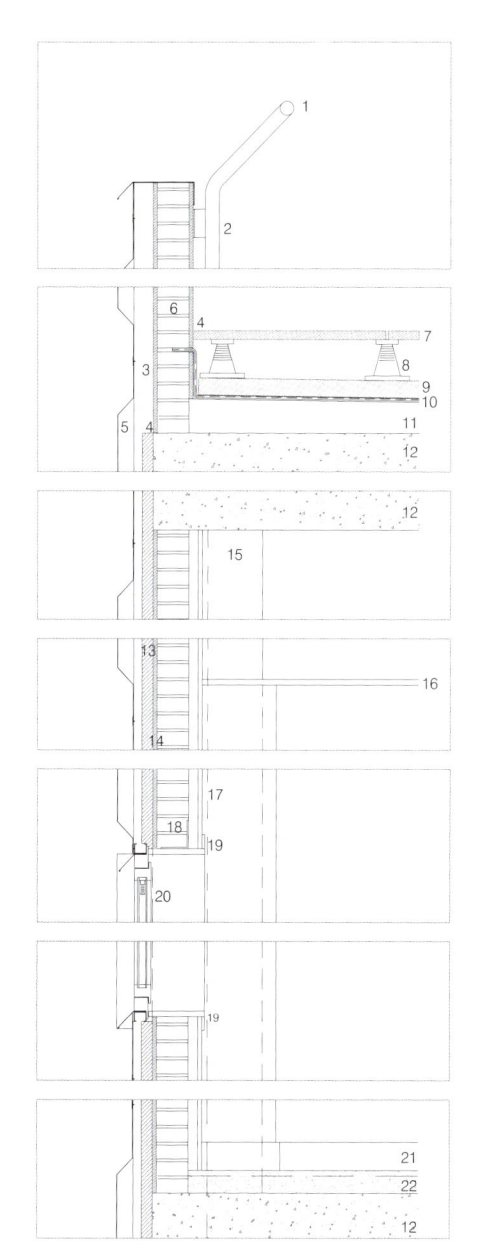

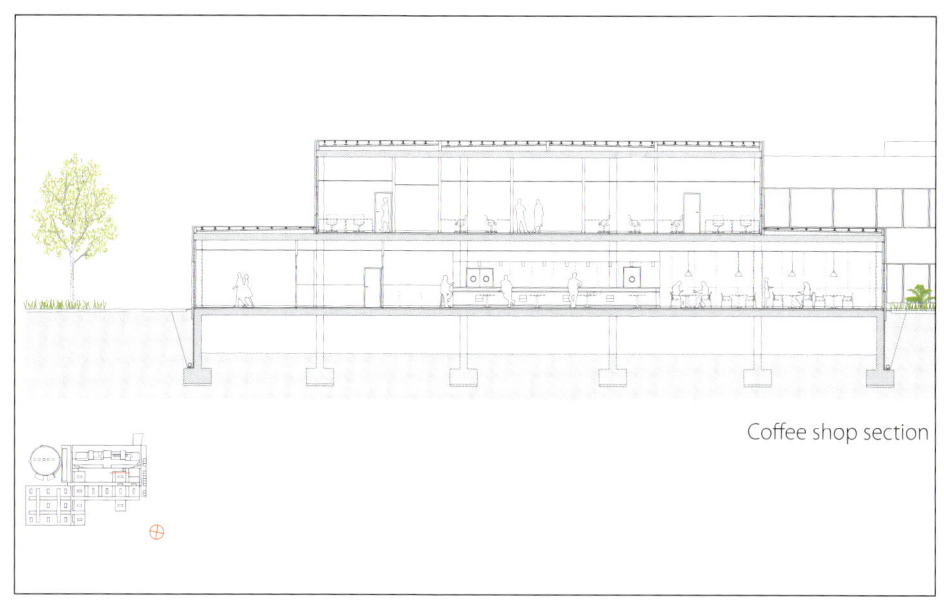

Detail of cut AA

1. Rail: metal tube
2. Anchoring foot of railing
3. Auxiliary structure for anchoring panel
4. Rendering
5. Stainless steel sheet
6. 1/2 solid p.l.
7. Floor tiles, prefabricated reinforced concrete. 70x30
8. Graded support
9. Insulation, as defined, 60mm
10. Waterproof sheet. double, 4 kg
11. Fixing mortar.
12. Slab: reinforced concrete. 30cm
13. Insulation, sprayed. 40mm
14. Rendering: water-resistant mortar
15. Pillar reinforced concrete. 40x40 cm
16. Suspended ceiling: plaster
17. Plaster board 1,5+1,5 on angles 70mm
18. L 100. 100. 5
19. Mouth of opening, lacquered DM board
20. Carpentry: lacquered aluminum with in-built blind
21. Baseboard: resin
22. Terrazzo, in situ, with brass grouting

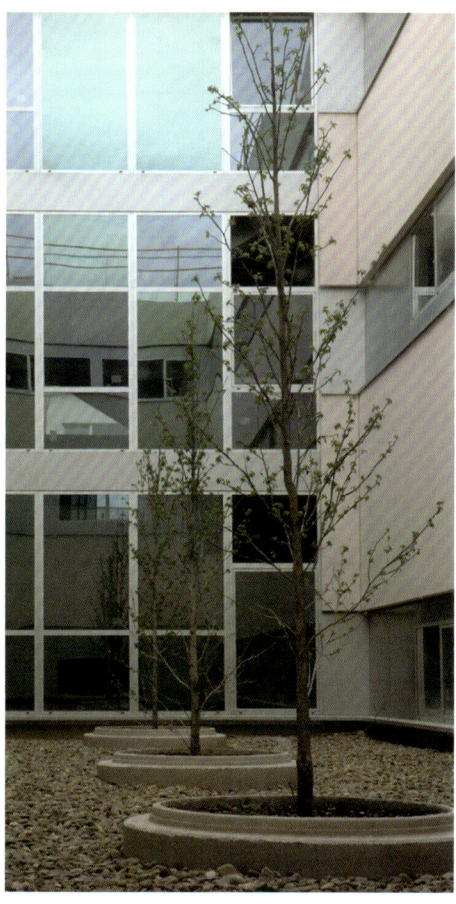

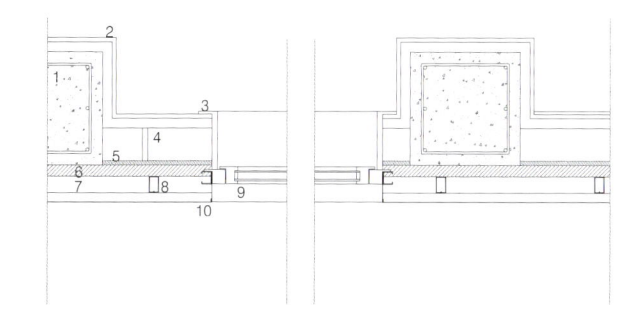

Detail of floor plan

1. Pillar reinforced concrete. 40x40 cm
2. Plaster board 1,5+1,5 on angles 70mm
3. Mouth of opening, lacquered DM board
4. 1/2 solid p.l.
5. Rendering: water-resistant mortar
6. Insulation, sprayed. 40mm
7. Auxiliary structure
8. Anchoring for sheet
9. Carpentry: lacquered aluminum
10. Stainless steel sheet

81

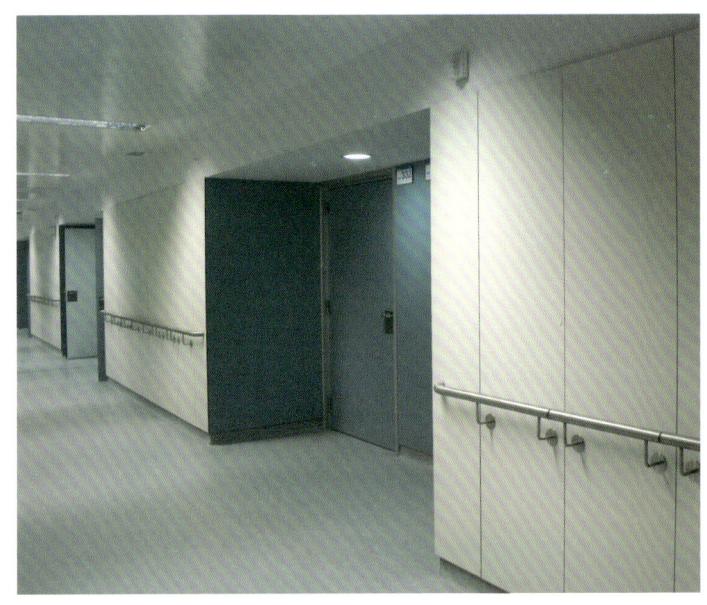

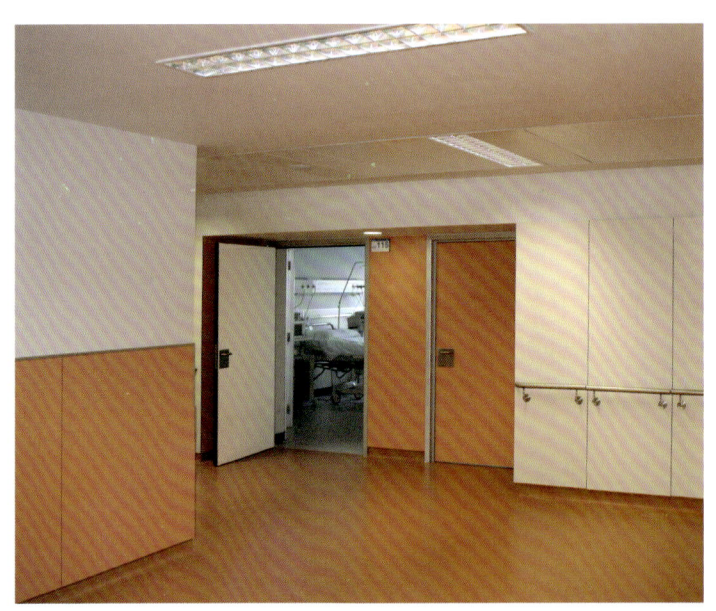

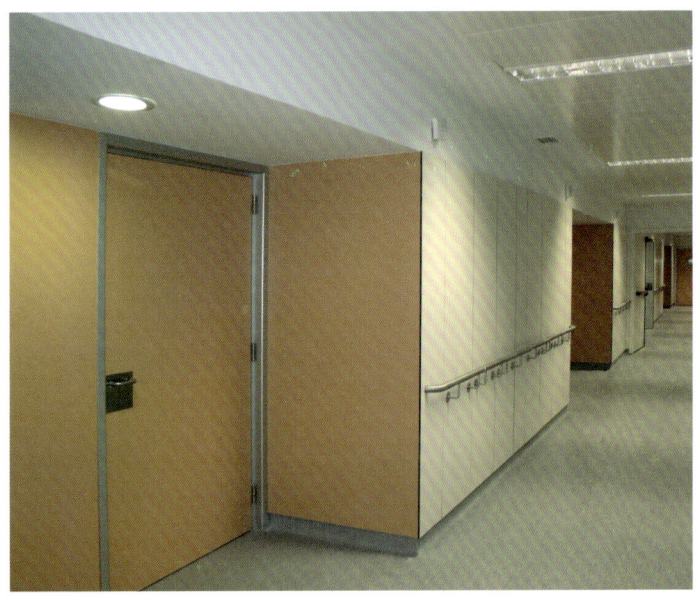

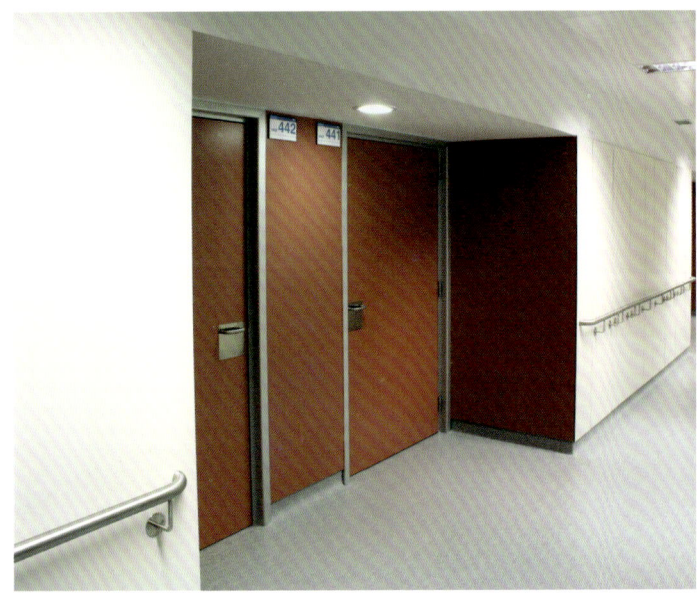

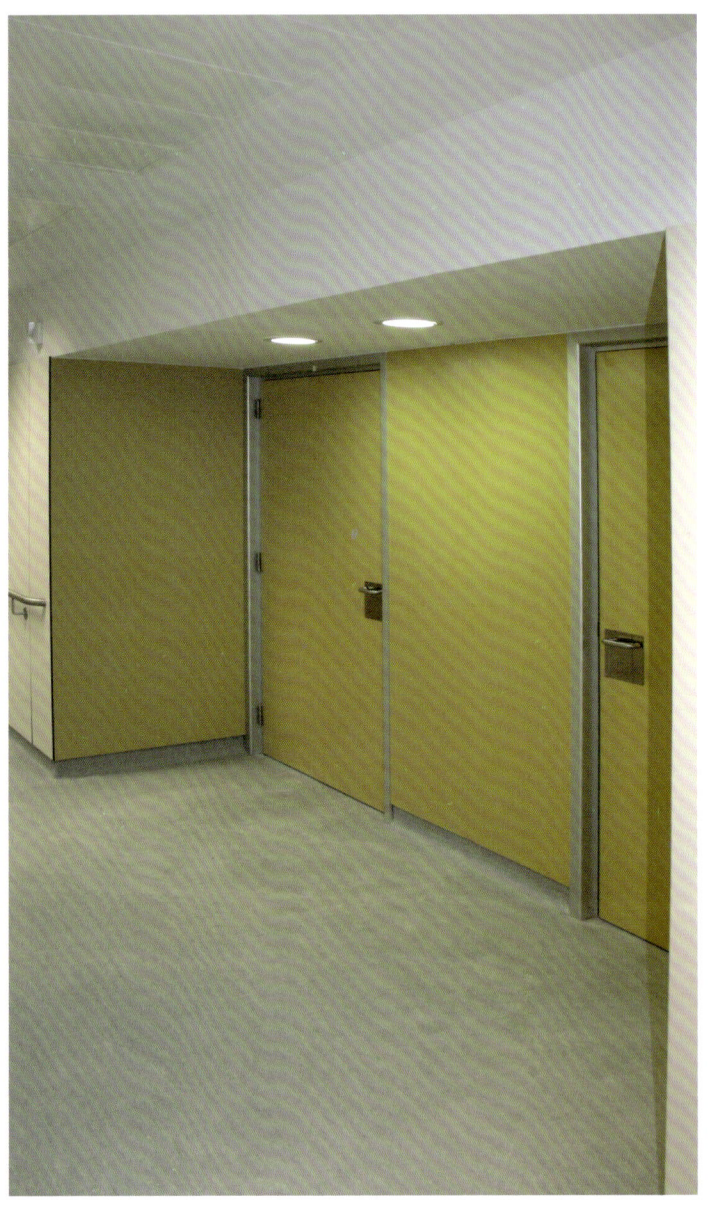

83

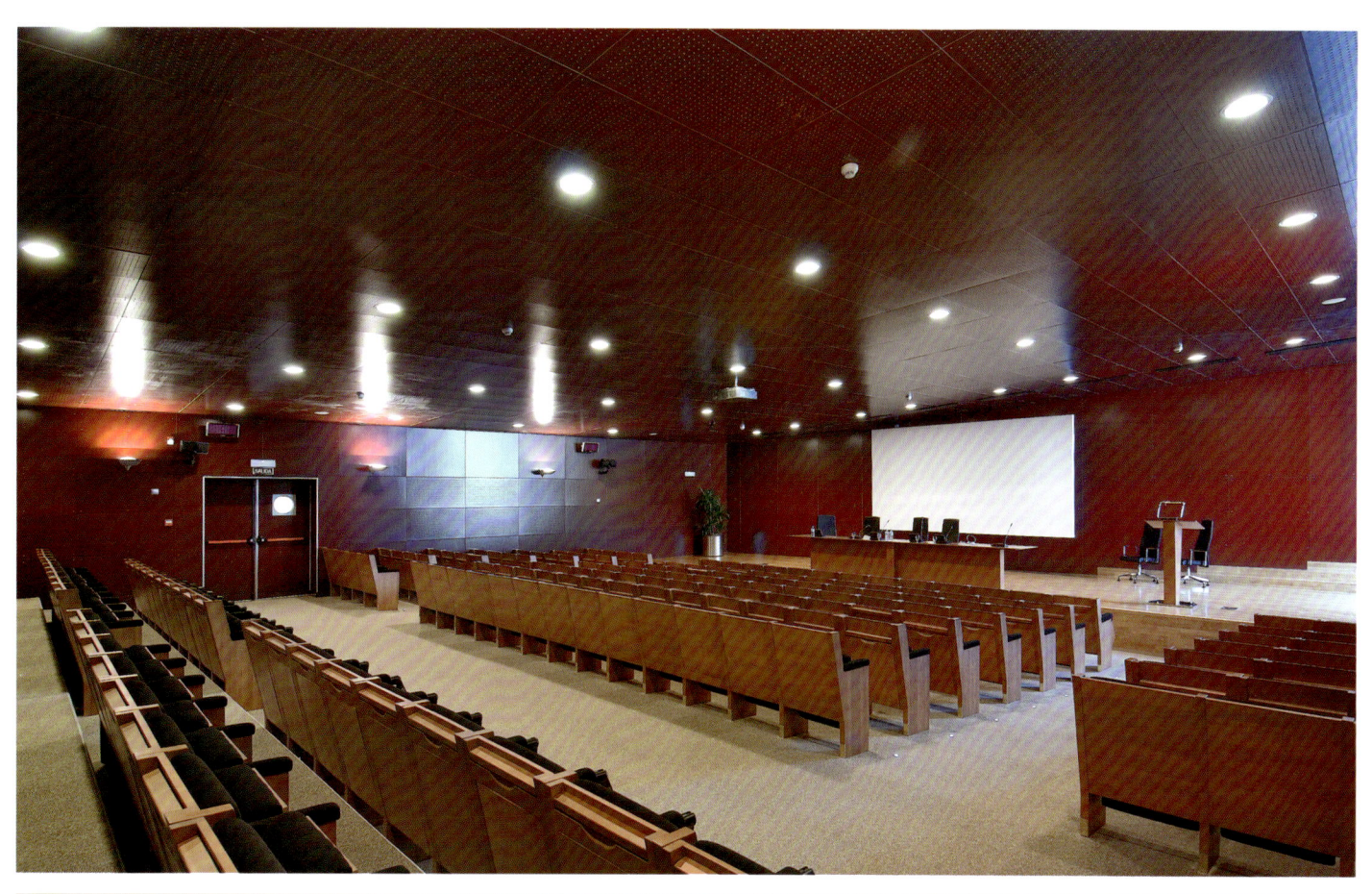

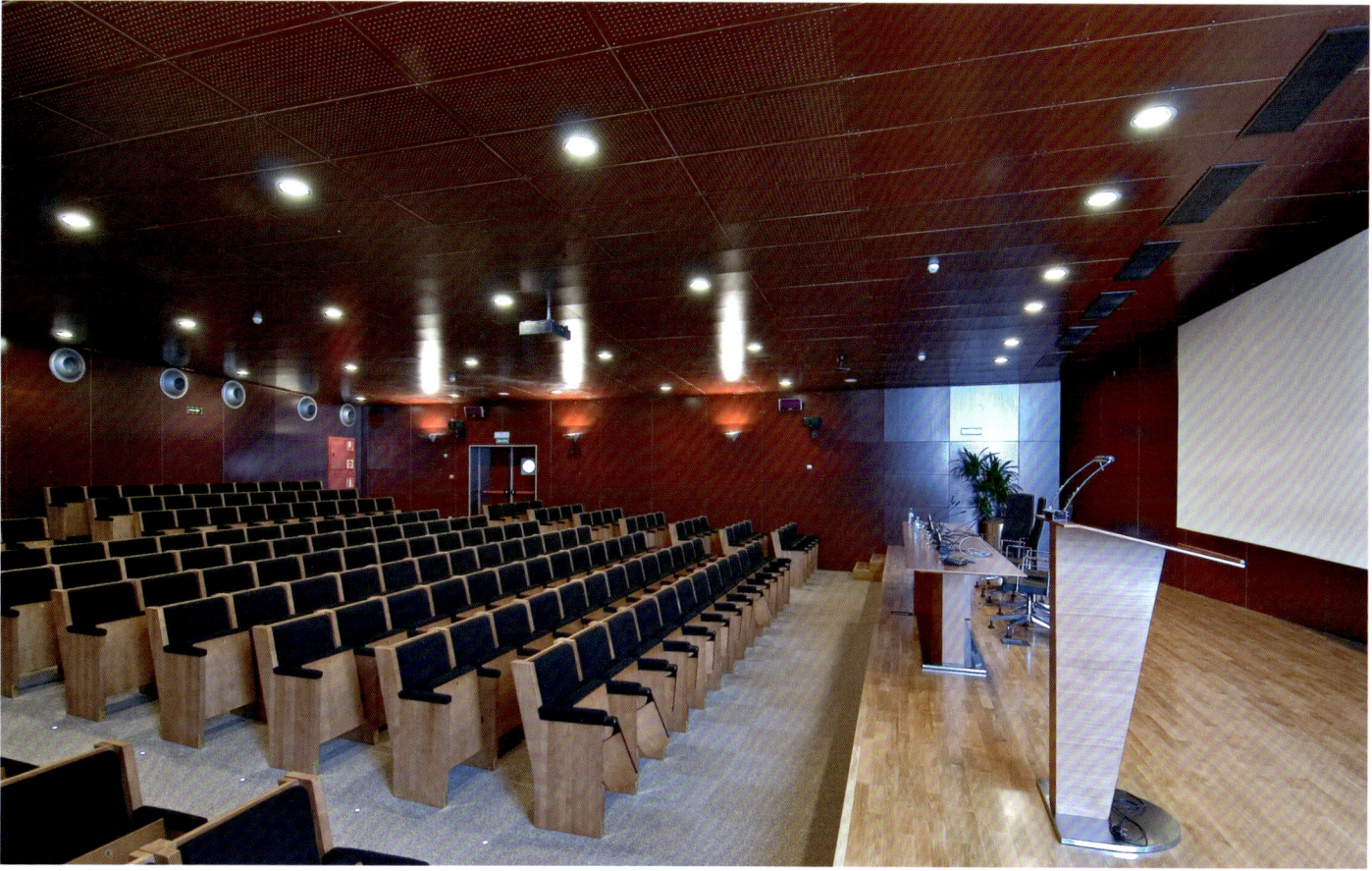

Perkins Eastman

Queens Hospital Center: Ambulatory Care Pavilion

New York, USA

Photographs: Paúl Rivera, ArchPhoto

The Pavilion at Queens Hospital Center represents the culmination of an extensive project to replace one of New York City Health and Hospital Corporation's oldest facilities. Taking into consideration the specific needs of this vibrant New York City borough, the Health and Hospital Corporation devised a master plan that brings to Queens a medical facility equipped to support its community well into the 21st century – as well as creating a signature landmark for the hospital campus at its northern edge. With the divestment of properties and demolition of outmoded facilities, this project reassembles essential healthcare and administrative components in a more compact, convenient, and cost effective adjunct to the Queens Hospital Center. The Pavilion houses primary care, pediatrics, behavioral health, dental, diabetes, and eye care functions; in addition to housing administrative, educational, and training facilities for the entire hospital center.

In order to accommodate all of these expectations, the planning process adhered to design principles that included maintaining separation of patient areas from staff areas, providing separate access for patients and staff, maximizing the use of natural sunlight wherever possible, placing patient circulation along day-lit corridors, creating memorable spaces to facilitate wayfinding, planning for operational efficiencies, and building in flexibility for the future.

The elegant 13,400 sqm (144,000 sqft) five-level building is organized by a 90 m (300 ft) long glazed public concourse along the southern perimeter. This cantilevered circulation spine links all clinics to the staff and service elevator core on the west and the public elevator core to the east. Composed of pre-cast concrete and a glass curtain wall, the building also provides a light-filled two-story atrium and public entry plaza at the eastern end and a staff/service entry on the west.

In addition to its functional requirements, the Pavilion exceeds the goals of welcoming outpatients in a dignified and life-affirming context; being operationally efficient; accommodating changing functions over time; attracting physicians and other practitioners; reducing patient anxiety levels and staff stress levels; and serving as an attractive and inviting entry point for the entire hospital center.

Client:
Queens Hospital Center
Surface area:
13,400 sqm (144,000 sqft)
Start date:
January 2004
Finish date:
June 2006
Design team:
Jonathan Stark, Duncan Reid, Robert Adler, Maria Jelinek, Shane Walton, Zeynep Aydin, Cristobal Mayendia, Matthew Tether

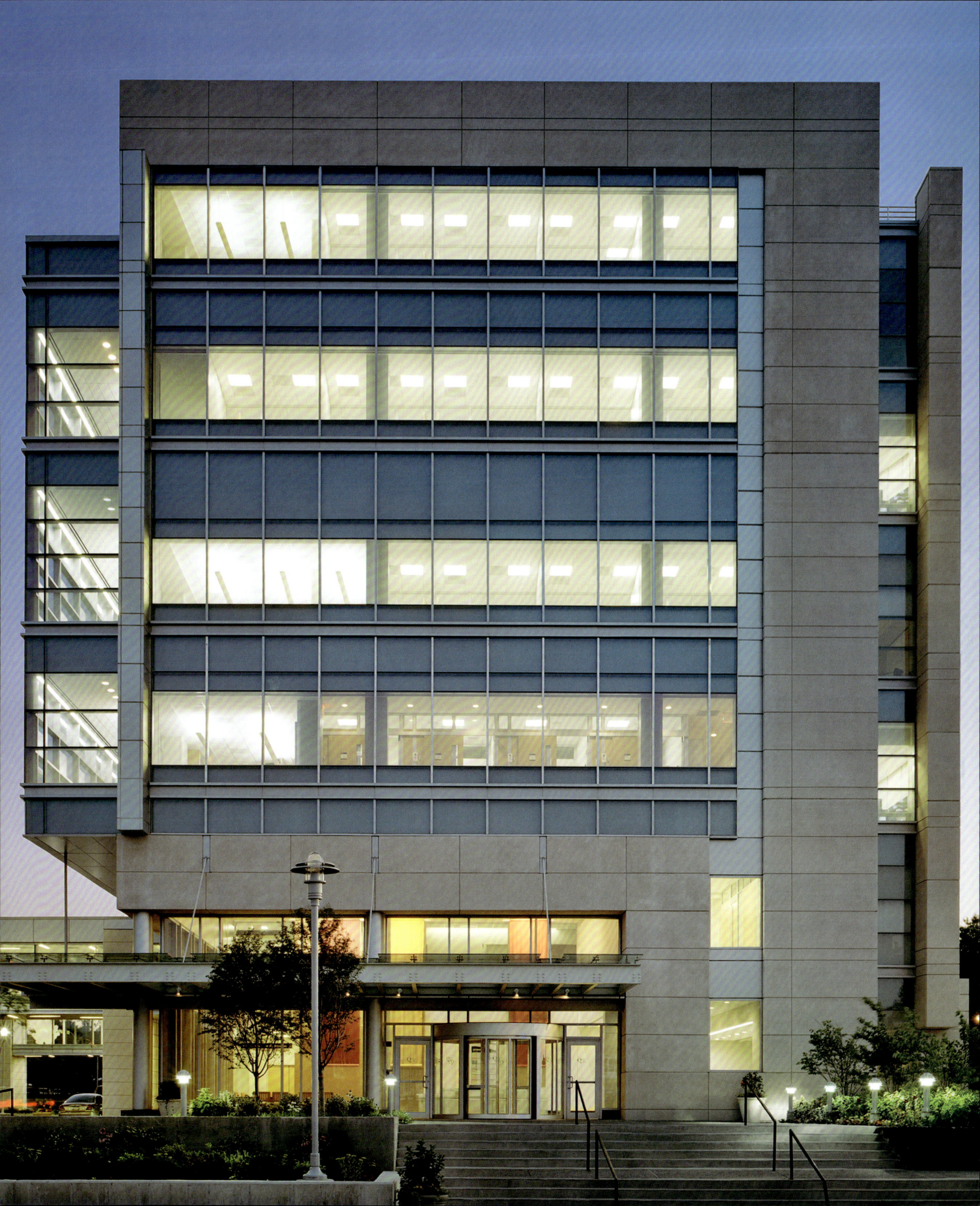

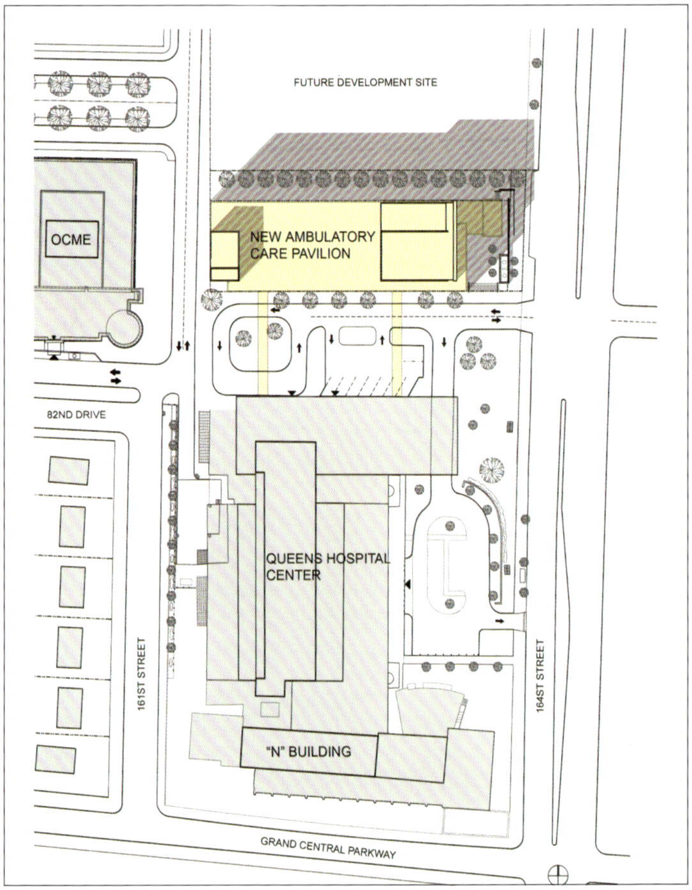
FUTURE DEVELOPMENT SITE
OCME
NEW AMBULATORY
CARE PAVILION
82ND DRIVE
QUEENS HOSPITAL
CENTER
161ST STREET
164ST STREET
"N" BUILDING
GRAND CENTRAL PARKWAY

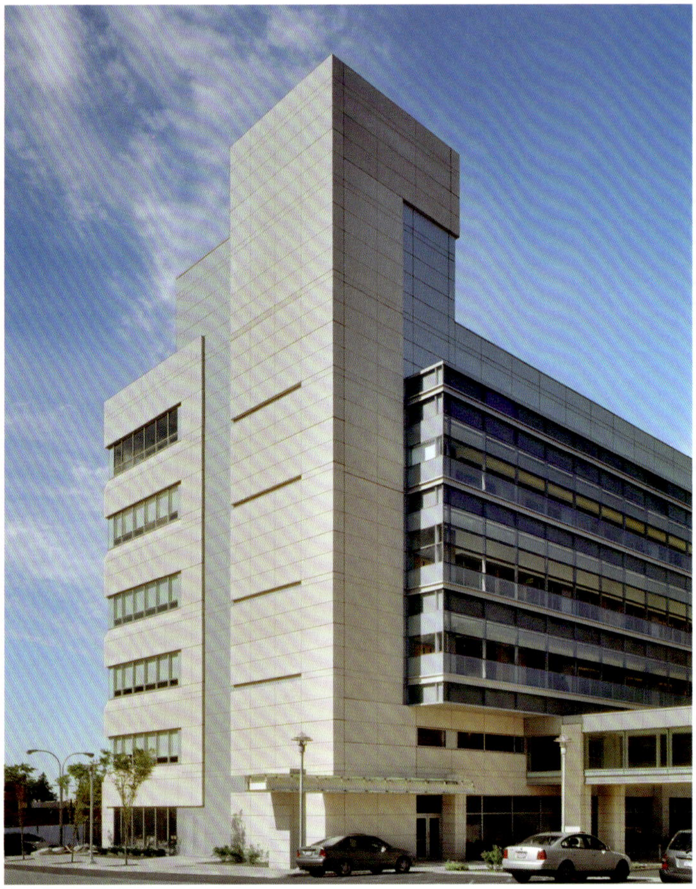

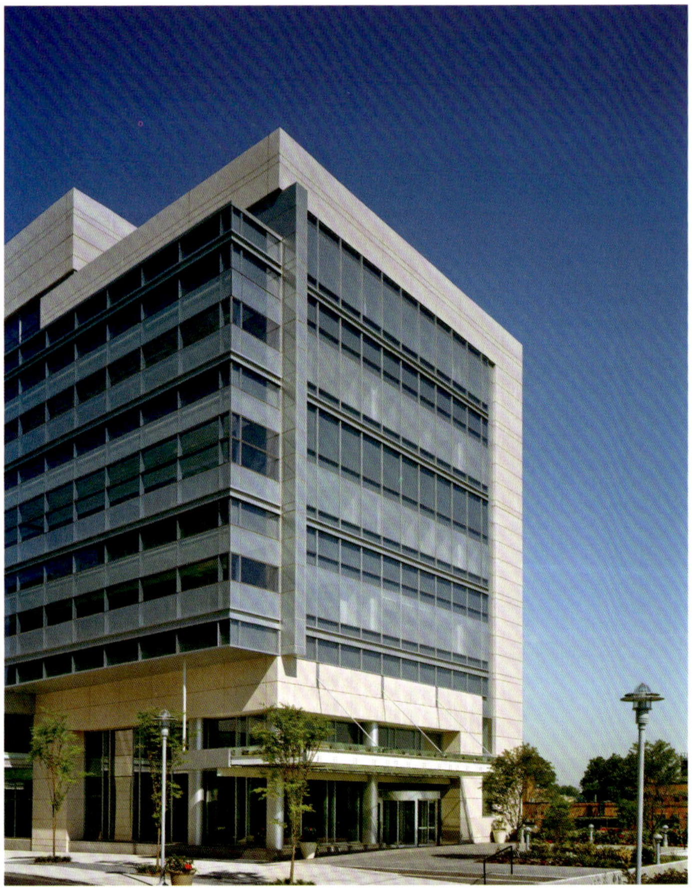

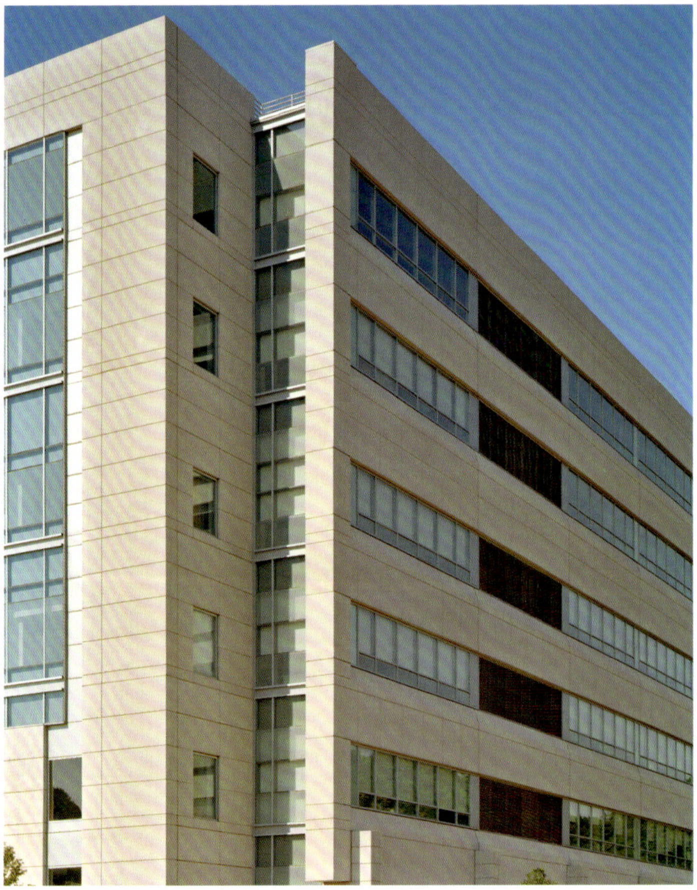

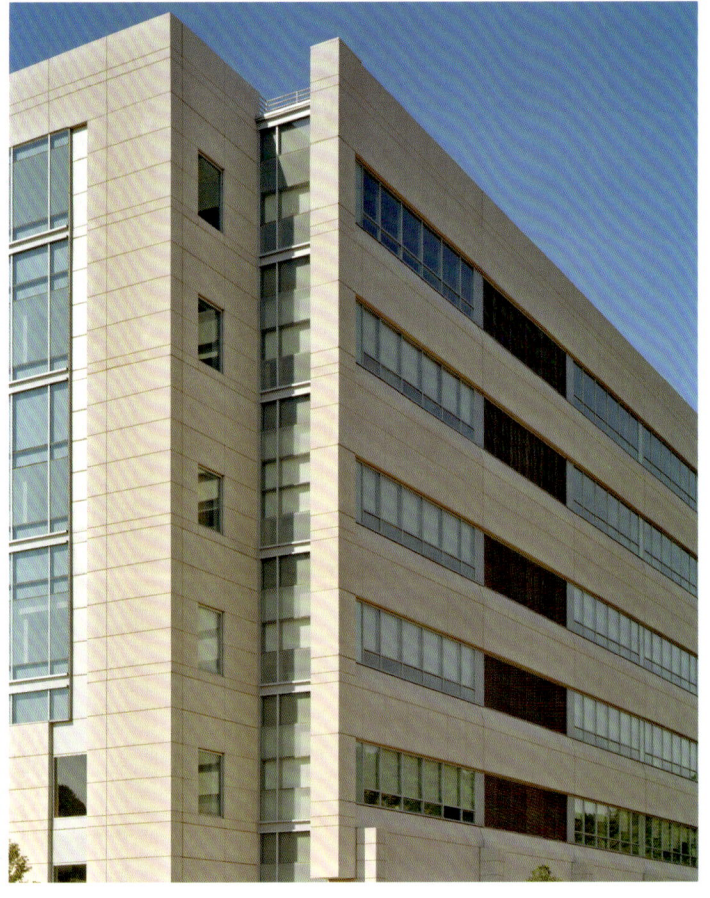

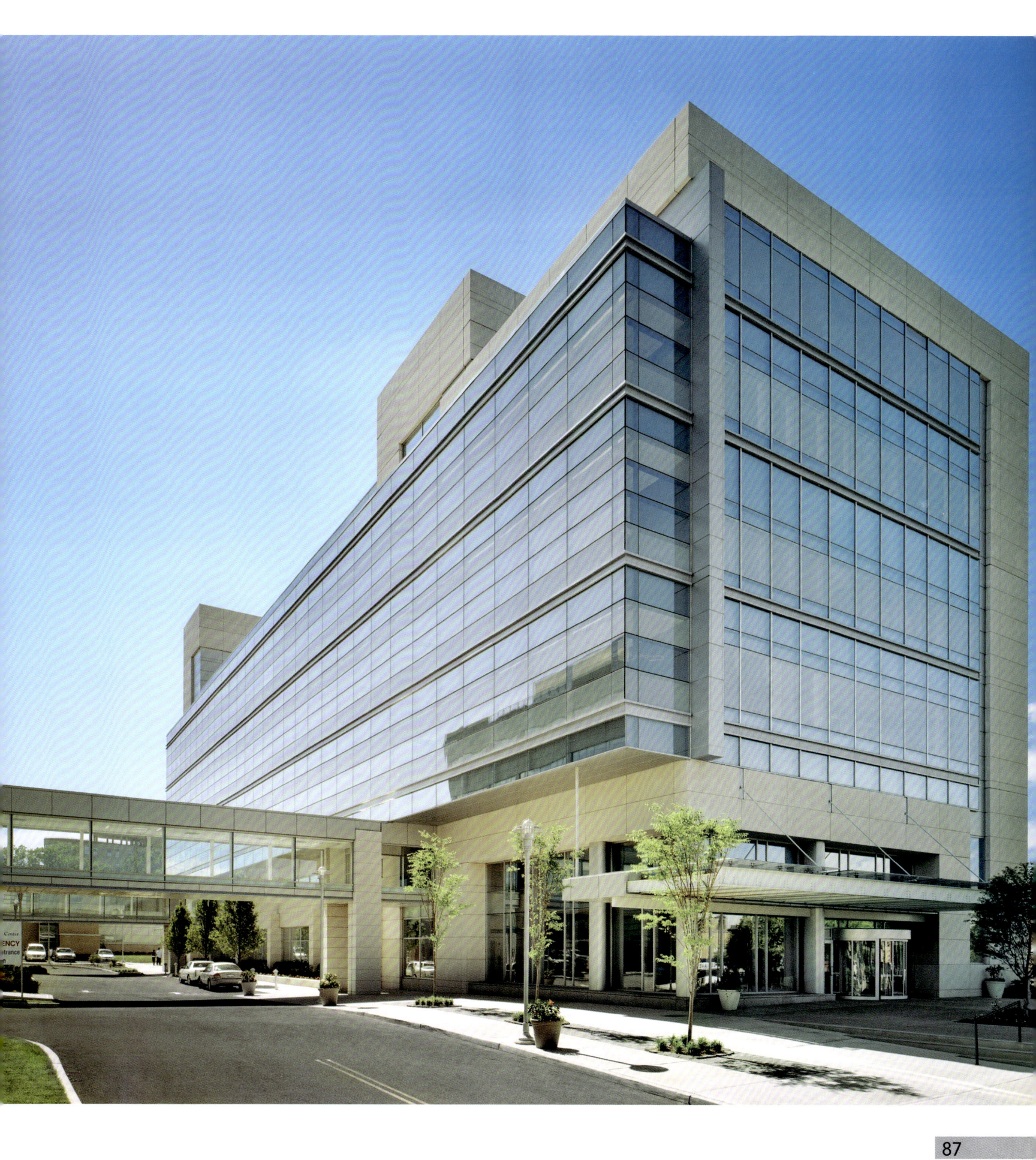

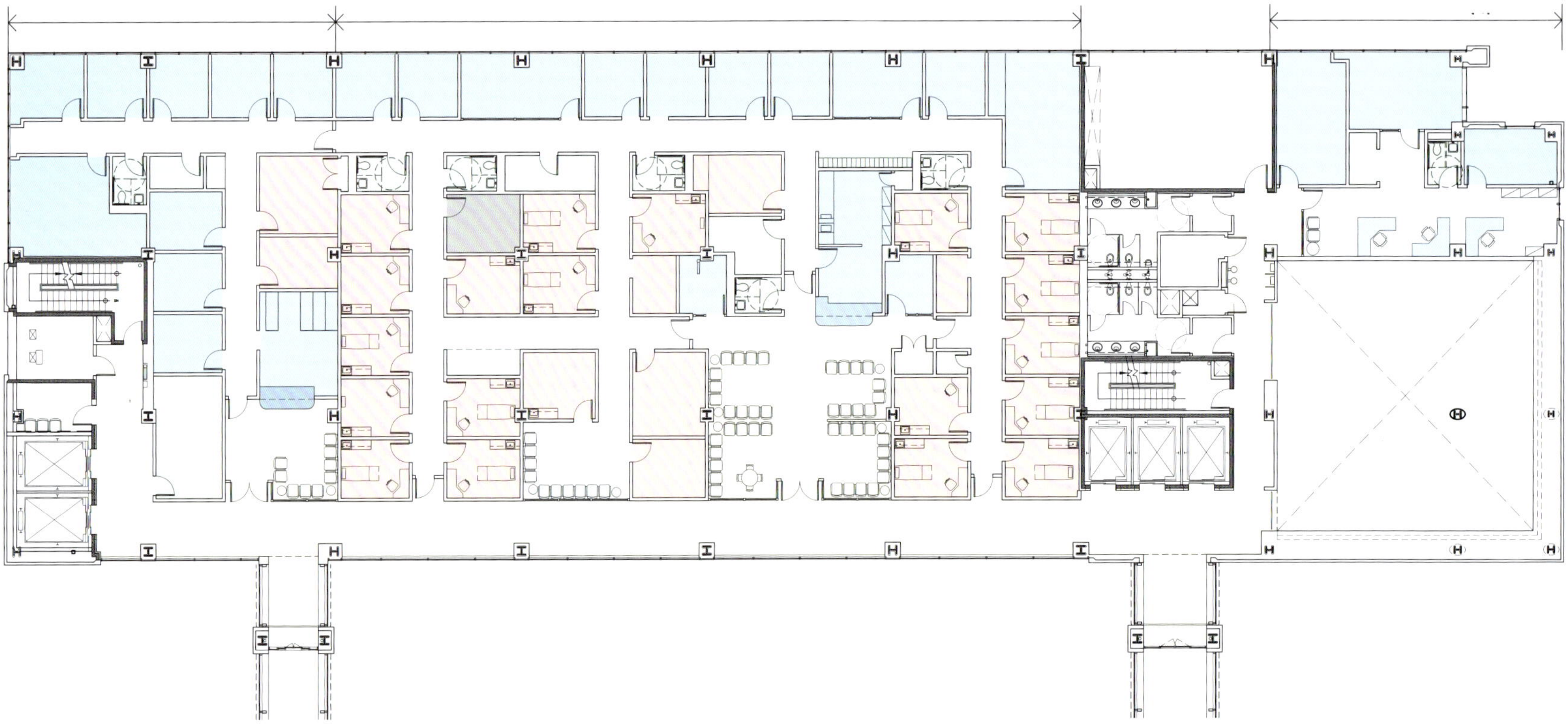

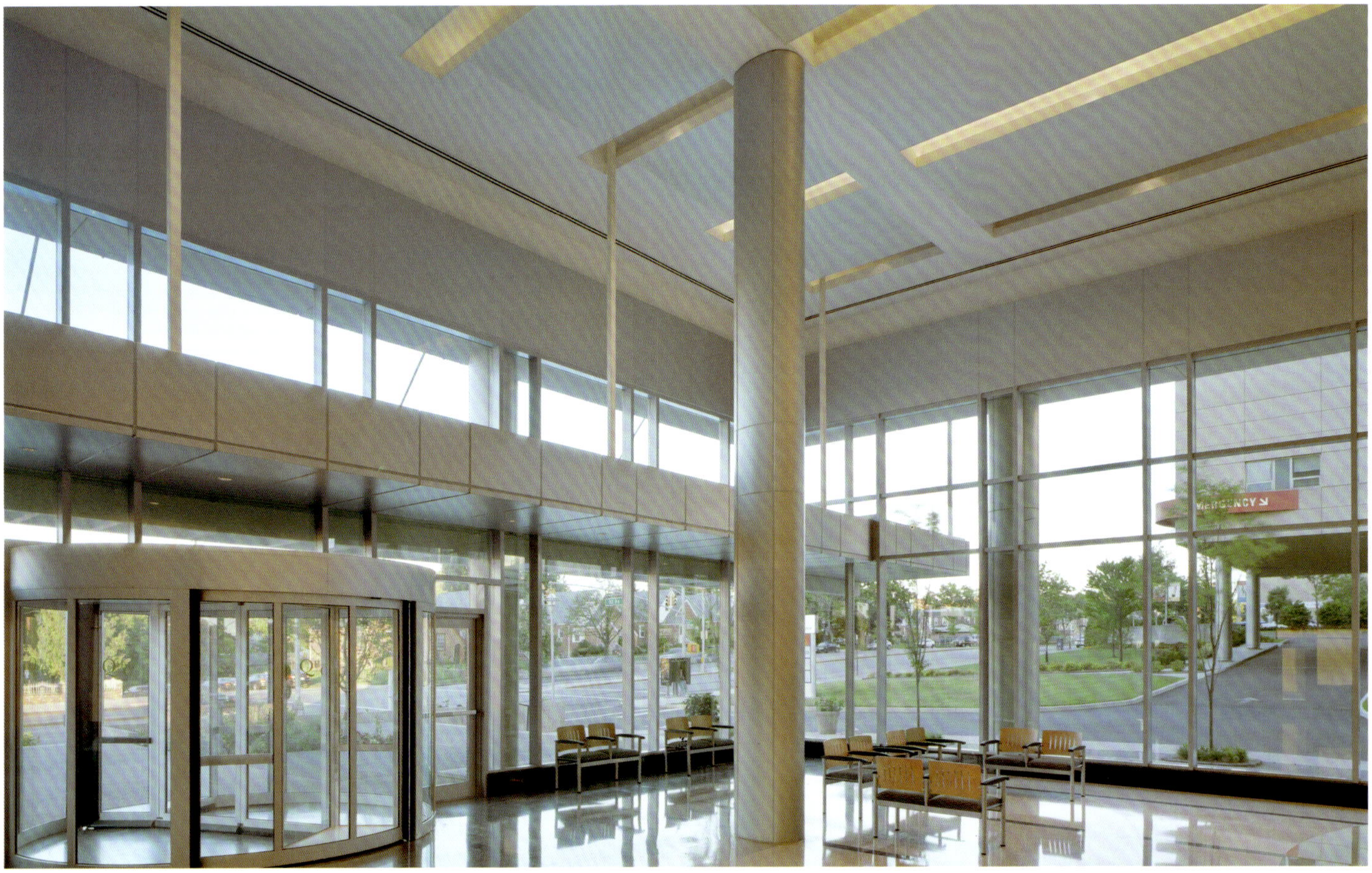

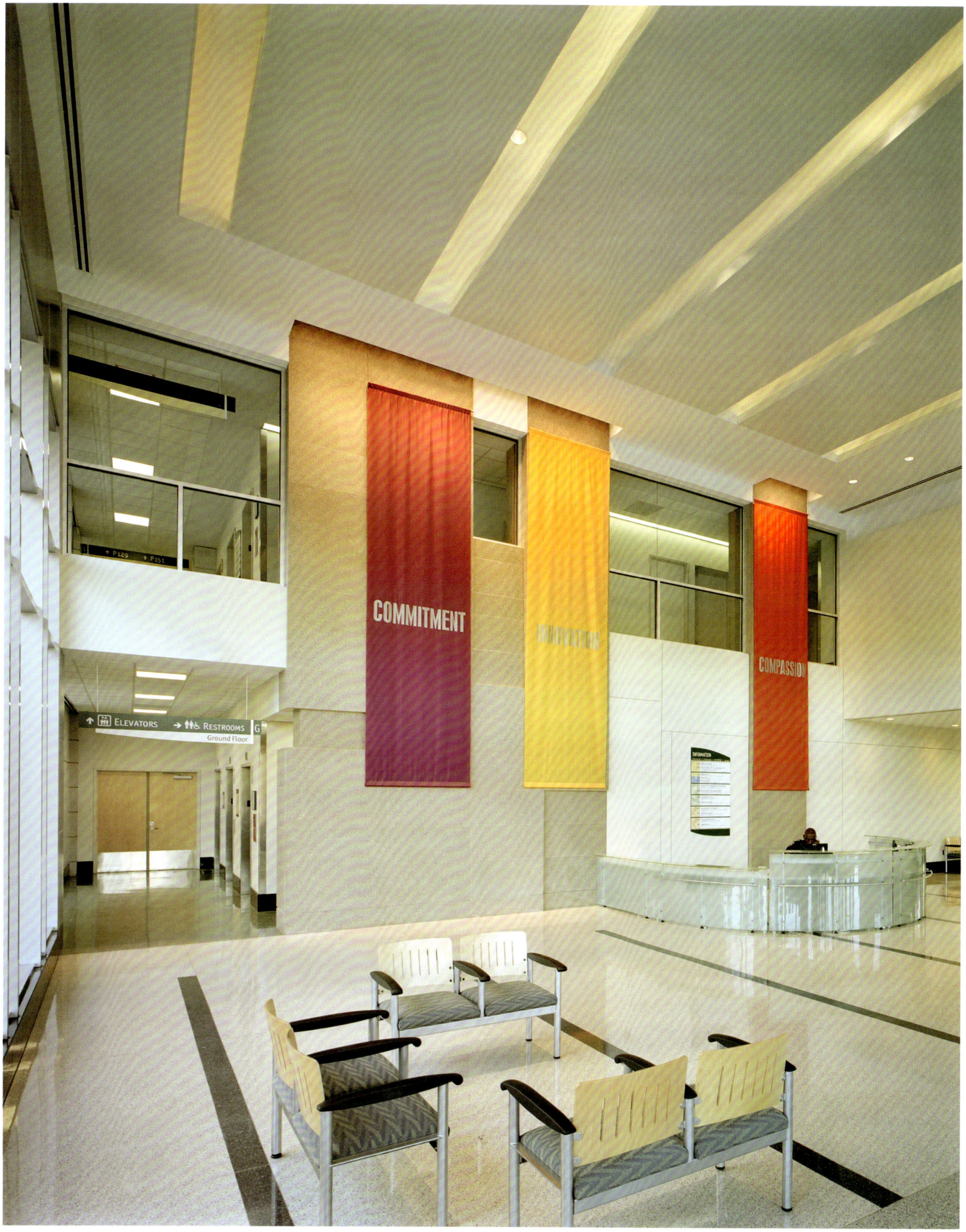
COMMITMENT
COMPASSION
ELEVATORS
RESTROOMS
Ground Floor

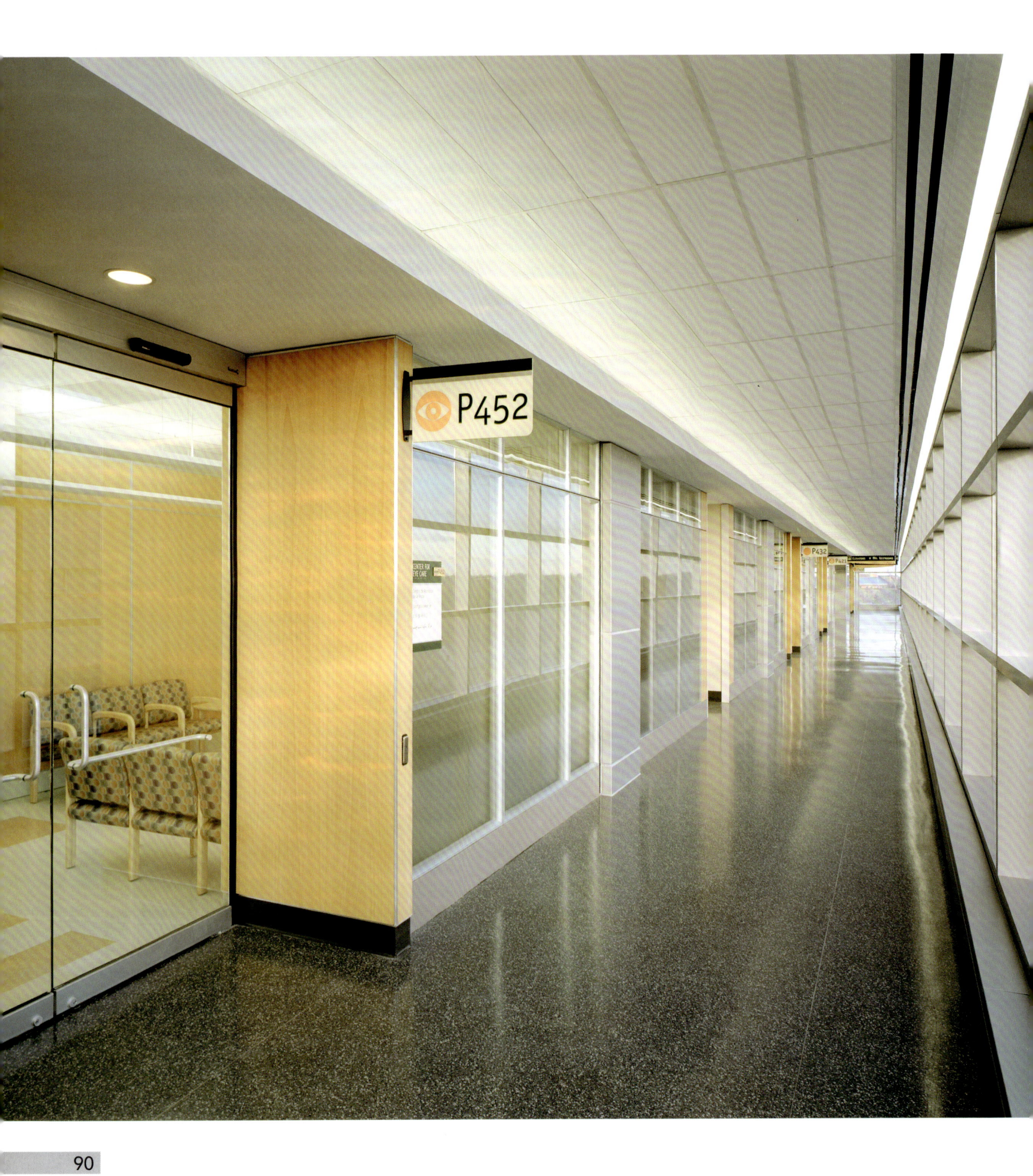

91

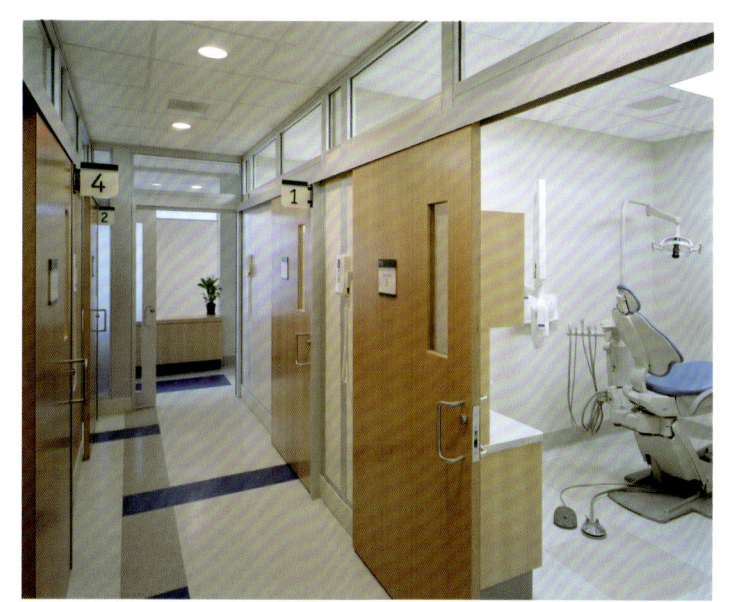

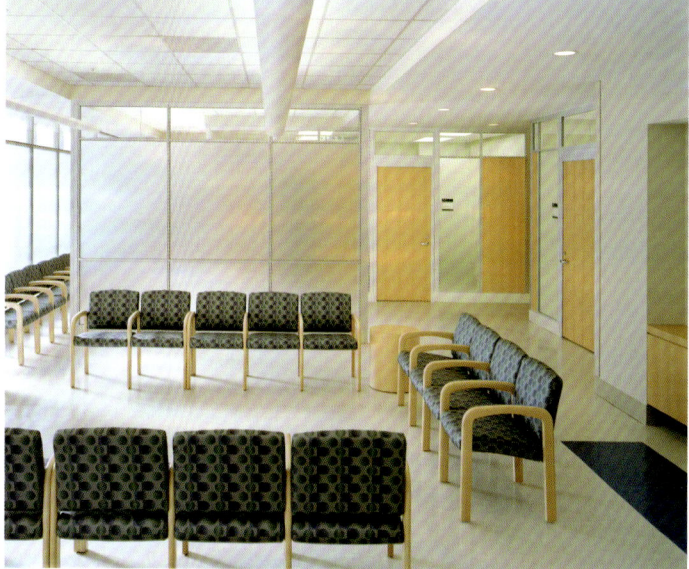

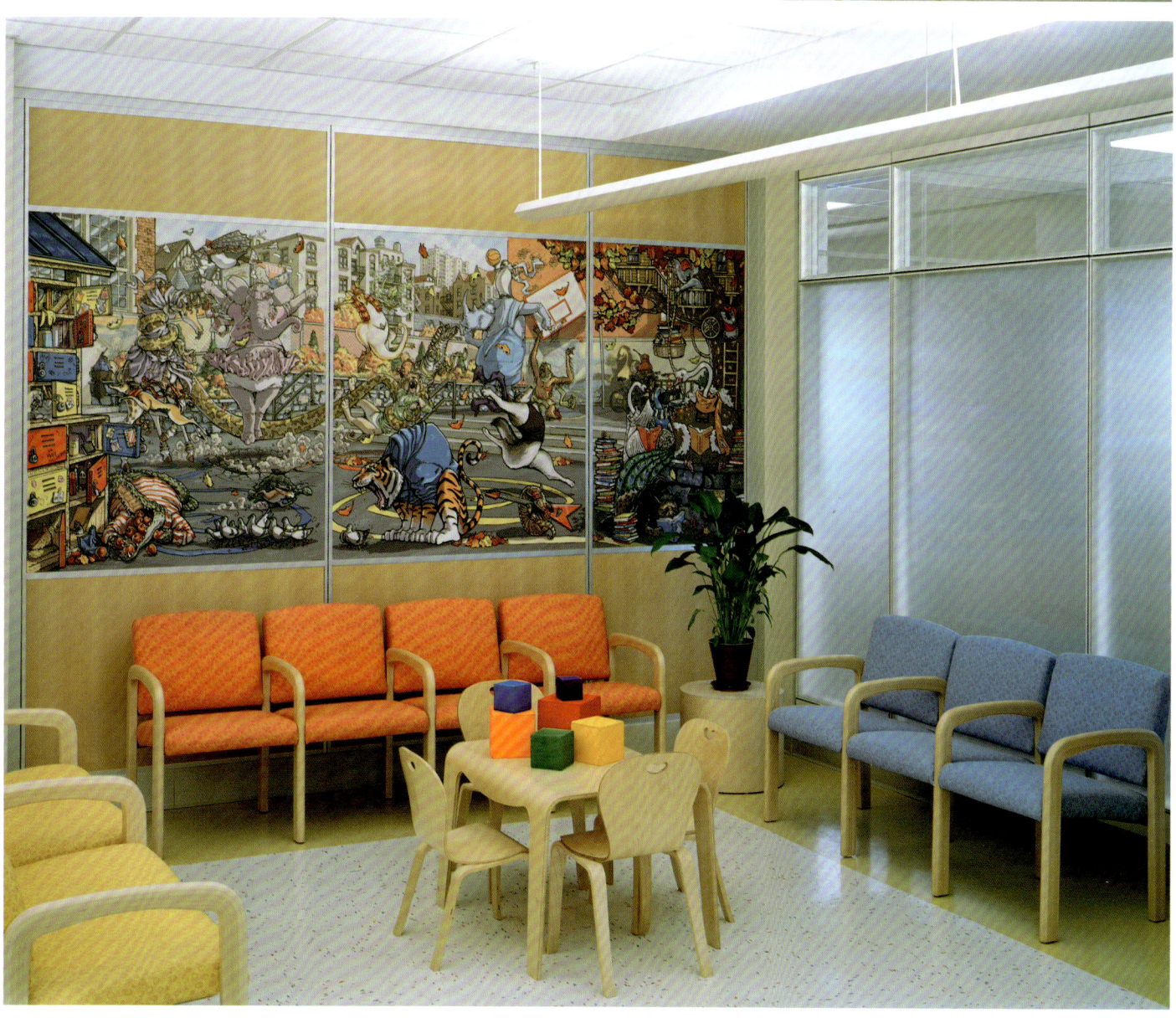

Pinearq. S.L

Quirón Hospital

Barcelona, Spain

Photographs: Fernando Guerra

The Quirón Hospital is located in Barcelona's Gracia district, next to the Pere Virgili Medical Park and with a direct connection with the Ronda de Dalt (the periphery road to the north of the city). The site has a floor surface area of 6,937 sqm (74,669 sqft) and is situated on the Alfonso Comín square. The building includes a ground floor, 6 floors above grade and 7 below.

The volumes have been designed around the site's topography, whose primary characteristic is the pronounced north-south slope that creates a 16 m (52 ft) level change. The building also responds to a very specific urban environment (the Alfonso Comín is a major circulation node) and a complex and specific functional hospital program.

The volumes of the upper floors of the building are configured in an L-shape in order to situate the six ward units. The floors located between the access to the hall and the ward levels are intended for external consultations and special examinations, intensive care and outpatient care. The morphology of these floors does not respond directly to the needs of the functional plan, but instead is intended to relate with the topography and morphology of the site.

The ground floor fulfills entrance hall functions and contains the public access points for both pedestrians and vehicles. This floor relates with the square outside and the landscaped area, which has been created in the northeastern corner of the site. It therefore accommodates all of the hospital building's more public functions, such as the cafeteria, the conference room, the admissions area and lastly a large shopping area which can function independently of the hospital.

The two floors immediately below the hall accommodate the emergency department, radiology, operating theatres, obstetrics, recovery, sterilization and laboratories. Due to the slope of the plot and its topography, and to the way in which the courtyards connect, these floors have direct access from the street at different levels. Beneath here is the floor for general services and the parking.

The hospital's three main entrances, the public, emergency and goods entrances, have been installed independently of each other at the lower part of the site.

Client:
Grupo Hospitalario Quirón, S.A.
Surface area:
57,775 sqm (621,880 sqft)
Start date:
2004
Finish date:
2007
Project team:
Albert de Pineda Álvarez, Manuel Brullet Tenas
Collaborators:
Xavier Llambrich, Alfonso de Luna, Marc Gomà, Juan García, Gerardo Solera, , Silvia Salueña, Albert Vitaller, Patricio Martinez, Pau Calleja
Contractor:
Dragados - Vías
Cost:
€ 49,894,838

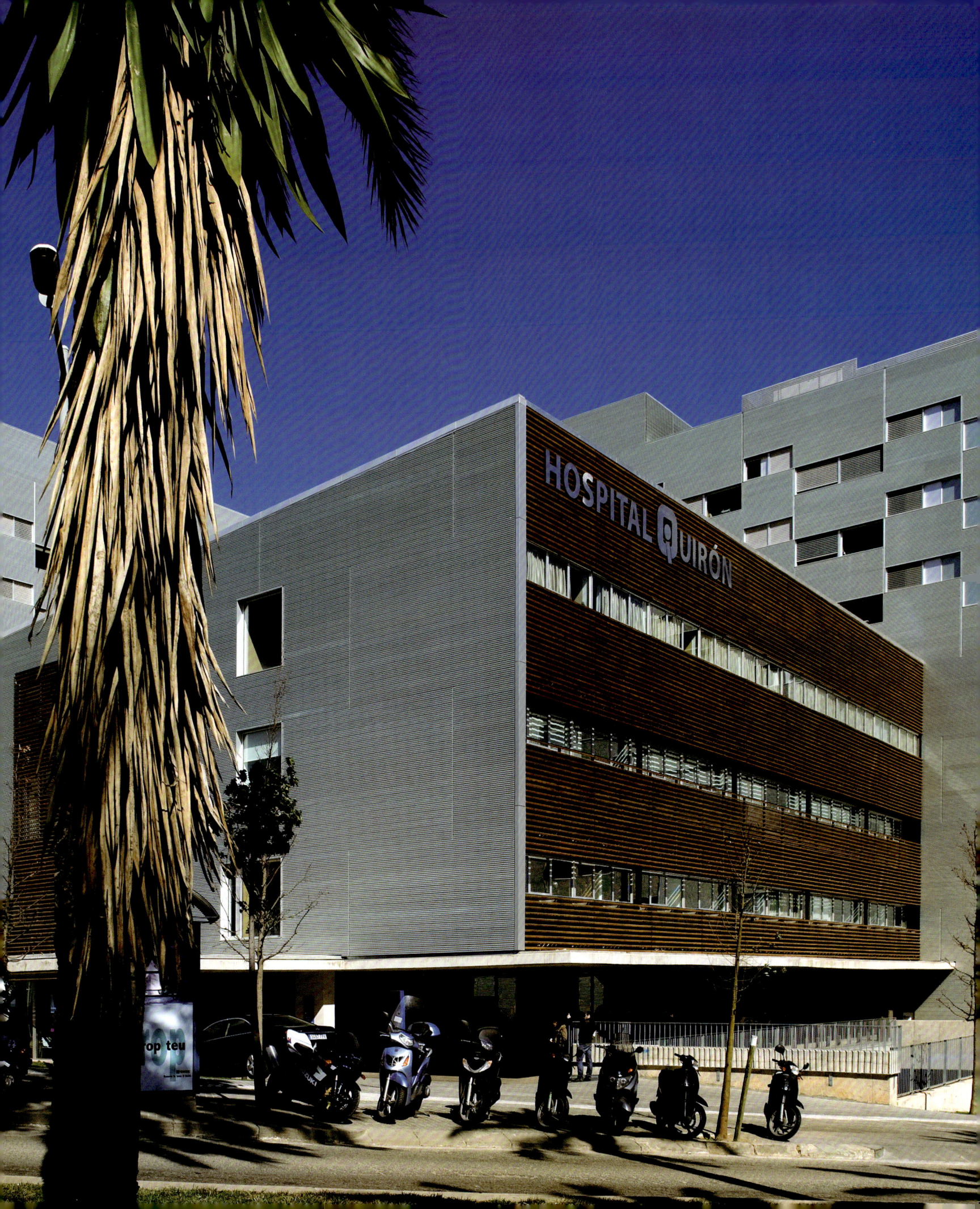

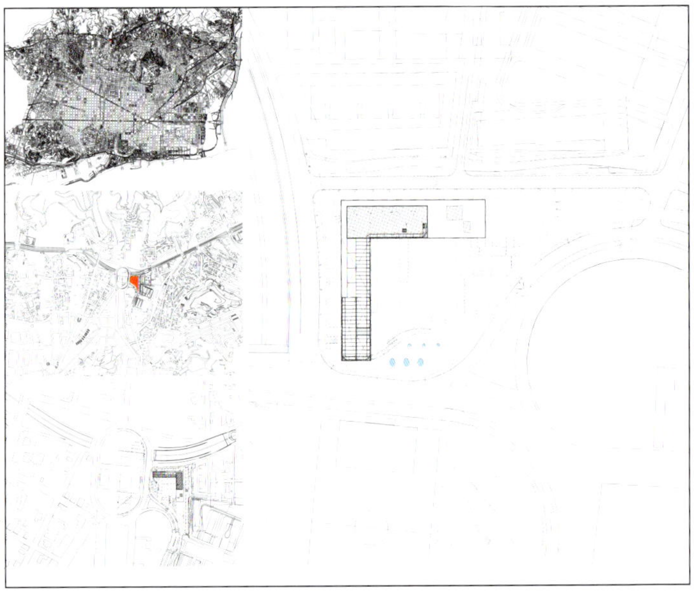

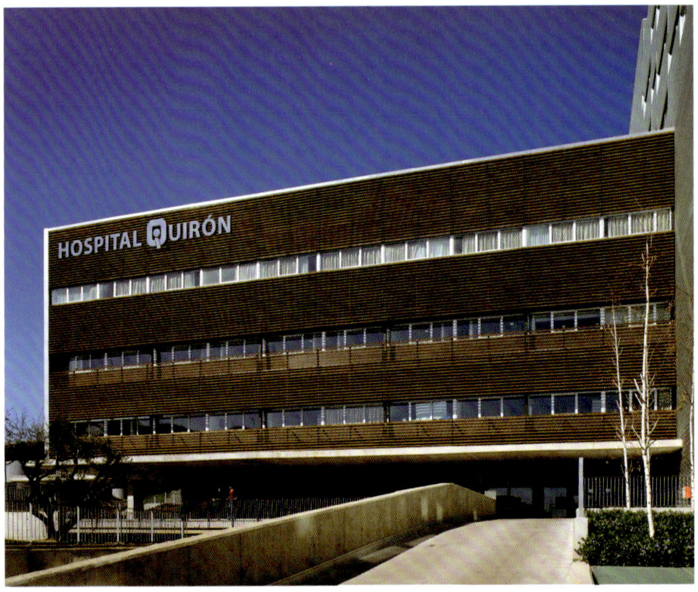
HOSPITAL QUIRÓN

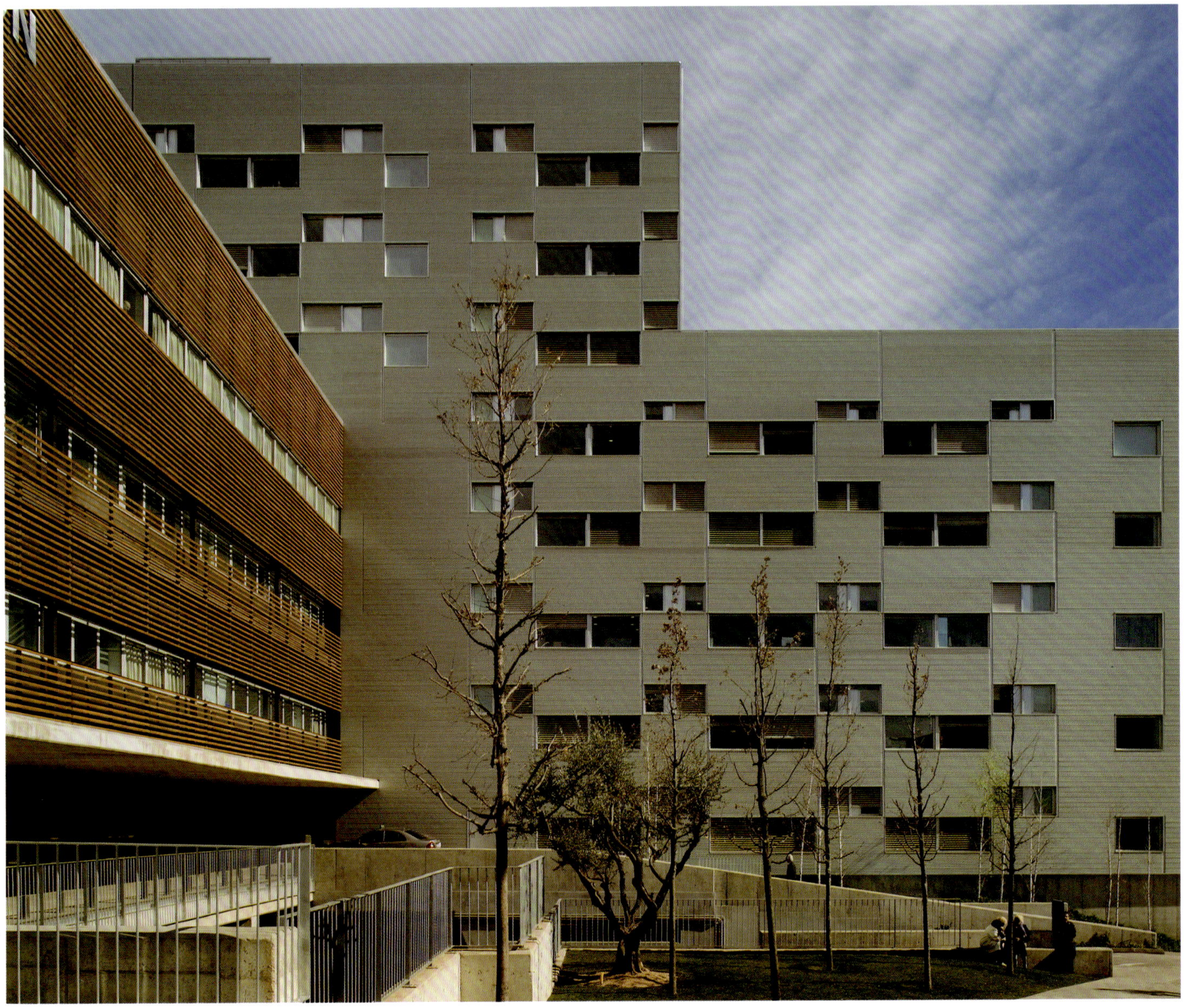

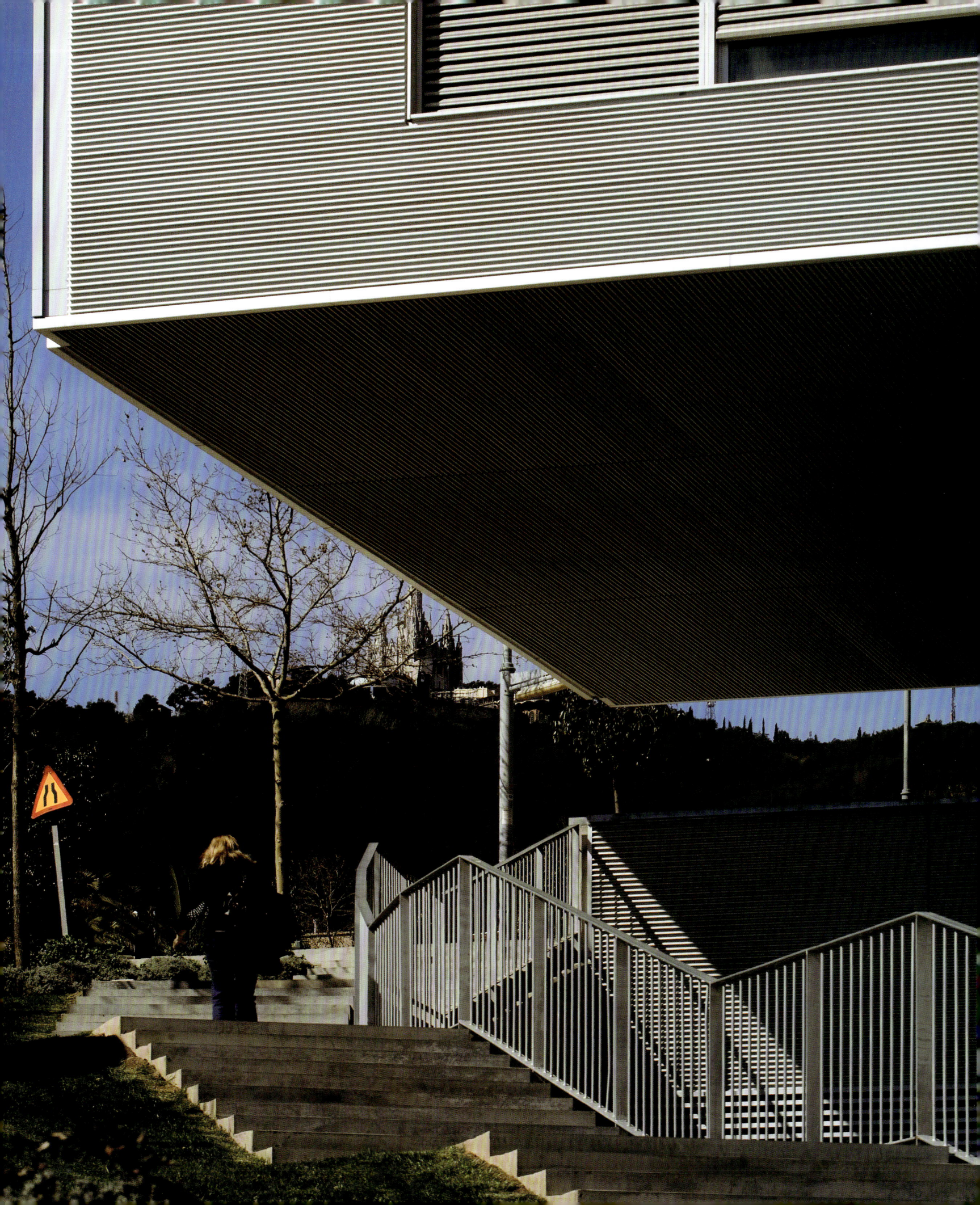

96

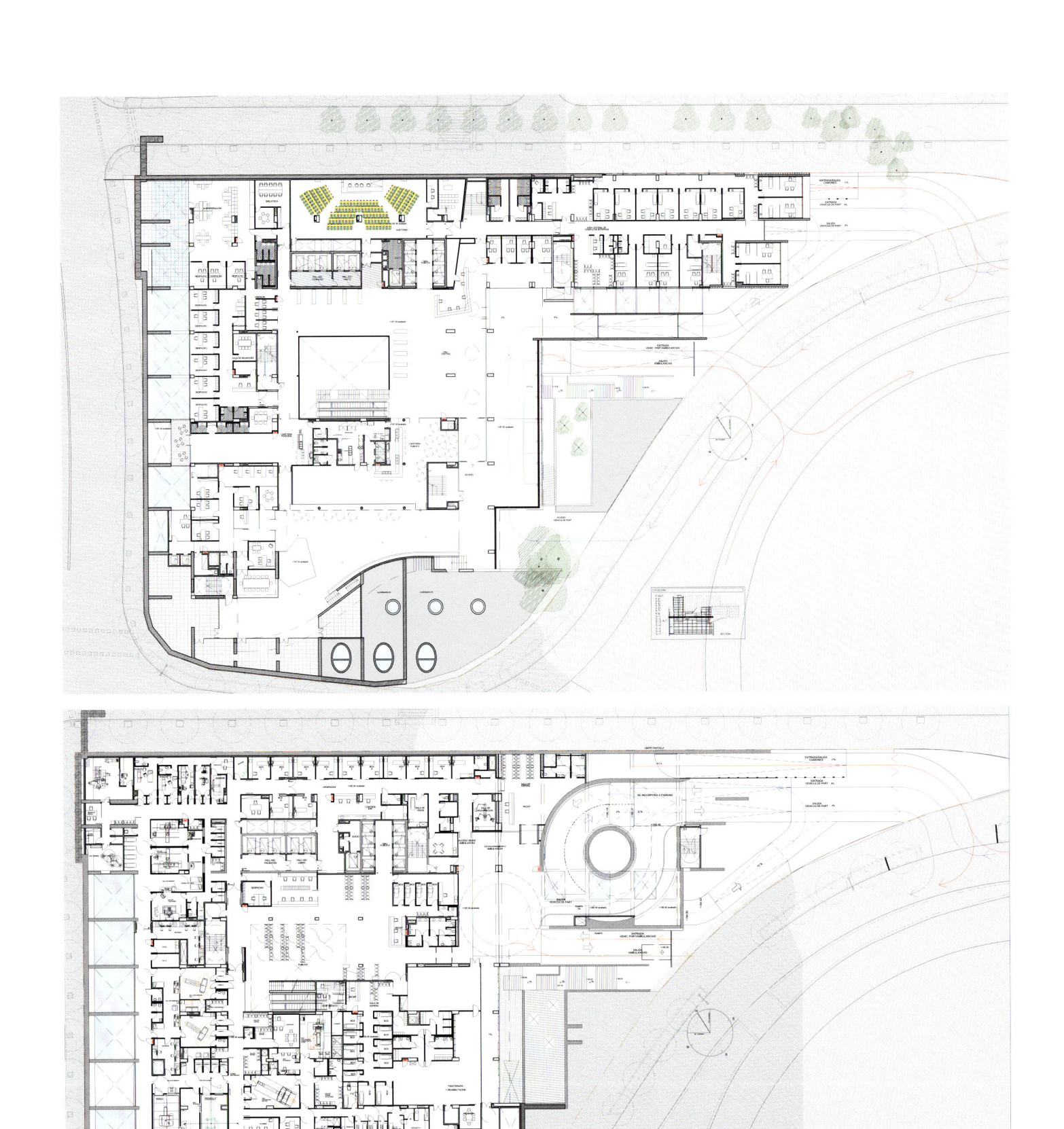

97

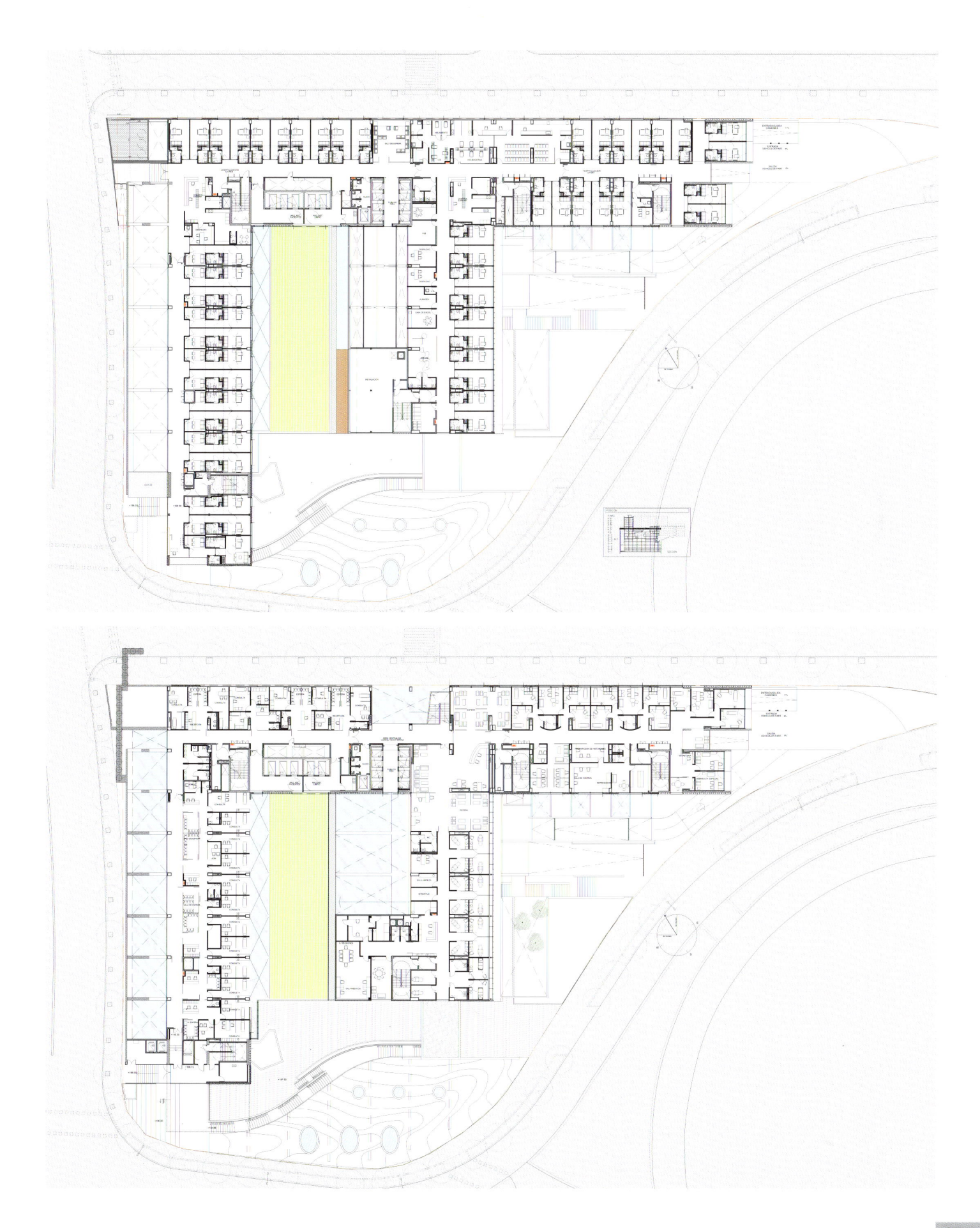

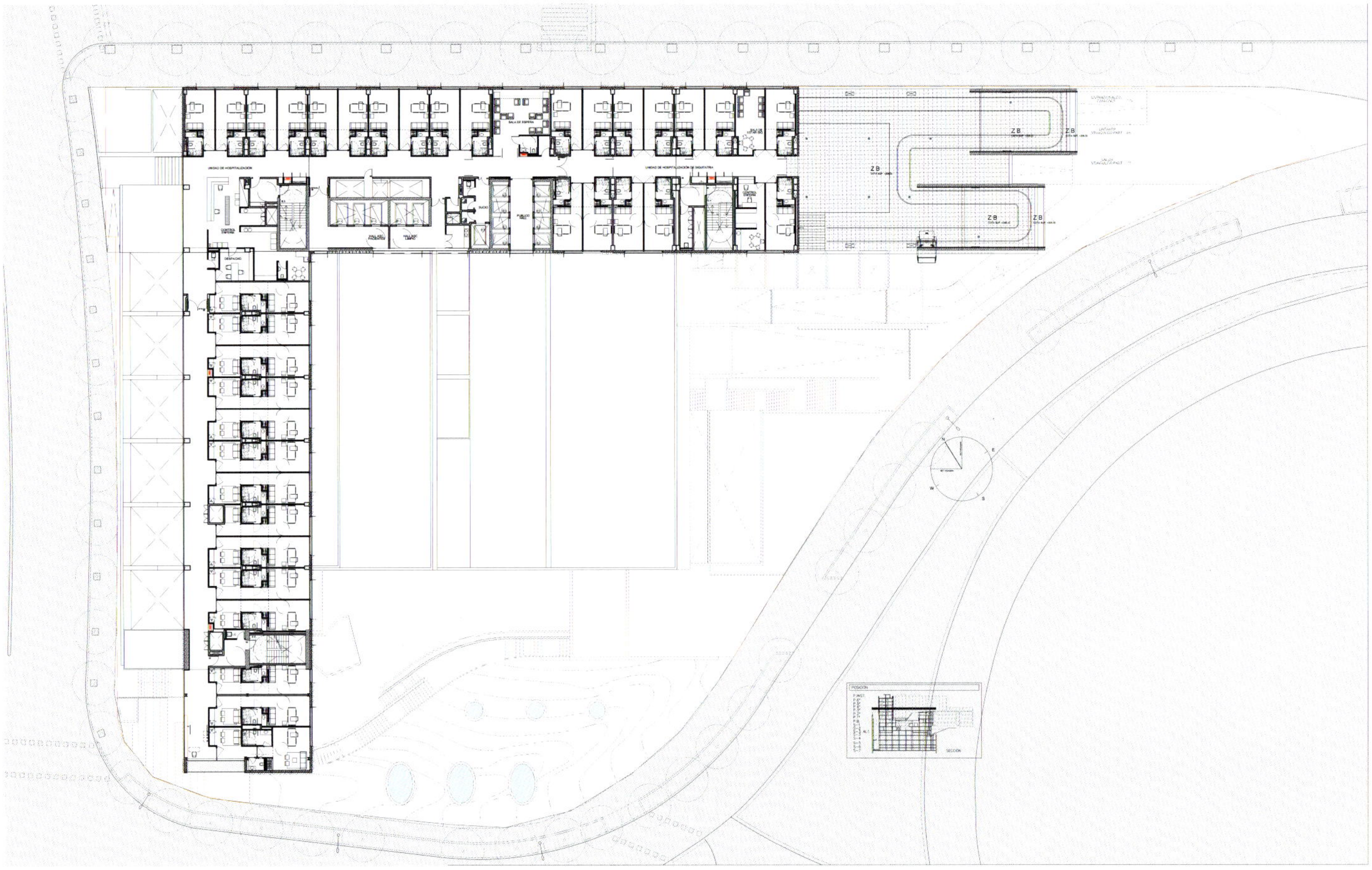

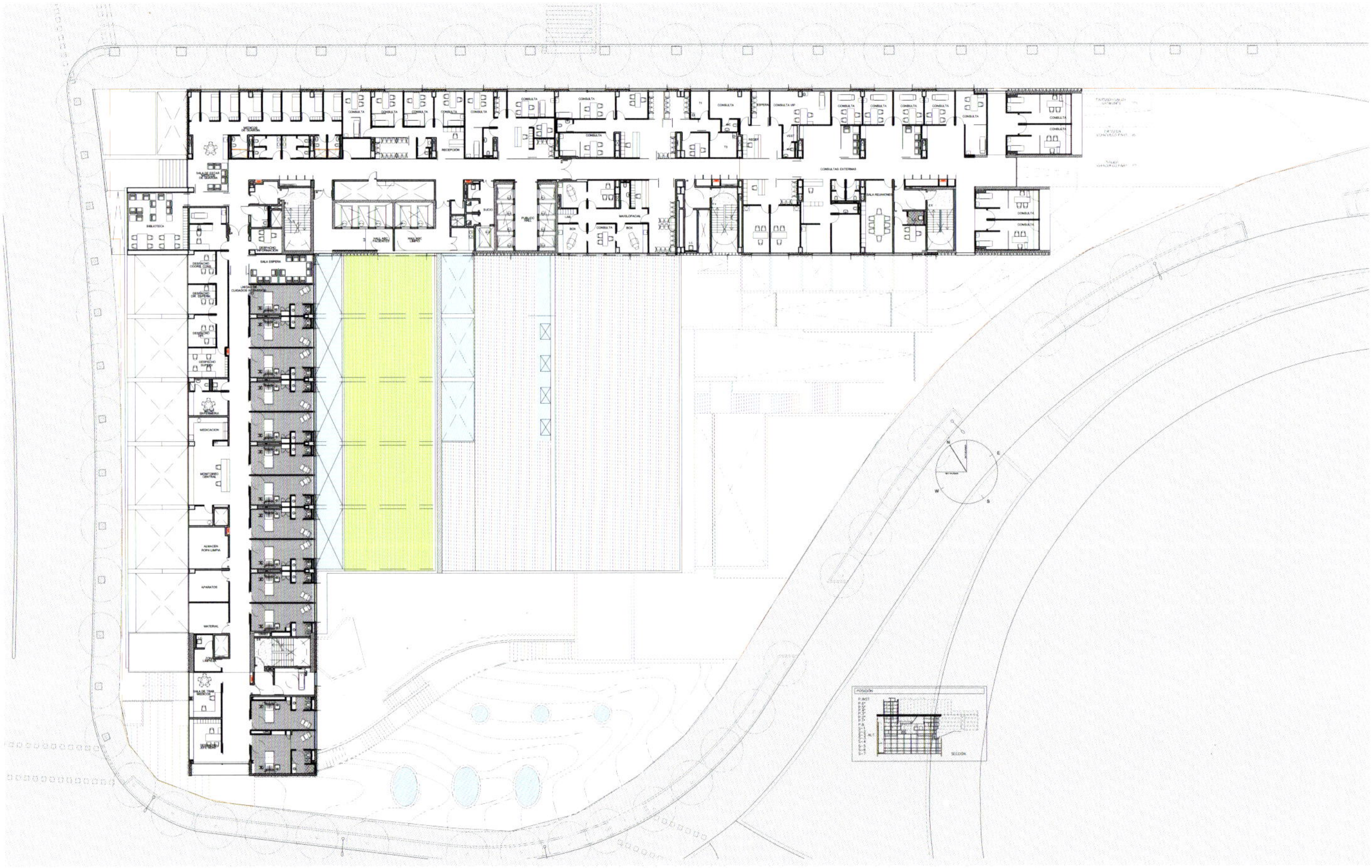

99

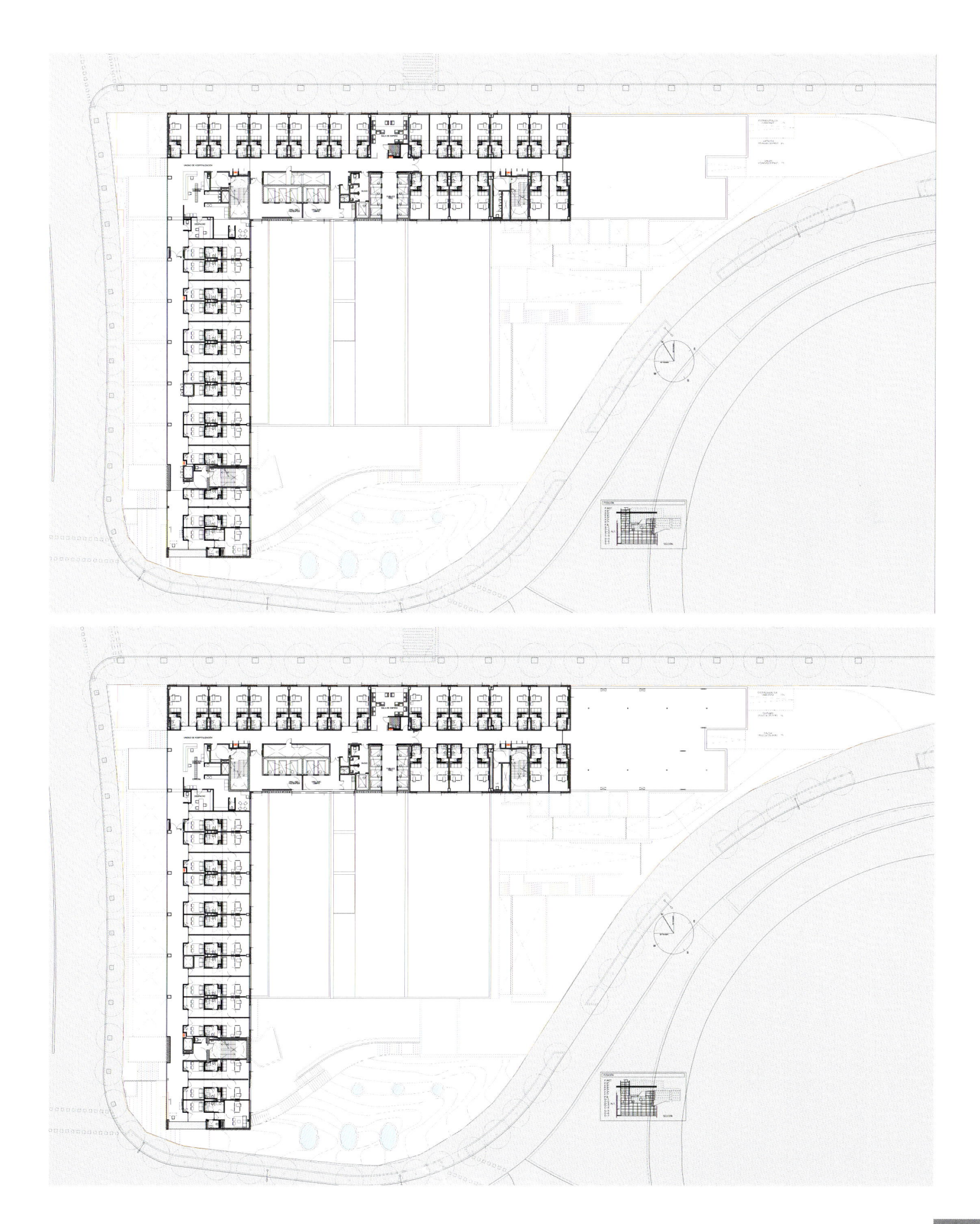

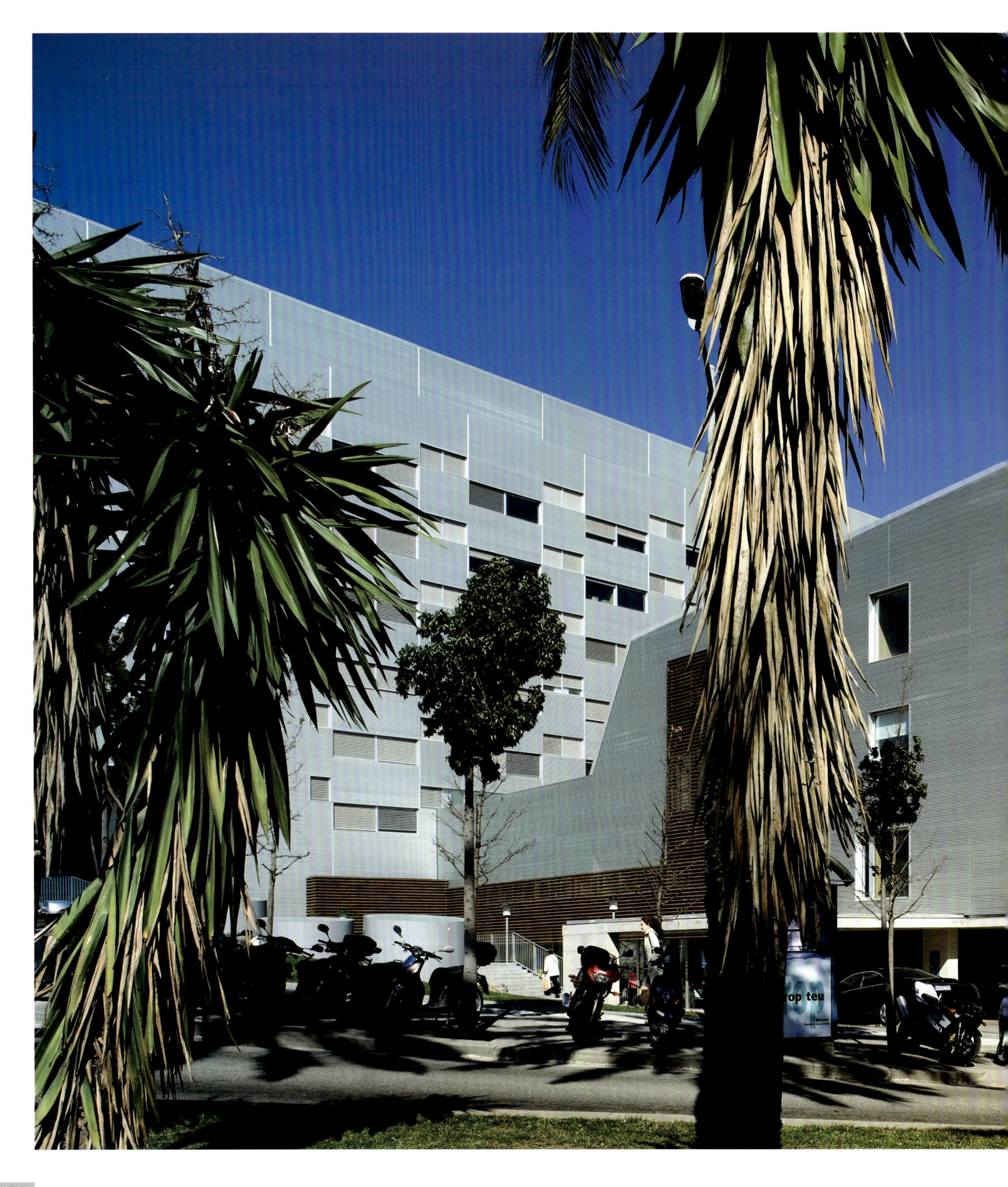

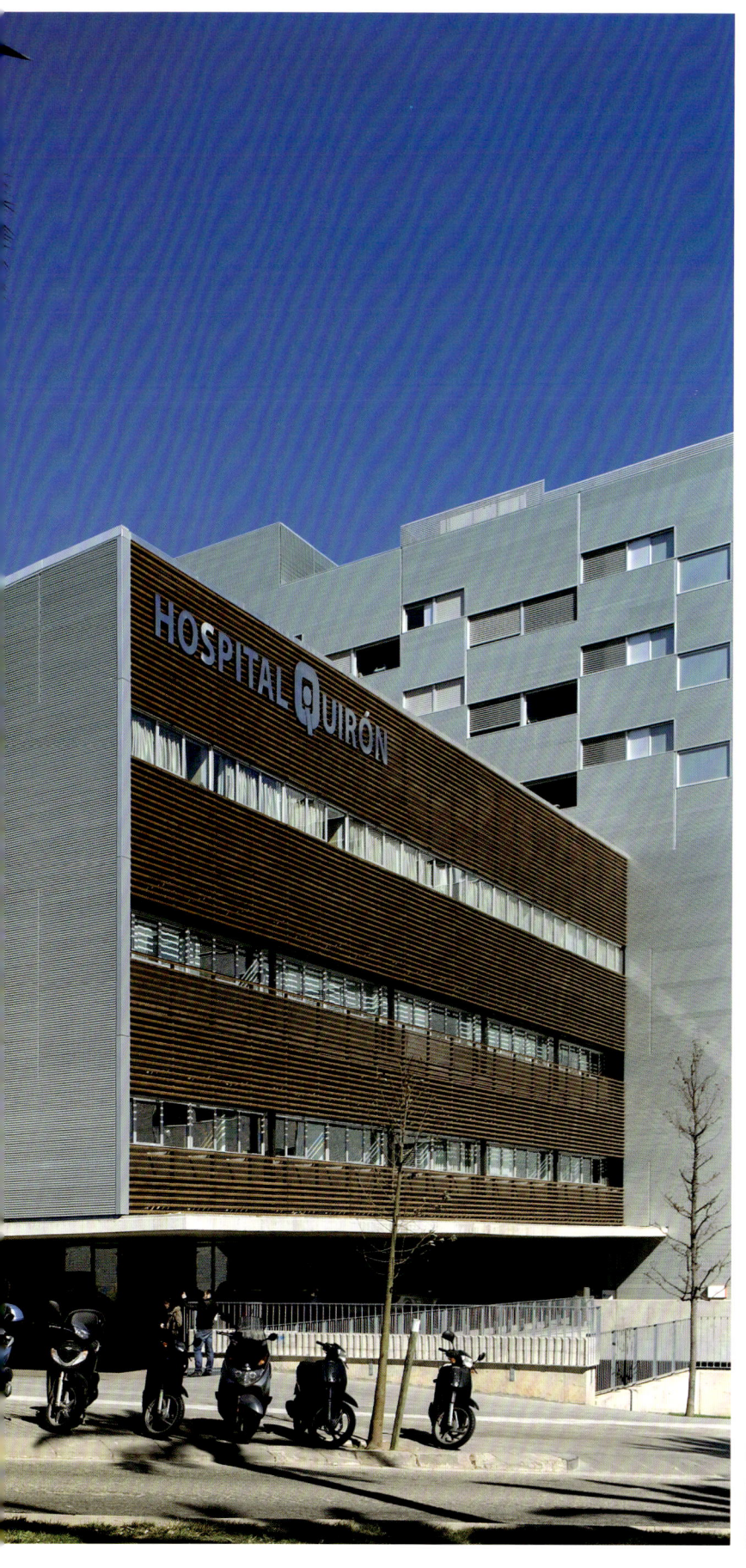

The volumes have been designed around the site's topography, whose primary characteristic is the pronounced north-south slope that creates a 16 m (52 ft) level change. The building also responds to a very specific urban environment (the Alfonso Comín is a major circulation node) and a complex and specific functional hospital program.

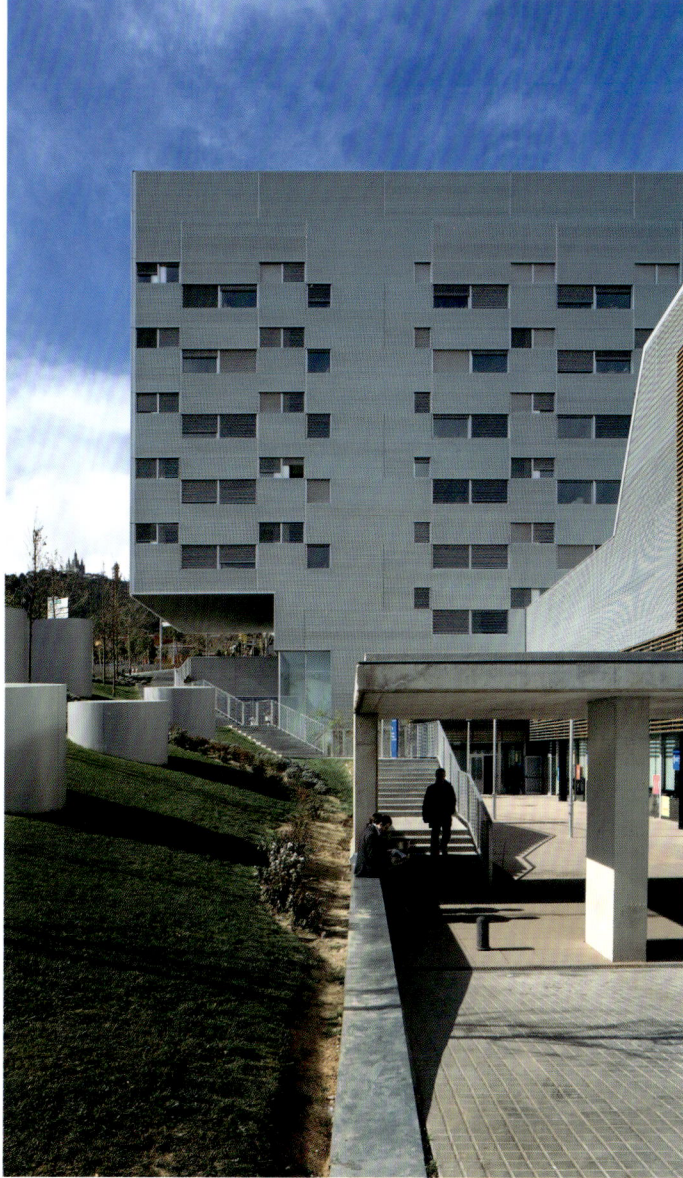

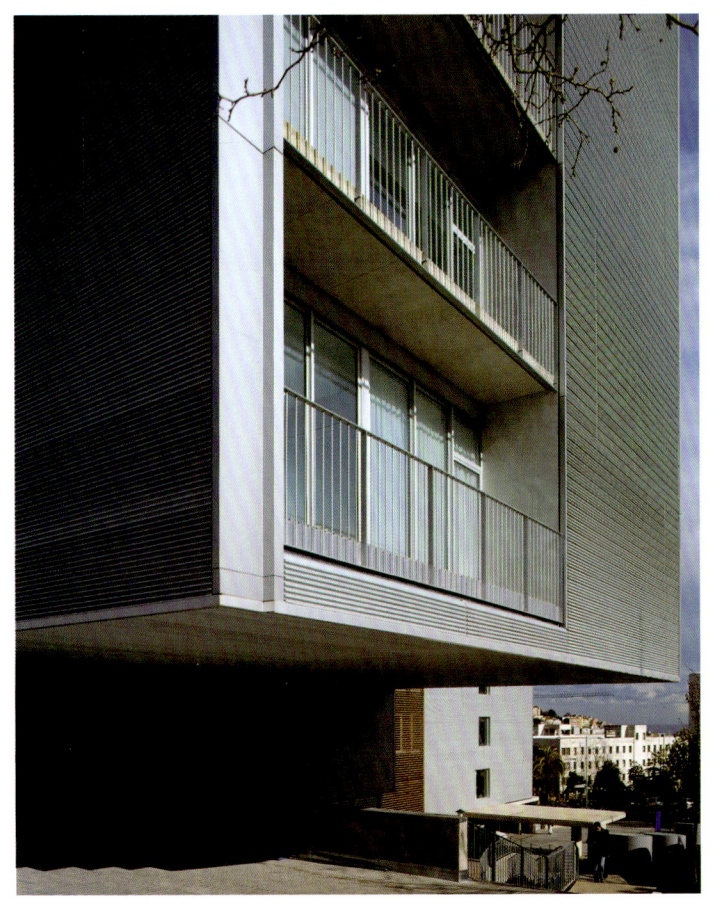

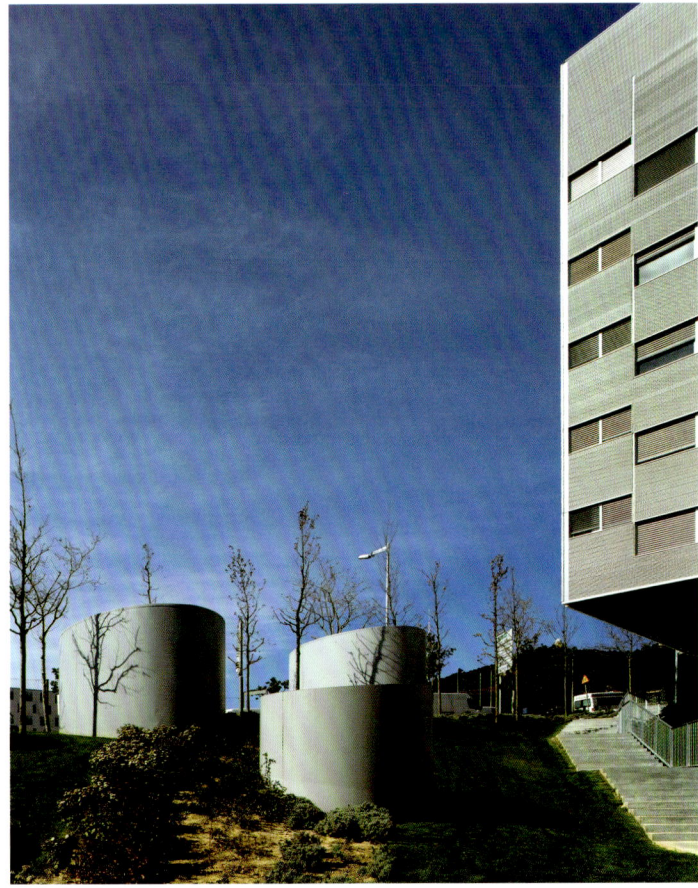

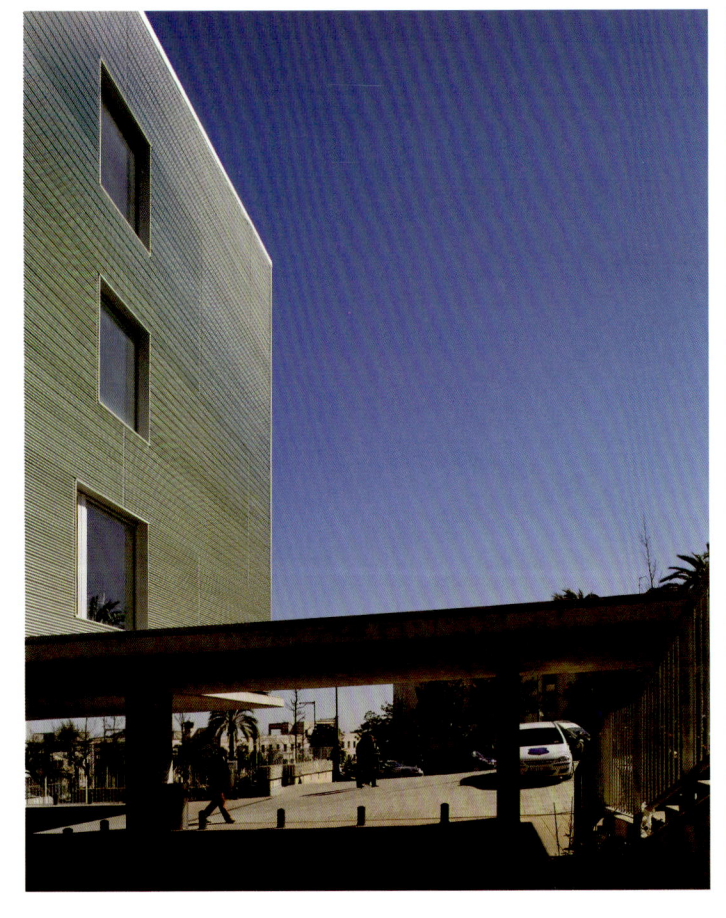

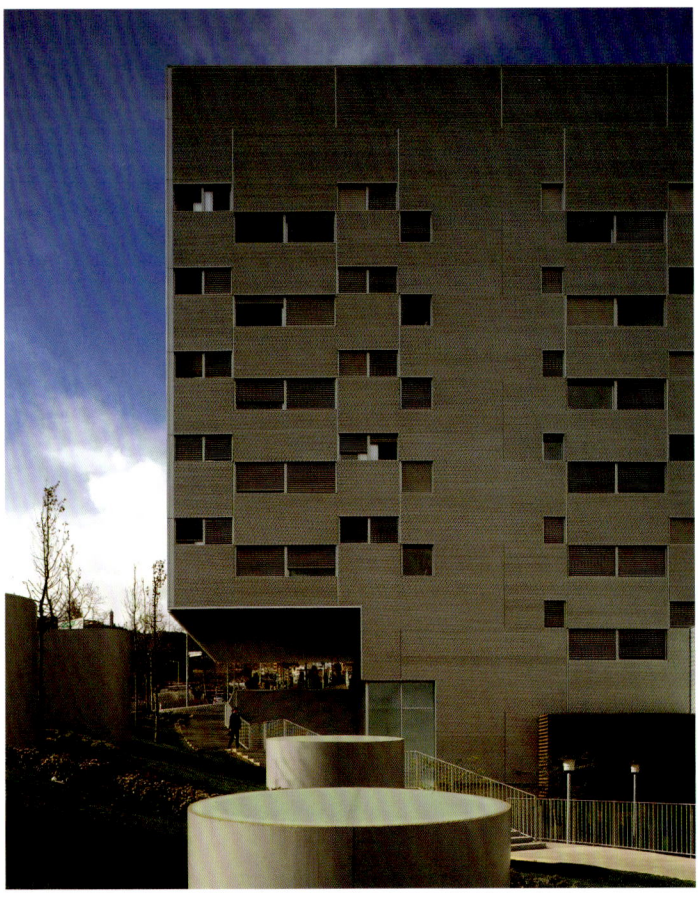

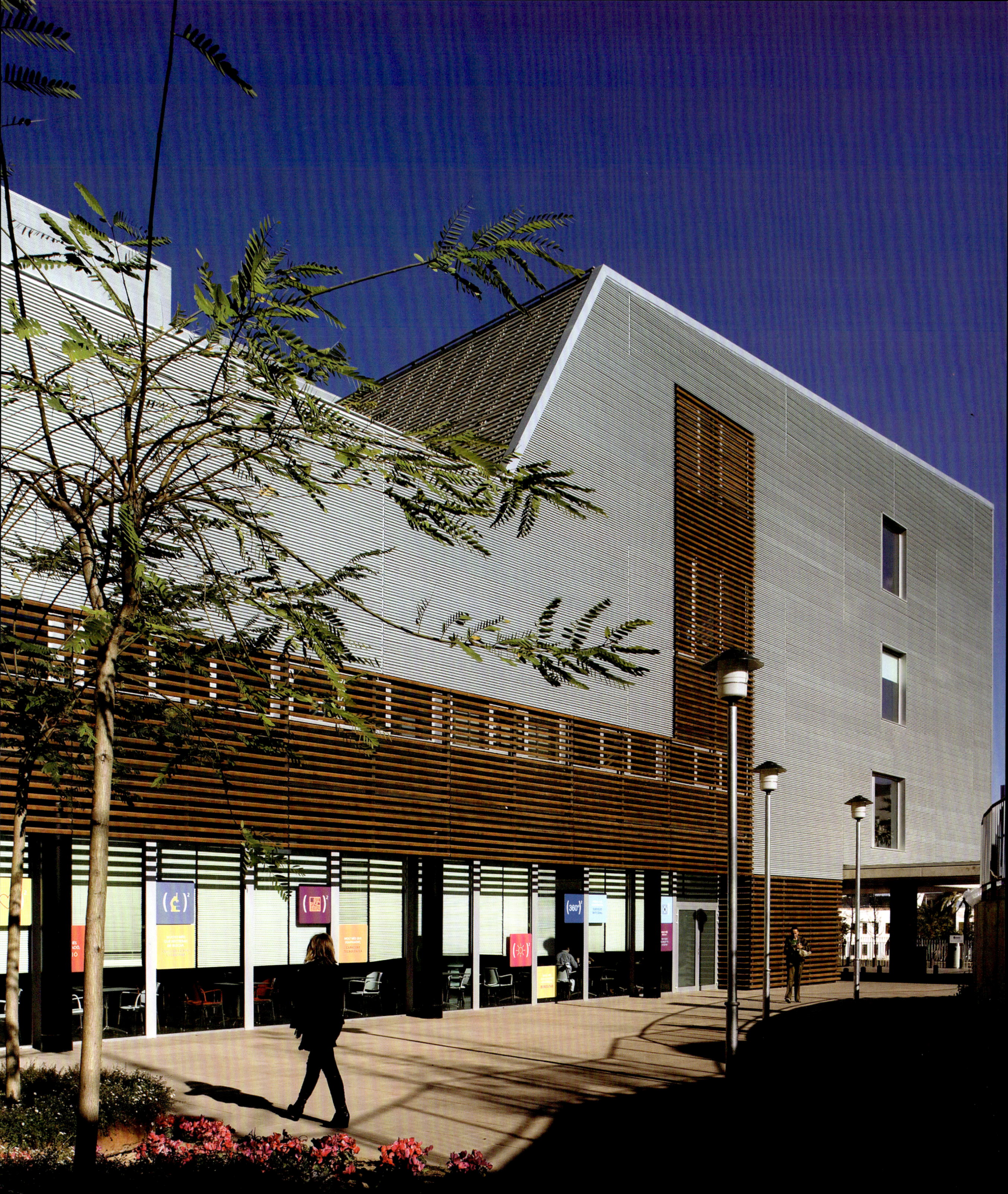

104

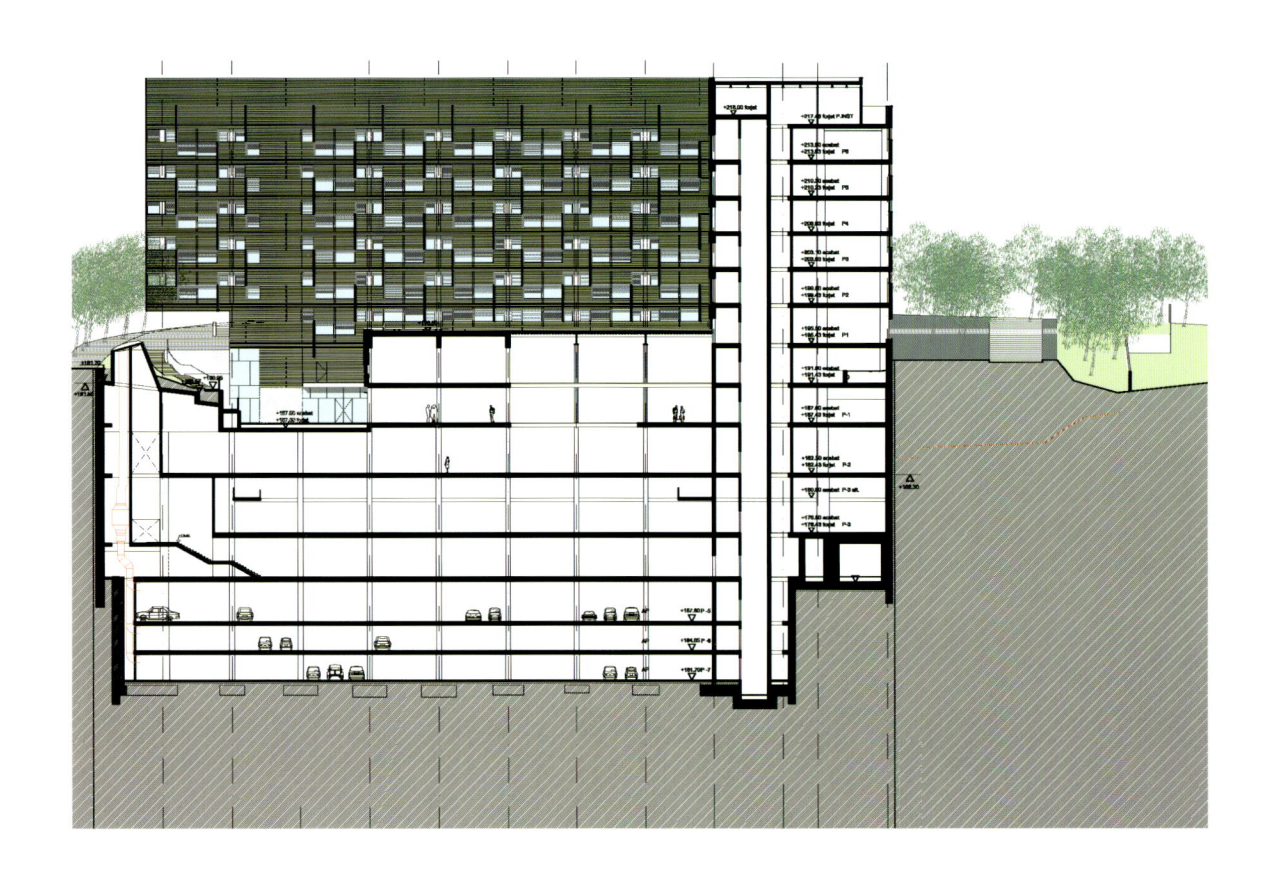

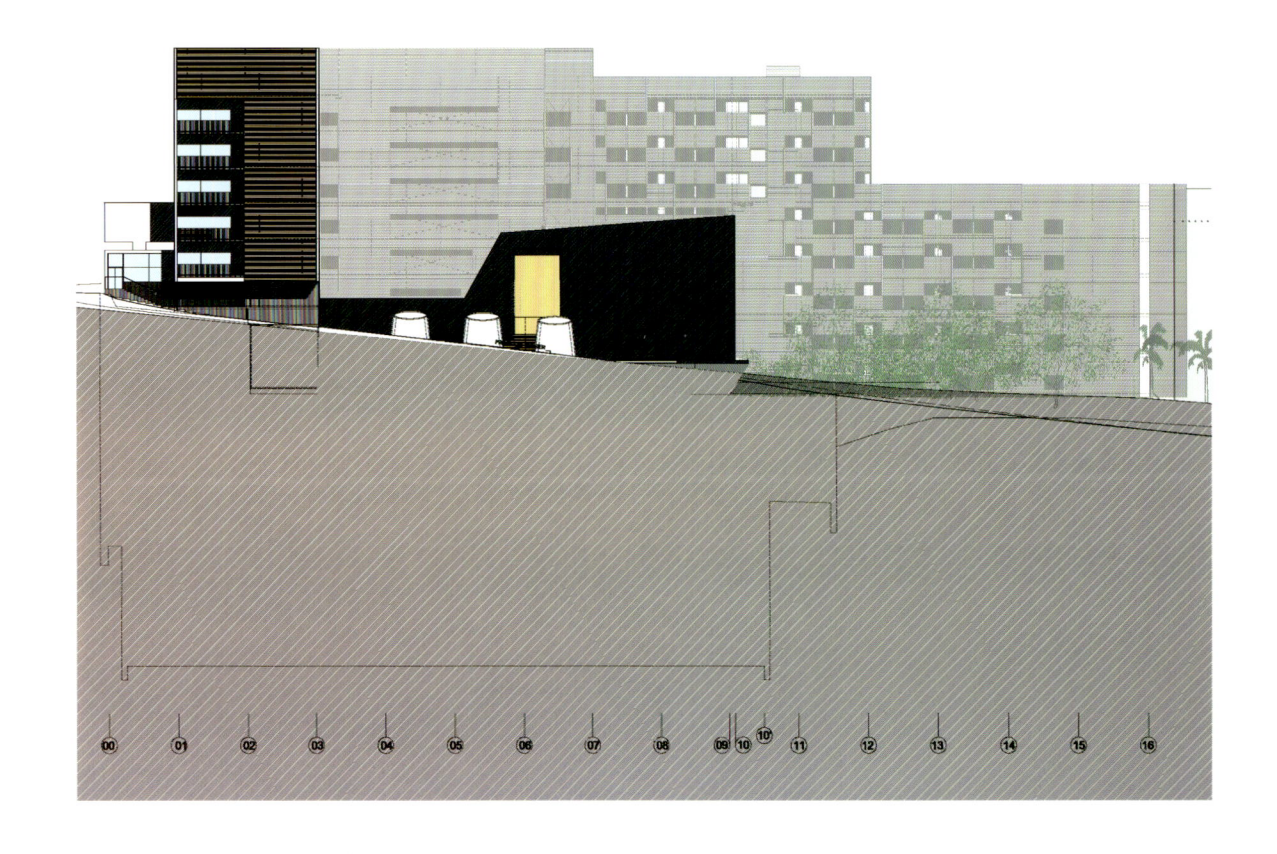

105

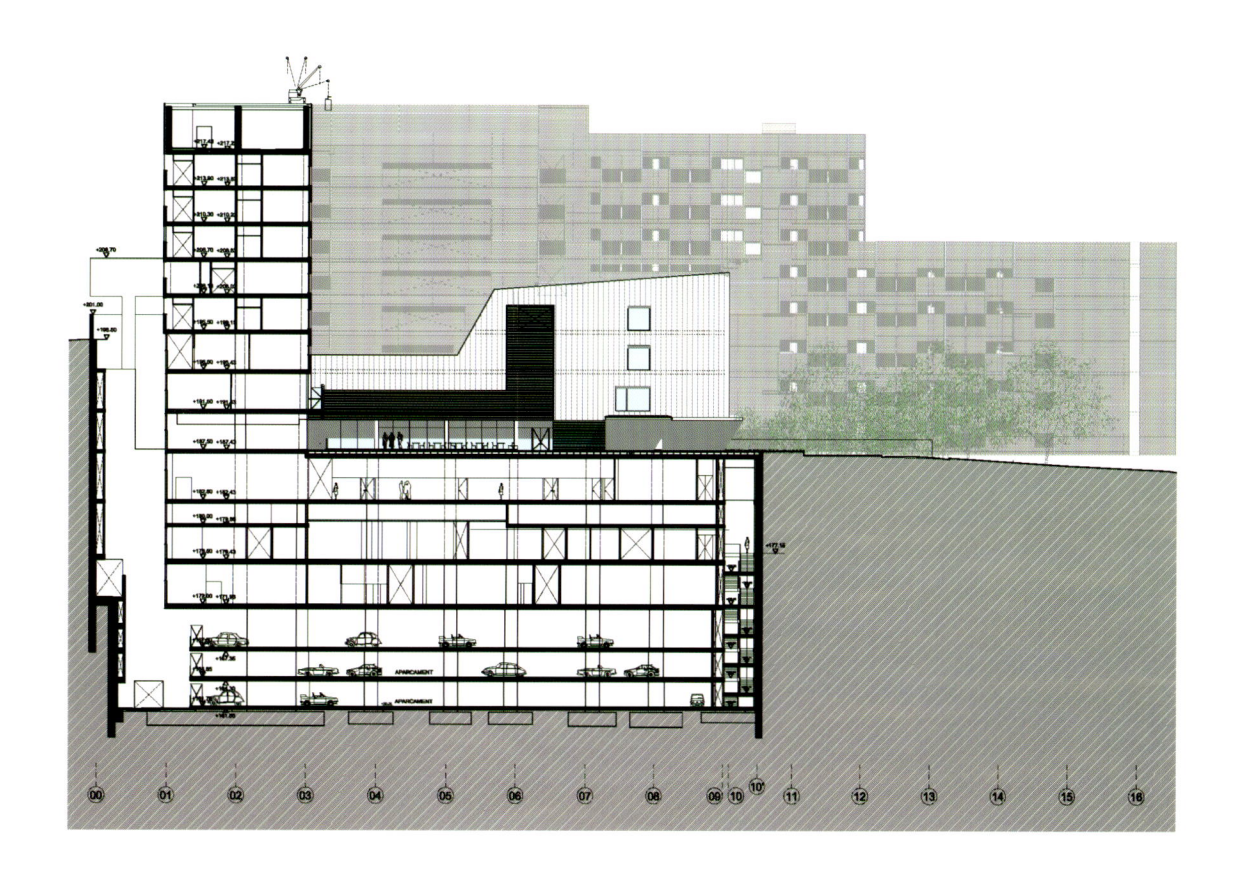

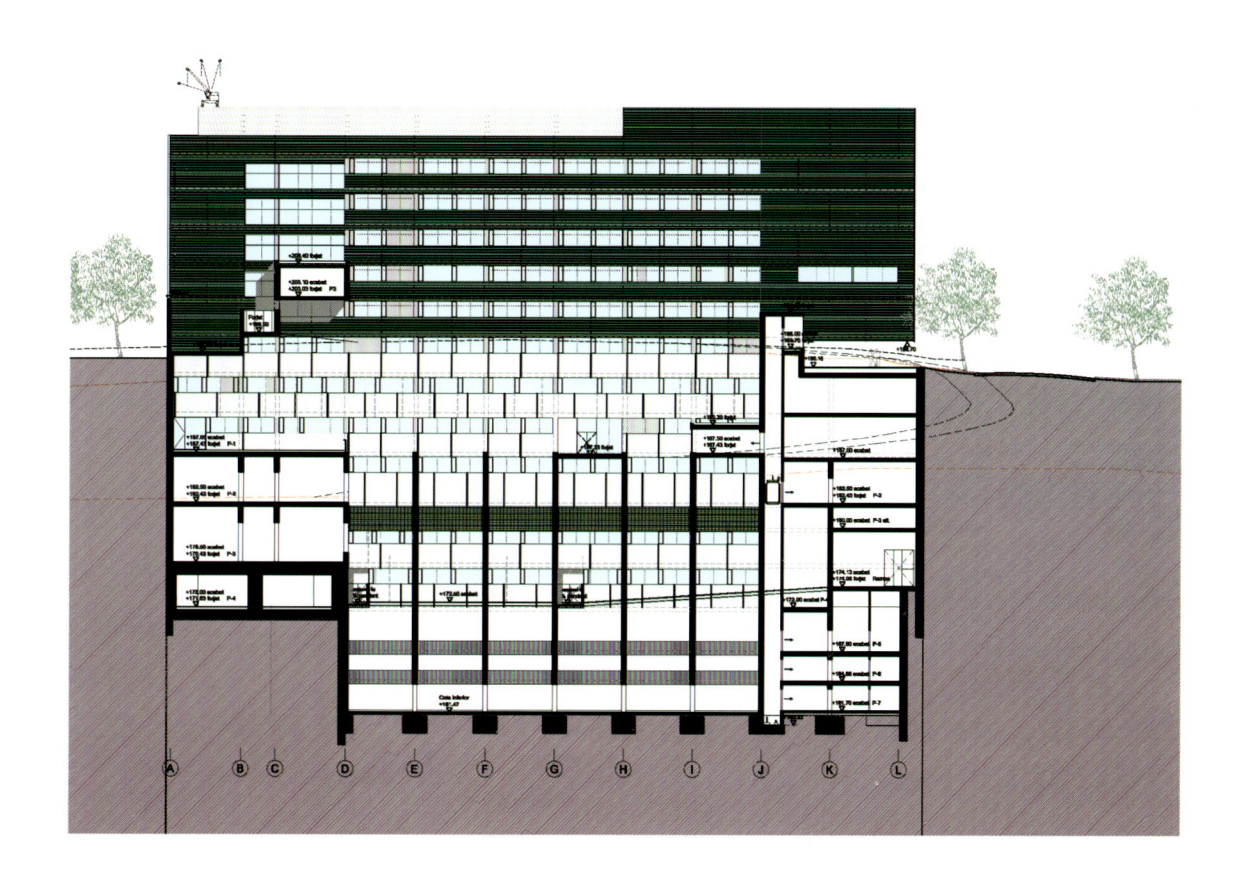

106

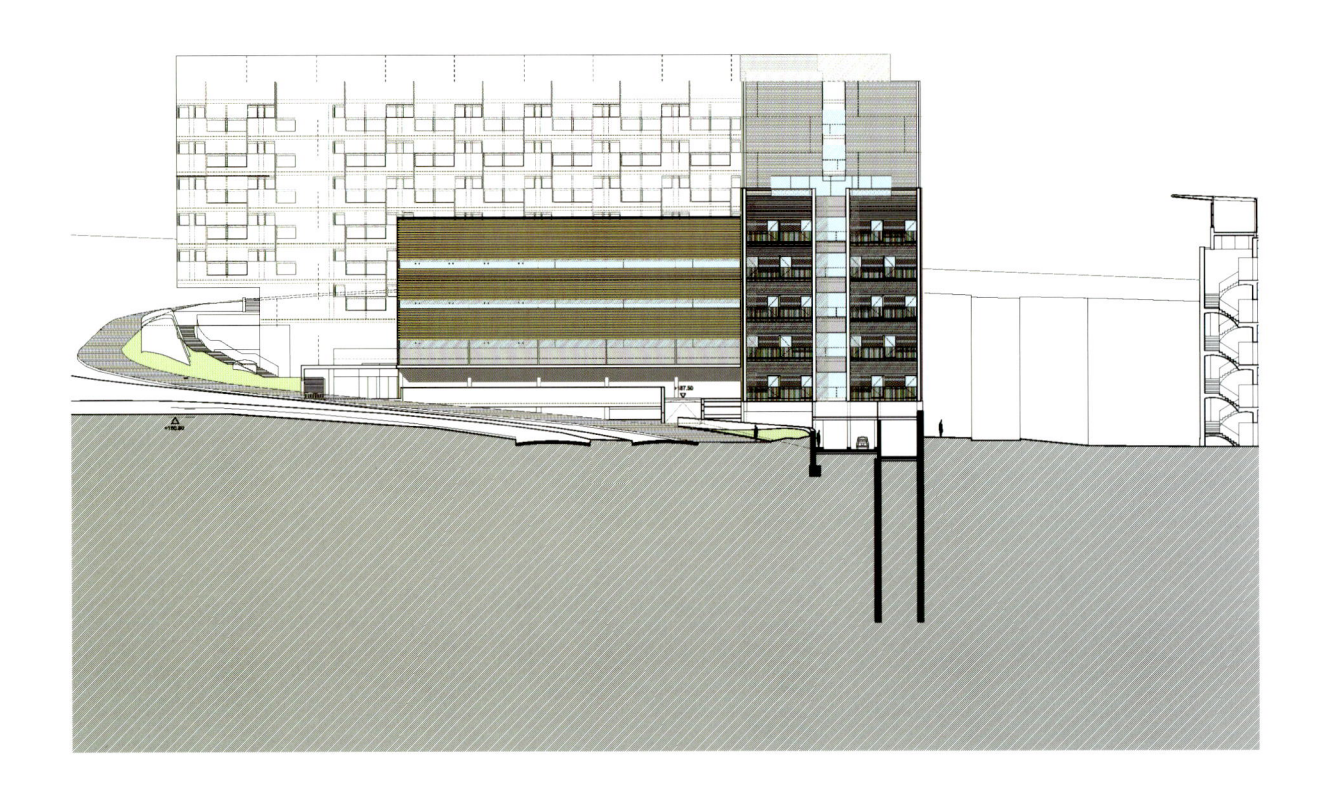

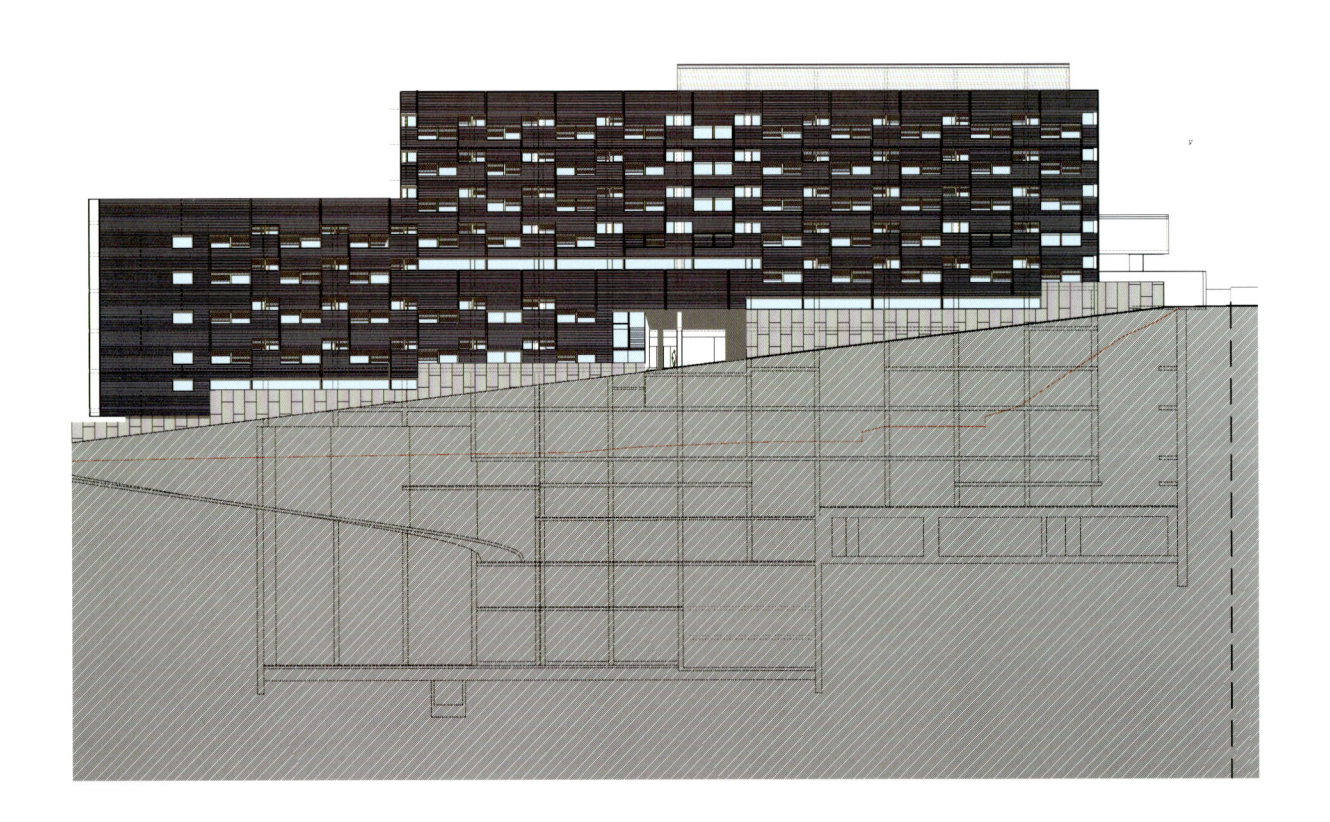

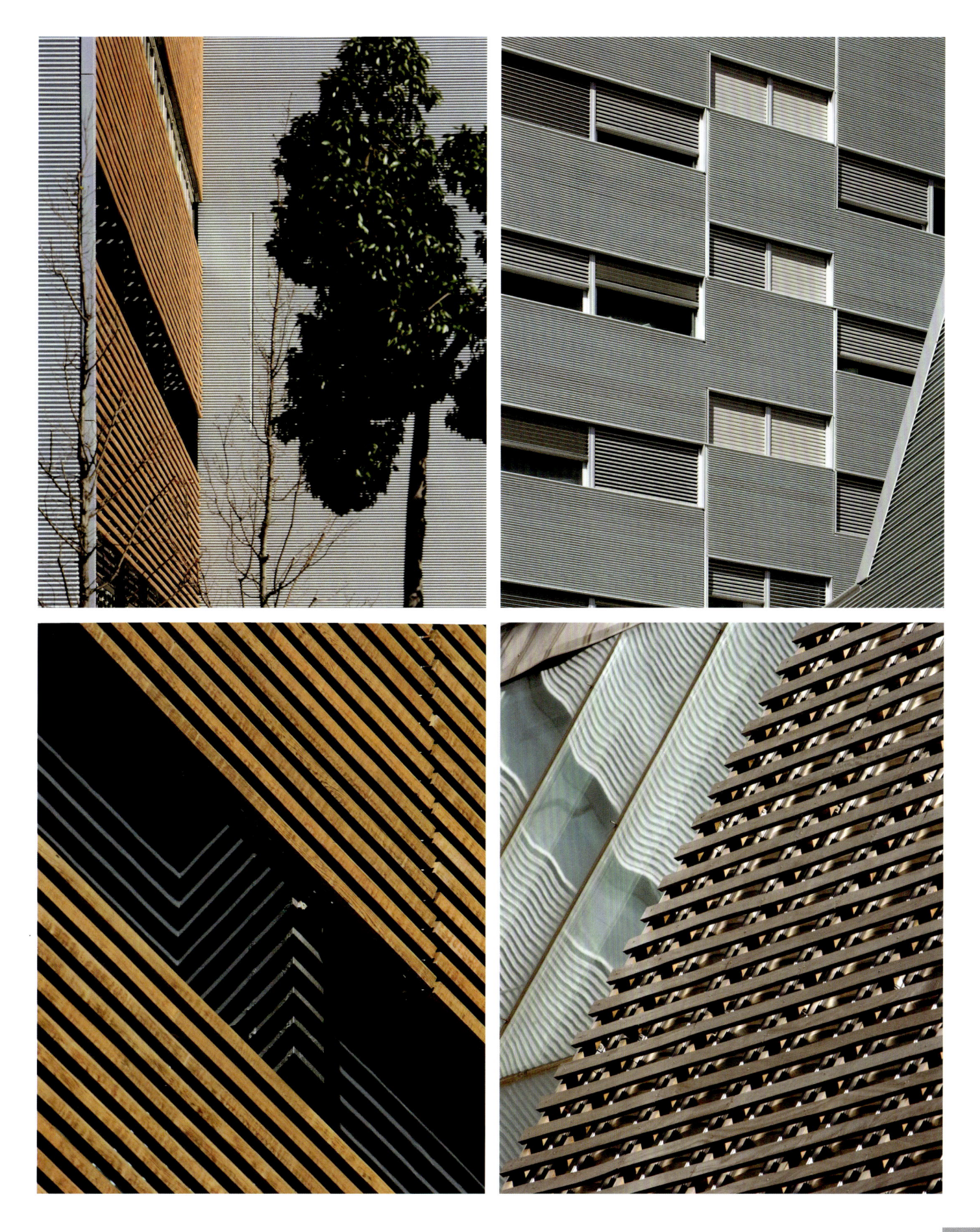

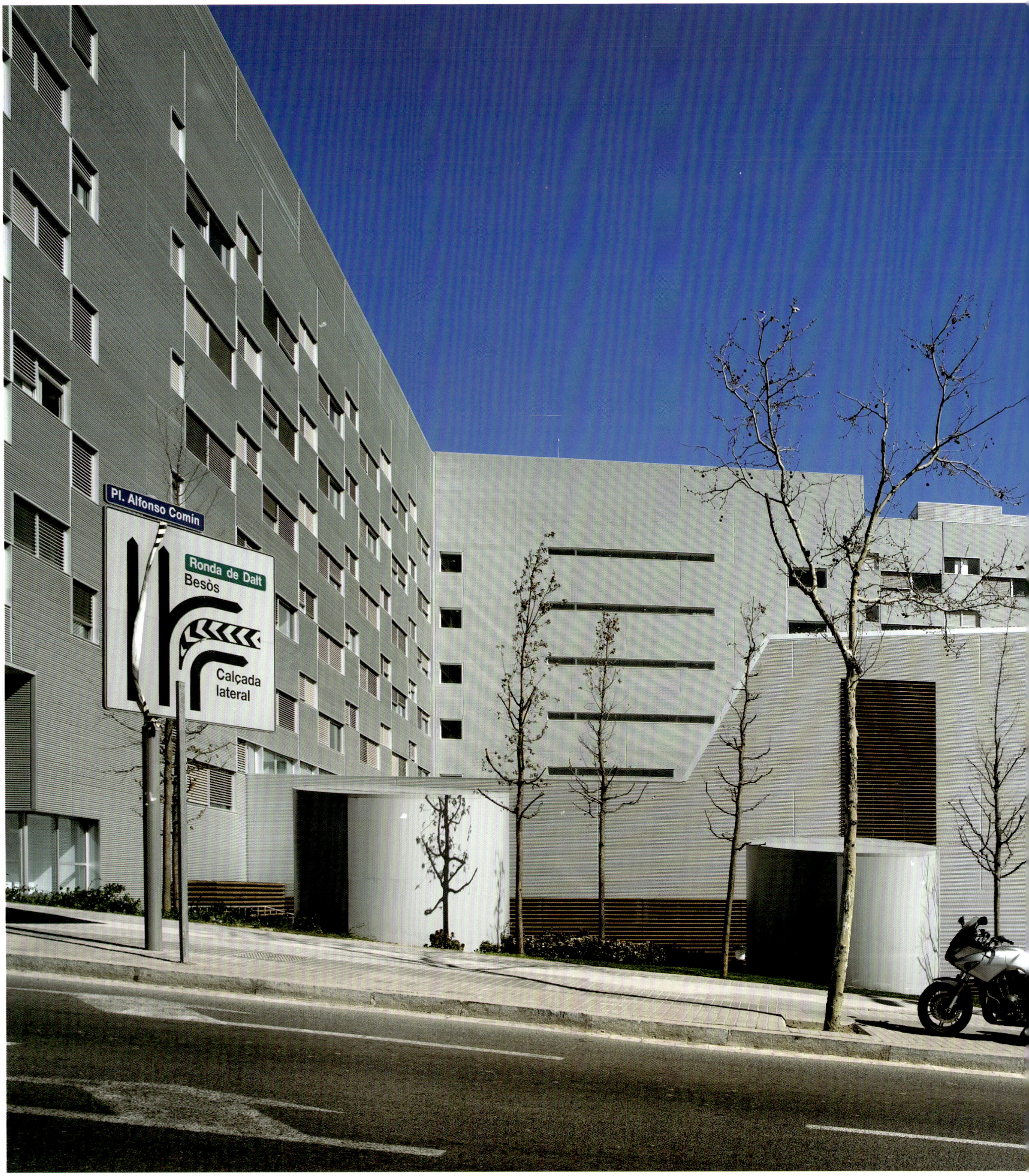
Pl. Alfonso Comín
Ronda de Dalt
Besòs
Calçada
lateral

109

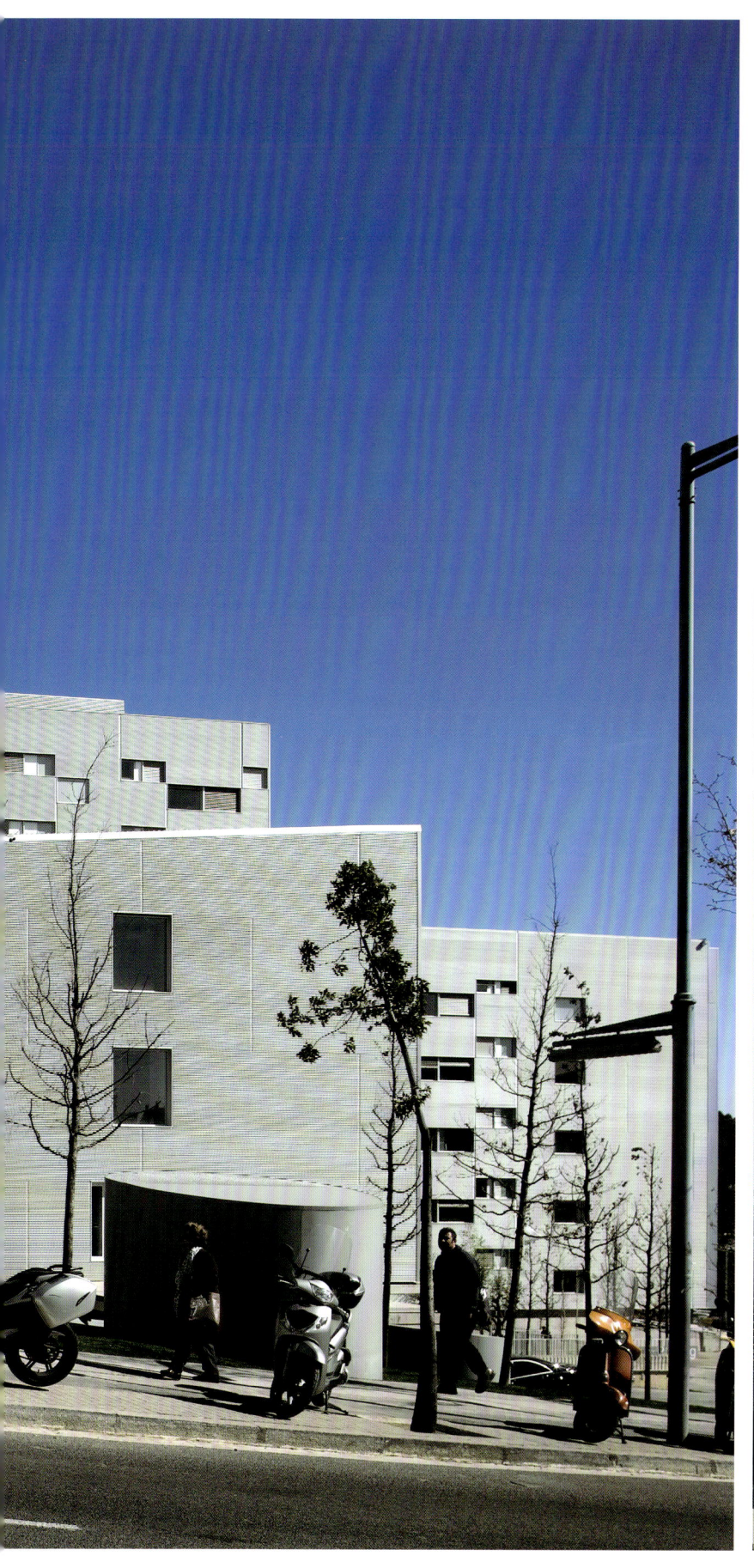

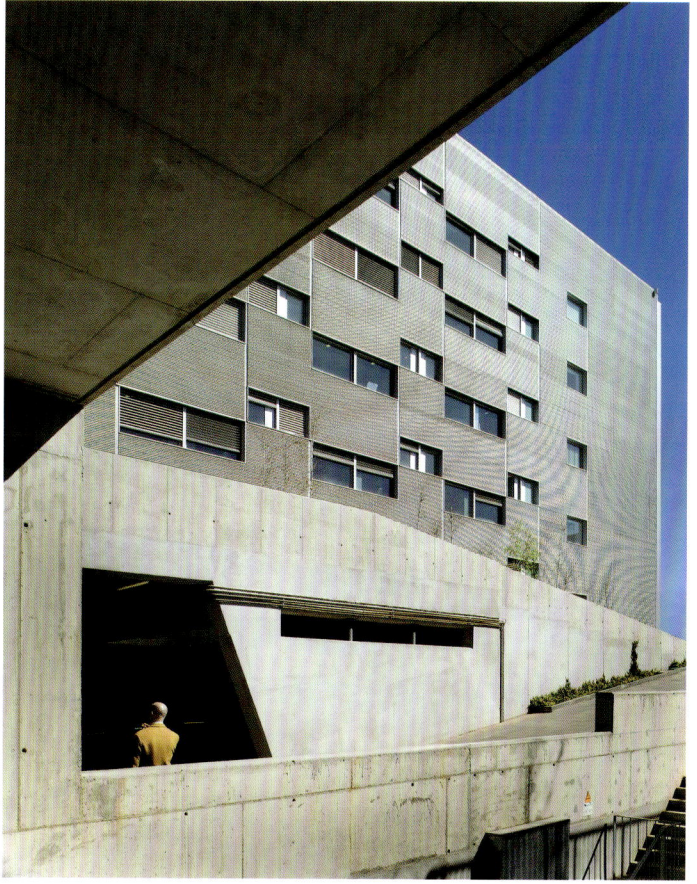

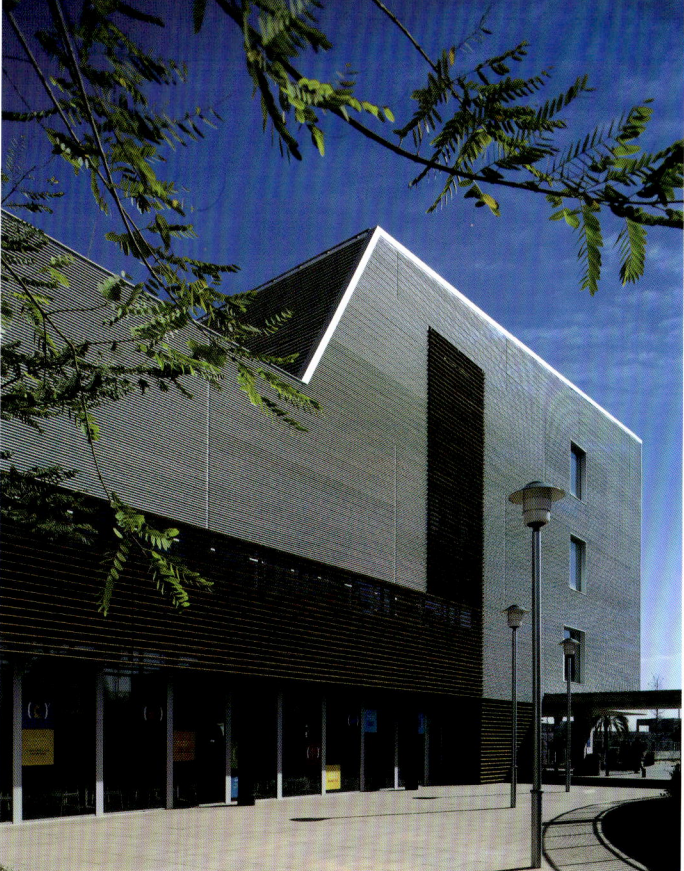

Corea, Quijano, Codina.
Secretaria Salud Pública Rosario

Clemente Alvarez Emergency Hospital

Rosario, Argentina

Photographs: *Gustavo Frittegotto, Sebastián Martínez*

The project for the new Clemente Álvarez Emergency Hospital (HECA) forms part of the strategy of Rosario's town council to renovate its health-care network and to adapt the general system to contemporary technological standards. Having been subject to repeated modifications, the original hospital had been rendered obsolete and it was no longer capable of responding to the needs of the citizens of the metropolitan area of Greater Rosario. A new building was therefore proposed whose design was based on flexibility, in order to be capable of absorbing and adapting to medical advances in the 21st century, thereby ensuring future growth and development.

The project developed from a network of 7 x 7 m (23 x 23 ft) modules which can be subdivided and interconnected. The modular approach allows the hospital to meet its current requirements while at the same time being adaptable to any necessary modifications in the future. This system implies that any changes would involve minimal physical alterations and the circulation systems and façade would not need to be altered in any way. The mechanical system is located on an intermediate floor that runs through the entire building in order to facilitate repairs as well as the installation of new services with minimal interference in the daily running of the hospital.

Pellegrini Avenue, one of Rosario's major arteries, was chosen for the location of the hospital to facilitate access, particularly for ambulances. The building is organized in a series of bar-shaped volumes, two of which run parallel to the avenue. On the first floor of the front volume are the main entrances as well as the spaces for admissions, the waiting room for emergencies and the cafeteria; while the first floor accommodates the teaching areas, chapel, conference room and administration offices. The offices and service areas for the medical staff are located in the volume at the back of the building. In between and perpendicular to these two volumes, there are three bars that are separated by two internal courtyards, providing natural light and ventilation. The function of each of these spaces is differentiated in both plan and section. On the ground floor are the areas dedicated to emergency treatment, laboratories, x-ray rooms and surgery. The in-patient rooms are located on the first floor and are organized according to the level of care required by the patients: intensive care, medium-level care and those who are almost ready to be discharged.

Given its scale – the hospital occupies nearly an entire city block – the design for the HECA was understood as a predominantly horizontal mega-structure developed on two levels and capable of consolidating its urban surroundings.

Client:
Rosario Town Council
Surface area:
18,350 sqm (200,000 sqft)
Start date:
2000
Finish date:
2007
Head architects:
Mario Corea, Silvana Codina, Francisco Quijano
Collaborators:
Miguel Antezza, Marcelo Brunetti, Alejandro de Stefano, Alfredo Llusa, Jorgelina Paniagua, Antonio Muiño
Contractor:
IECSA
Cost:
€ 21,000,000

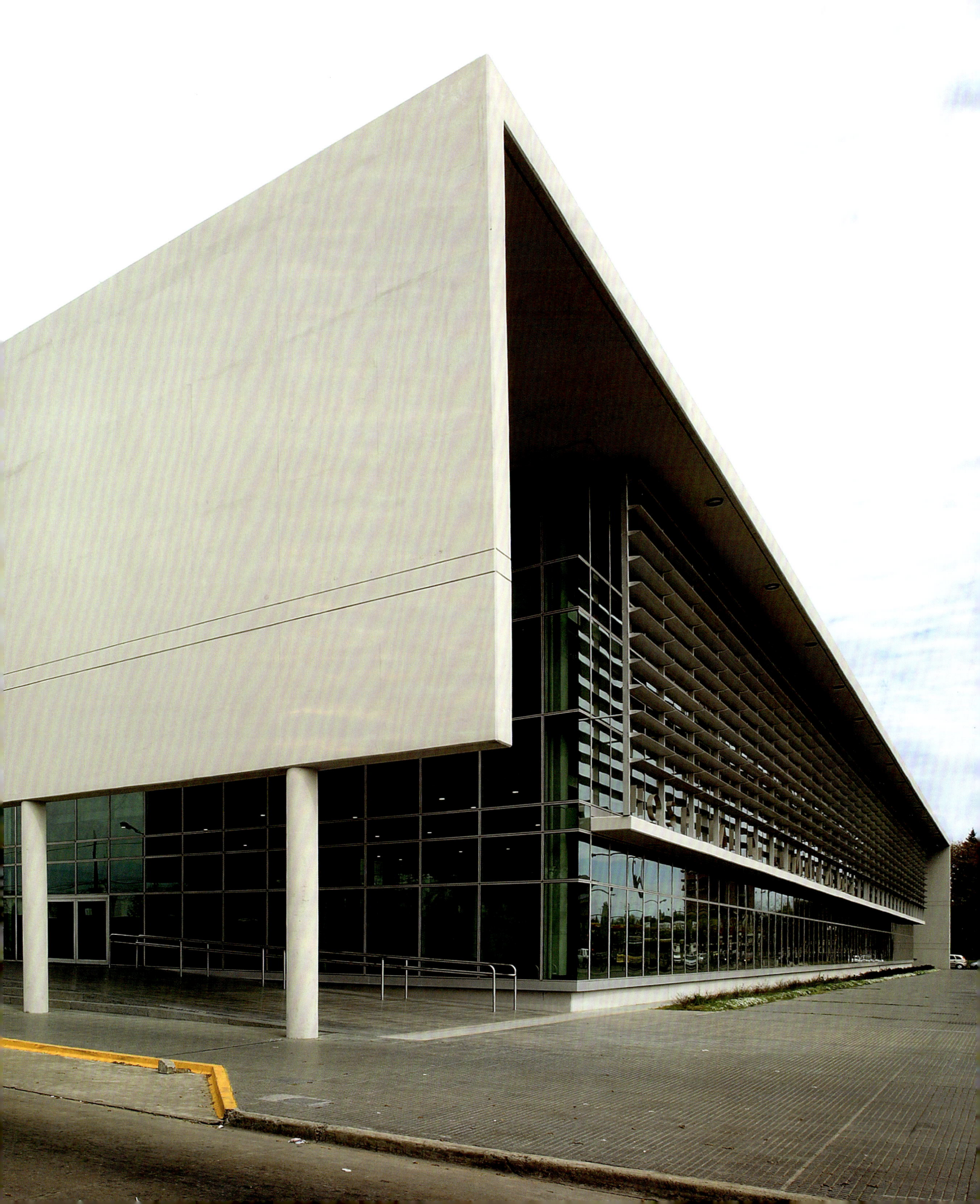

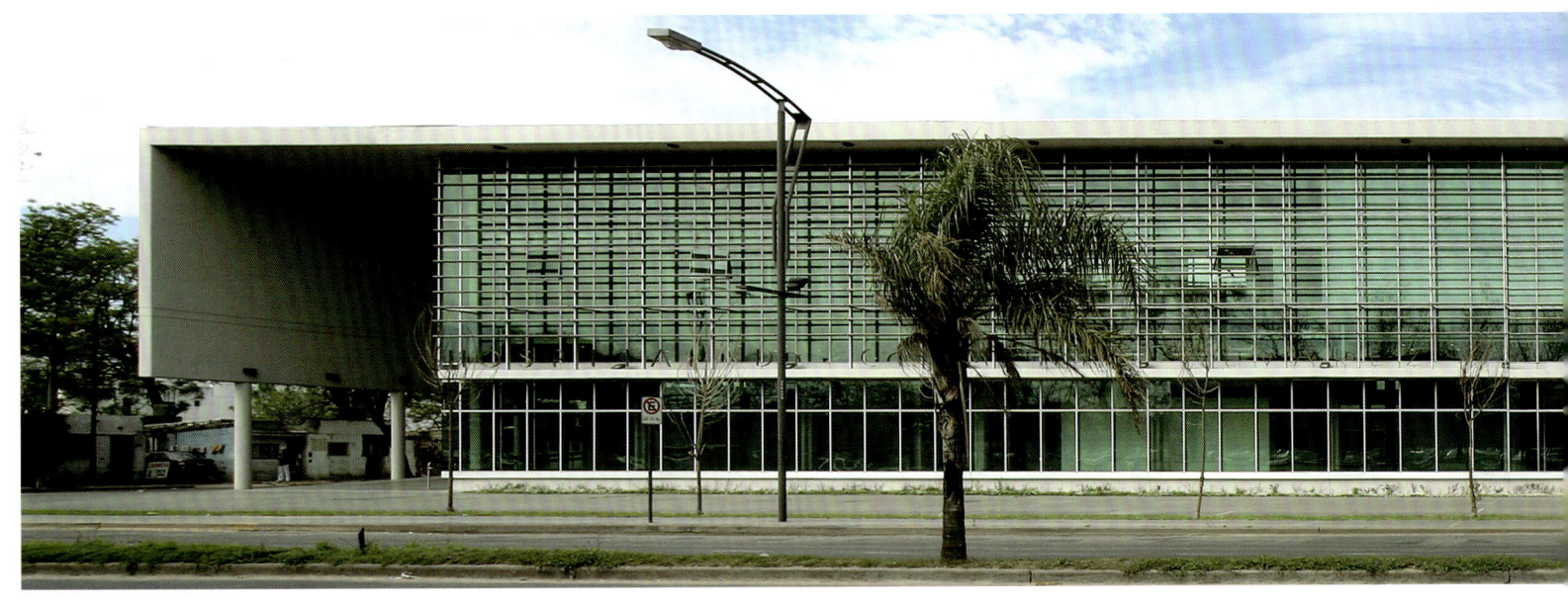

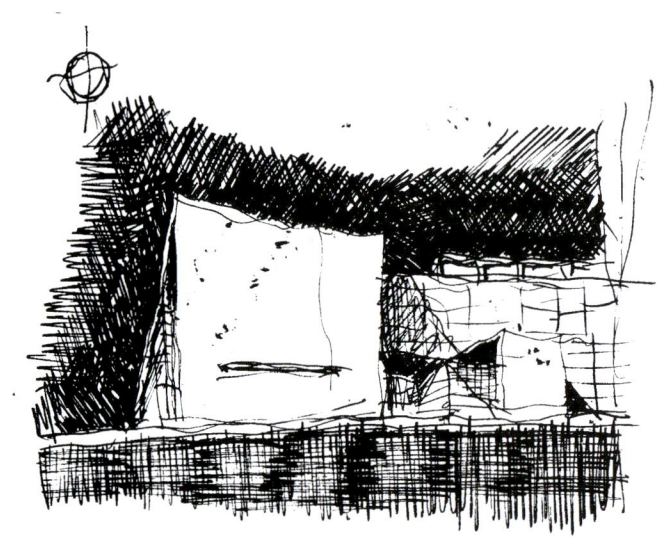

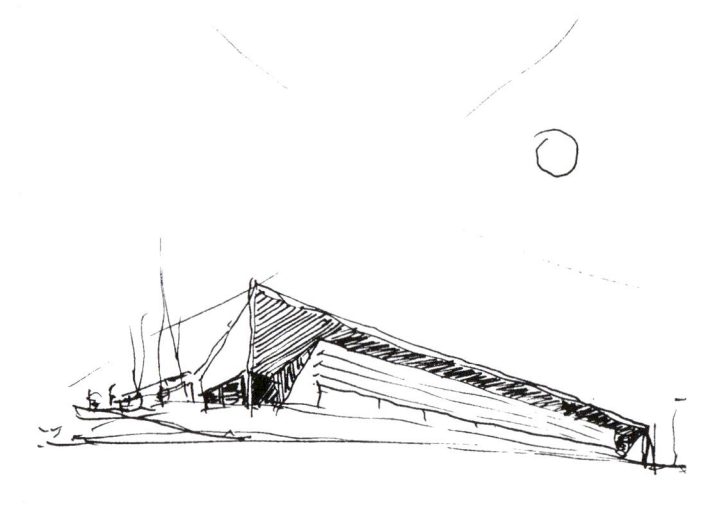

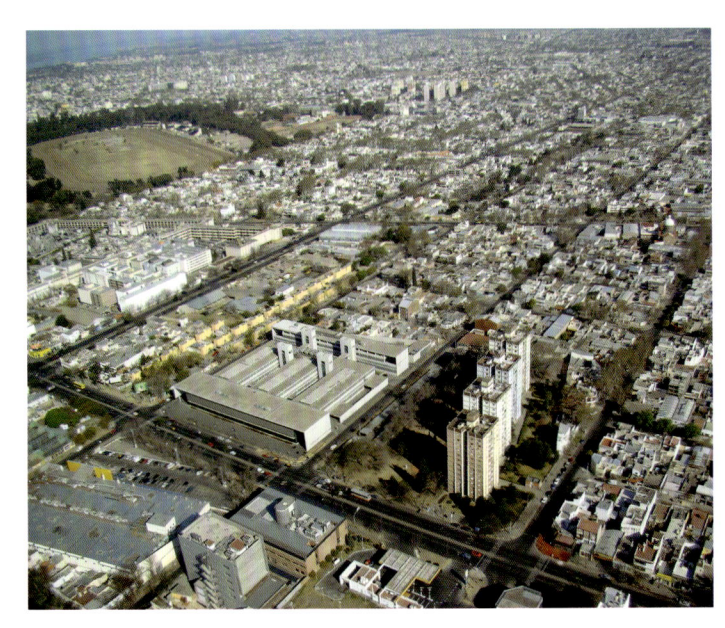

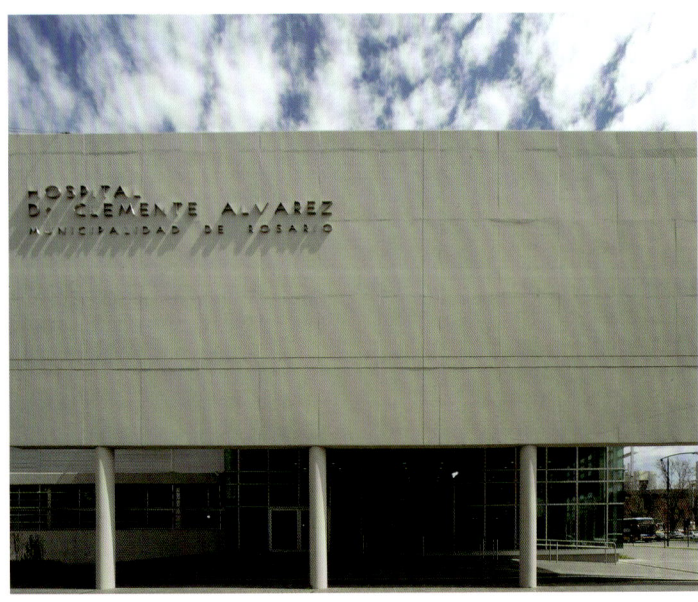

113

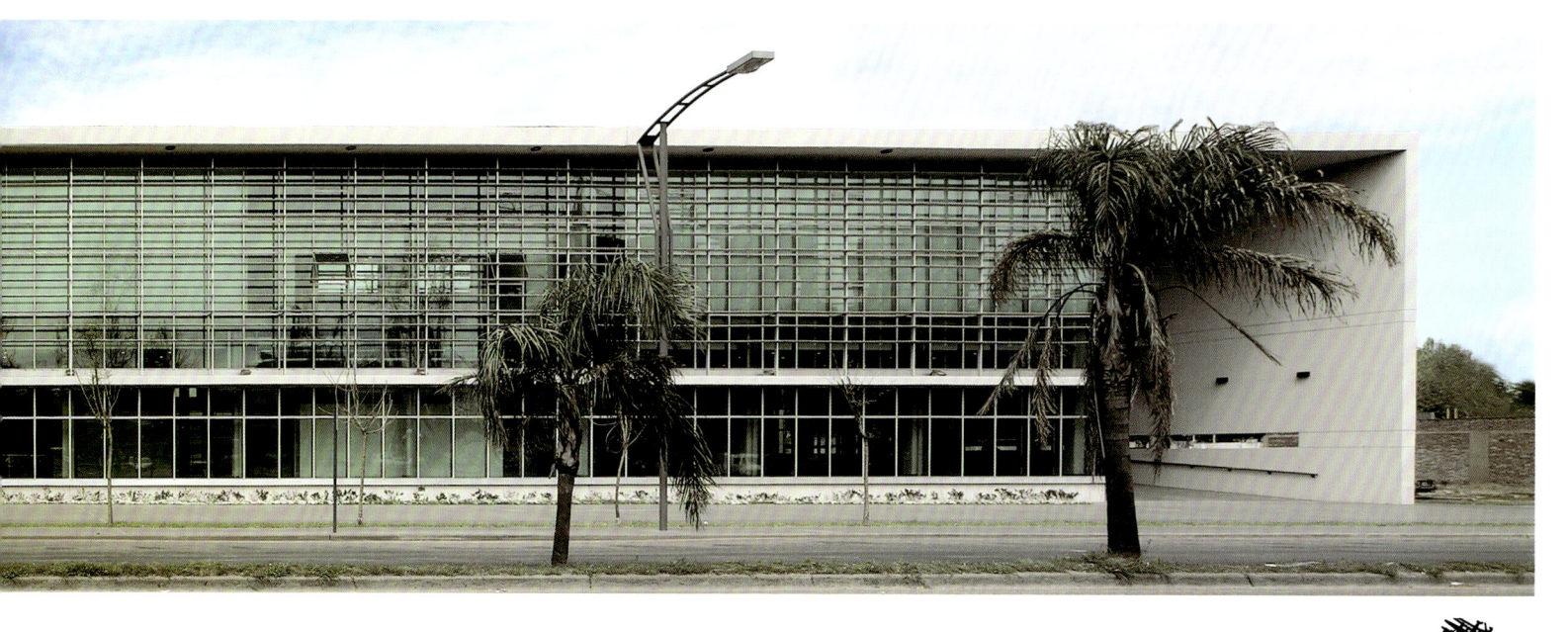

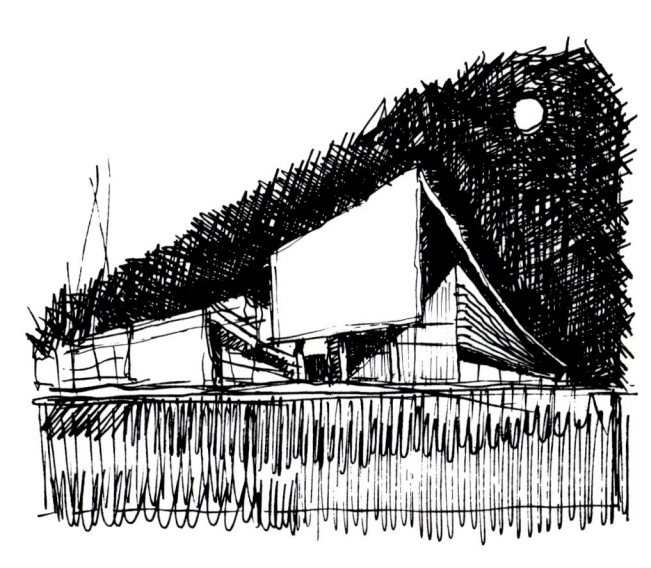

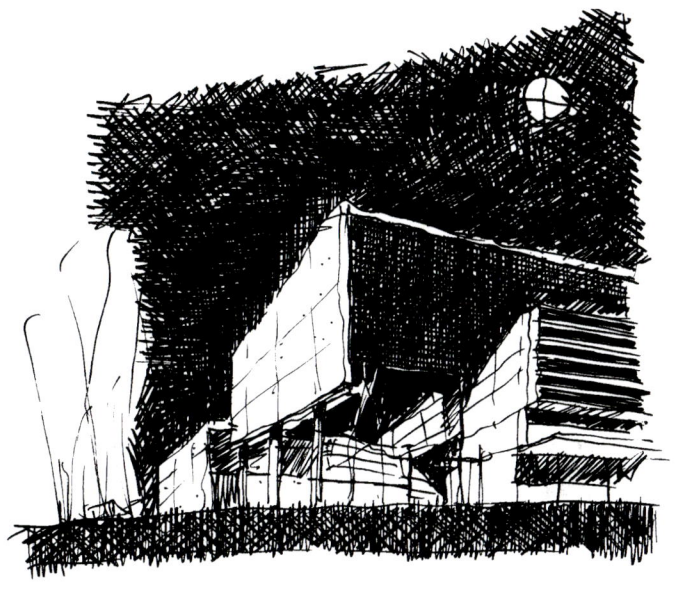

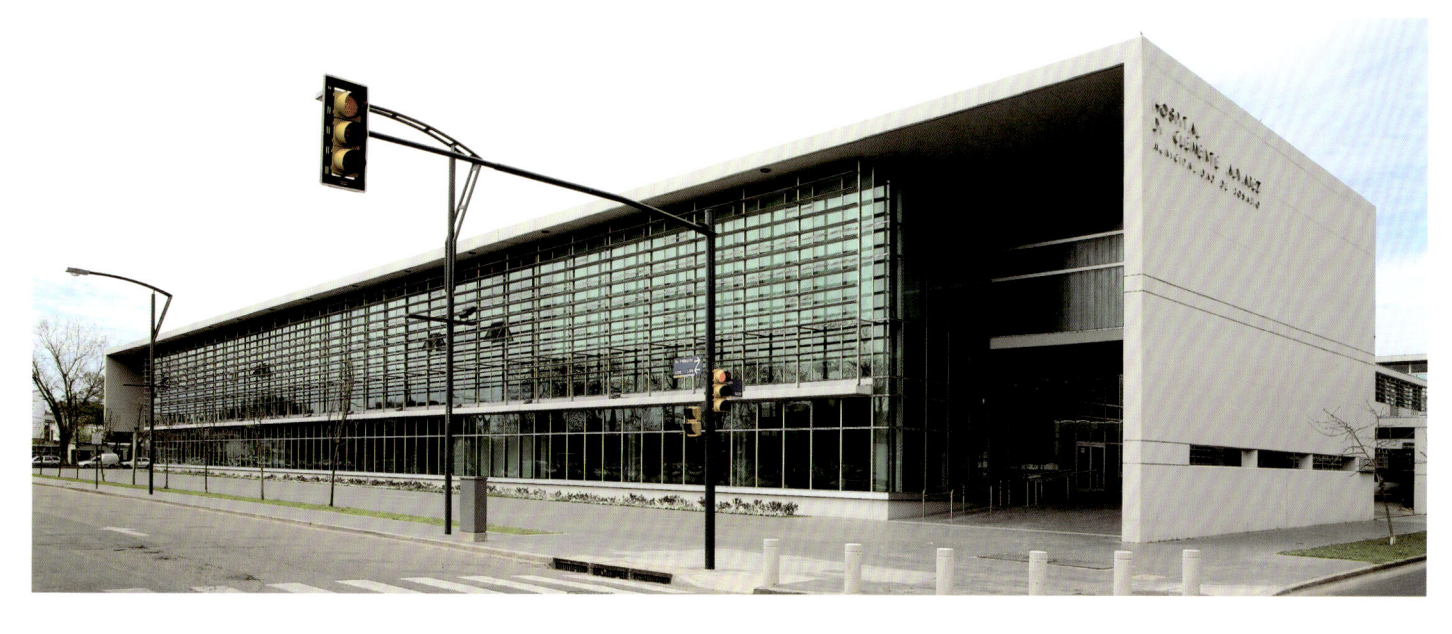

Ground floor plan

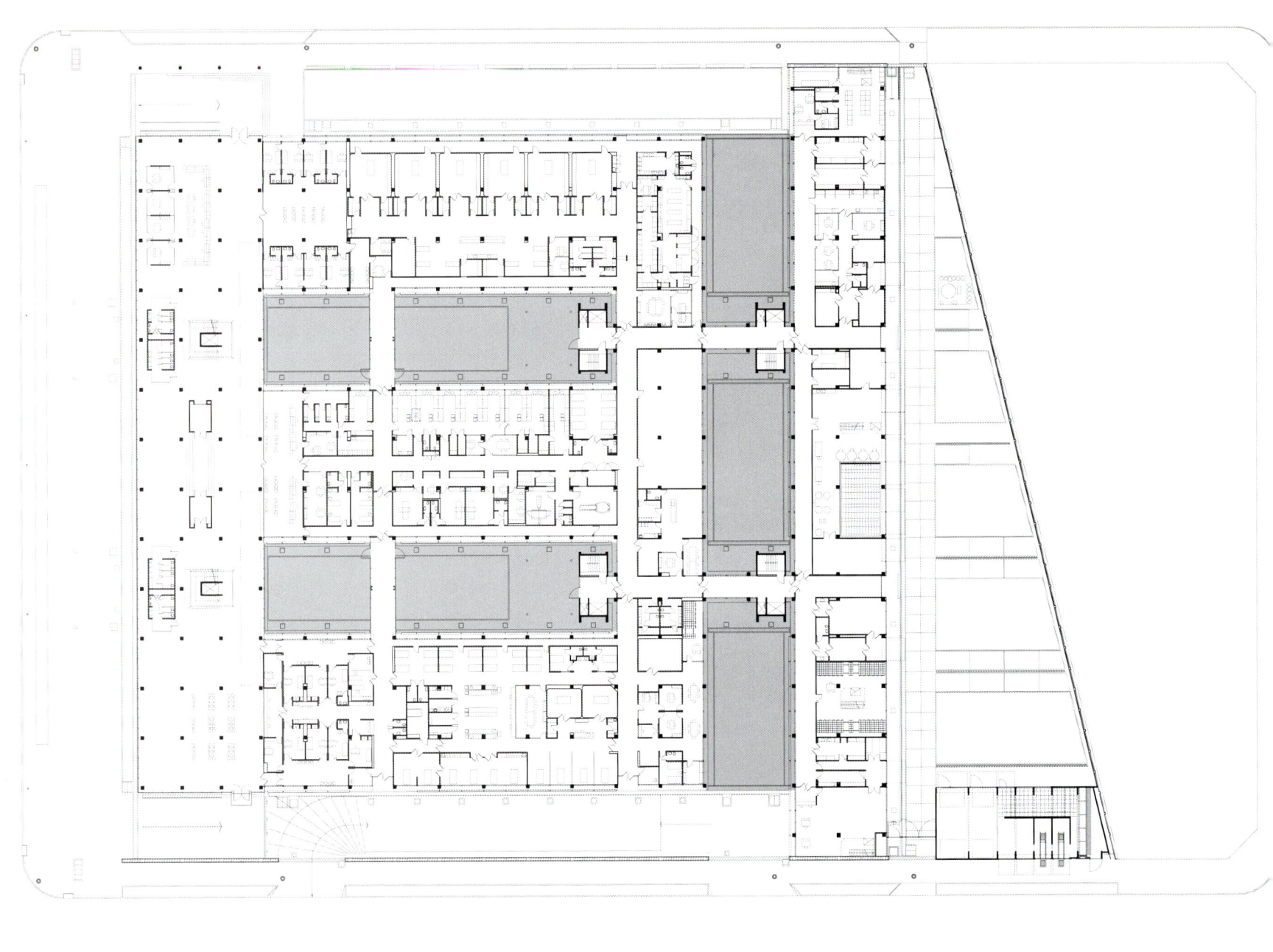

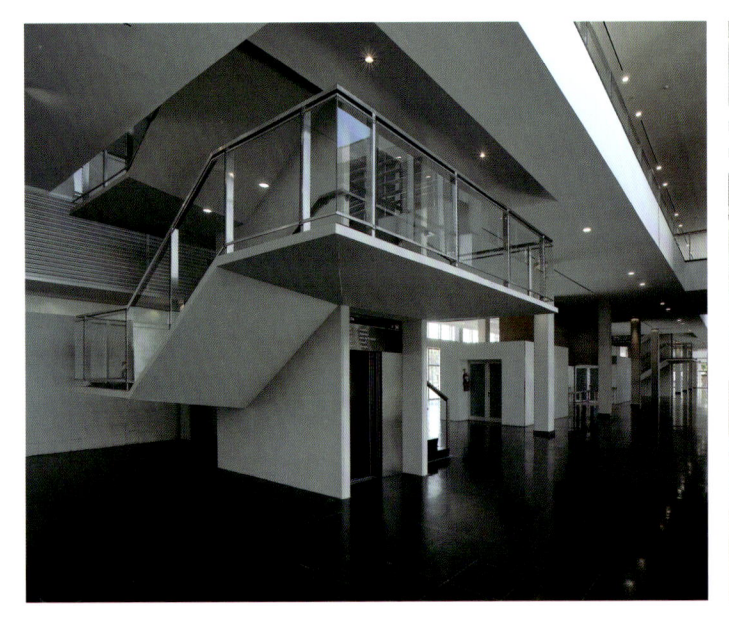

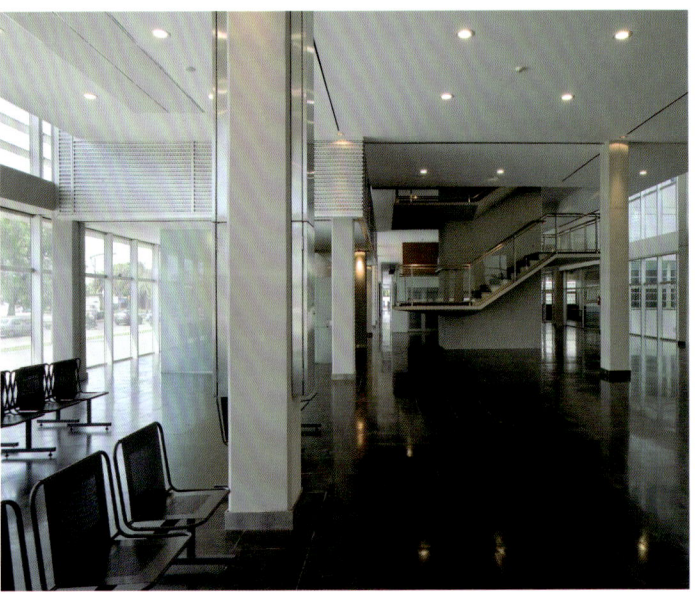

114

First floor plan

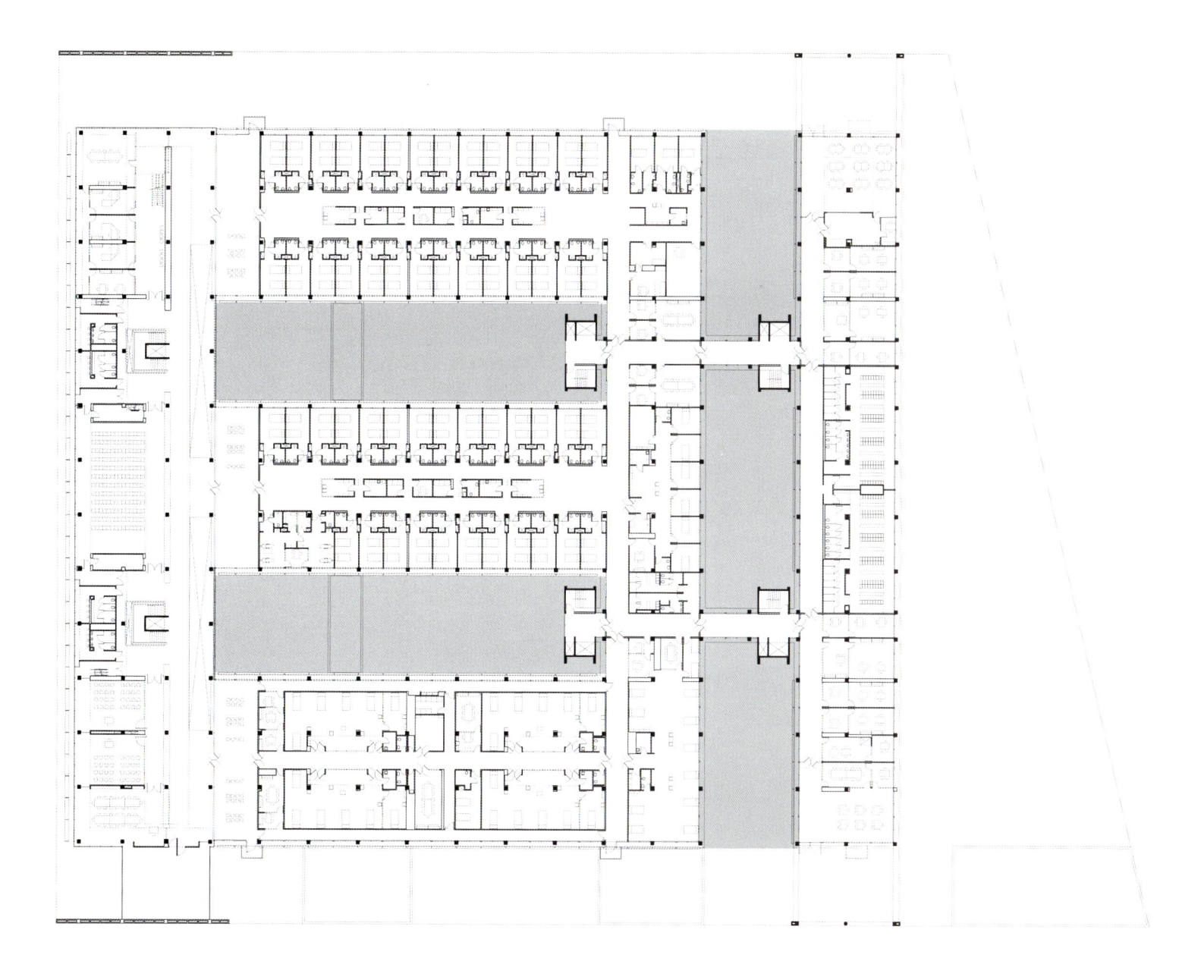

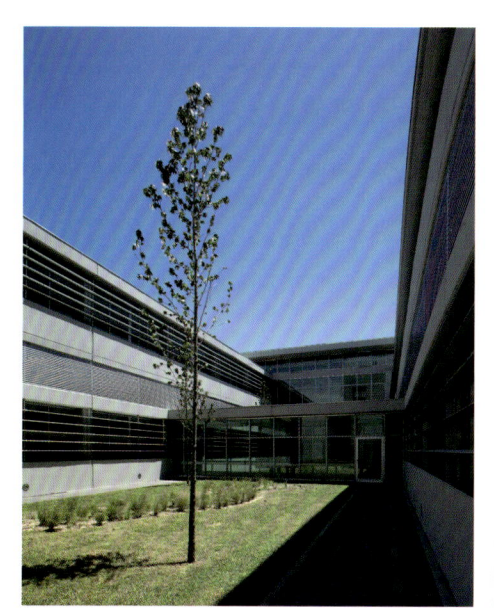

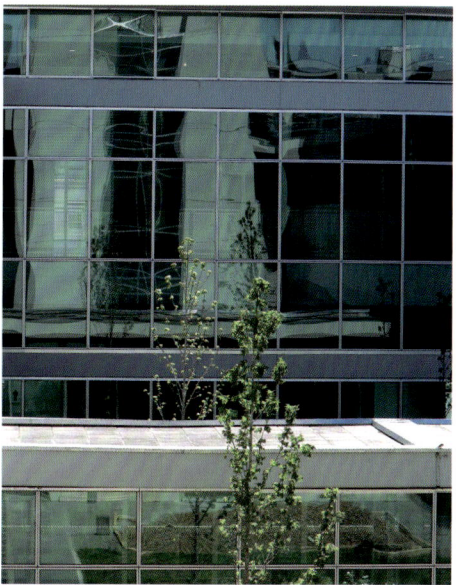

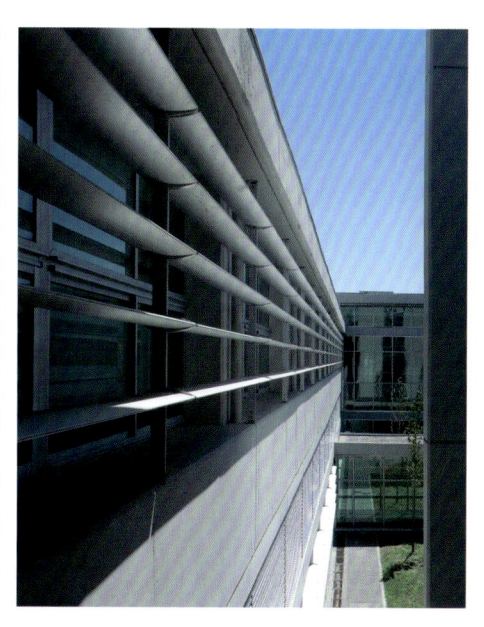

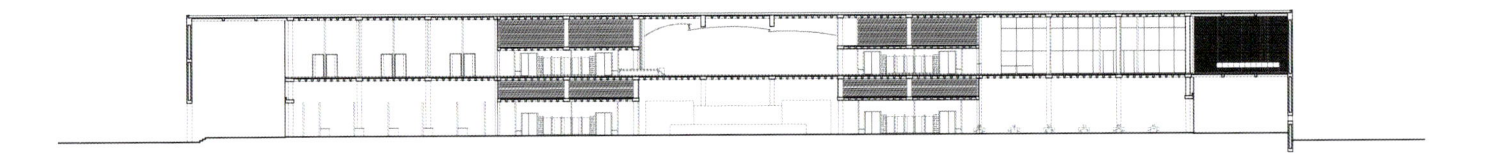

Section 1-1

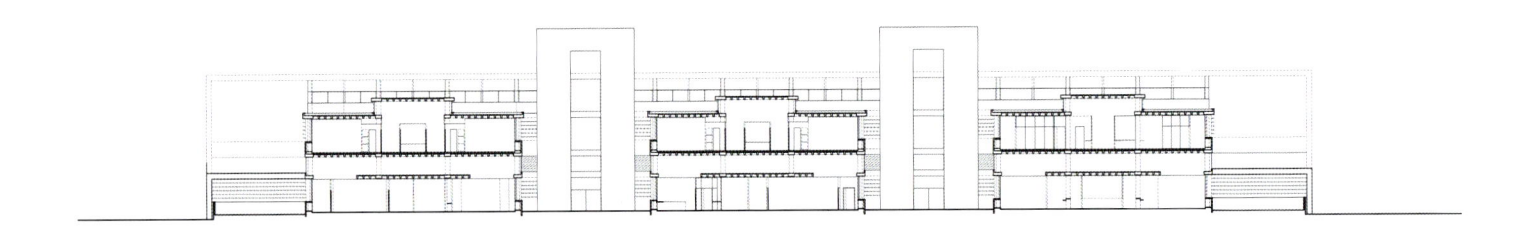

Section 2-2

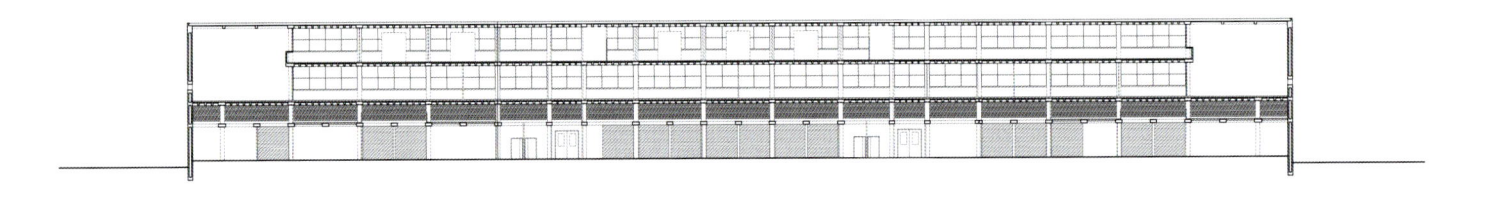

Section 3-3

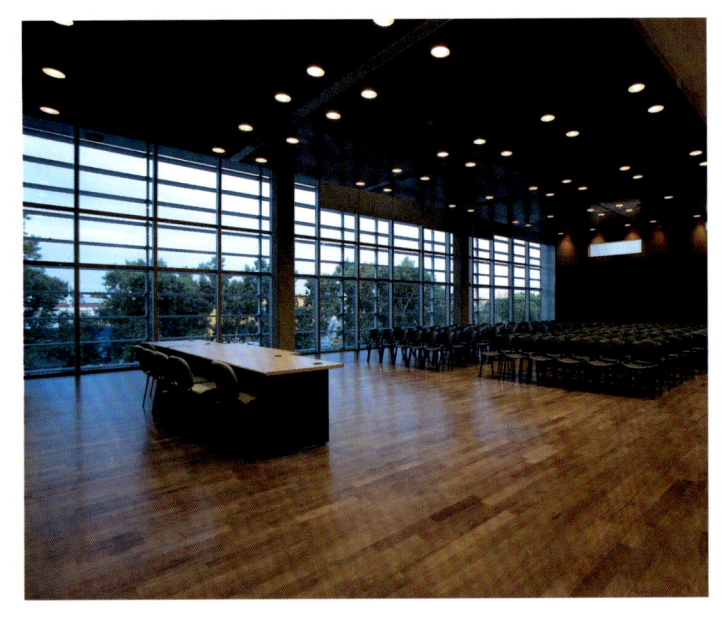

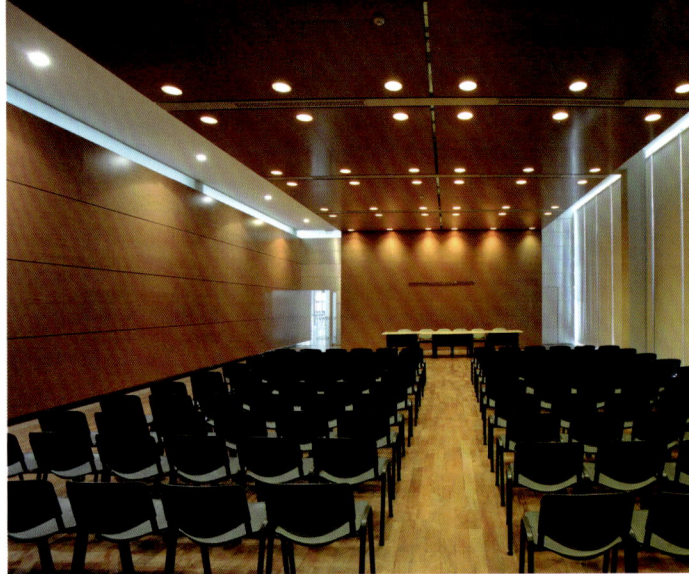

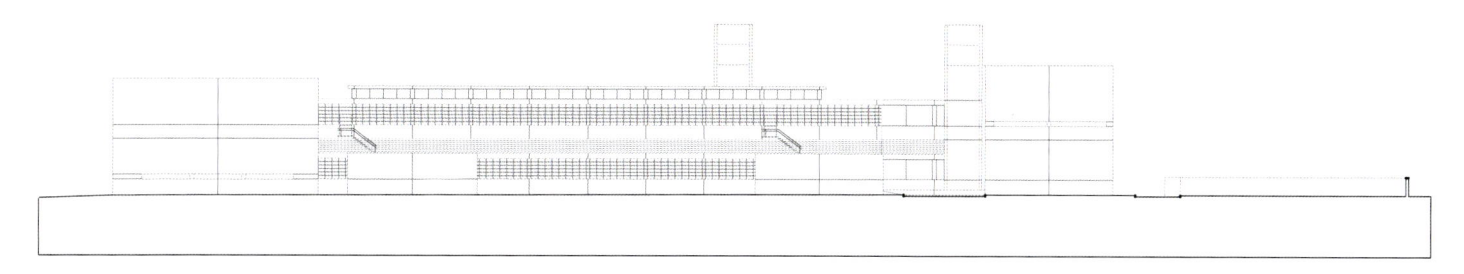

West elevation

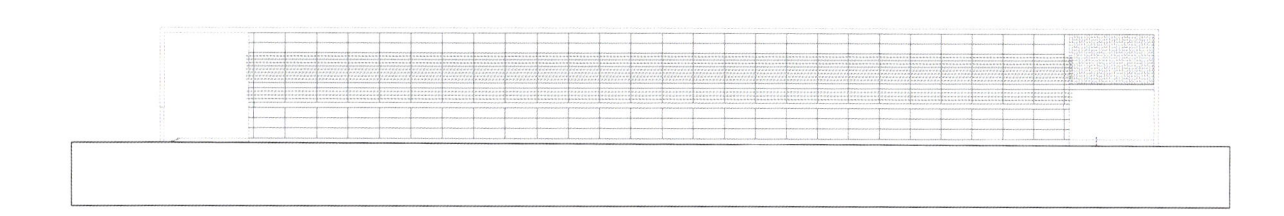

North elevation

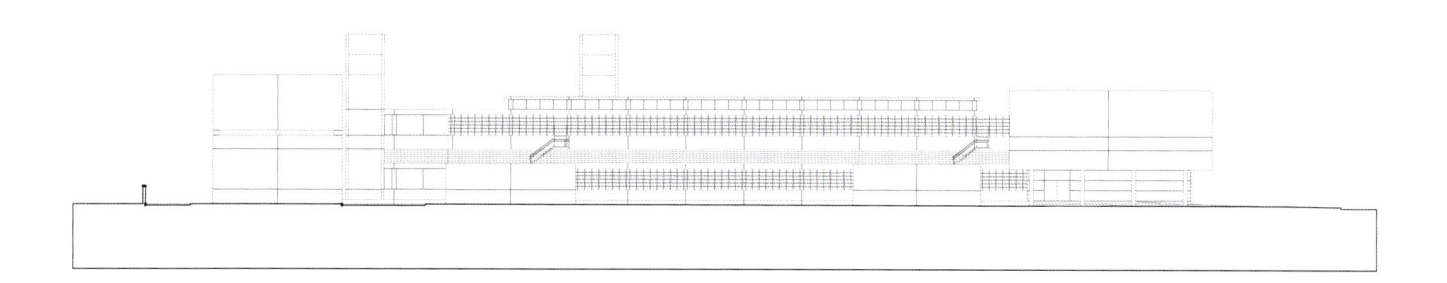

East elevation

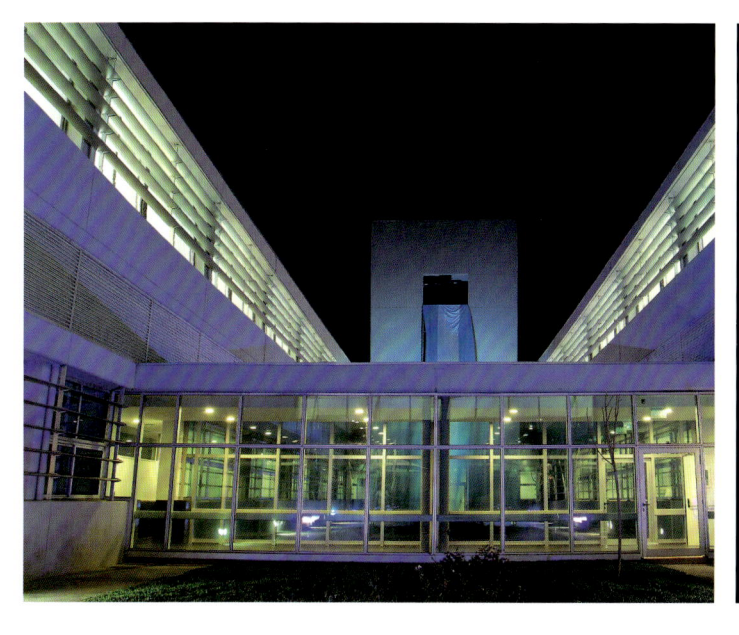

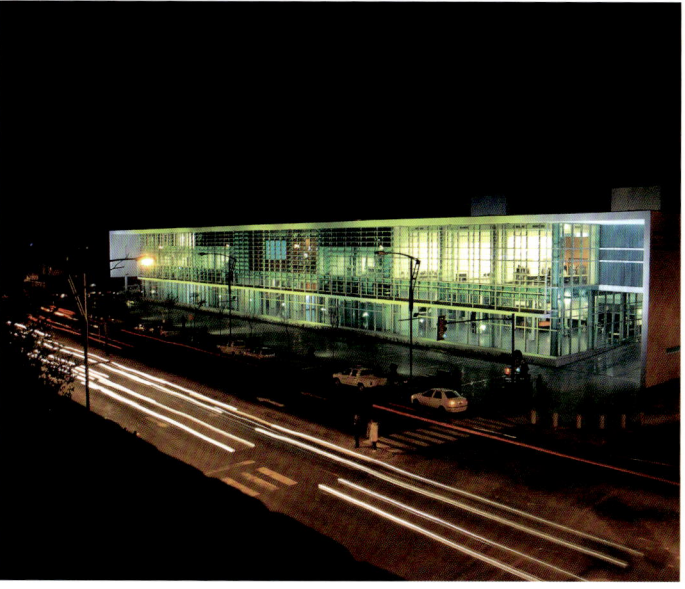

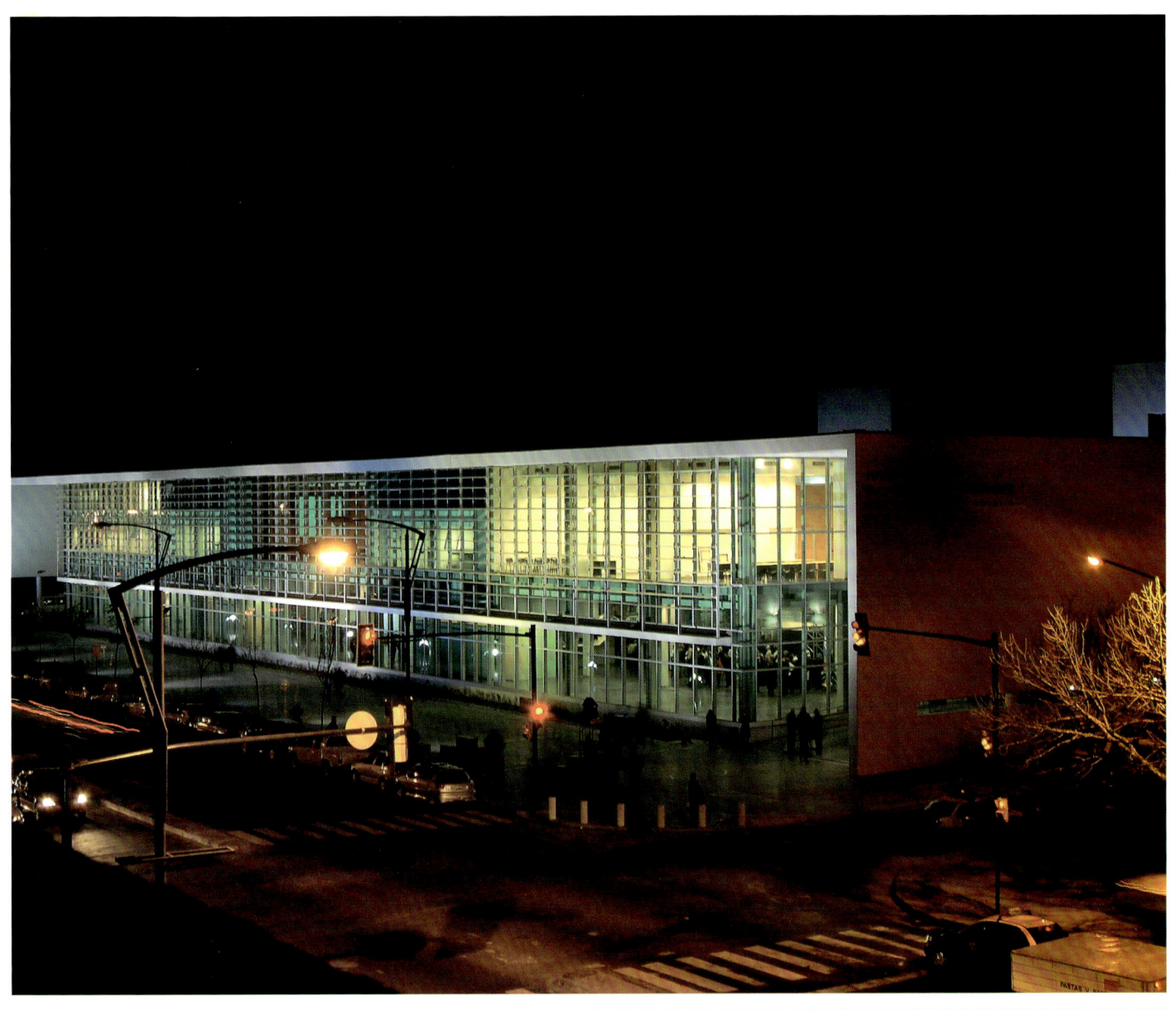

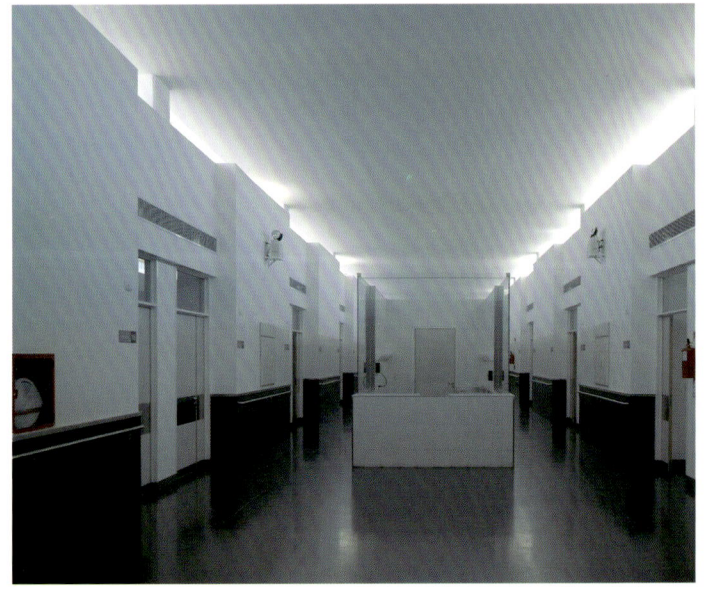

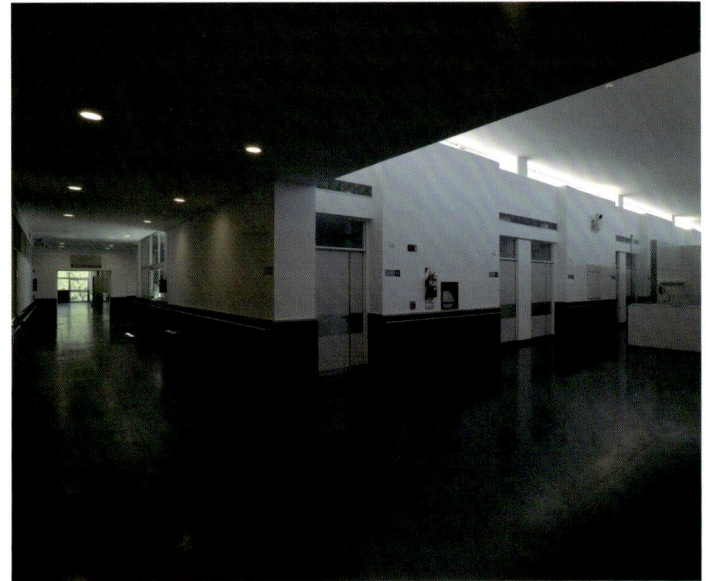

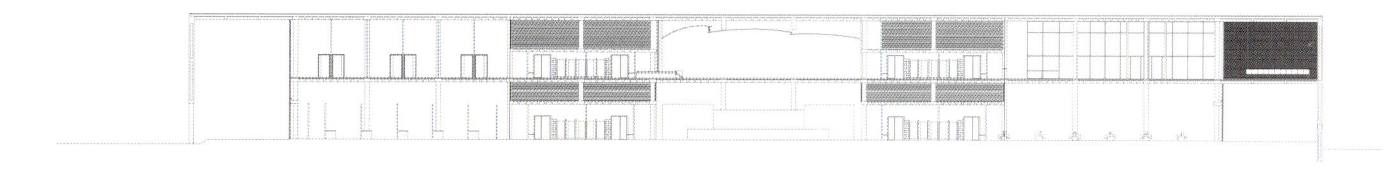

Section 1-1

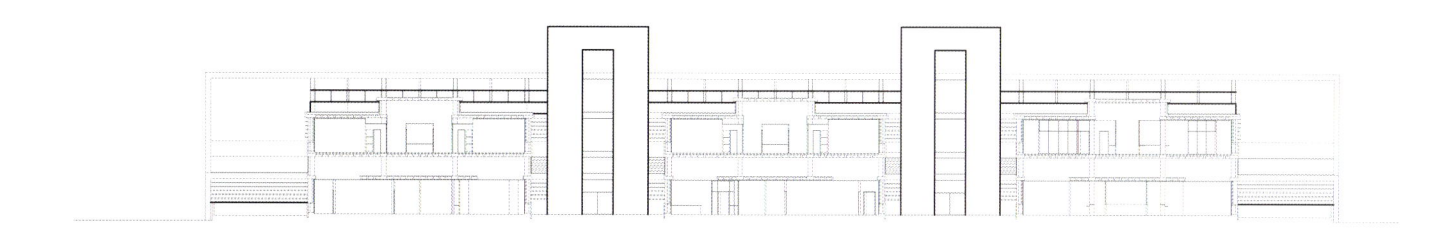

Section 2-2

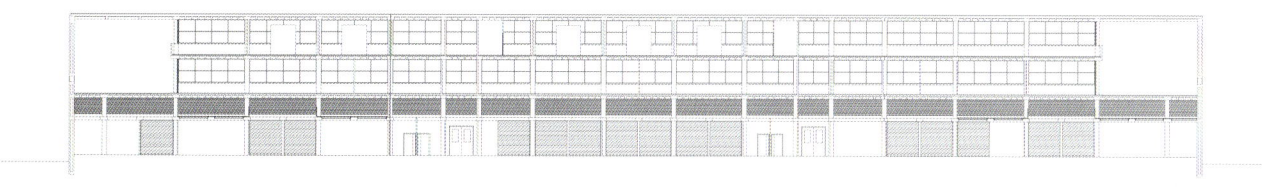

Section 3-3

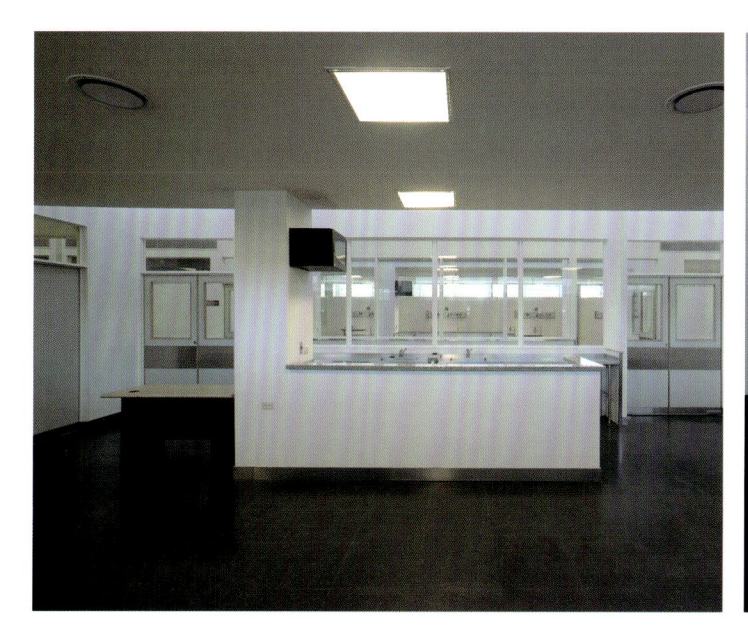

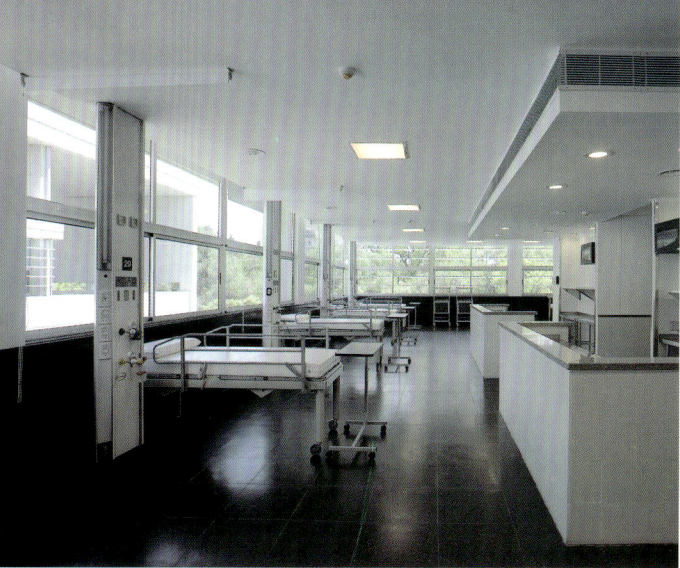

Argola Arquitectos

Tajo Hospital

Aranjuez, Spain

Photographs: *contributed by the architects*

The new Tajo Hospital is located in Aranjuez, to the south of Madrid, on a site measuring 147,000 sqm (1,582,000 sqft). The plot's irregular shape presents an upward incline, rising as it moves away from the main road. Where the building is positioned there is a level change of approximately one floor. It was decided that the hospital would develop horizontally, taking advantage of the level changes to situate entrances at either end of the building on different levels.

The hospital has a modular structure set within a clear orthogonal layout. Landscaped courtyards serve to separate the individual buildings and allow natural light and air to penetrate the interiors. They establish a rhythm and generate visual variation inside the hospital, breaking up the long corridors. Their design aims to produce a calming atmosphere.

A two-story block houses the outpatients department and contains the hospital's main entrance, where the public vertical circulation core is situated. The ground floor accommodates admissions, file storage, rehabilitation services and the cafeteria, while external consultations and a laboratory area are located on the first floor. The consulting rooms are spread across the two floors. Three wings form the next section, which run parallel to the previous building and are separated by courtyards. On the upper floors of two of the wings are the wards while the third contains central services. At either end of these modules run the hospital's main circulation routes. The technical block is positioned perpendicular to the wings and takes advantage of the level change housing logistics and other general services in the semi-basement. The ground floor contains the emergency department and pharmacy, and the operating theatres and obstetrics are located on the first. The installations block is a separate building at the northern end of the hospital. The circulation system is divided in two: an internal route for staff, supplies, beds etc. and an external route for visitors and outpatients.

Outdoor parking has a capacity for 265 cars and is arranged to connect with the access points of the different departments. An underground car park for 262 cars is located below the main entrance hall. The modules that comprise the hospital allow it to be flexible. Serving as "functional containers", the wings have equal dimensions so that their functions can be easily modified and exchanged. The system also allows the hospital to grow if required, through the addition of modules. An extra wing, for example, could be added to the north of the existing ones. In fact each area can be extended independently of the others.

Client:
Madrid Health Service
Surface area:
147,000 sqm (1,582,000 sqft)
Finish Date:
2007
Head architect:
Luis González Sterling
Engineer:
Rafael Muñoz
Collaborators:
Margarita Marqués, César Arribas, Vanesa Jalle Marco
Contractor:
Hispanica, Sando Construcciones, Inebensa

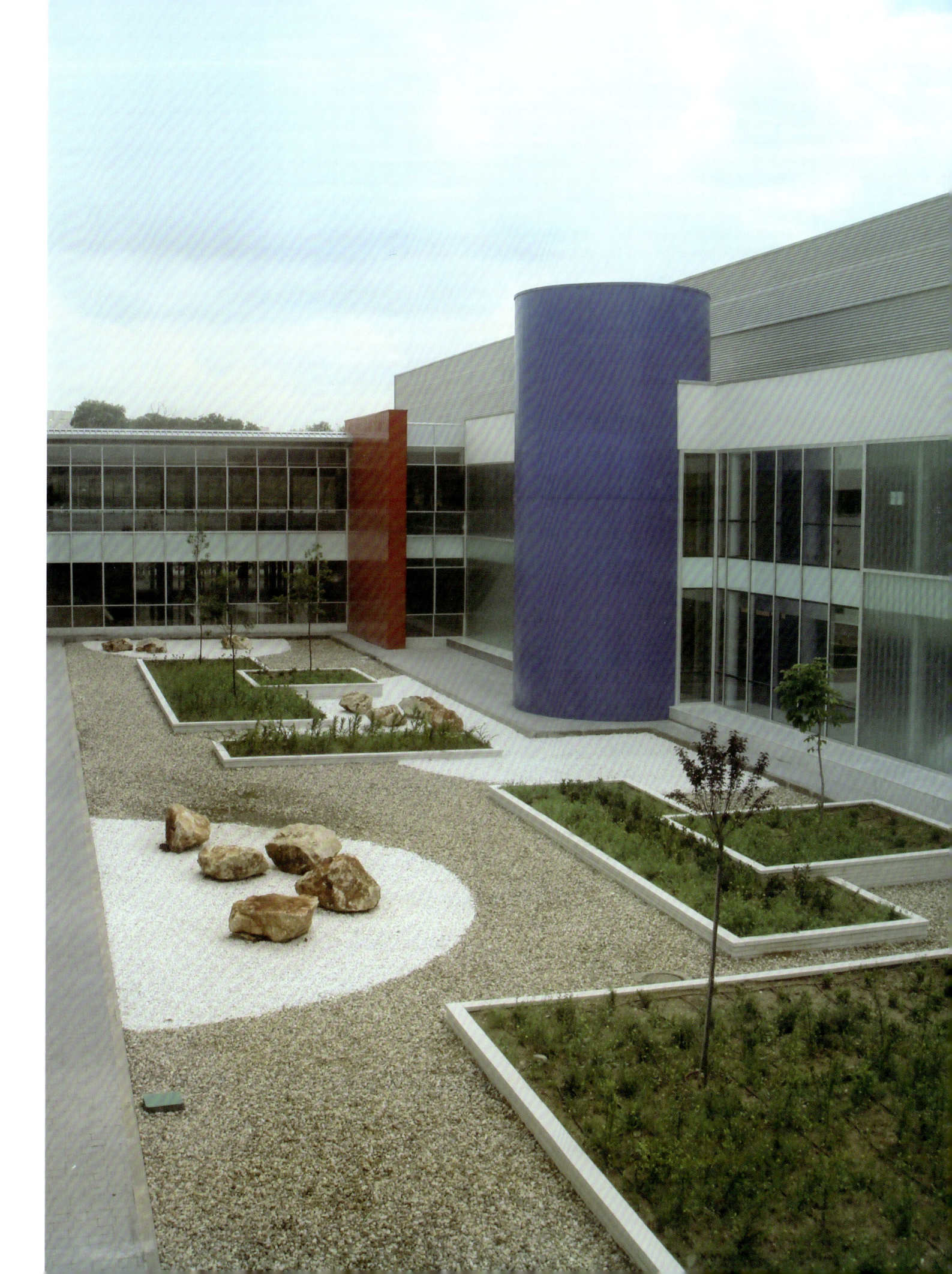

Site plan

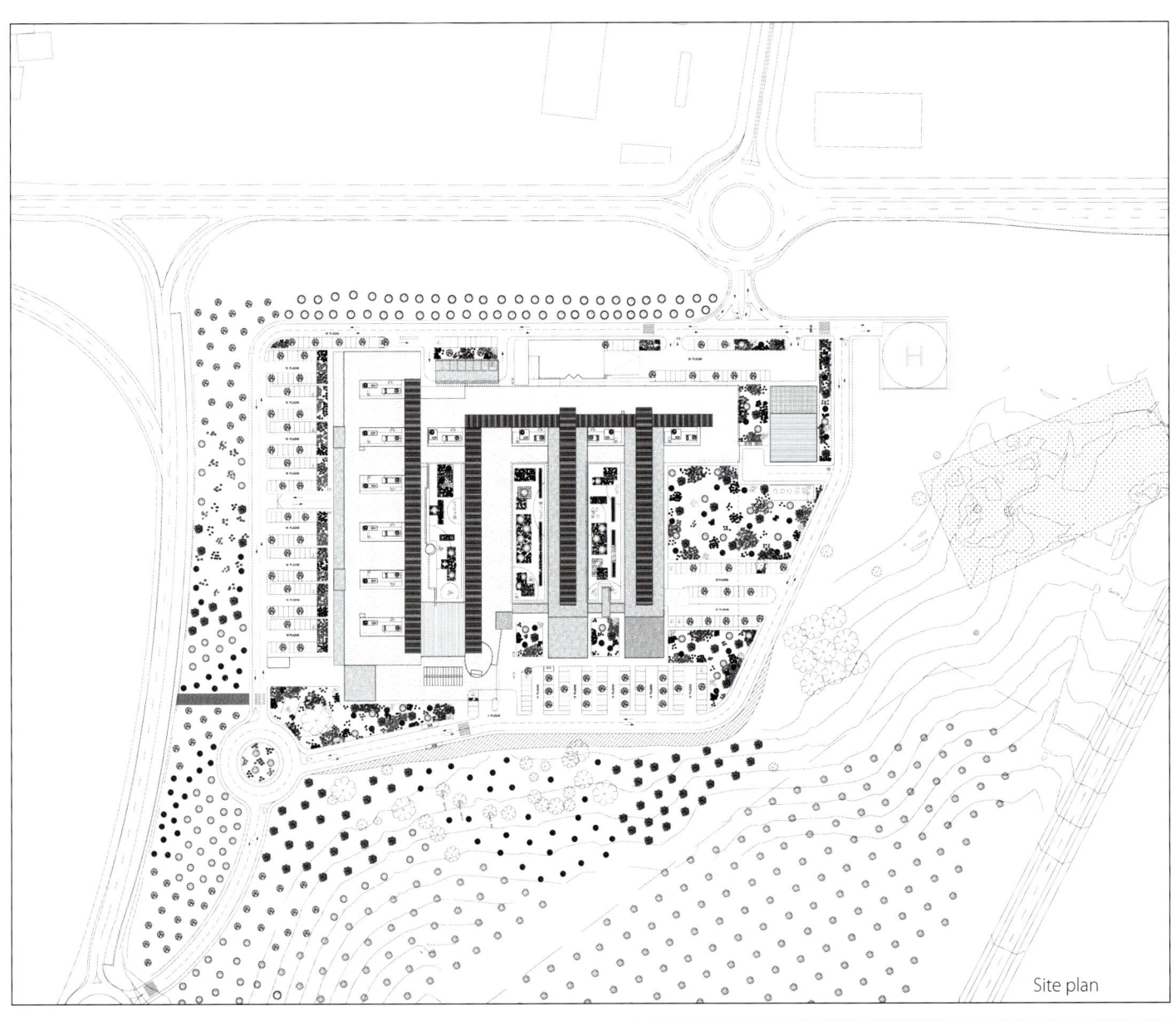

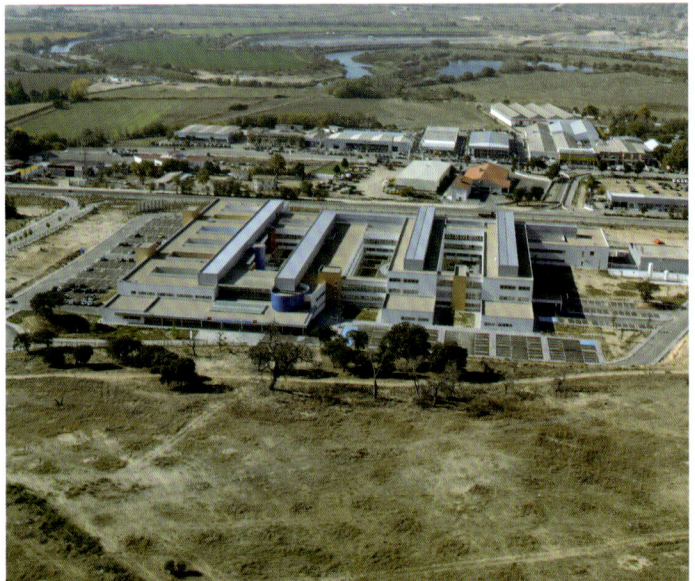

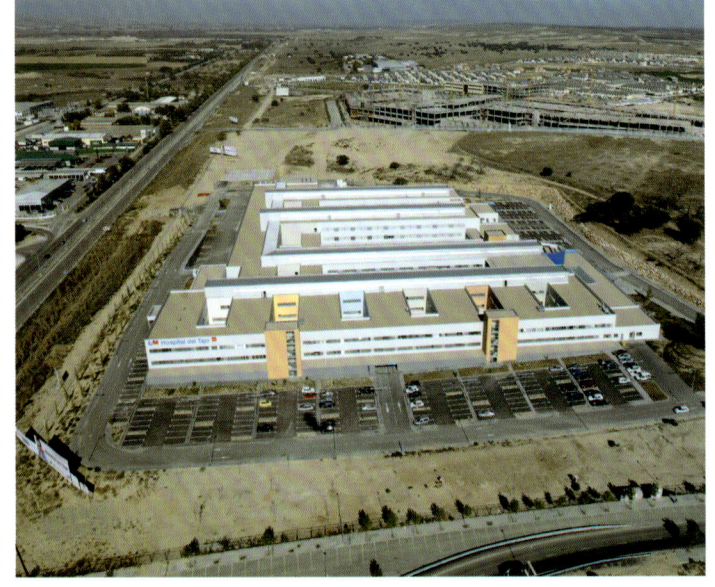

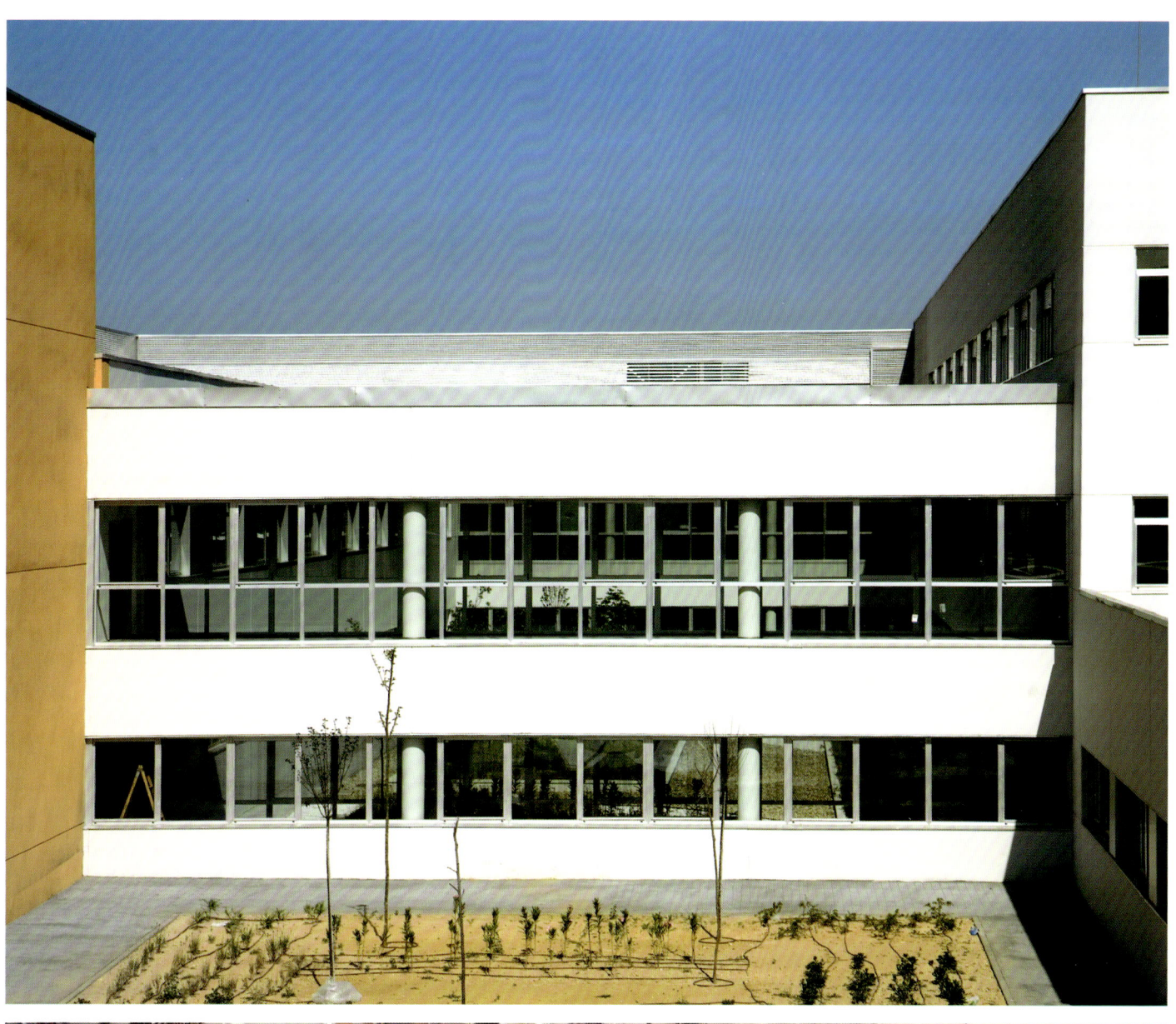

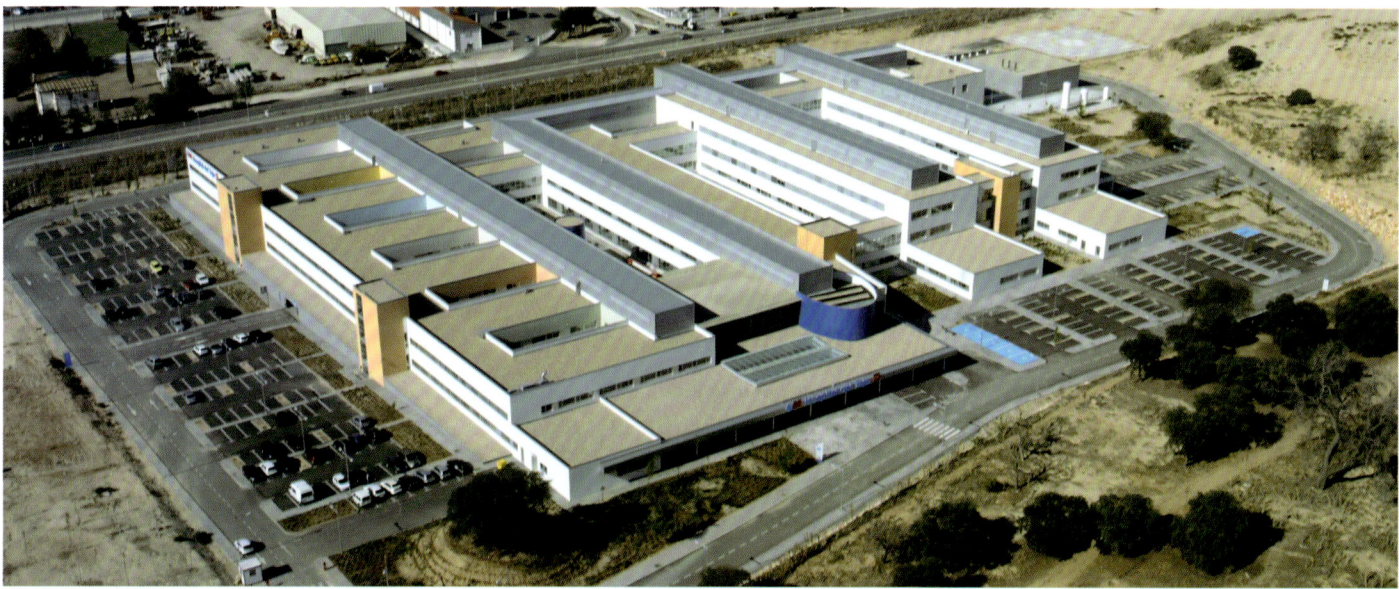

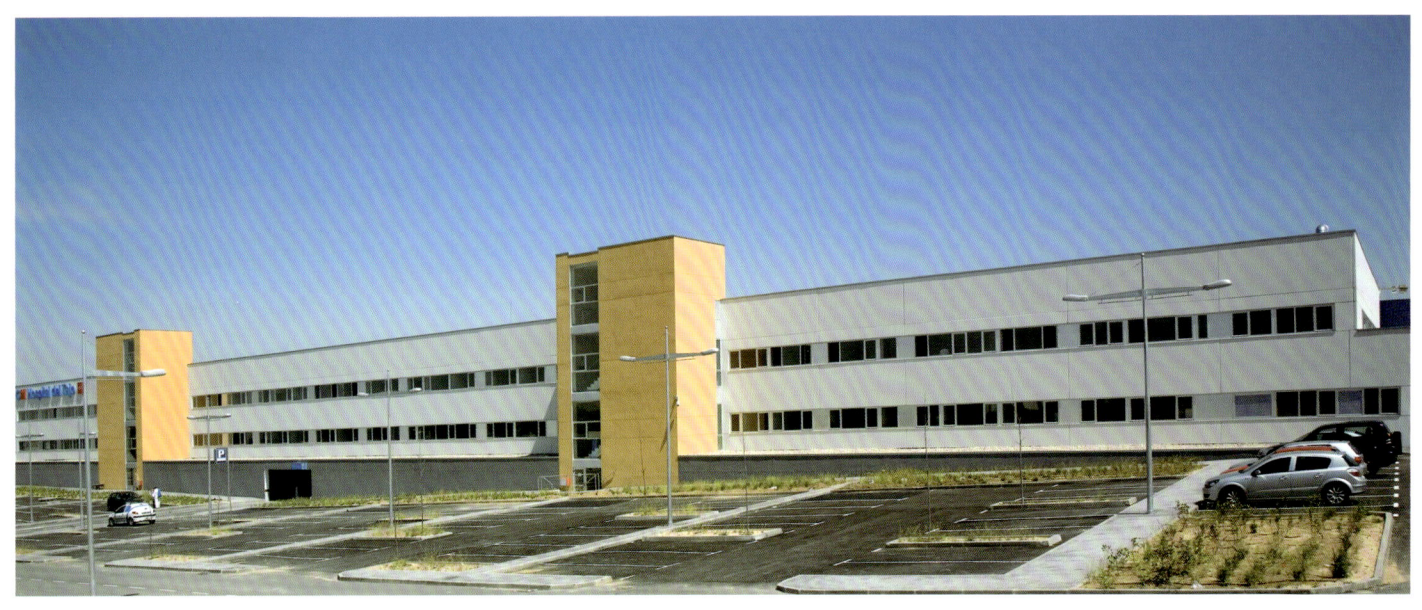

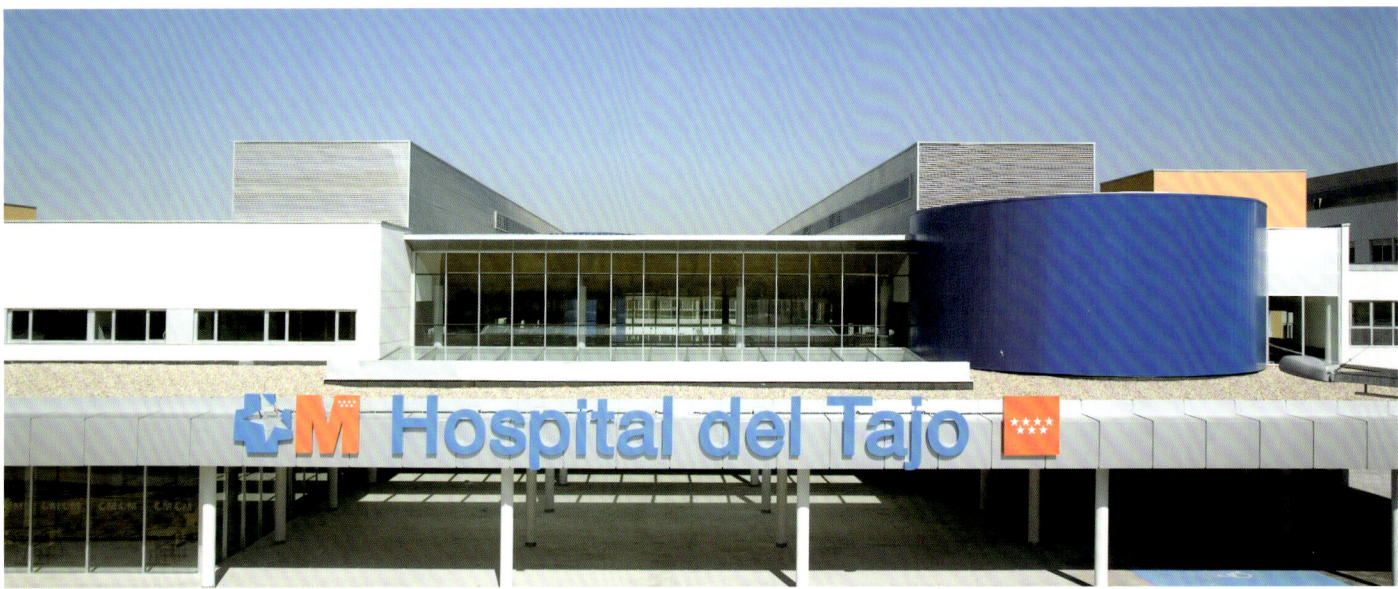

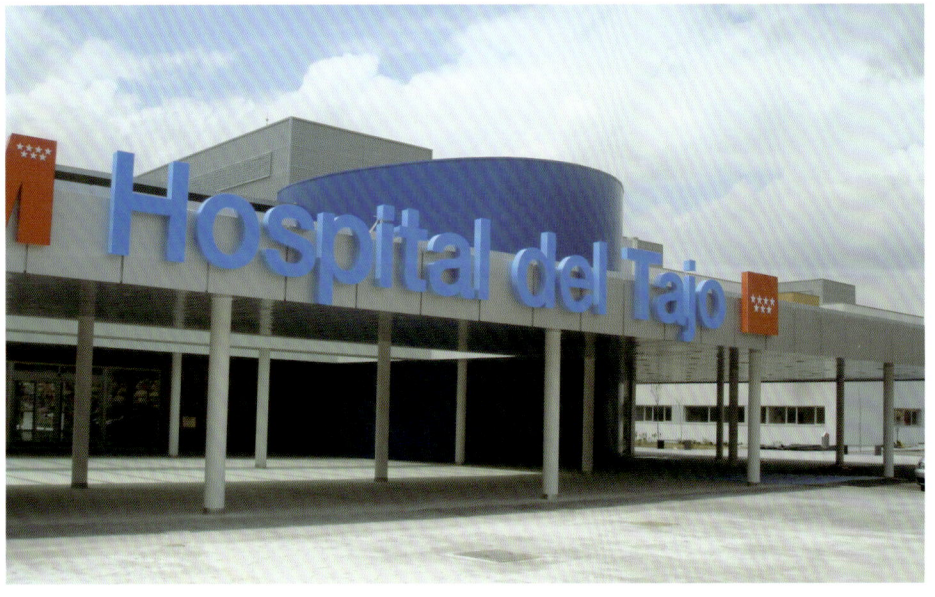

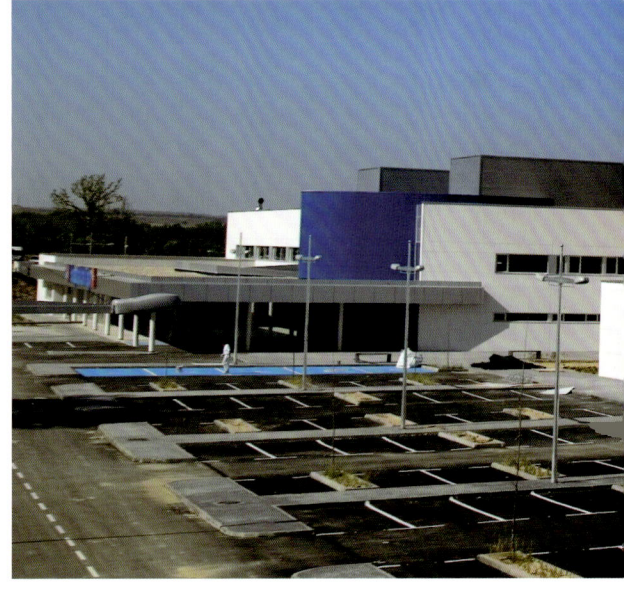

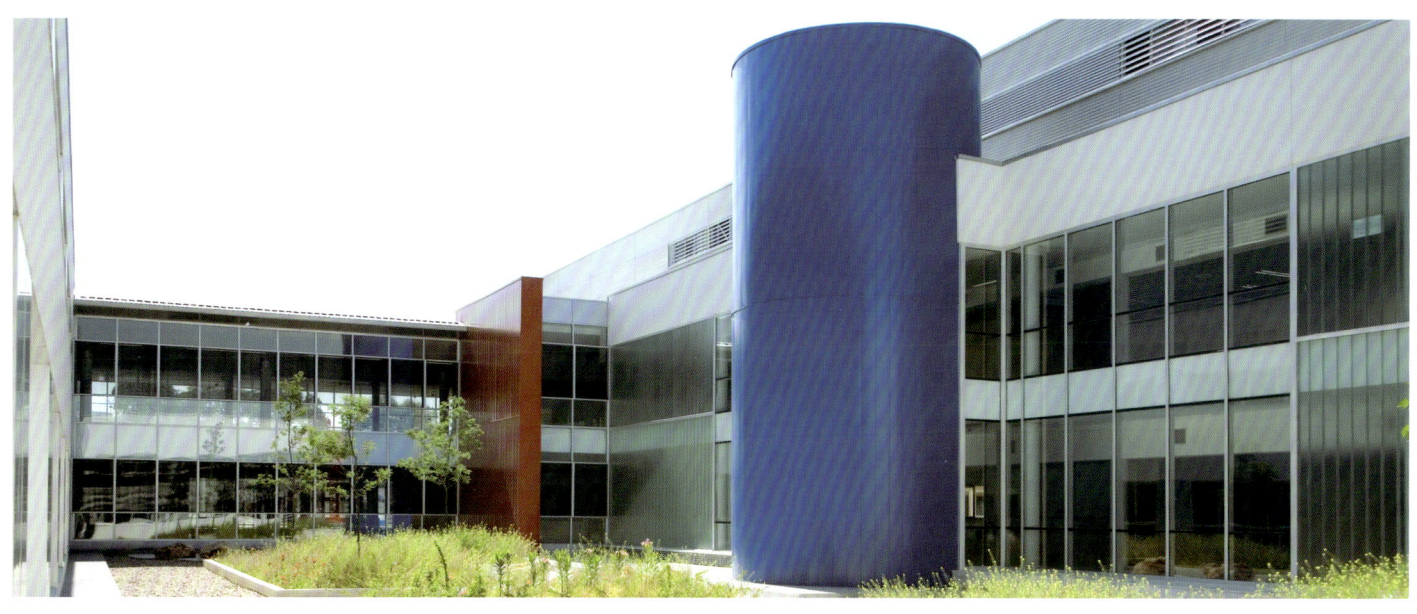

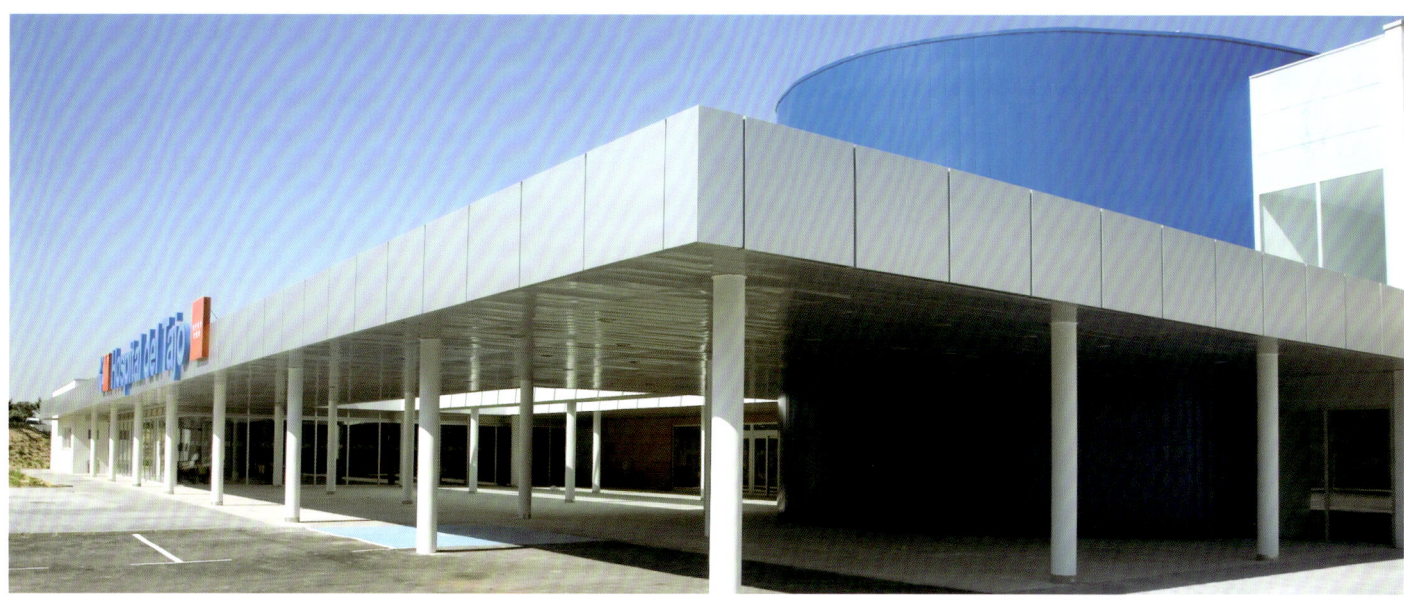

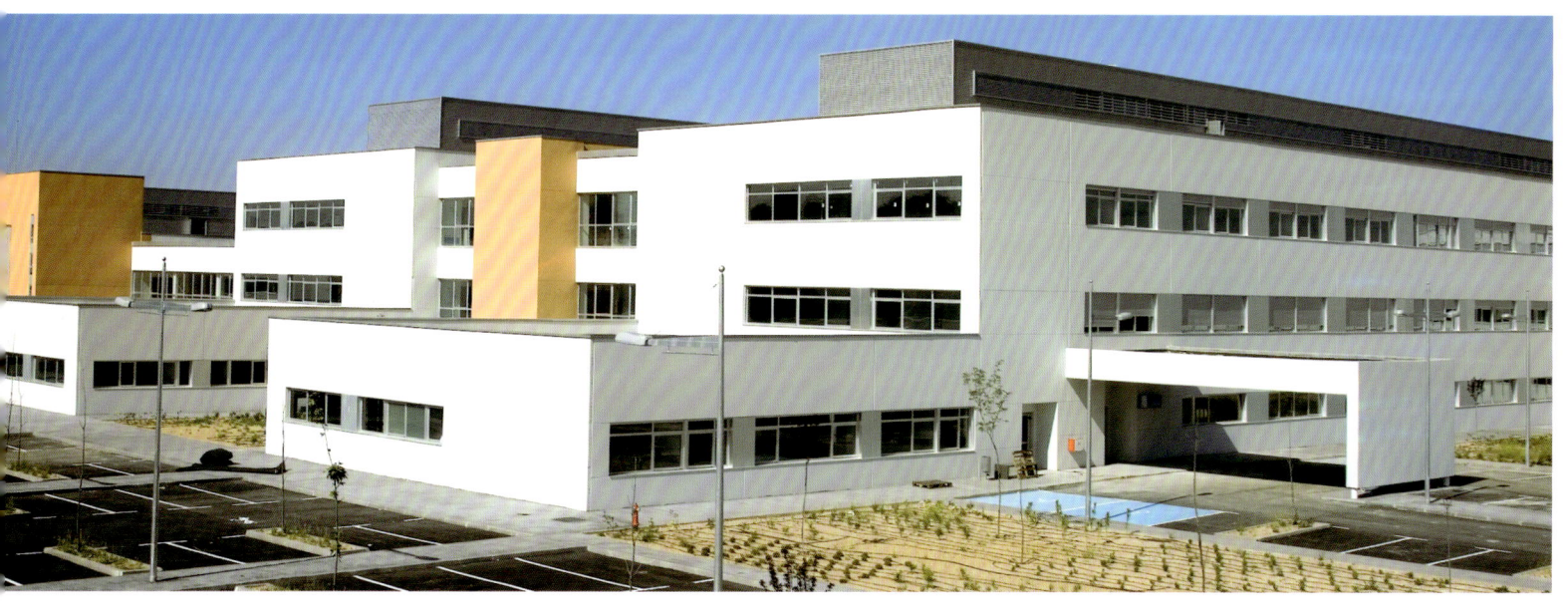

Basement plan

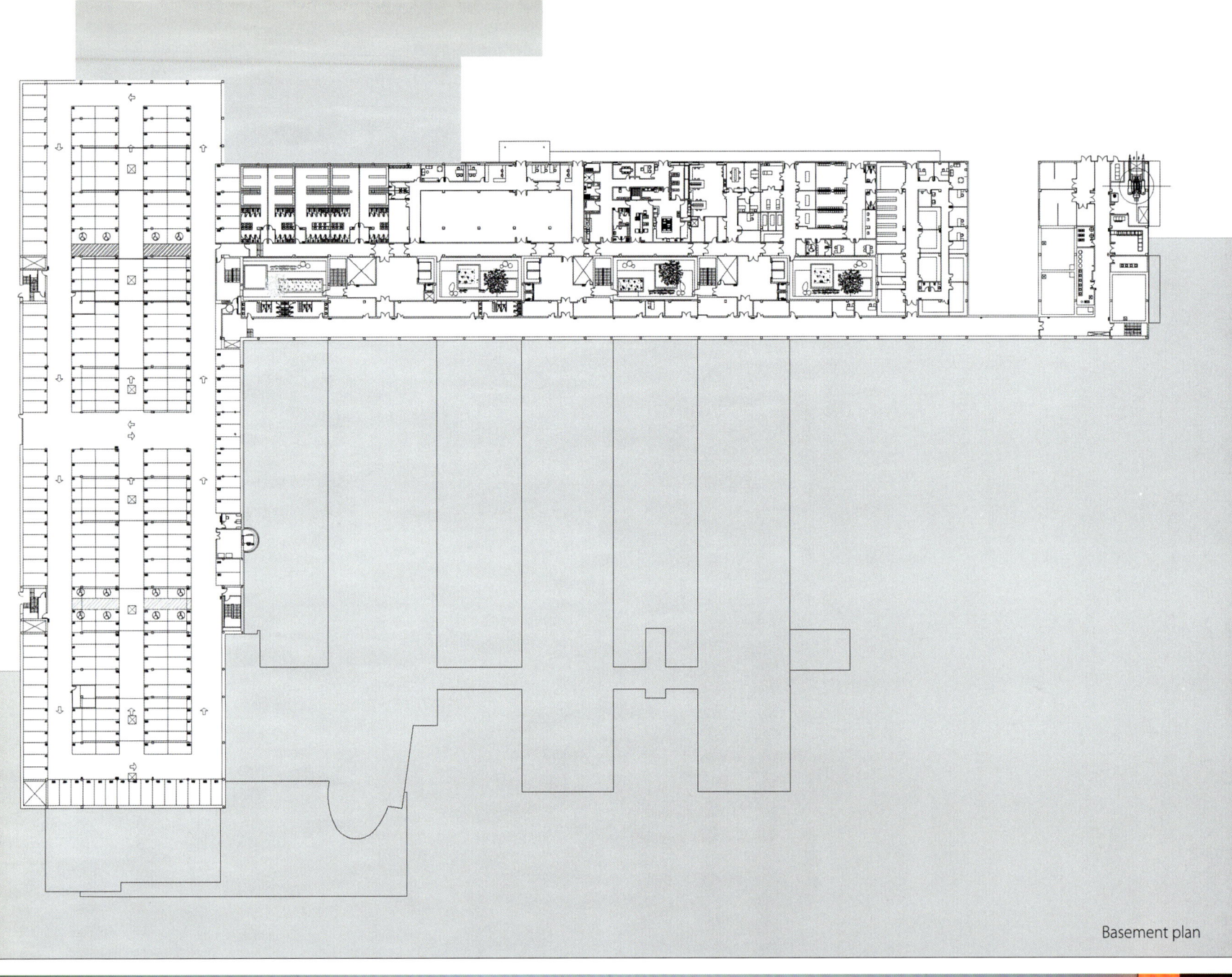

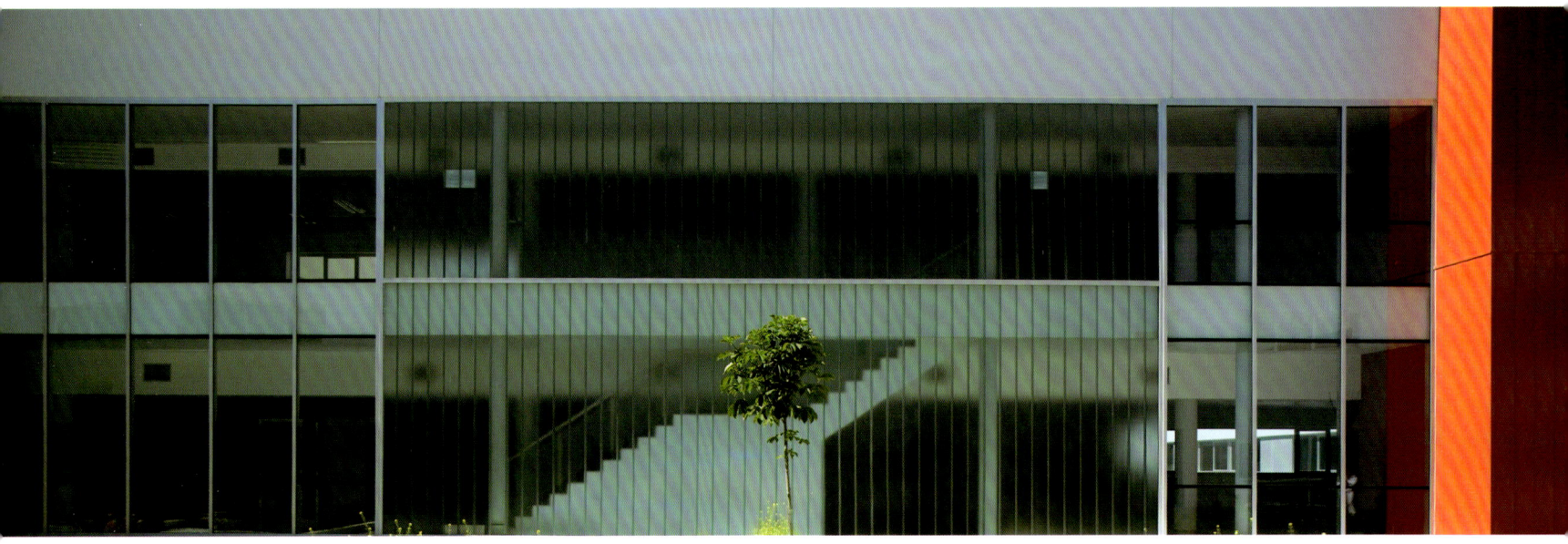

126

Ground floor plan

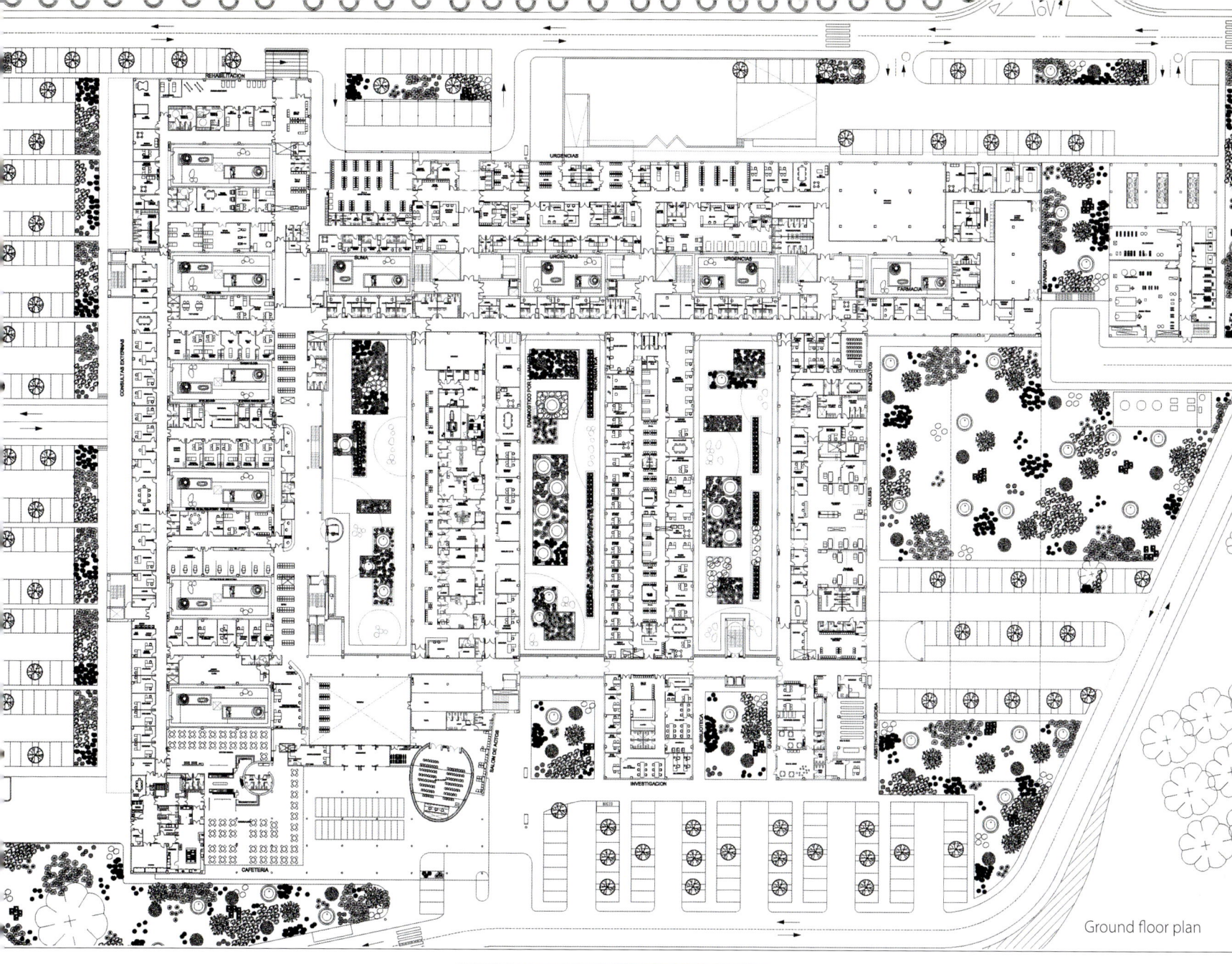

The hospital has a modular structure set within a clear orthogonal layout. Landscaped courtyards serve to separate the individual buildings and allow natural light and air to penetrate the interiors. They establish a rhythm and generate visual variation inside the hospital, breaking up the long corridors. Their design aims to produce a calming atmosphere.

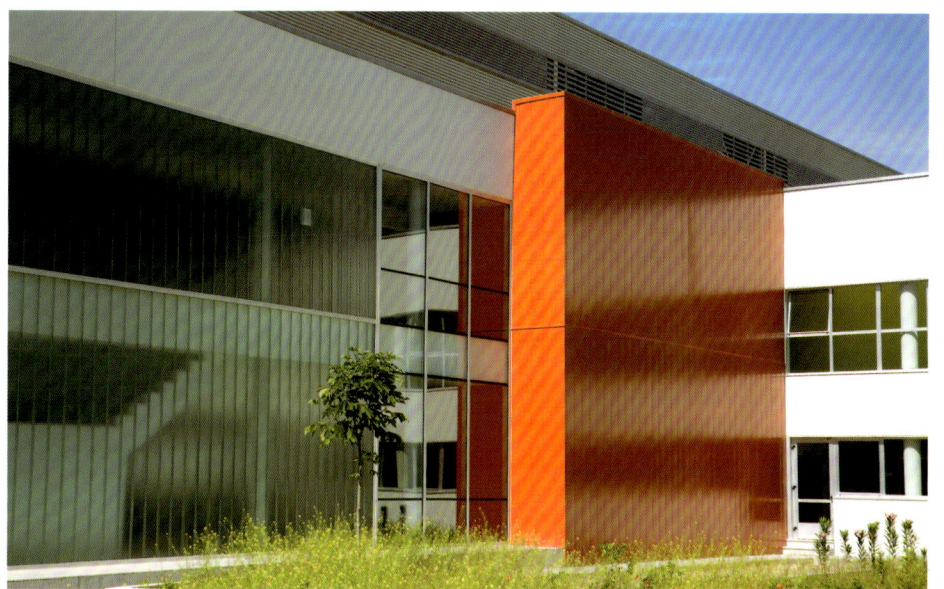

First floor plan

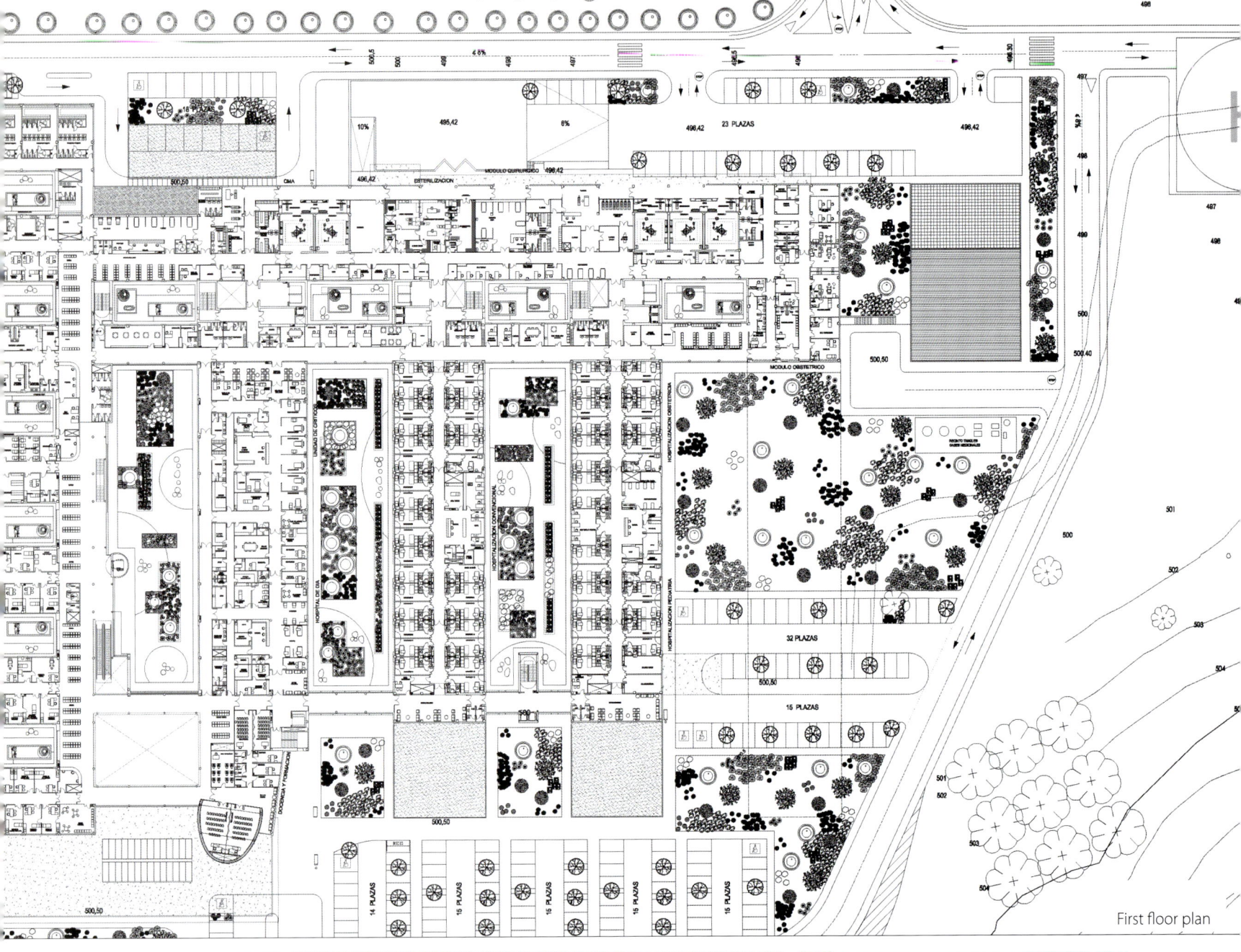

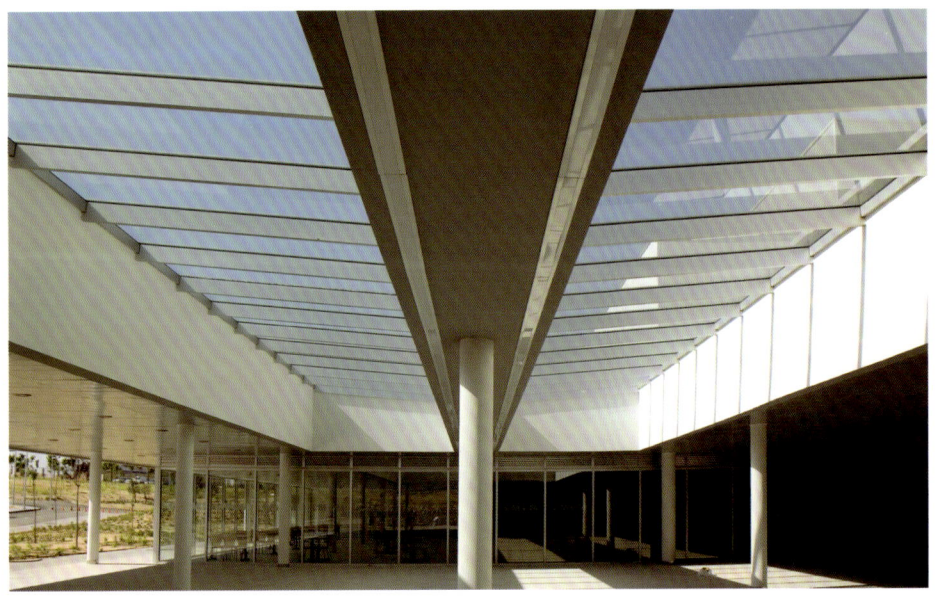

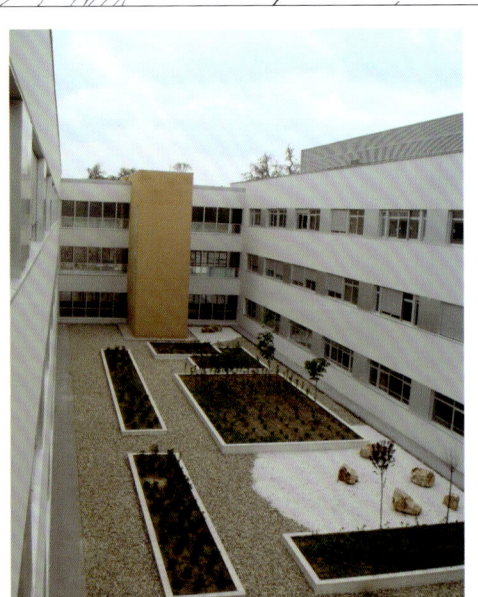

128

Second floor plan

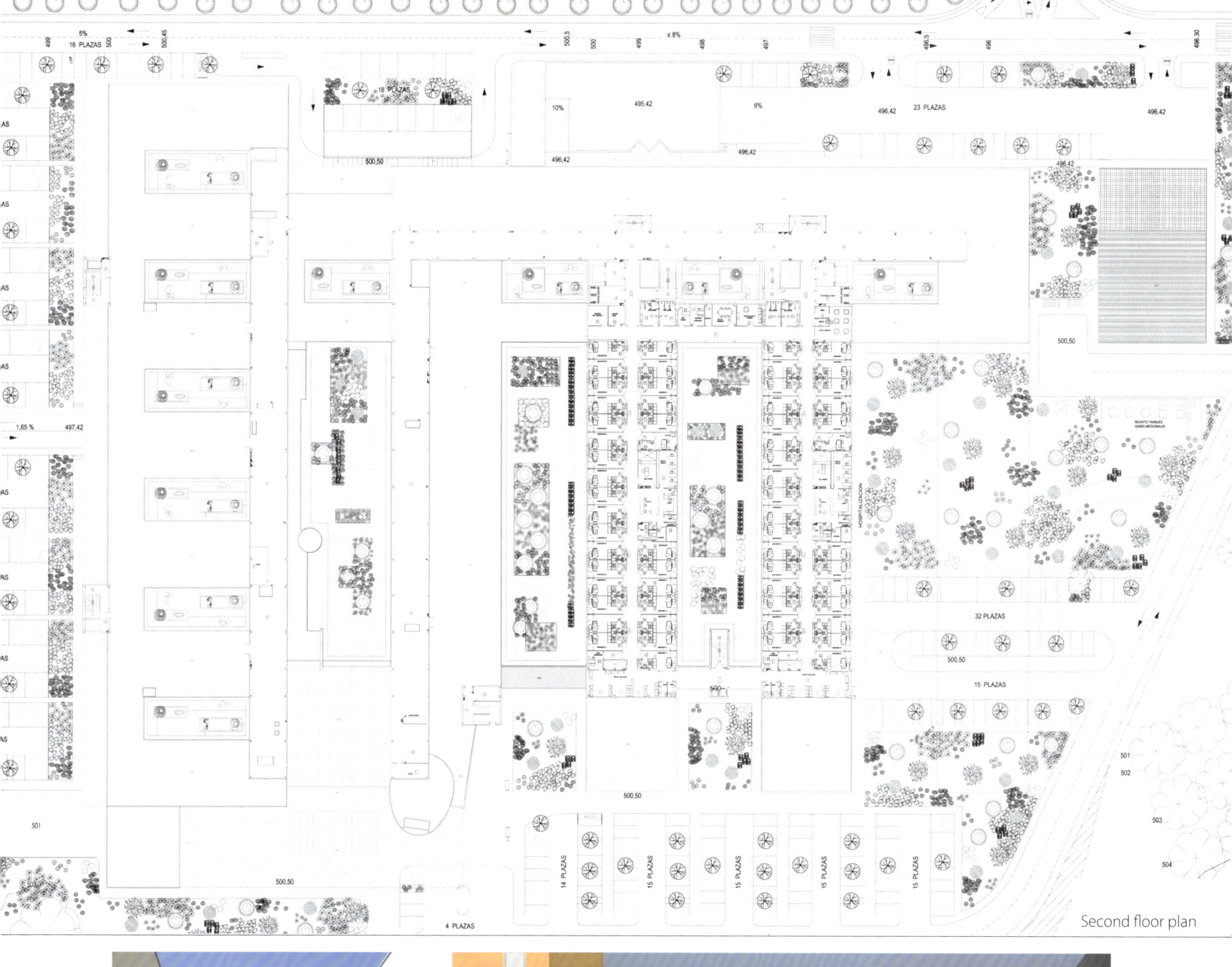

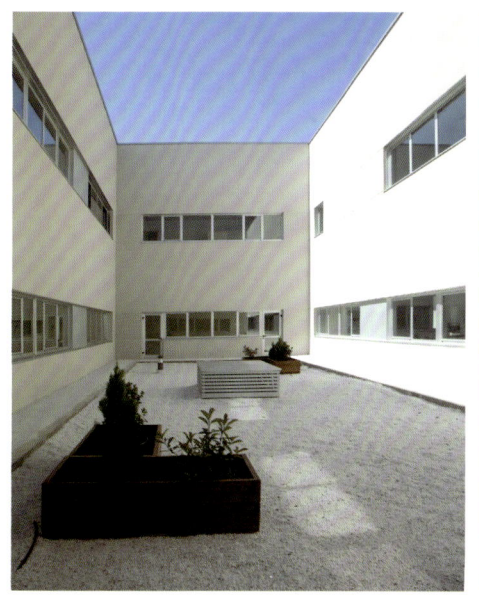

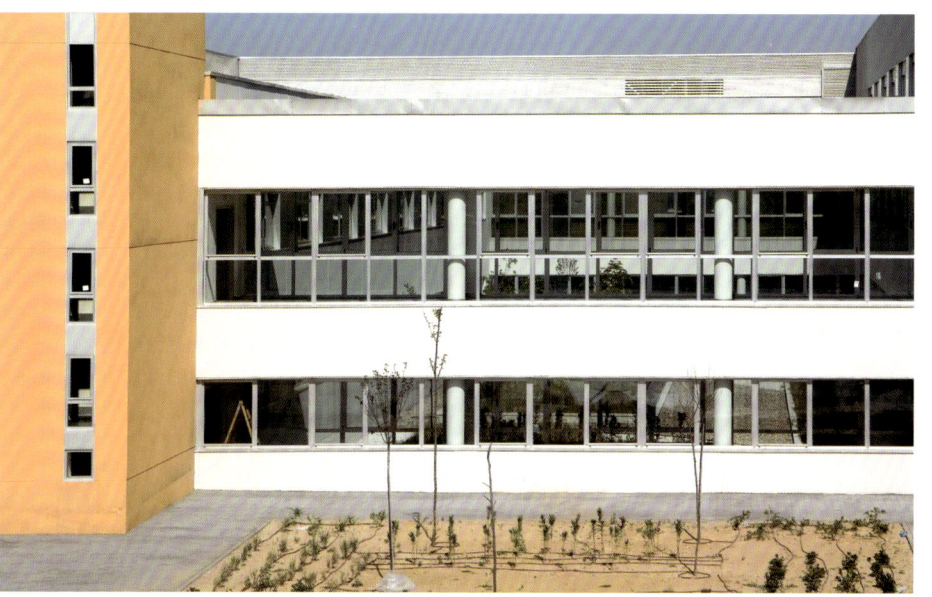

129

Roof plan

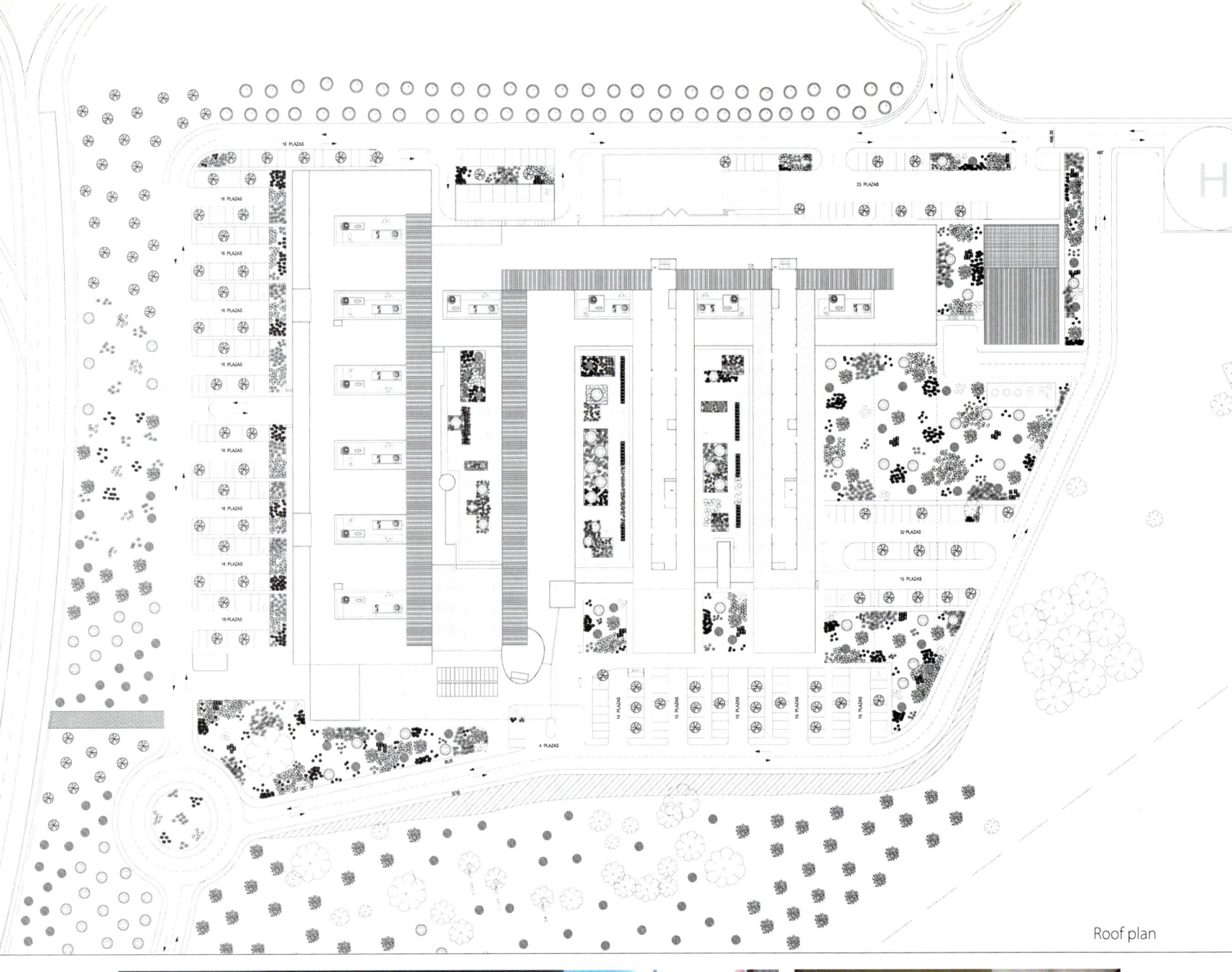

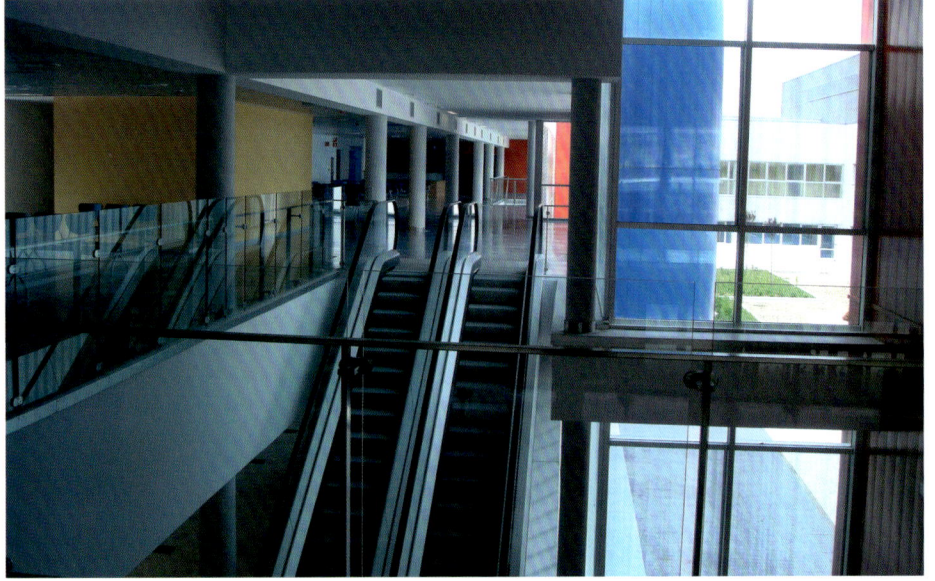

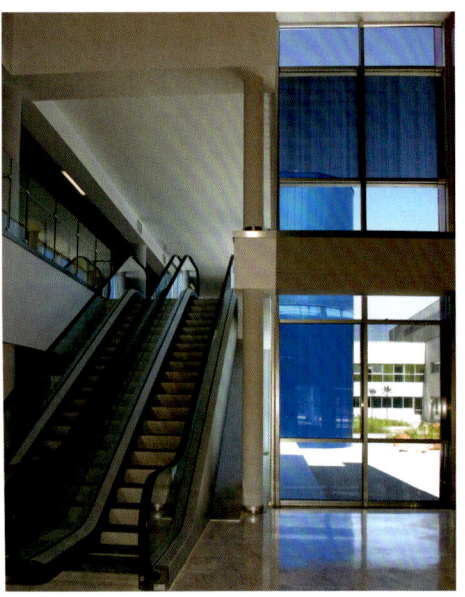

130

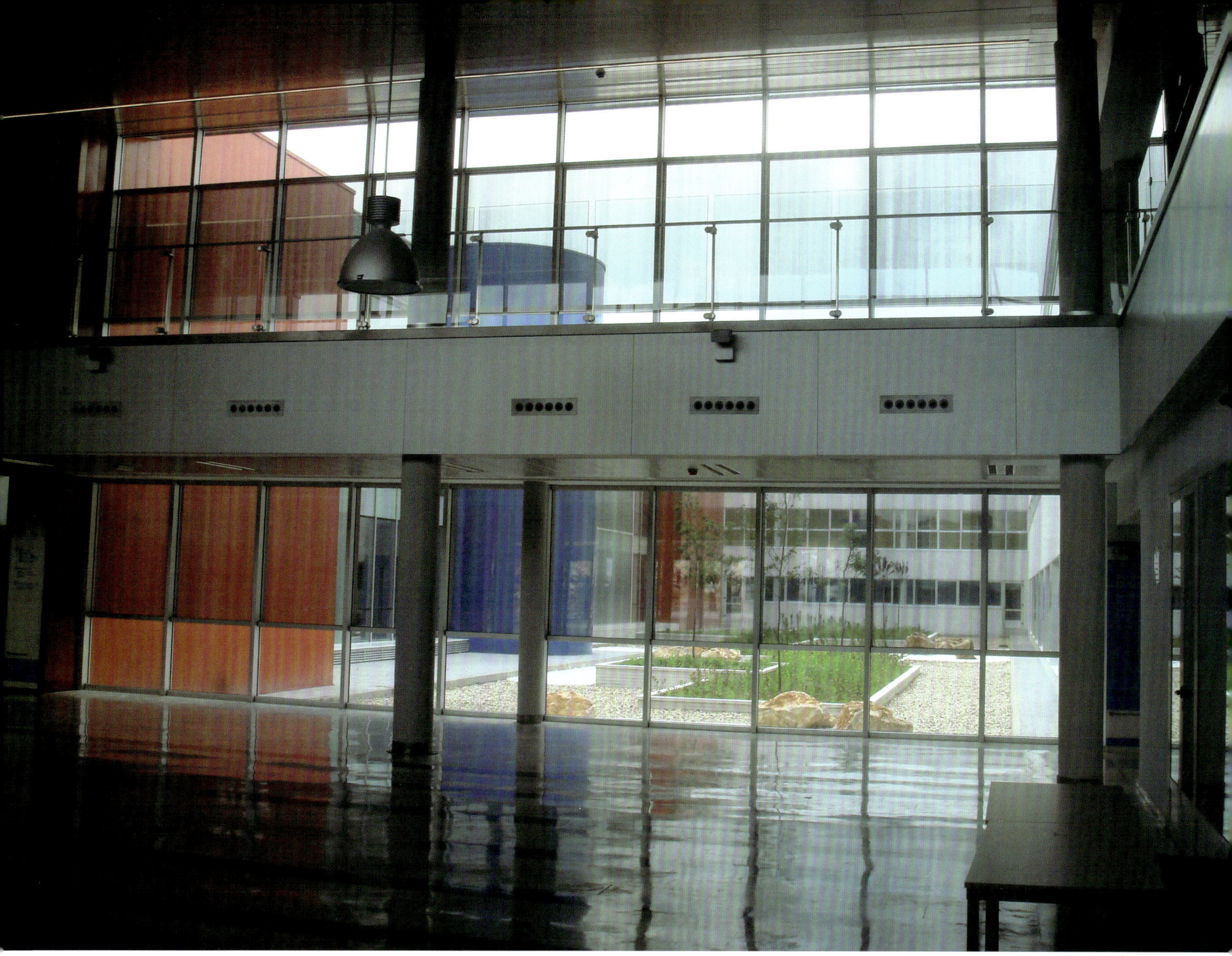

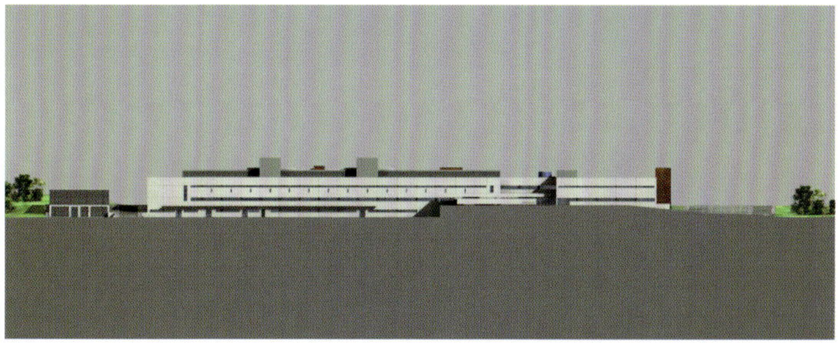

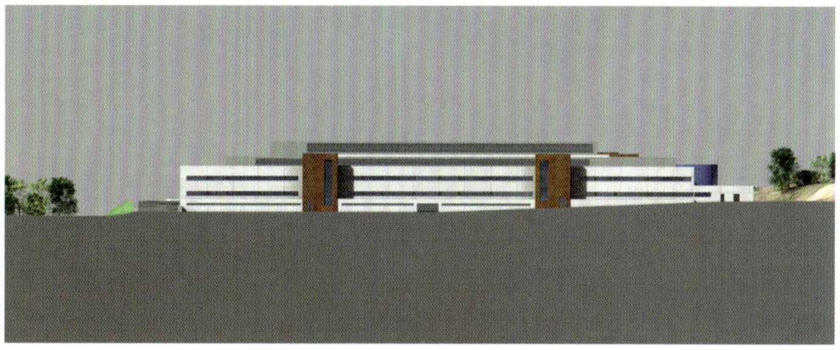

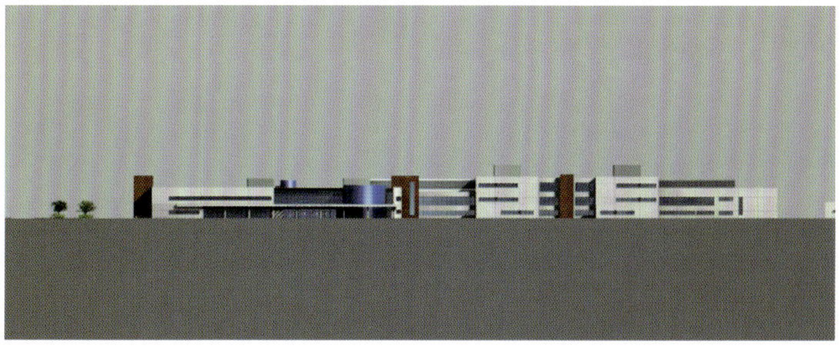

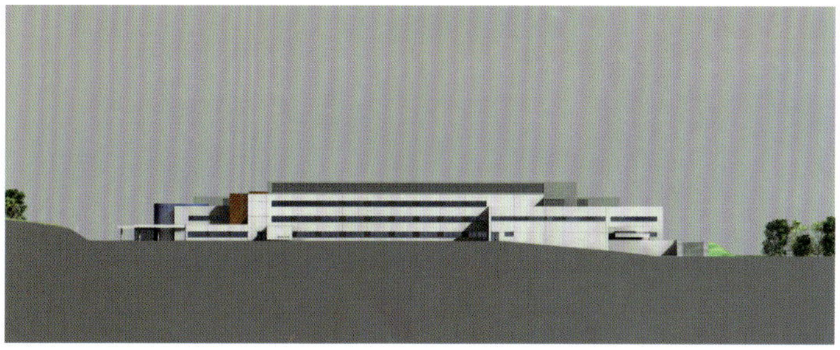

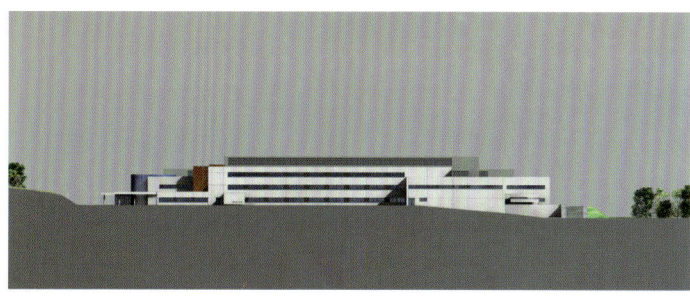

Section 1

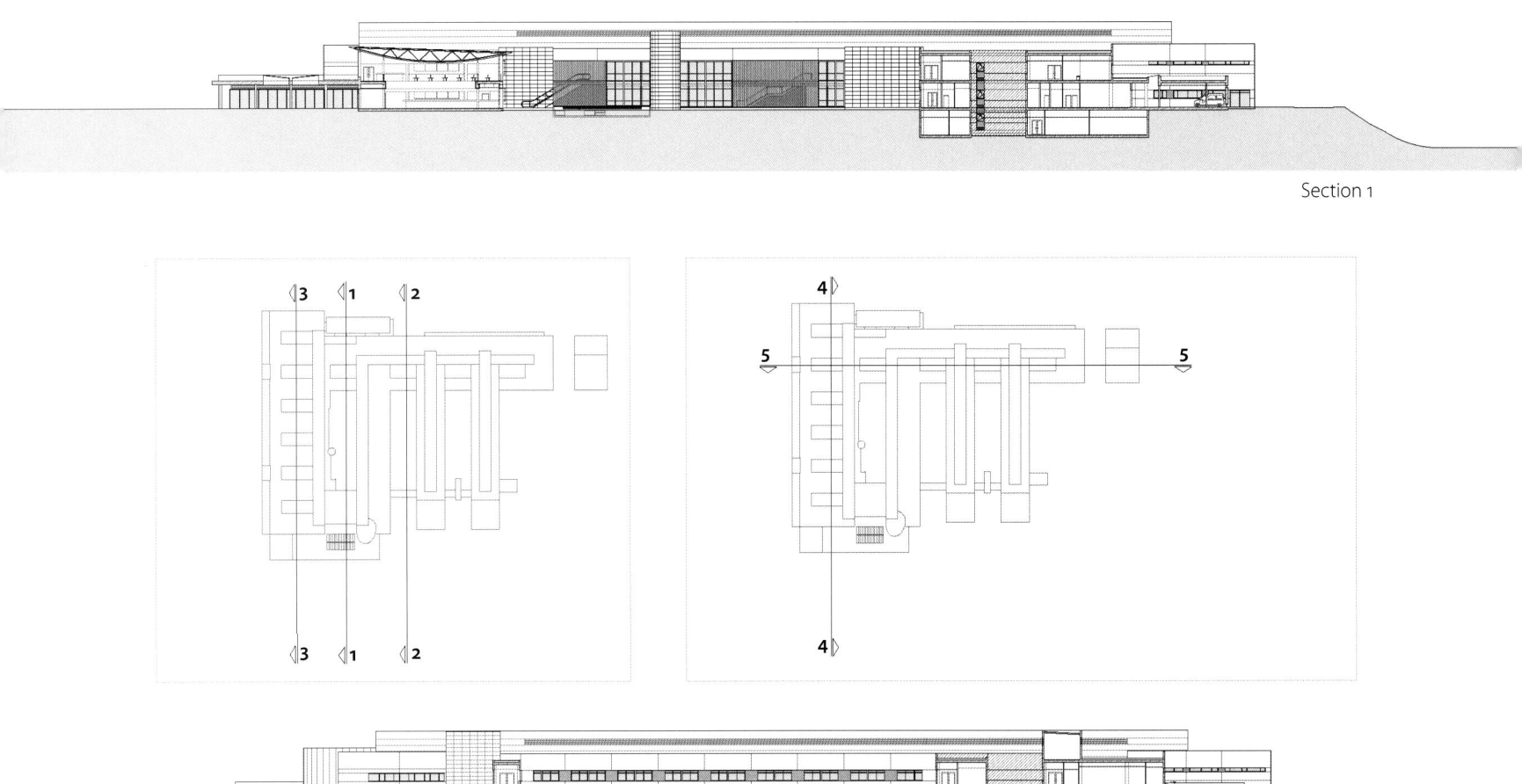

Section 2

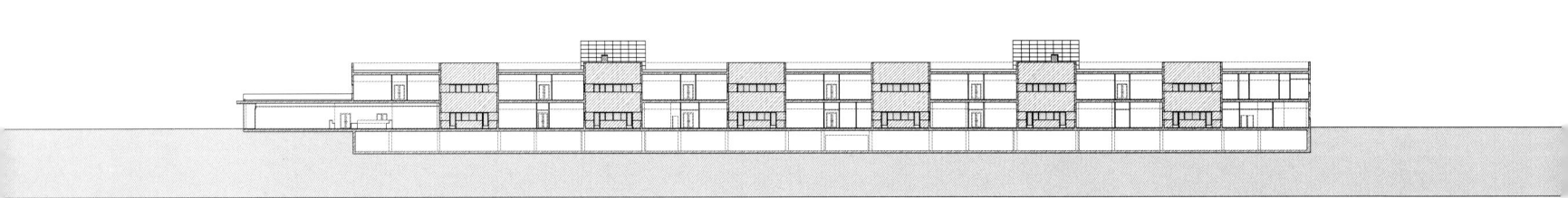

Section 3

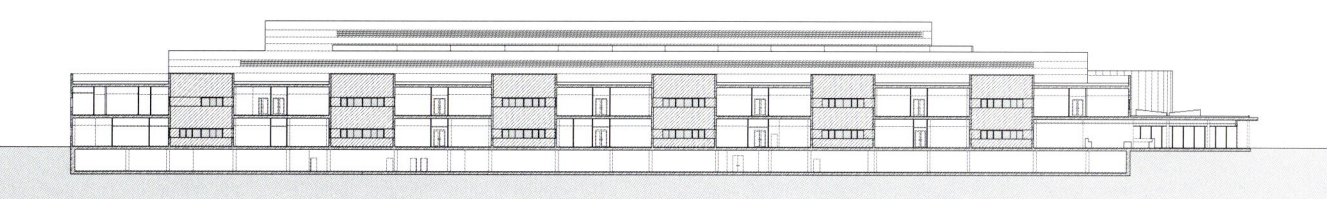

Section 4

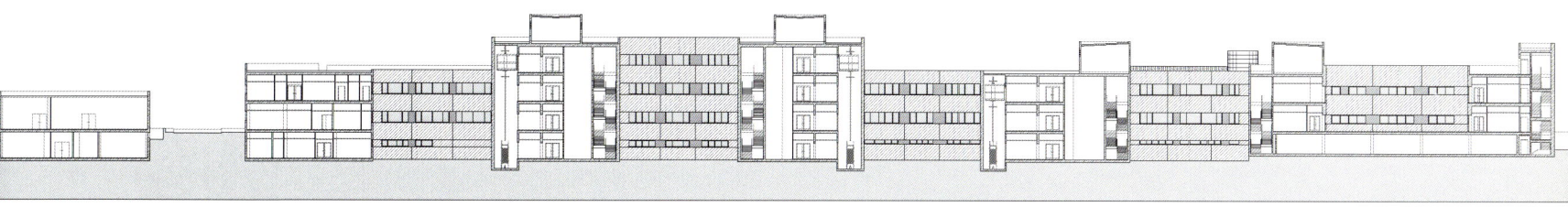

Section 5

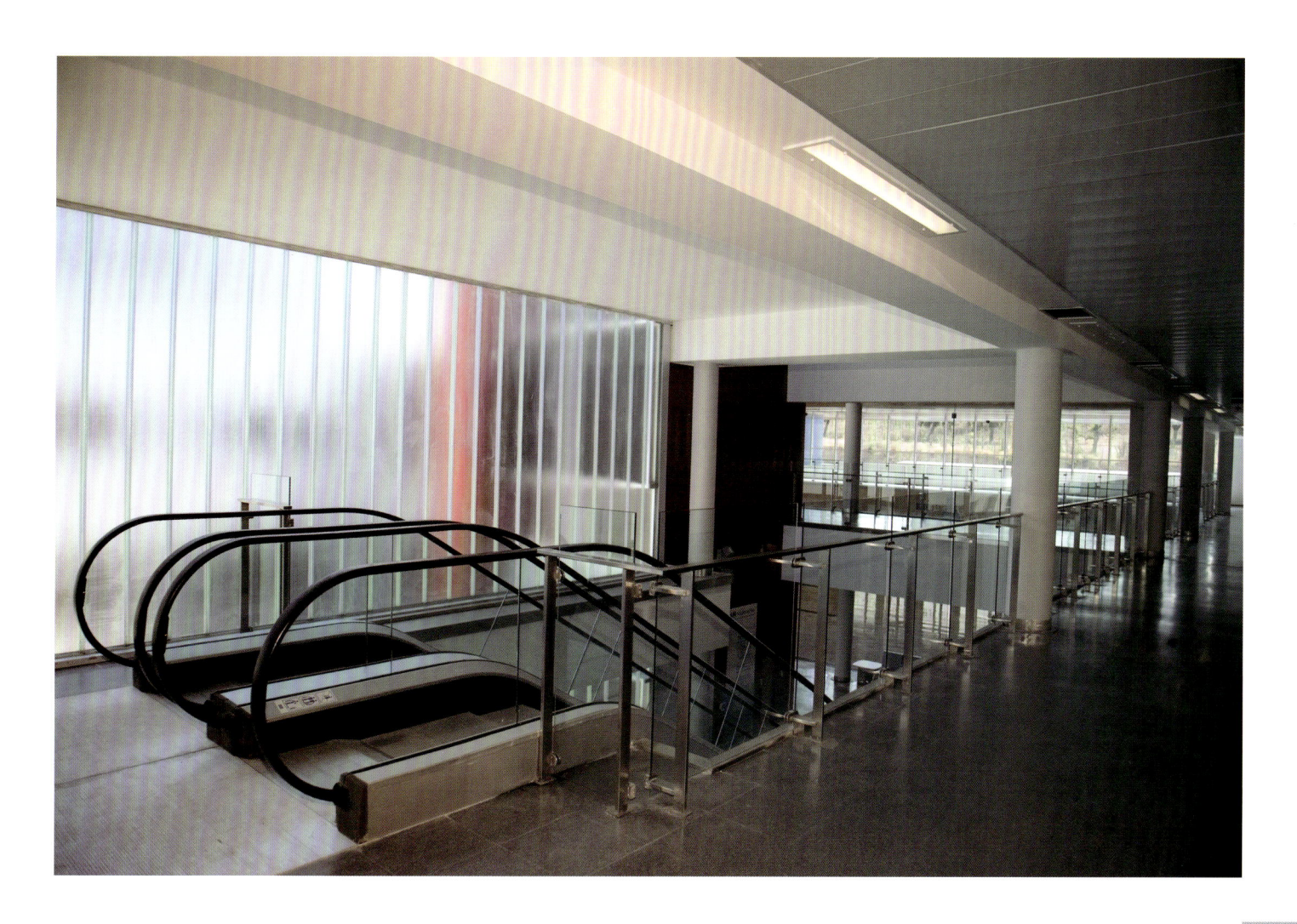

133

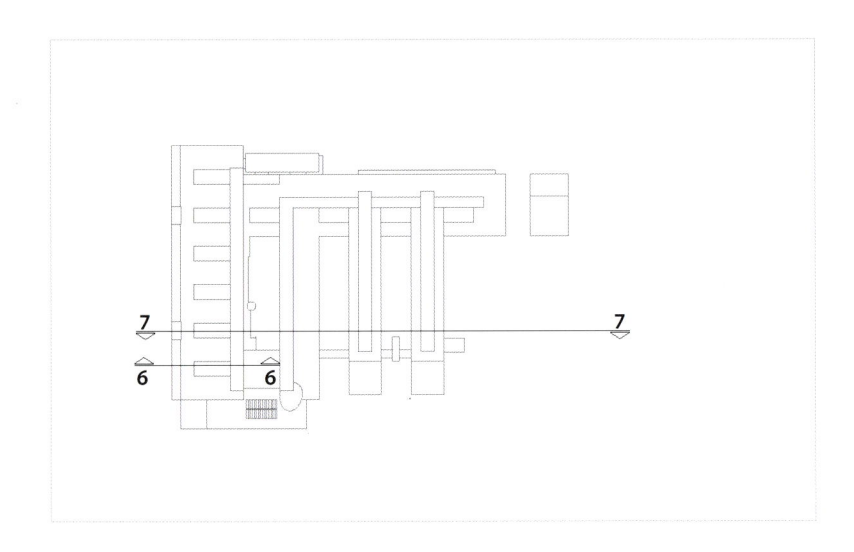

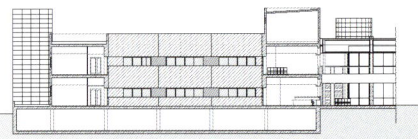

Section 6

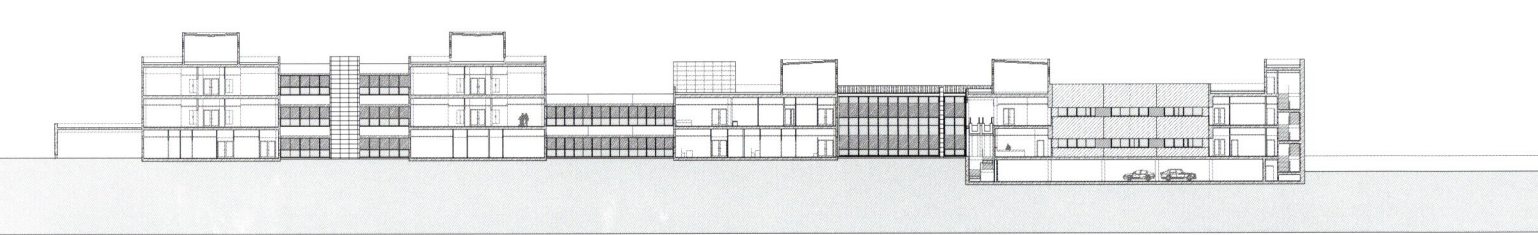

Section 7

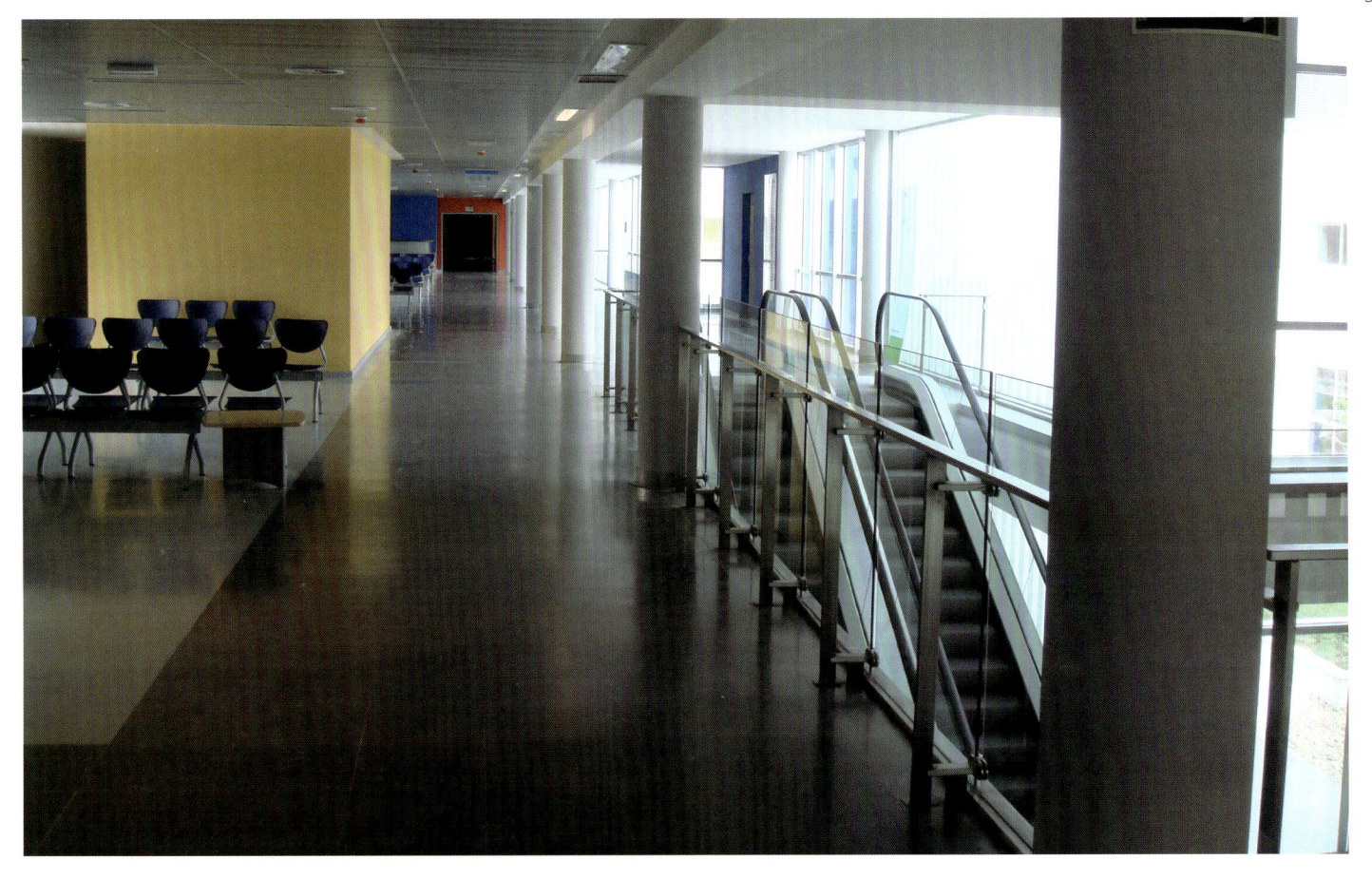

134

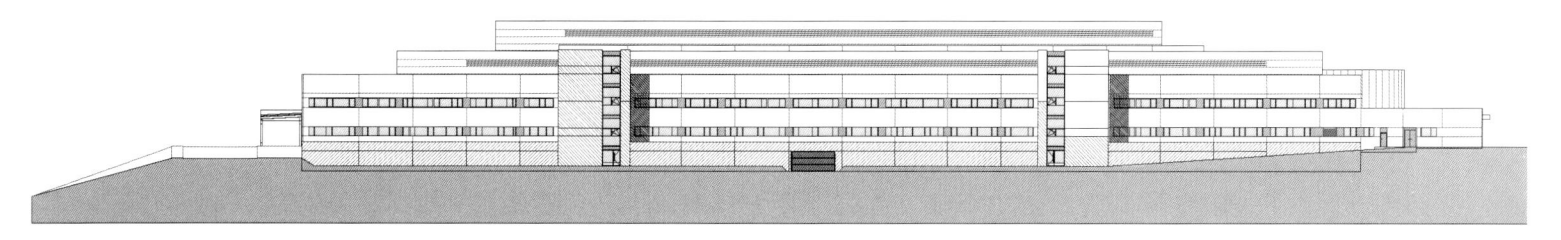

Façade 1

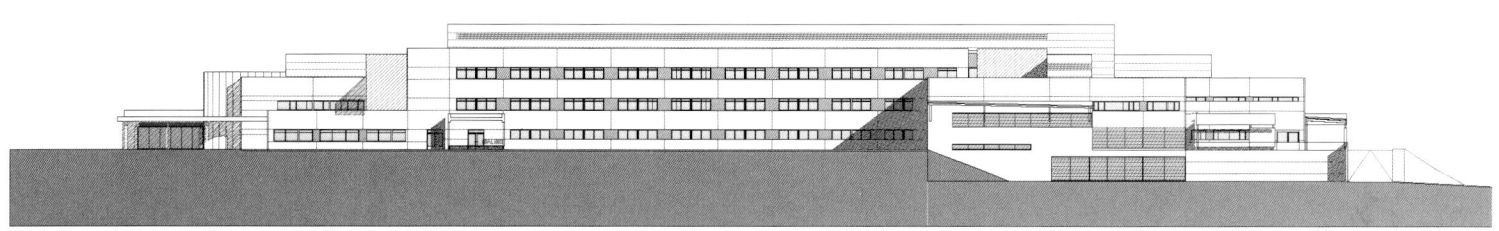

Façade 2

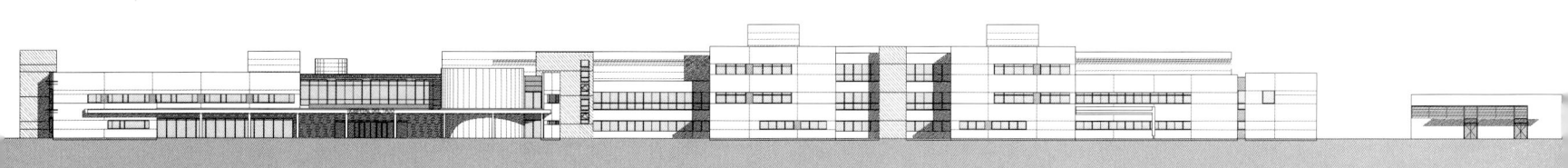

Façade 3

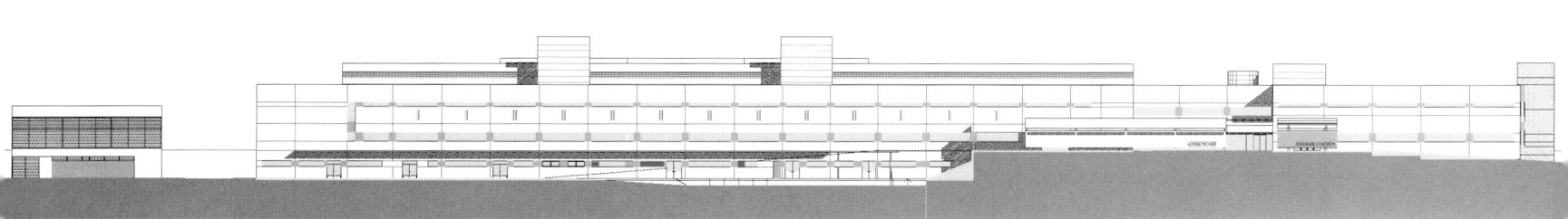

Façade 4

135

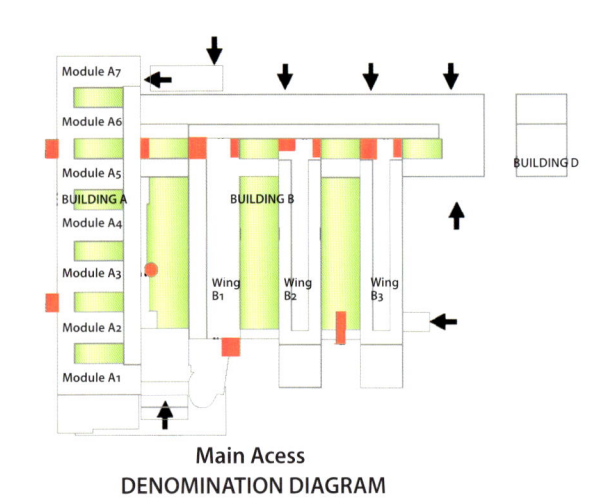

Main Acess
DENOMINATION DIAGRAM

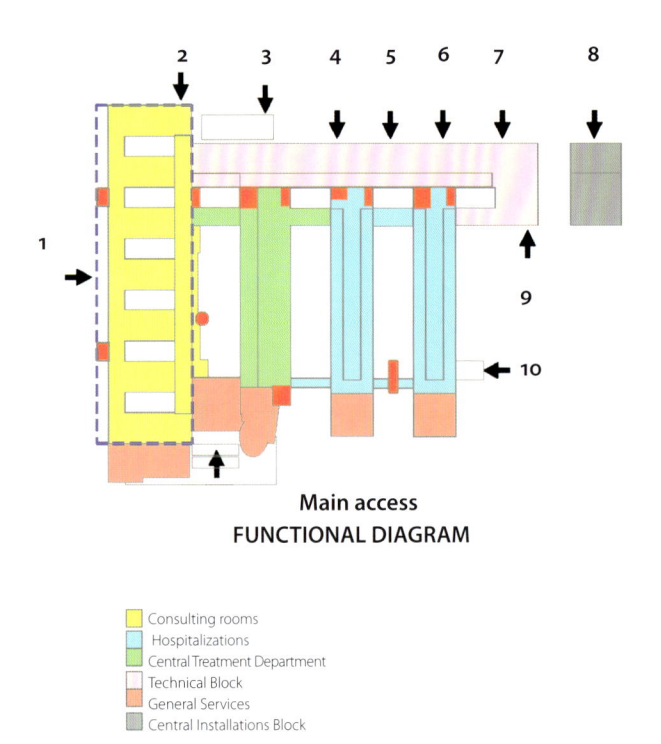

Main access
FUNCTIONAL DIAGRAM

- Consulting rooms
- Hospitalizations
- Central Treatment Department
- Technical Block
- General Services
- Central Installations Block

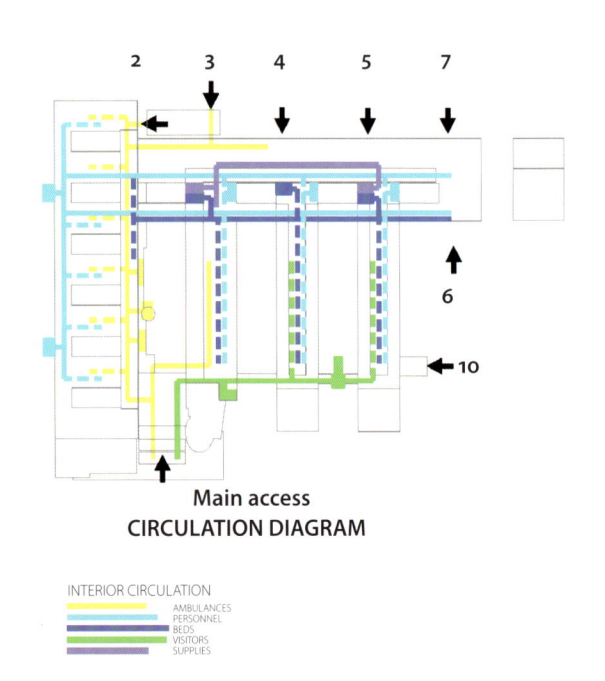

Main access
CIRCULATION DIAGRAM

INTERIOR CIRCULATION
- AMBULANCES
- PERSONNEL
- BEDS
- VISITORS
- SUPPLIES

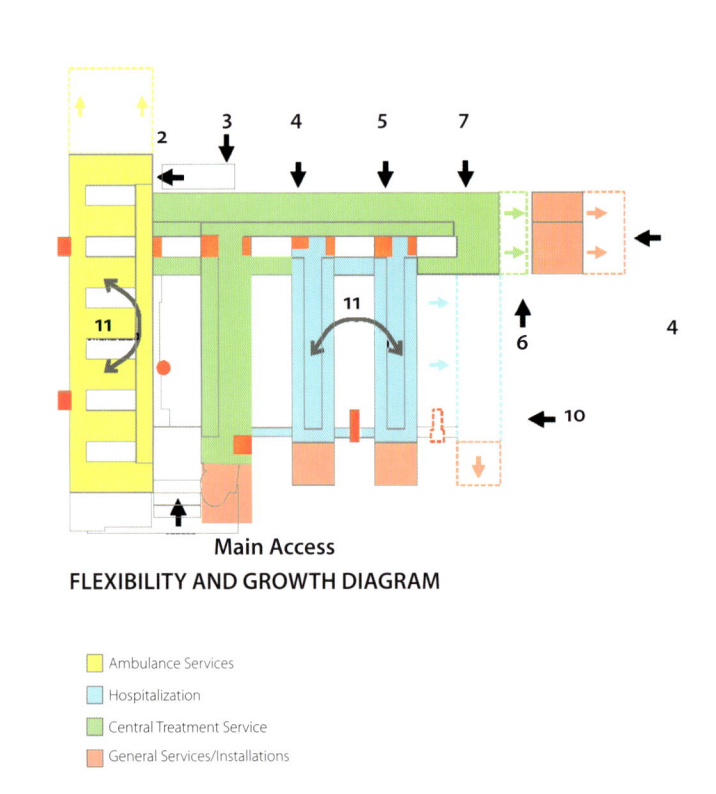

Main Access
FLEXIBILITY AND GROWTH DIAGRAM

- Ambulance Services
- Hospitalization
- Central Treatment Service
- General Services/Installations

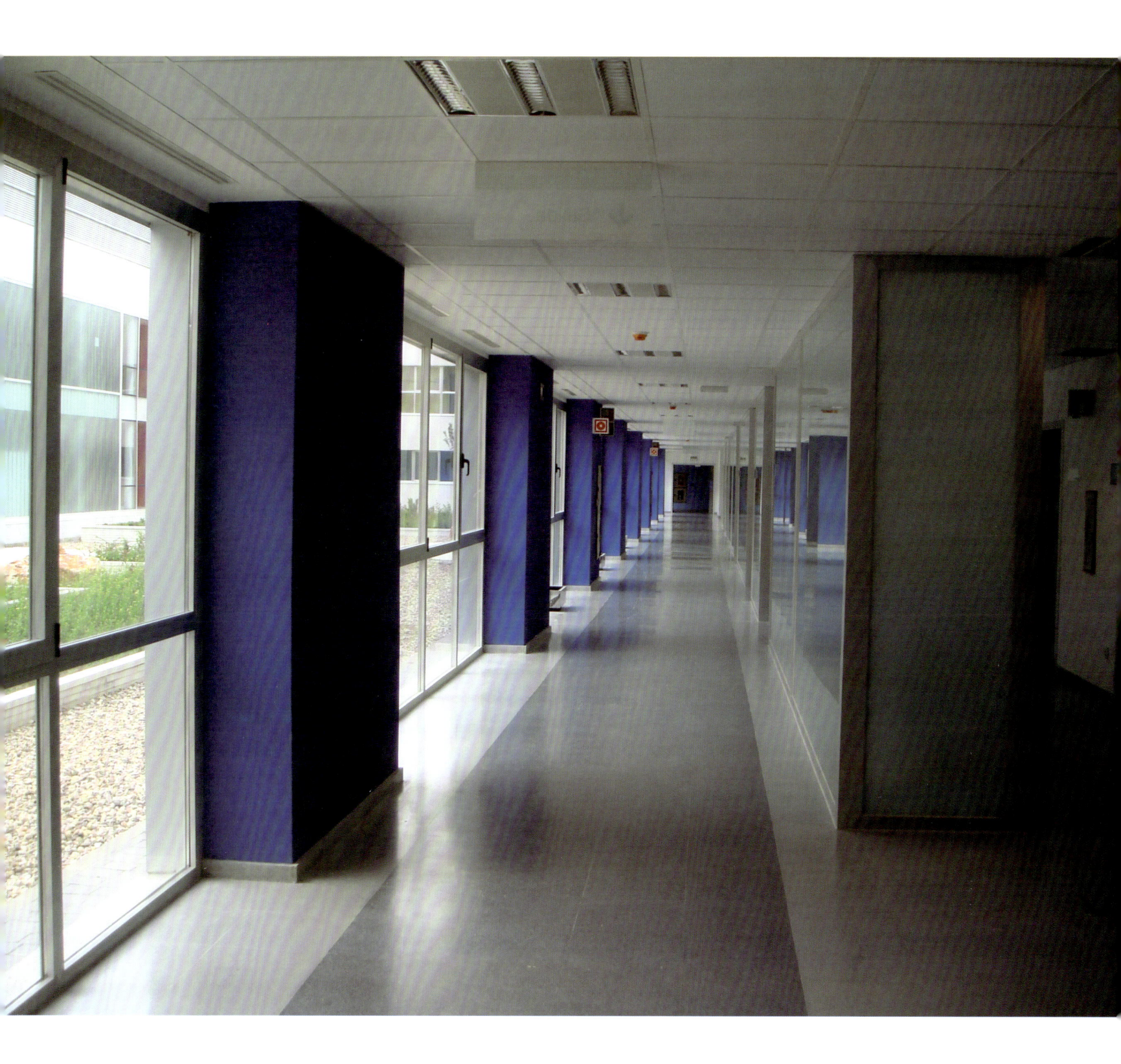

Section 1

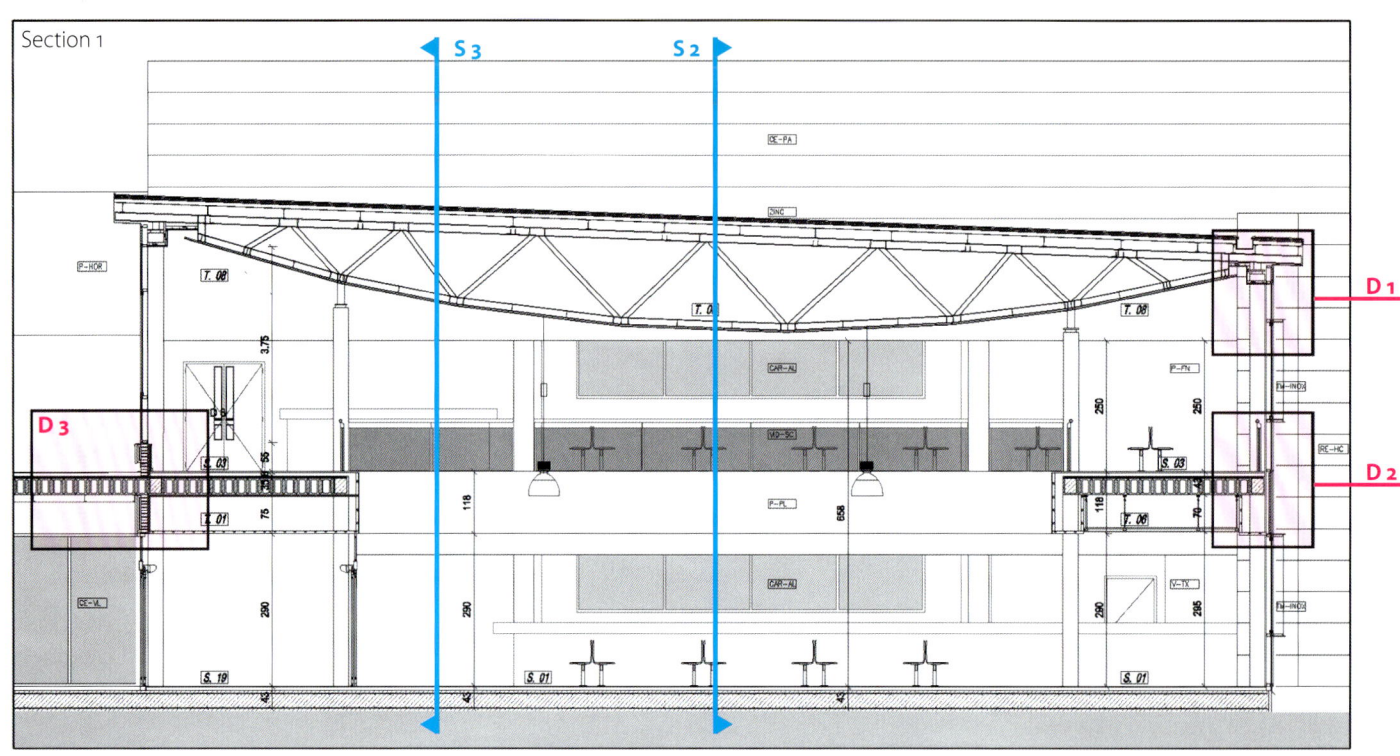

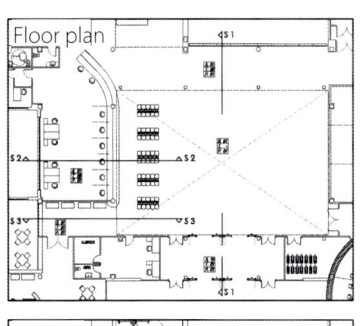

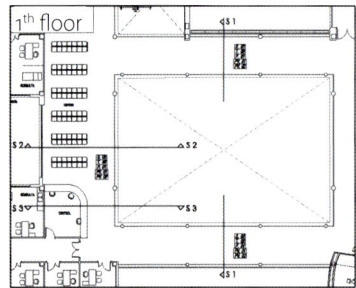

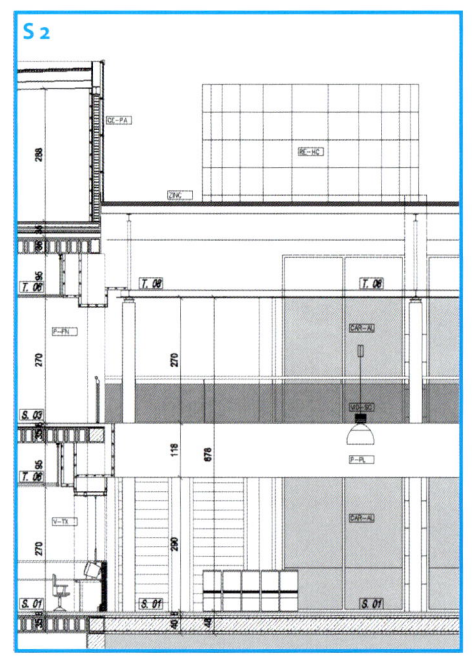

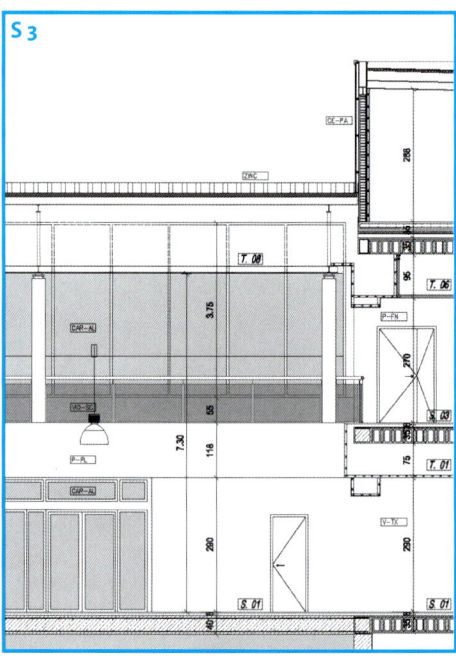

Floor plan

1th floor

S2

S3

CEILINGS:
1. Suspended ceiling-panel of fibre-reinforced plaster
2. Ceiling of micro-perforated metal 120/150x30, and anchoring piece
3. Acoustic ceiling, wood, and anchoring piece

FLOORS:
4. Polished marble floor tiles 60x40x2cm
5. Fine-grain terrazzo floor tiles 60x40x3.5cm
6. Carpet of aluminium angles and PVC lamellae

WALLS:
7. Vinyl cladding, "Vescon" or equivalent type
8. Flat plastic paint on fibre reinforced plaster
9. Flat plastic paint on "veloglass" or equivalent material
10. Compact gres tiles, 20x20cm

VERTICAL PROTECTIONS:
11. High protection for trolleys and beds
12. Low protection for trolleys and beds

FAÇADE:
13. Oxy-lacquered aluminium carpentry
14. Concrete panel
15. Lamellae of galvanized steel
16. Oxy-lacquered aluminium panel
17. Stainless steel wire mesh
18. Security glass
19. Galvanized steel grating
20. Prefabricated concrete slab cladding, coloured
21. Zinc roofing, raised joint
22. Sandwich panel enclosure
23. Laminated glass enclosure
24. Plastic paint

CEILINGS:	FAÇADE:
T.01 1	CAR-AL 13
T.06 2	P-HOR 14
T.08 3	LAM-AG 15
FLOORS:	PL-AOX 16
S.01 4	TM-INOX 17
S.03 5	VID-SC 18
S.19 6	R-AG 19
WALLS:	RE-HC 20
P.01 7	ZINC 21
P.03 8	CE-PA 22
P.04 9	CE-VL 23
P.06 10	P-PL 24
VERTICAL PROTECTIONS:	
PV.1 11	
PV.2 12	

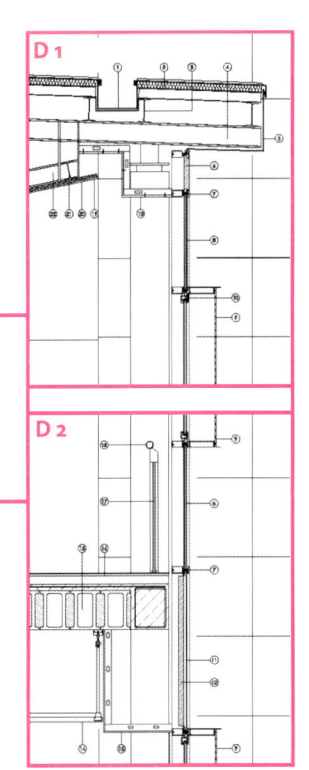

CAPTIONS: DETAILS D1 + D2:

1. Roof gutter.
2. Zinc roof over extruded polystyrene foam panel and vapour barrier.
3. IPE strap.
4. HEB 160.
5. Aluminium flashing
6. Sandwich panel.
7. Curtain wall, aluminium carpentry.
8. CLIMALIT glass 6/ 12/ 3+3
9. Wire mesh, galvanized steel.
10. Hinged aluminium carpentry.
11. Security glass.
12. Insulation panel.
13. Ceiling panel of fibre-reinforced plaster, suspended from auxiliary structure.
14. Ceiling of micro-perforated metal 120/150x30, with strap and auxiliary structure.
15. Two-way reinforced concrete, edge 30+5cm, kept light by prefab concrete arches20x70x28cm.
16. Terrazzo flooring 60x40x3,5cm, fine-grain.
17. Security glass.
18. Tube n6 mm.
19. Acoustic ceiling, wood, strap.
20. Thermo acoustic insulation, rockwool e=5cm.
21. HEB 140
22. HEB 140

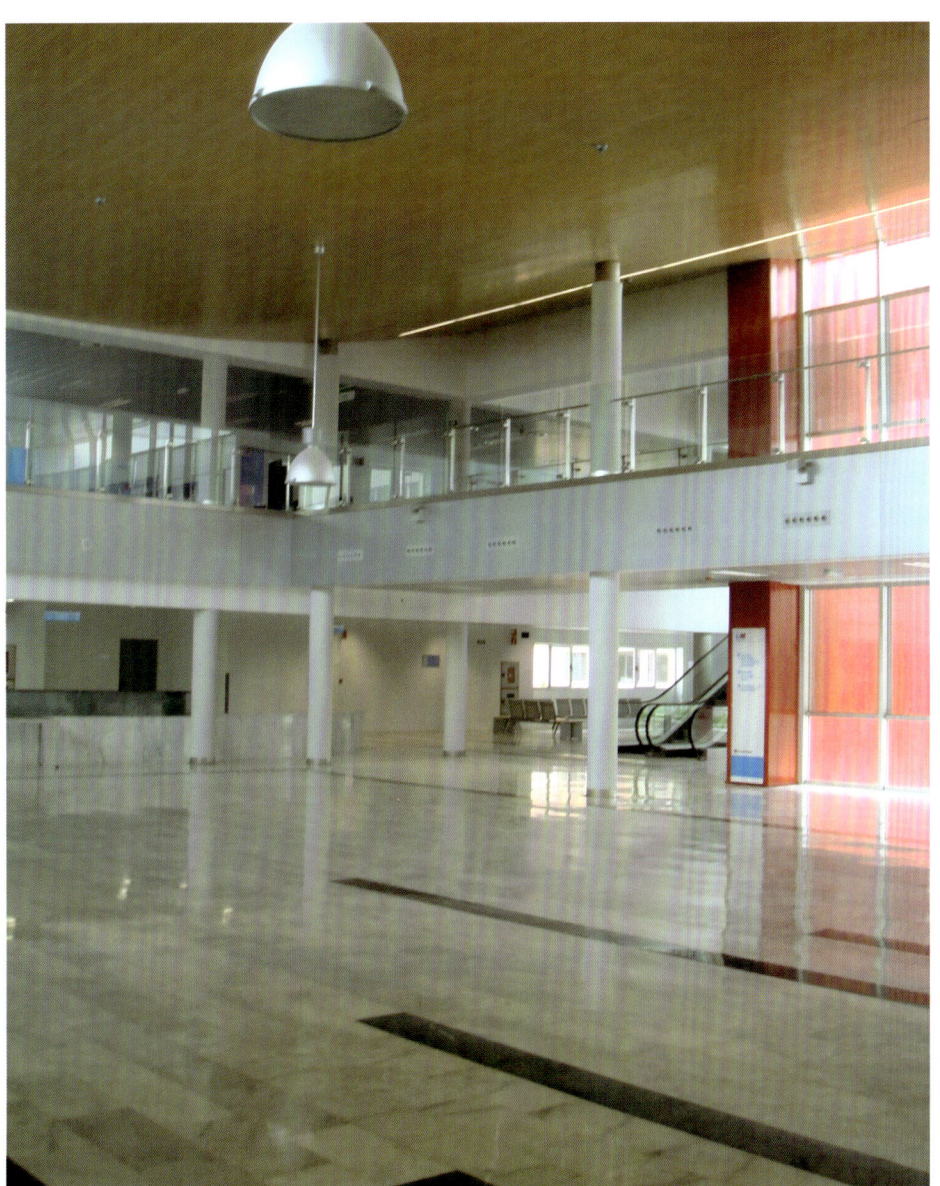

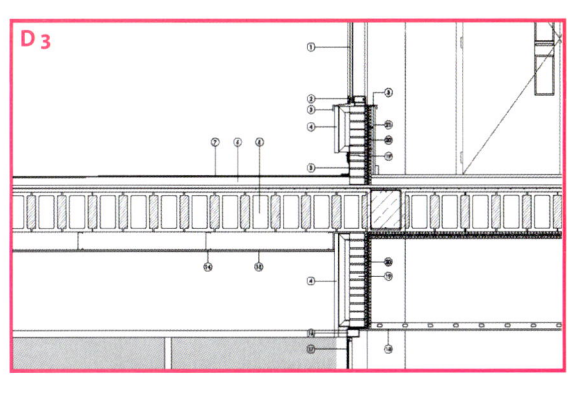

CAPTIONS: DETAILS D3:

1. CLIMALIT glass 6/ 12/ 3+3
2. Curtain wall, aluminium carpentry.
3. Aluminium flashing.
4. Wood cladding with auxiliary structure.
5. Two-way reinforced concrete structure, edge 25+5, kept light by prefab concrete arches 20x70x28 cm.
6. Cellular concrete for slope. Average e= 10 cm
7. Vynil-rubber finish
14. Metal angles.
15. Ceiling. Metal panels.
16. Metal frame
17. Aluminium carpentry
18. Ceiling panel of fibre-reinforced plaster, suspended from auxiliary structure
19. 1/2 foot hollow brick wall
20. Sprayed polyurethane, e=5cm
21. Rocksheet panel of "Pladur" or similar material, with auxiliary structure.

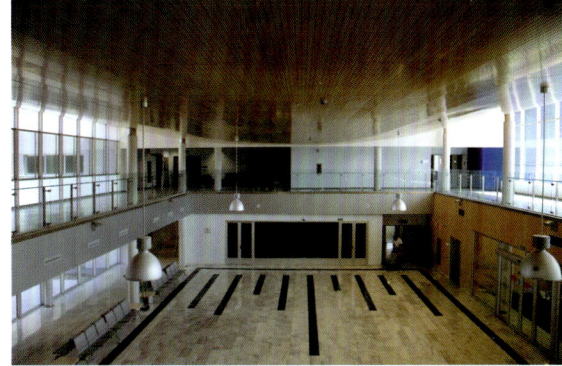

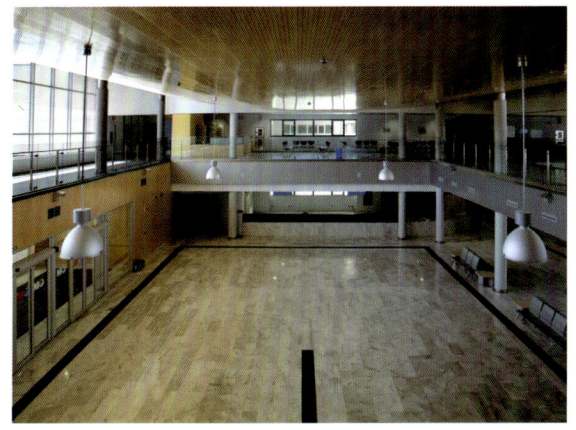

Carvajal + Casariego Baquerizo Cruz Petrement

Reina Sofia Hospital

Murcia, Spain

Photographs: Luis Asín and Carvajal Casariego

The building for this hospital has been erected on the site of the former hospital, which covers a floor surface area of 25,000 sqm (270,000 sqft). The hospital building has been positioned within the irregularly shaped site to integrate with its urban surroundings, while at the same time meeting all the requirements laid down by the client. Three parallel volumes were projected that define two intermediate courtyards completed by the maintenance and installations building, emplaced on the adjoining plot and connected to the main buildings through below grade passageways. There is also an underground car park with spaces for 1,000 vehicles.

Two service roads have been created on the main site running parallel to the nearby river, which fragment the built volume in three staggered bodies. The main façade overlooks the public square, set between the lightly curved building front and the river. The more internal services have been designated to the third volume. The sequence between the public spaces and outpatients department and the more technical hospital services therefore develops naturally, allowing for simple circulation routes.

The first eight-story body is essentially destined to administration and hospital wards, with all rooms on the upper stories positioned to maximize the sunlight and the views. Functions of a more public nature such as the cafeteria, shops and main entrances are also located in this volume. The building is crowned by a sloping roof that supports strips of solar panels. These create an interplay of reflections which form attractive contrasts with the gray stone used for the roof.

The regular orthogonal central volume defined on either side by the service roads houses the outpatient clinics and the examination rooms, supported by their complementary services. The gray sheet metal façade is enlivened by the continuous strip of windows. The modulation of this central block allows for the different parts that comprise it to have different sizes without this being visible from the outside.

The third body, which is smaller because of the need to maintain two existing buildings on the site, houses internal clinical functions with restricted access to the public. These include the emergency department, laboratories and operating theatres. Finishes here are similar to those of the central volume with a sheet metal façade, continuous openings and a flat roof.

The hospital's layout is supported by a clear circulation system and offers sufficient flexibility to meet future modifications. The network of passageways has been designed to take into account the different functions, guaranteeing intimacy in private areas and creating comfortable environments in the more public ones.

Client:
Murcia Health Service
Surface area:
95,000 sqm (1,023,000 sqft)
Start date:
2000
Finish date:
2004
Project team:
Pedro Casariego, Genaro Alas, Jose Manuel Baquerizo, Fernando Cruz, Carlos Petrement, Gádor de Carvajal and Juan Casariego
Collaborators:
Patricia Reznak, V.Aguilar-Amat, F.López, M.Pascual, A.Navarro, A.Montero, I.Prieto, O.Paz, P.Martínez
Contractor:
Ferrovial Agroman, S.A., FCC Construcción, S.A. U.T.E.

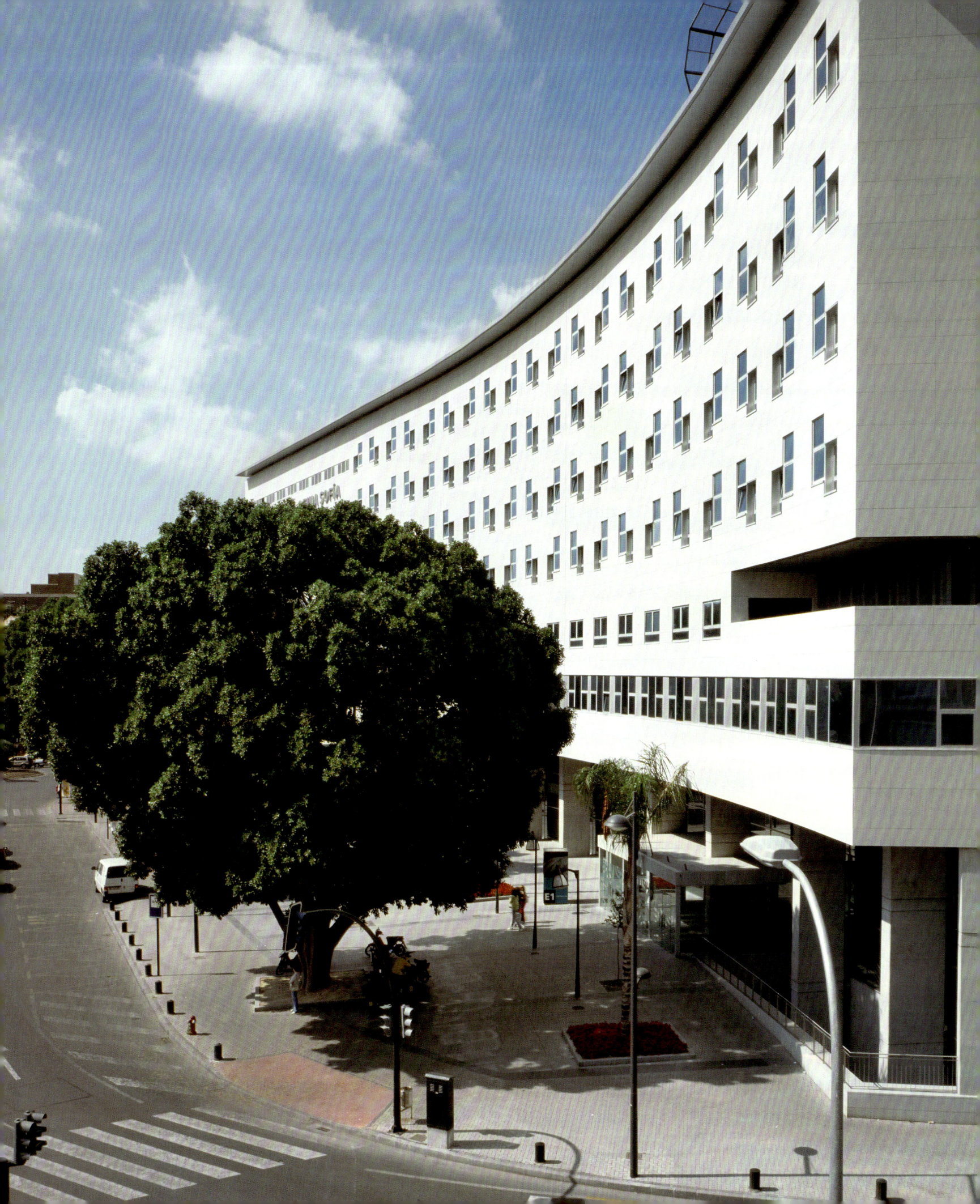

142

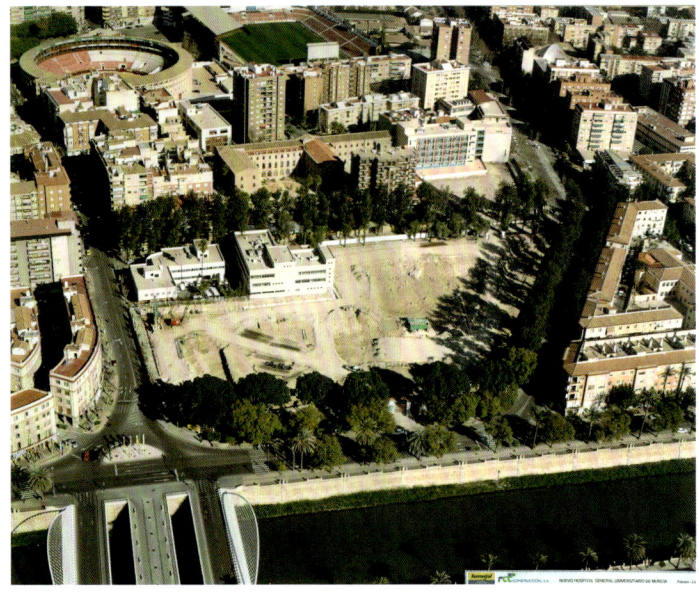

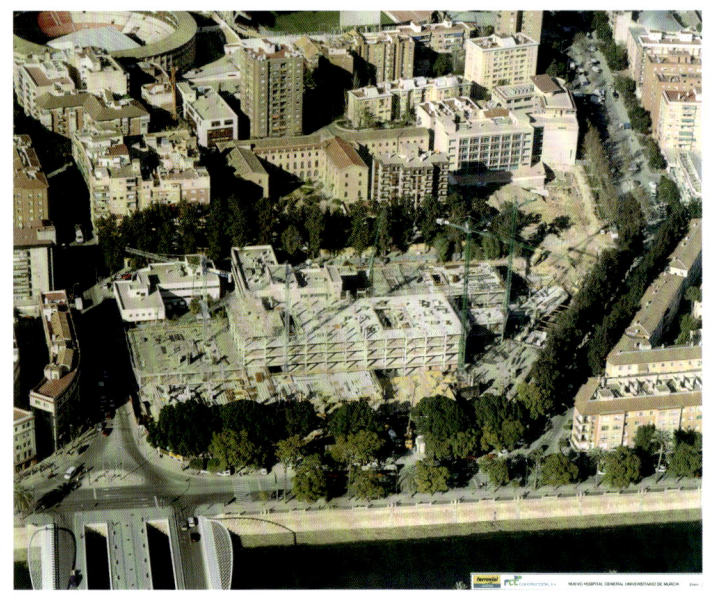

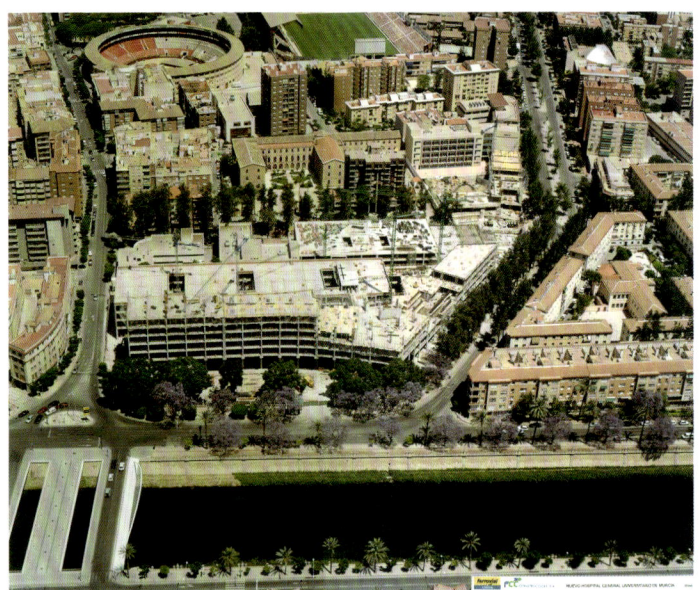

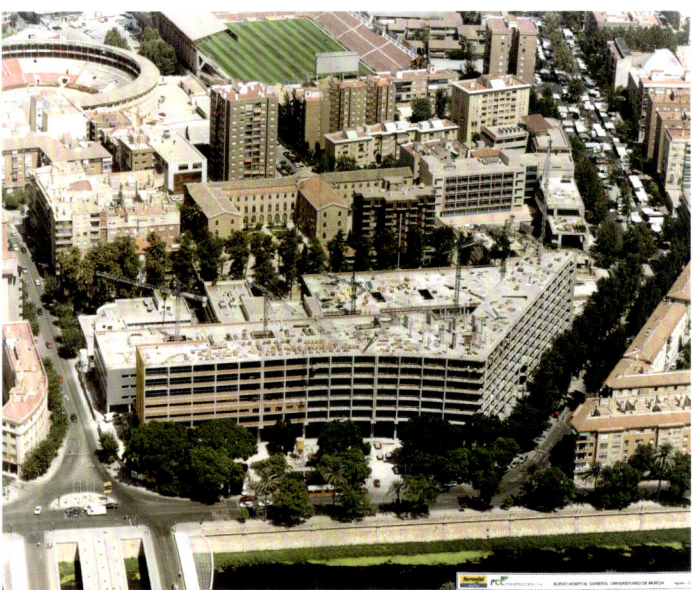

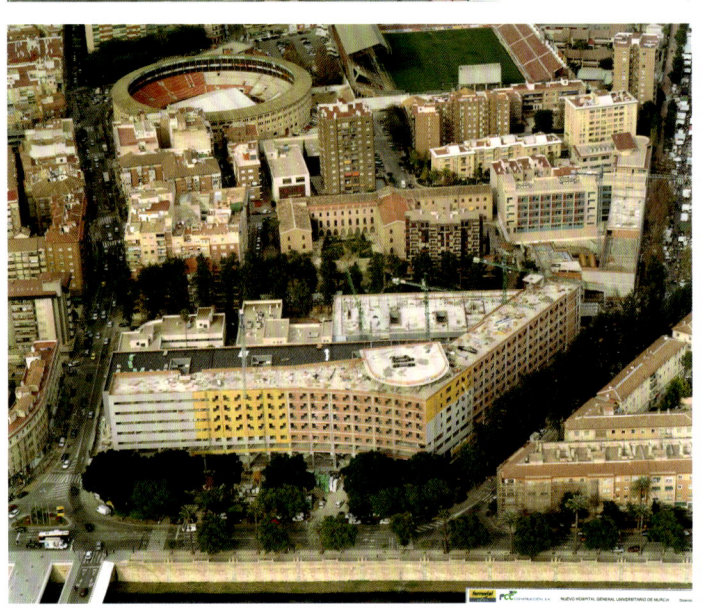

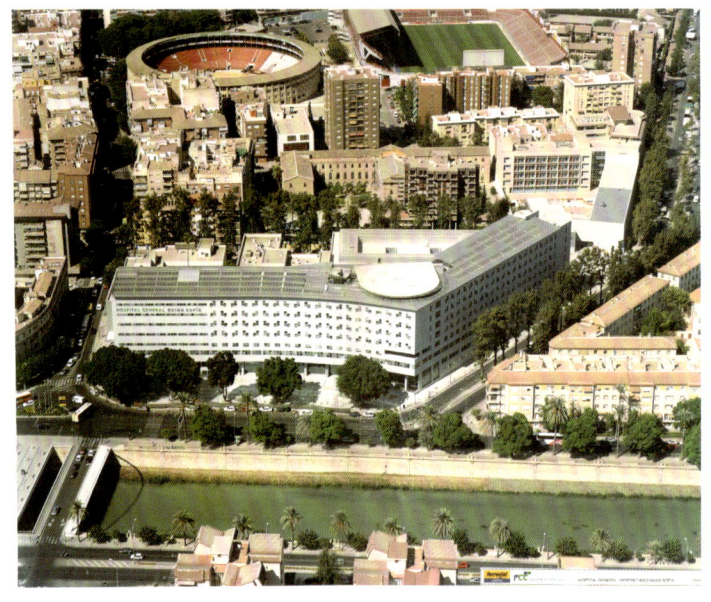

143

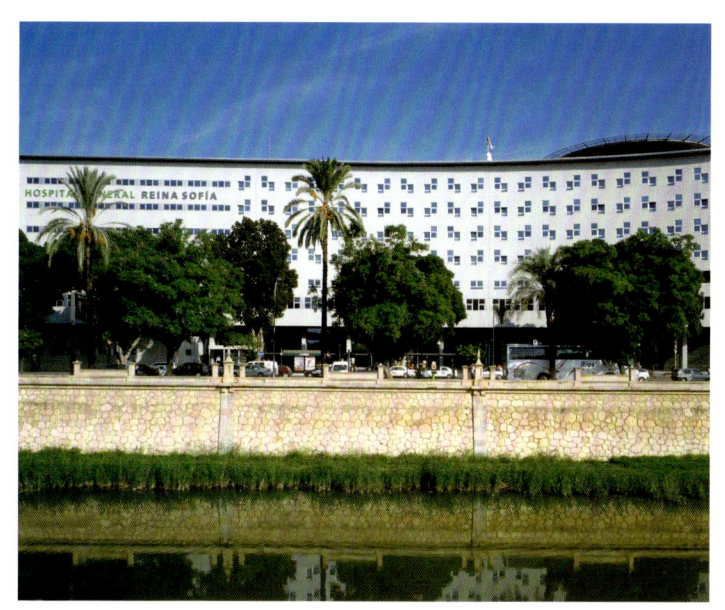

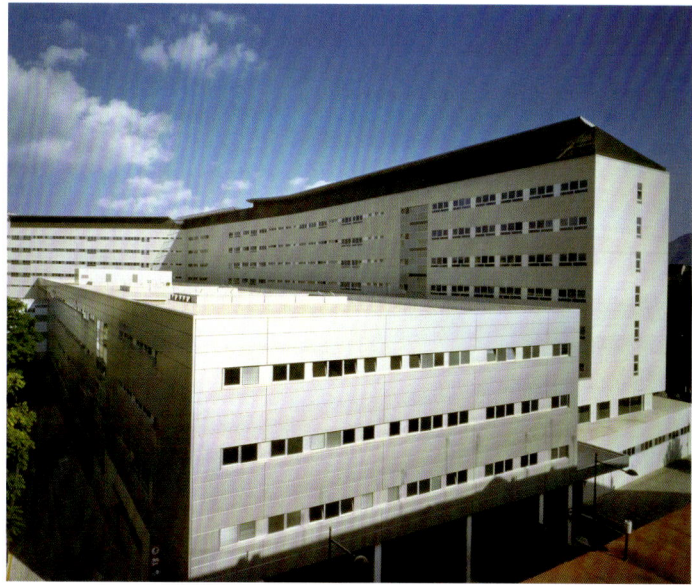

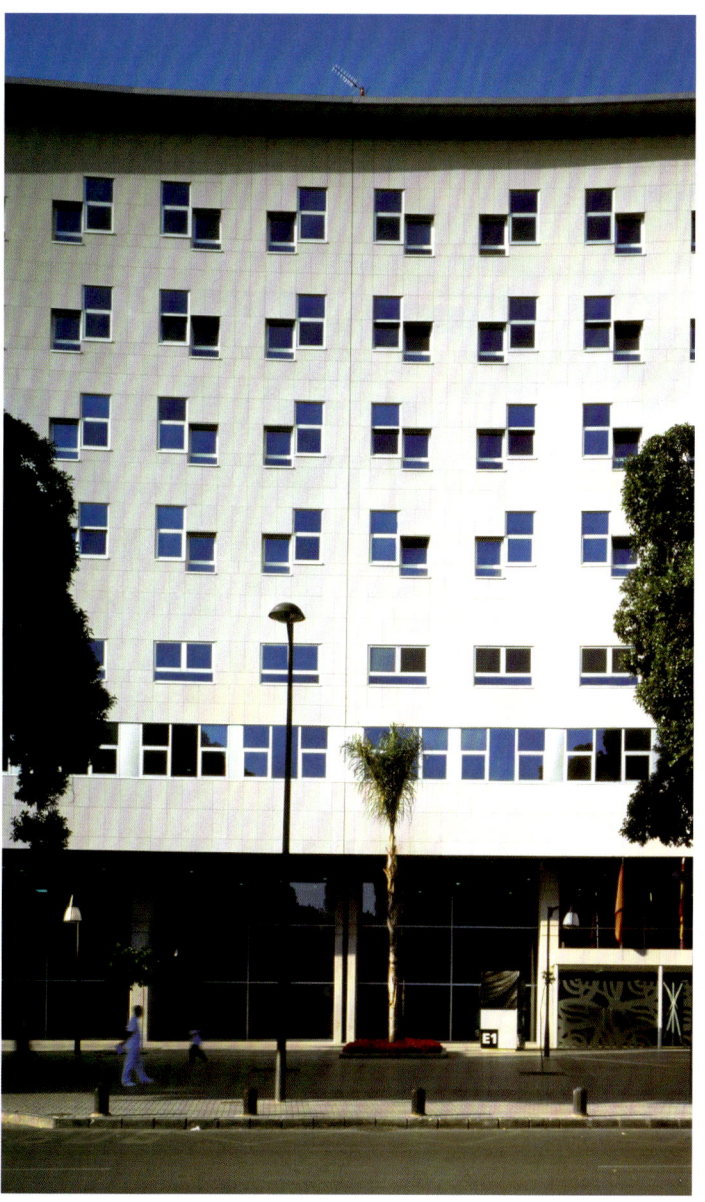

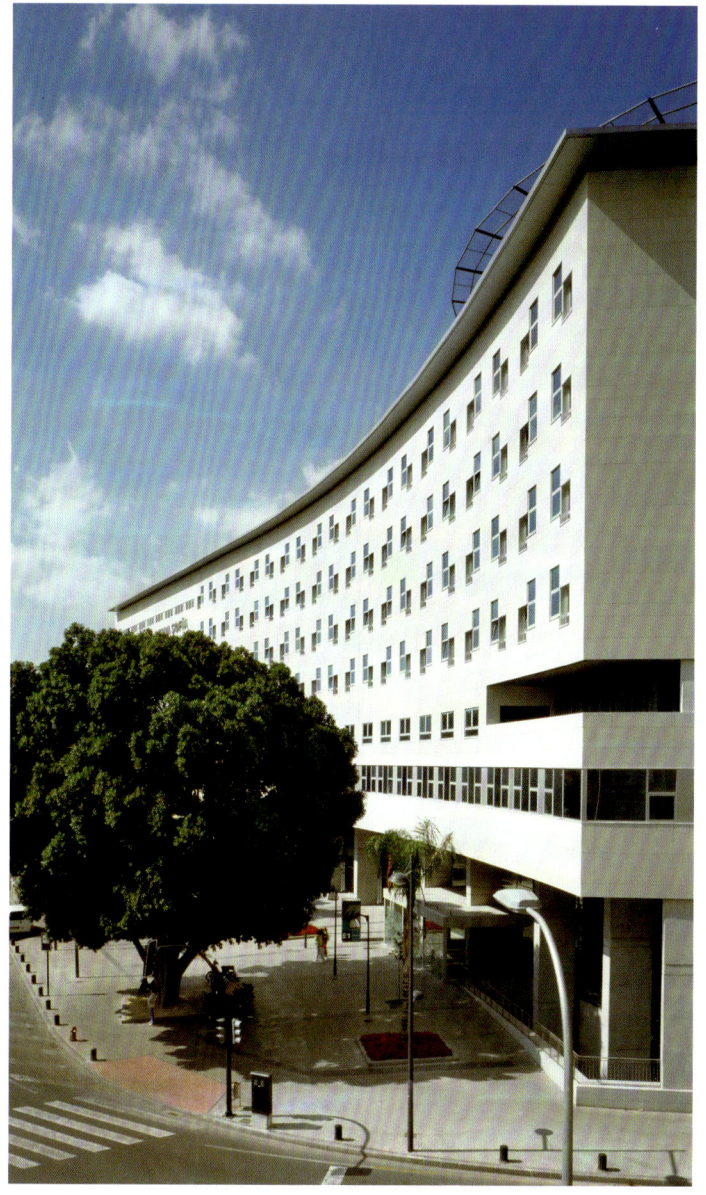

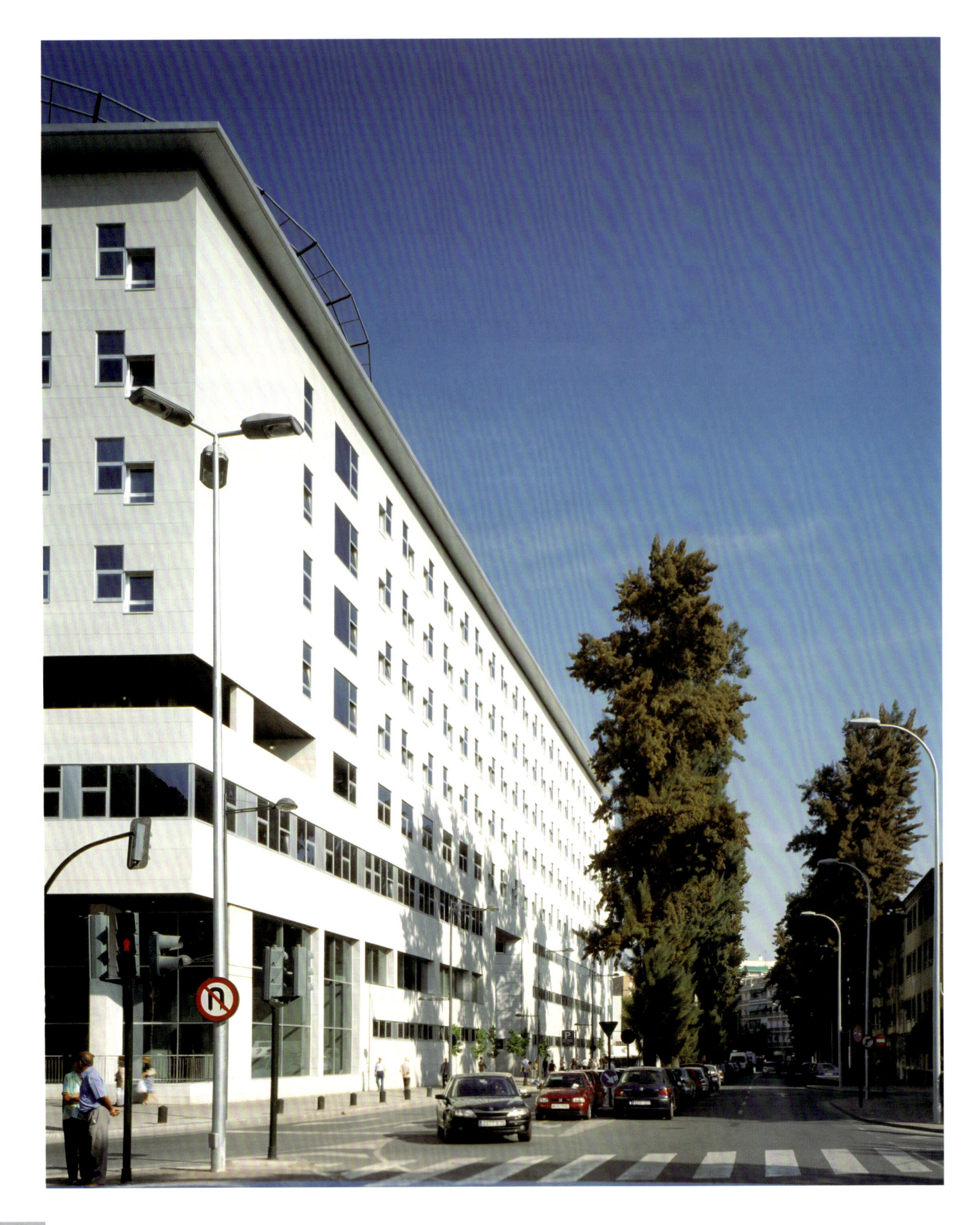

145

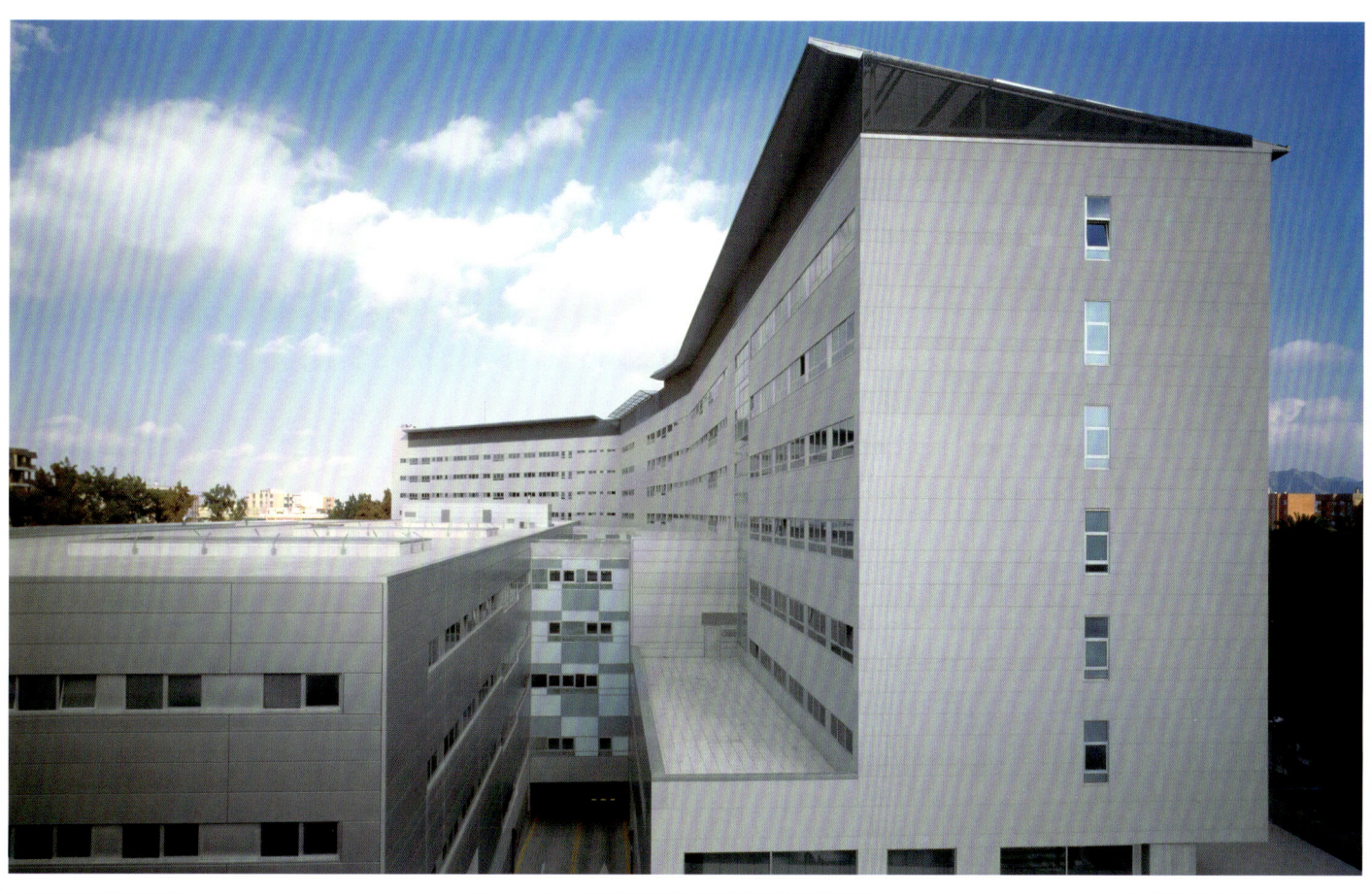

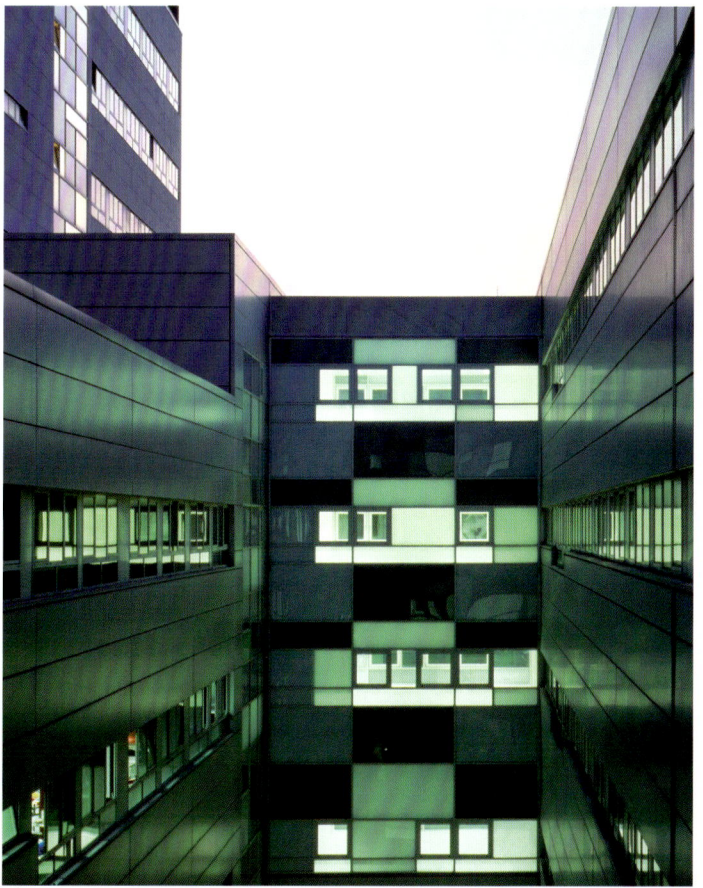

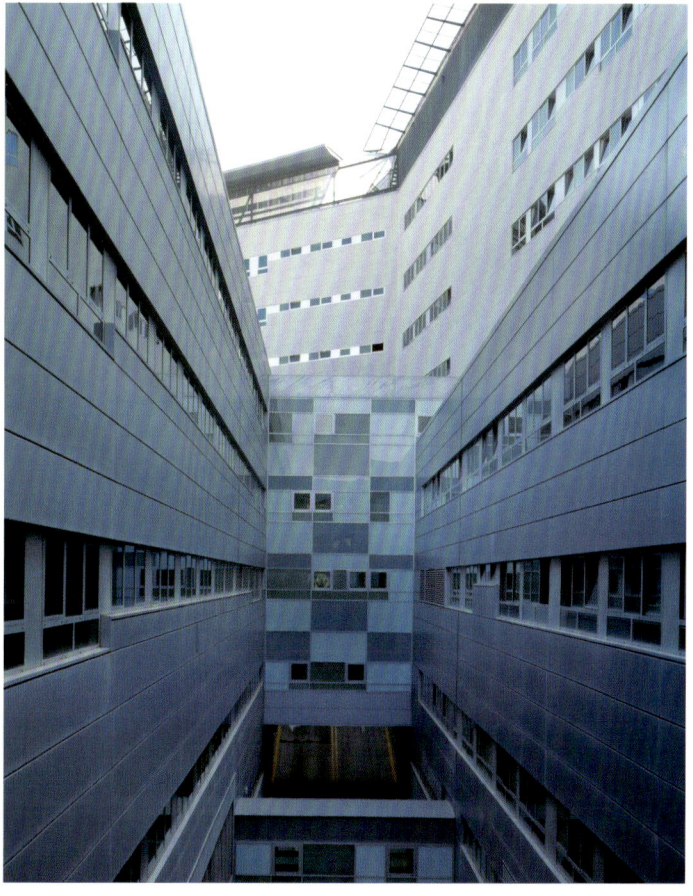

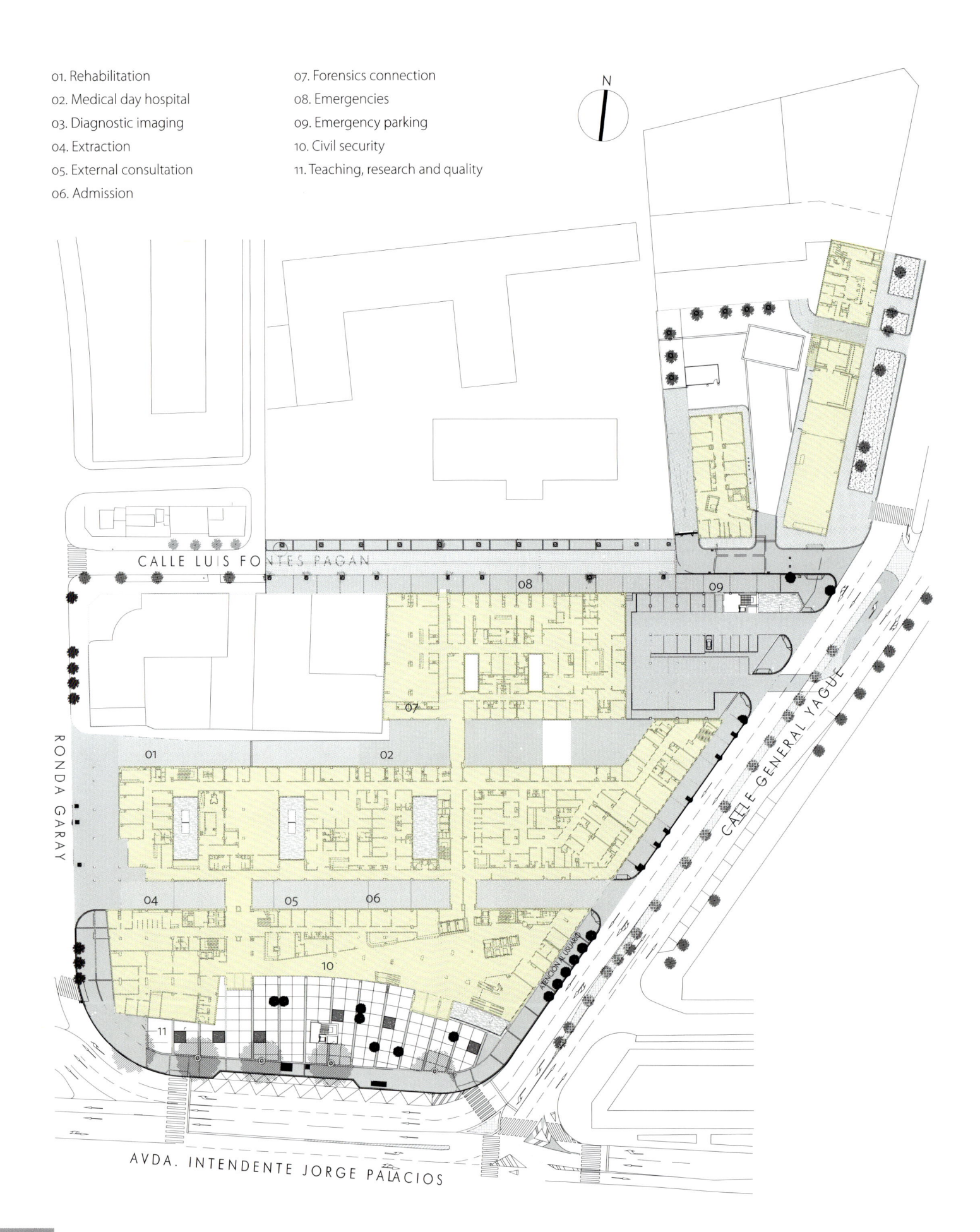

01. Rehabilitation
02. Medical day hospital
03. Diagnostic imaging
04. Extraction
05. External consultation
06. Admission
07. Forensics connection
08. Emergencies
09. Emergency parking
10. Civil security
11. Teaching, research and quality

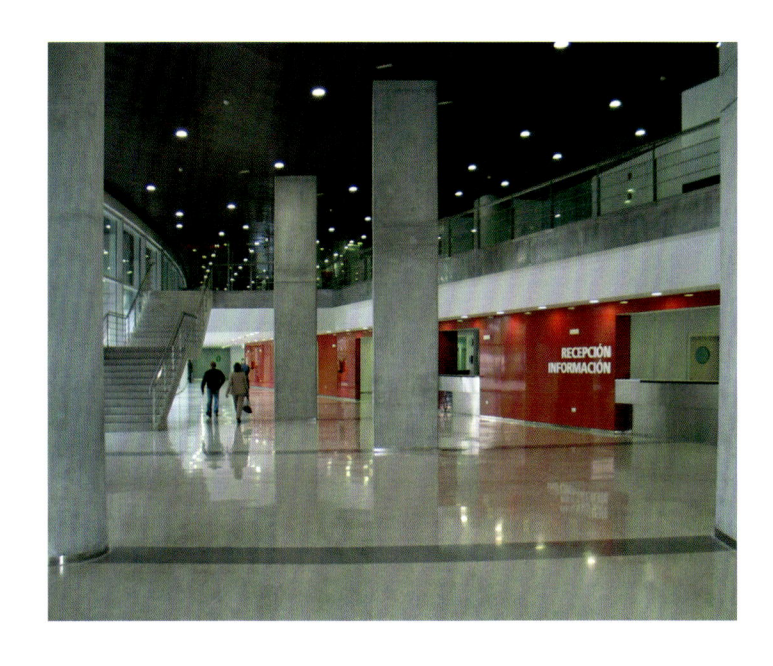

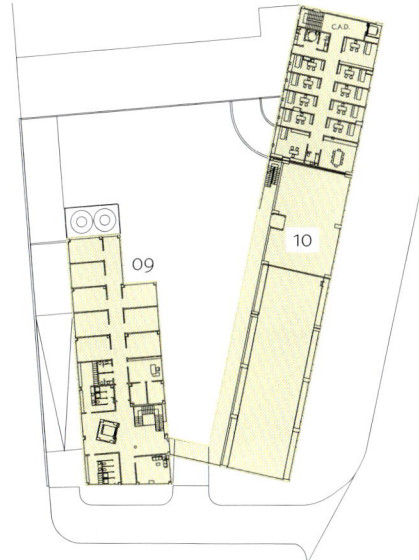

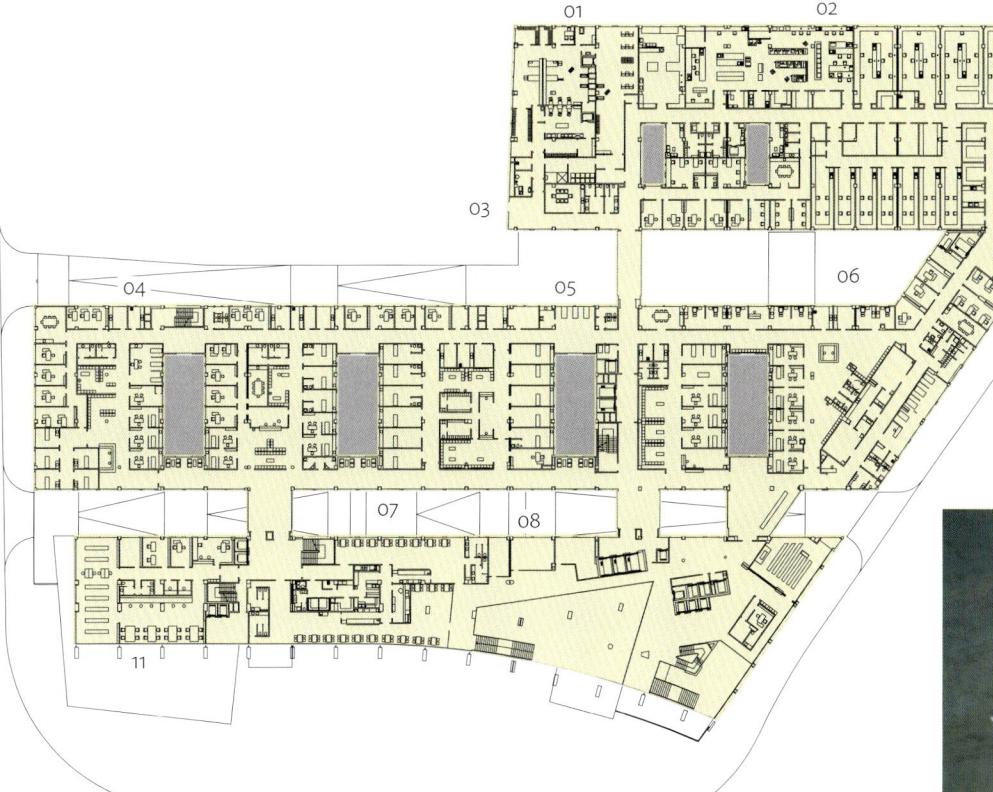

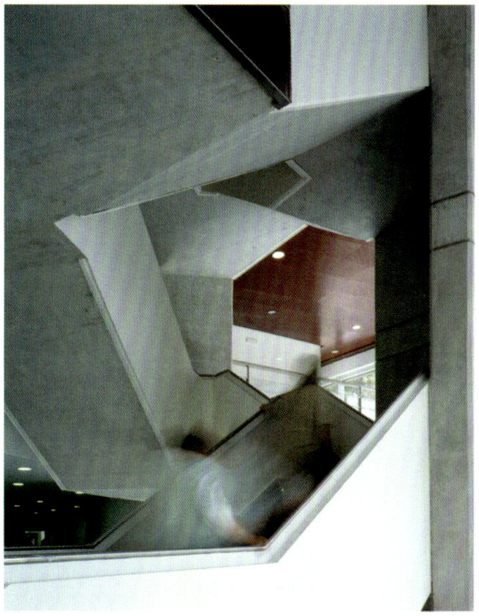

01. Sterilization
02. Laboratories
03. Forensics connection
04. External consultation & exploration
05. Medical day hospital
06. Ophthalmology
07. Cafeteria
08. Local
09. Workchops
10. Installations local
11. Library

147

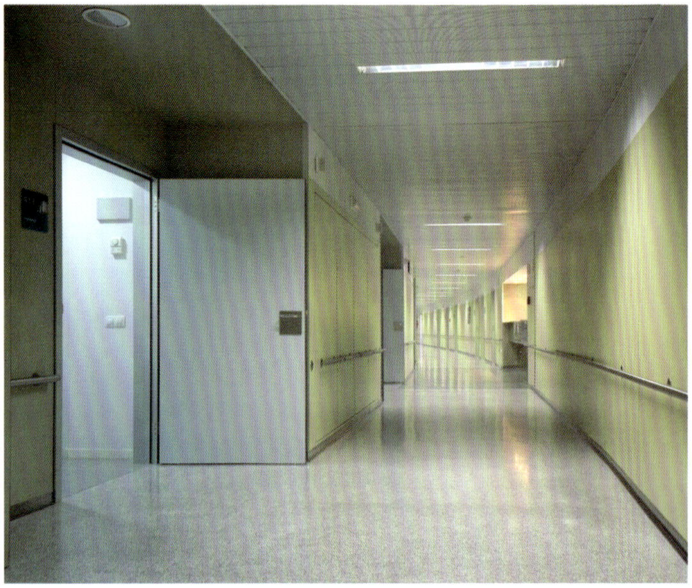

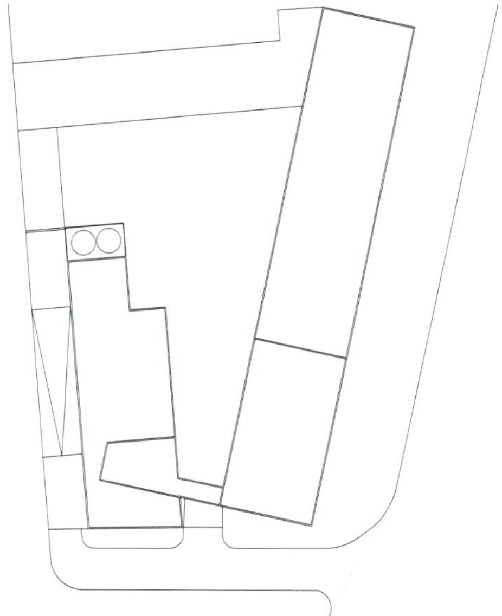

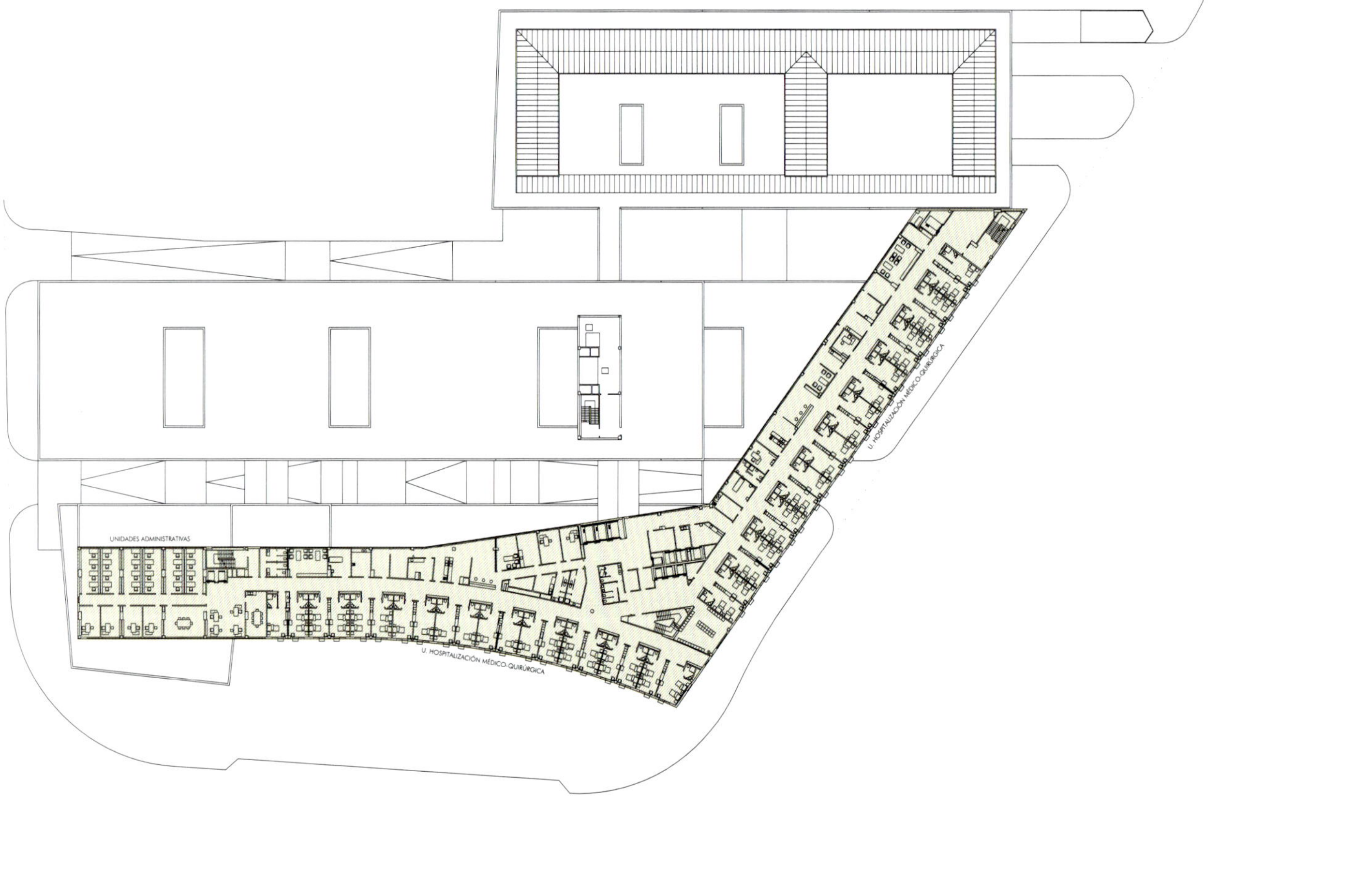
UNIDADES ADMINISTRATIVAS
U. HOSPITALIZACIÓN MÉDICO-QUIRÚRGICA
U. HOSPITALIZACIÓN MÉDICO-QUIRÚRGICA

149

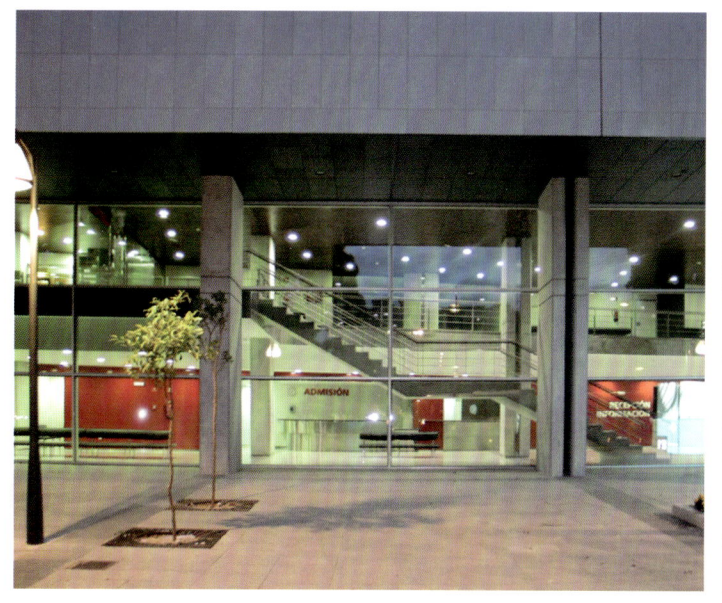

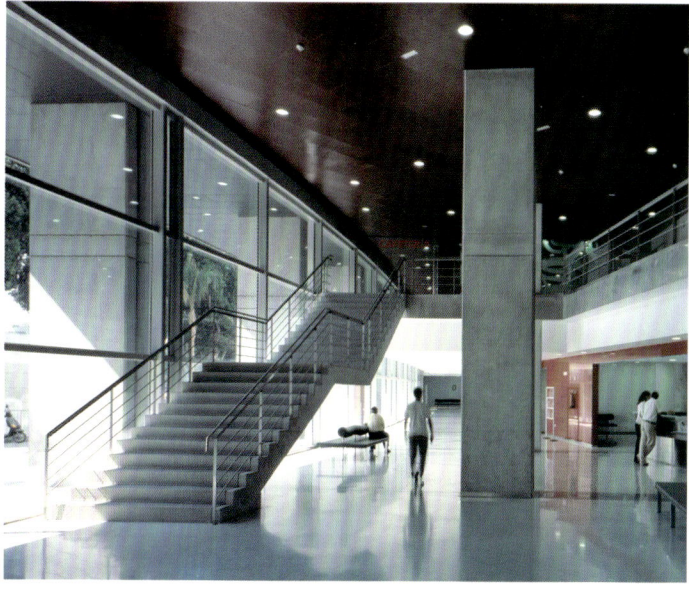

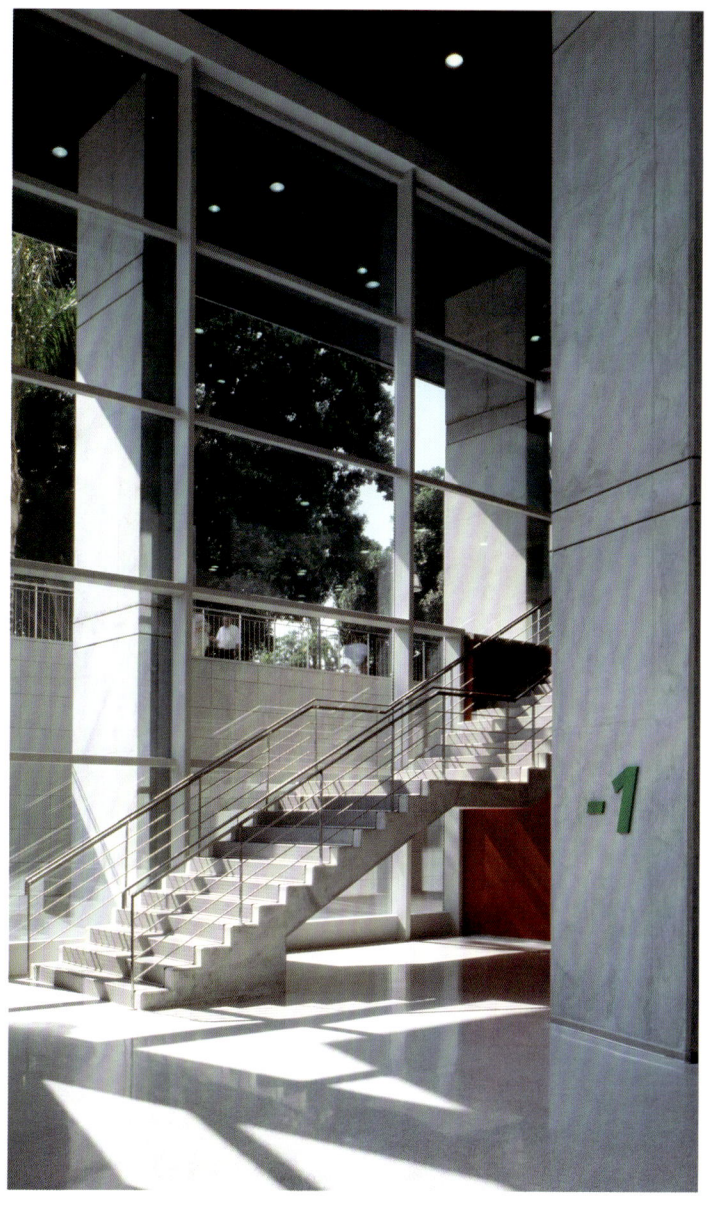

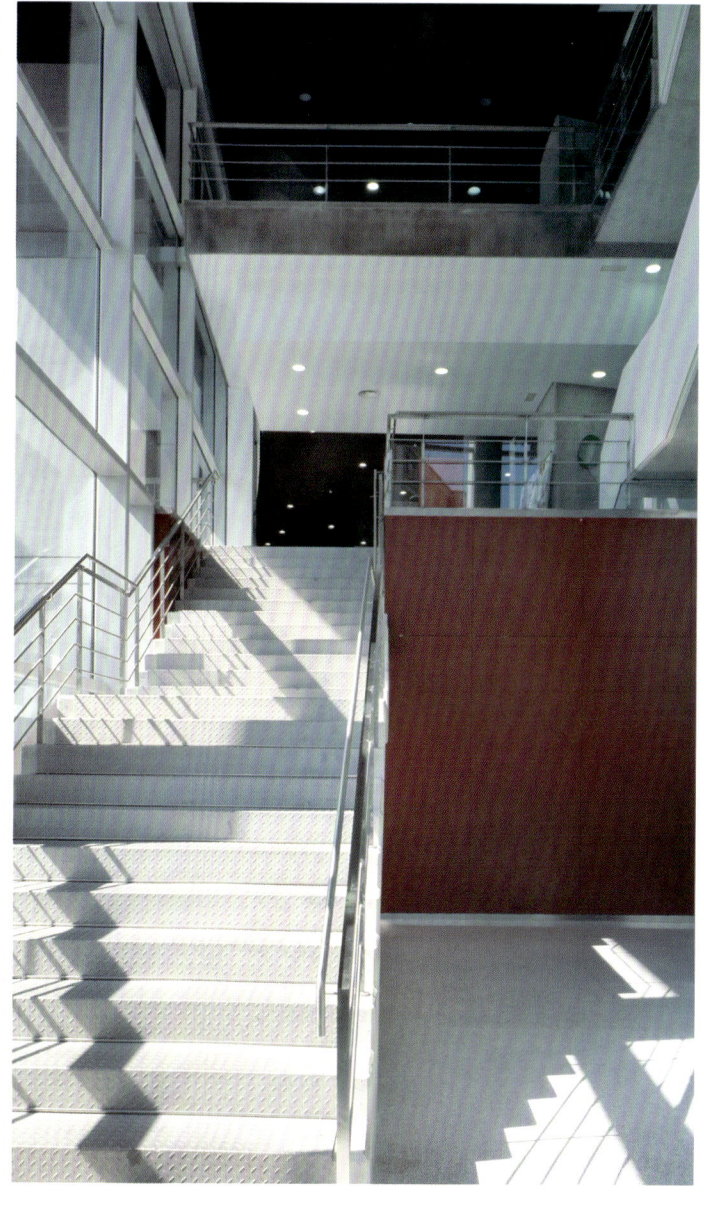

150

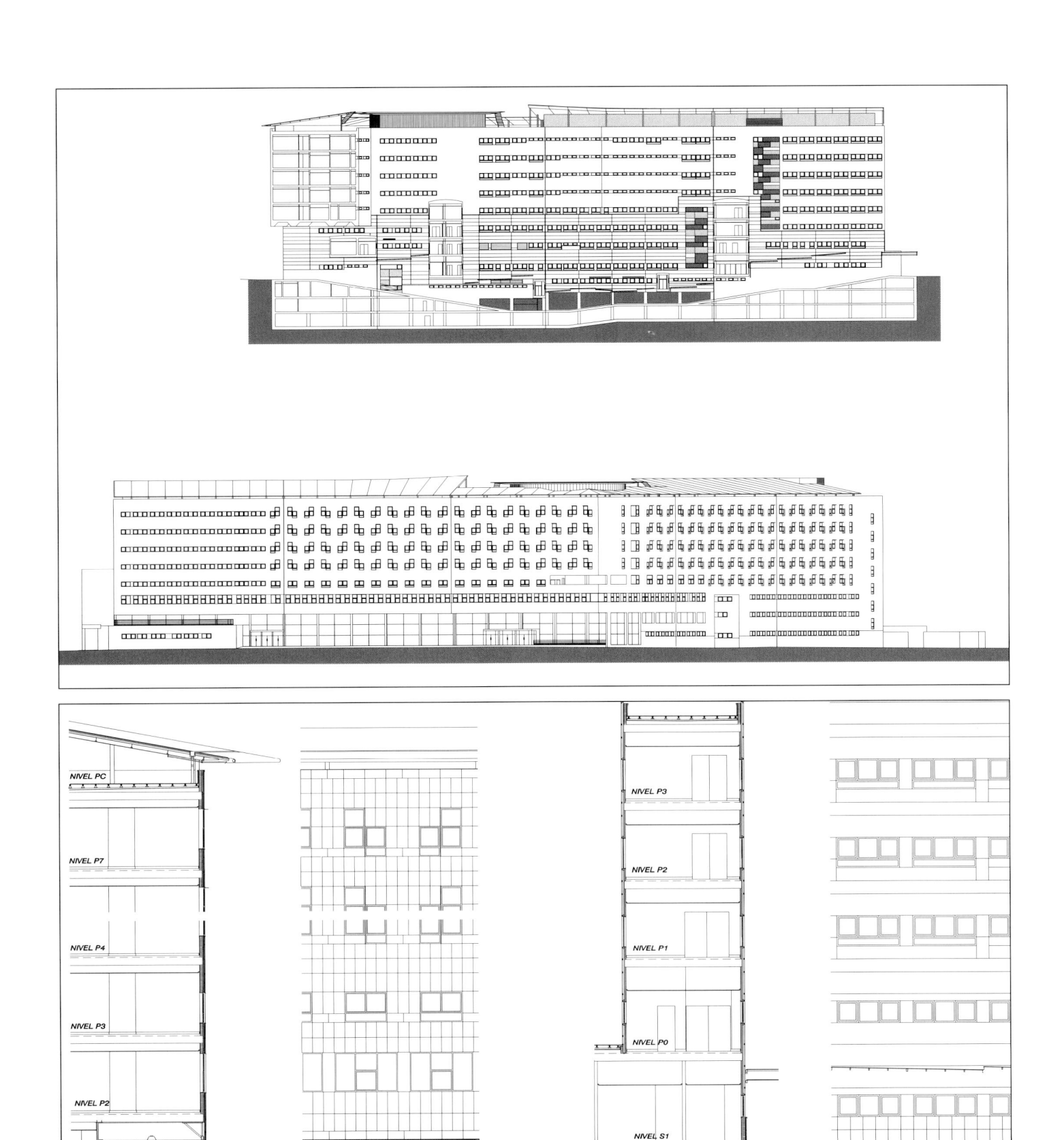

151

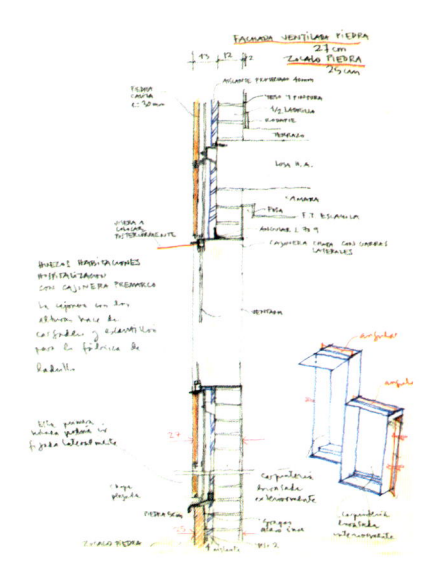

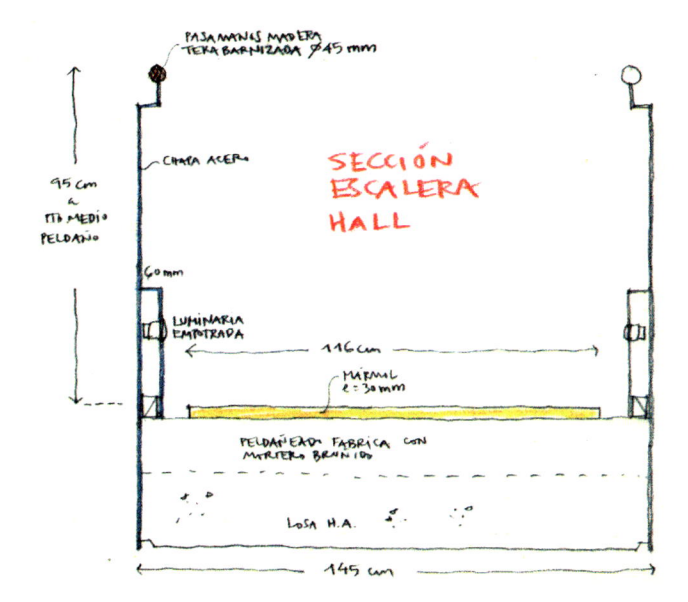

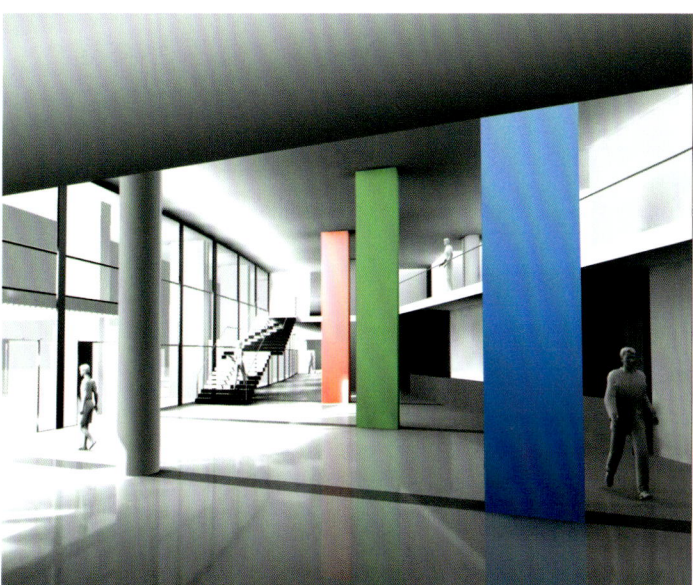

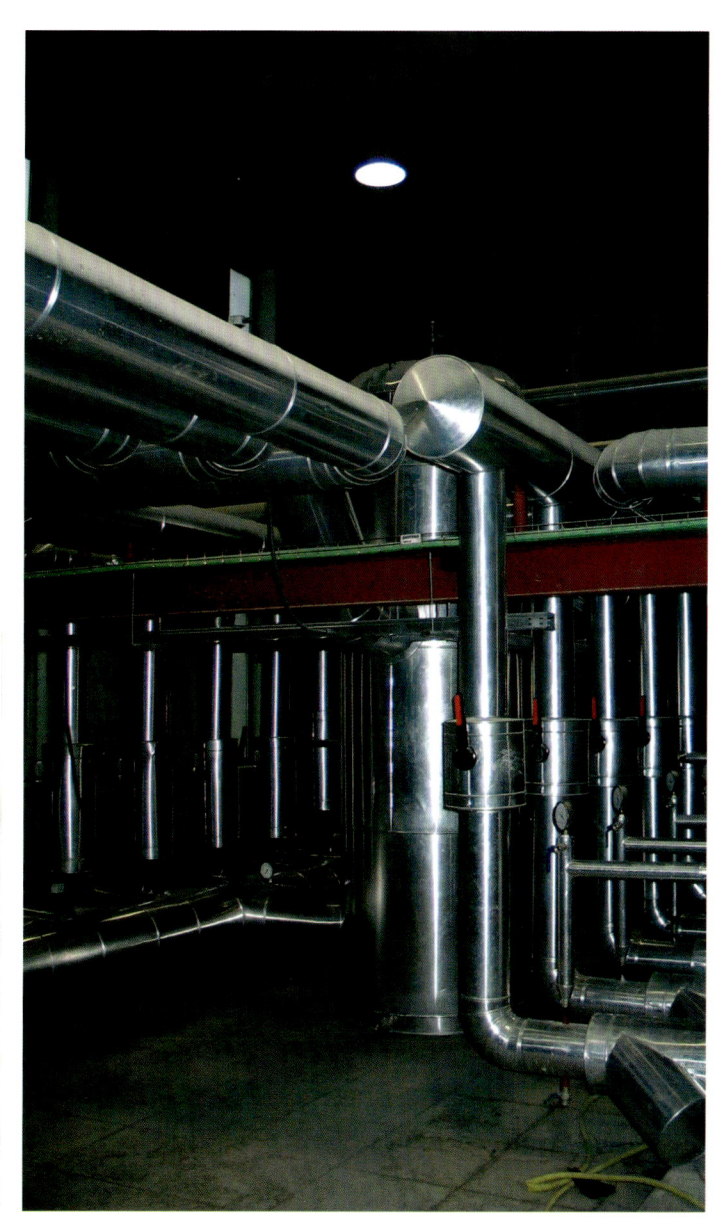

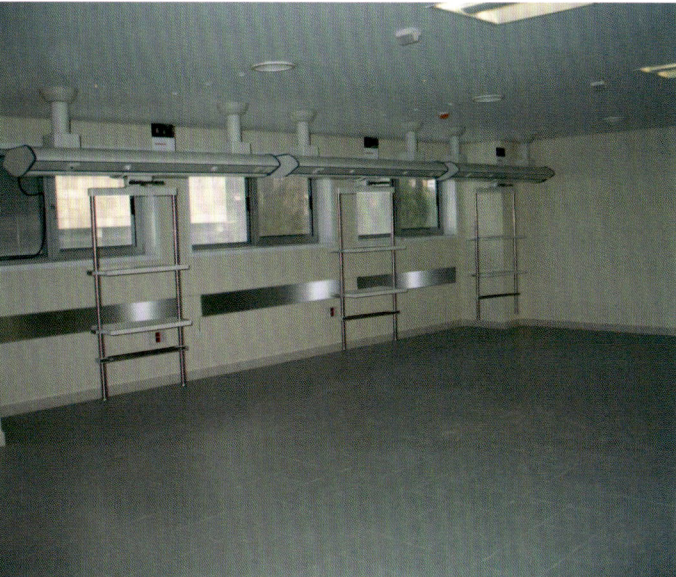

152

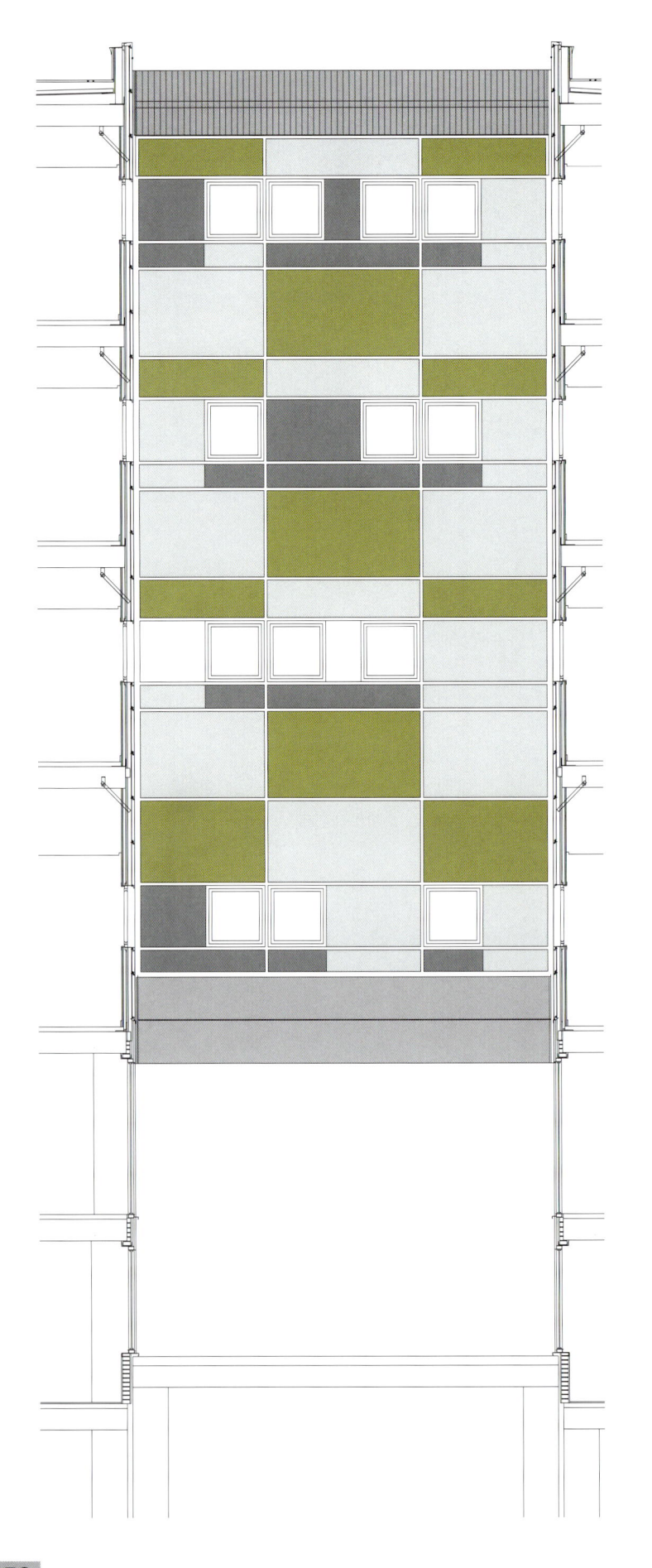

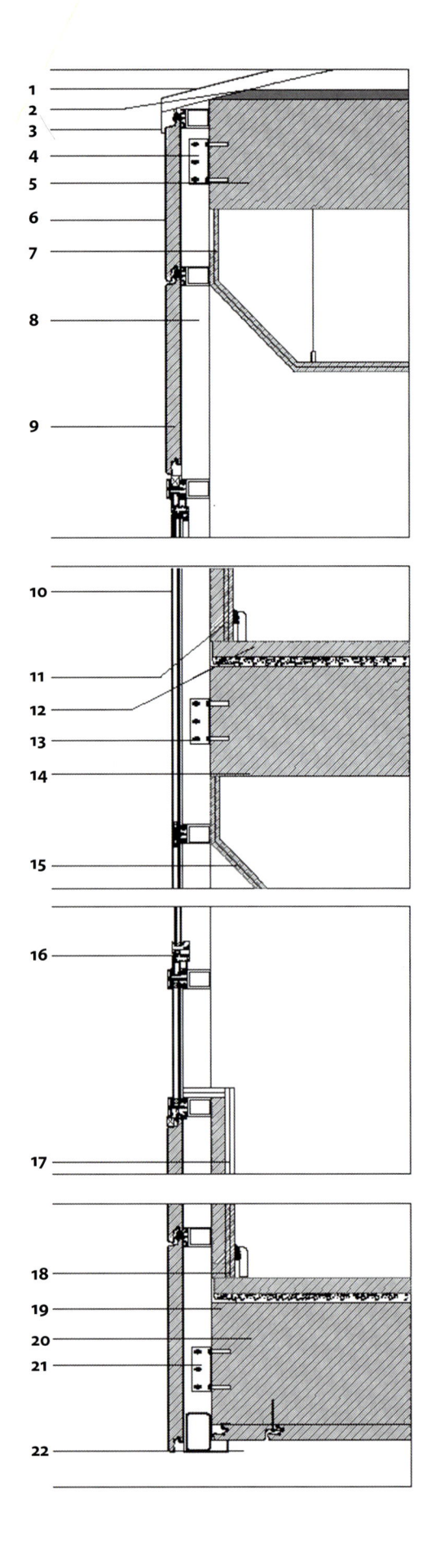

1. Corrugated curved sheet-metal for roofing
2. Insulation
3. Drip-board: lacquered sheet metal
4. Anchoring for substructure of slab
5. Slab, reinforced concrete 35 cm
6. Corrugated sheet metal
7. Suspended ceiling: Pladur
8. Metal substructure to anchor panels, carpentry and glass
9. Panel Robertson or equiv. Thickness=50mm
   2 Sheets of galvanized steel with injected polyurethane
10. Curtain wall system SVK60 by Schuco
11. Pladur panels 1.5 + 1.5mm., with angle of 4.6mm., backed with insulation.
    Baseboard finished in qualities as defined
12. Flooring
13. Anchoring substructure of slab
14. Slab, reinforced concrete 35mm
15. Suspended ceiling: Pladur
16. Curtain wall system SVK60 by Schuco or equivalent. See notes.
17. Pladur panels 1.5 + 1.5mm., with angle of 4.6mm., backed with insulation
18. Pladur panels 1.5 + 1.5mm., with angle of 4.6mm., backed with insulation
    Baseboard finished in qualities as defined
19. Flooring
20. Slab, reinforced concrete 35mm
21. Anchoring substructure of slab
22. Panel Robertson or equiv. Thickness=50mm
    2 Sheets of galvanized steel with injected polyurethane

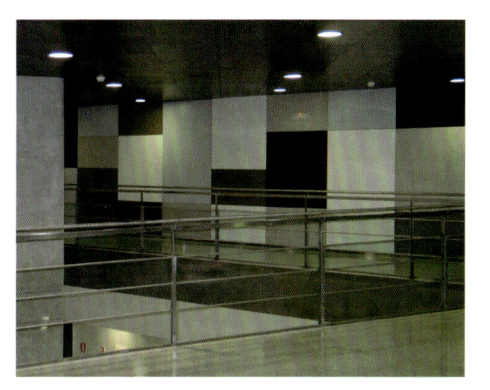

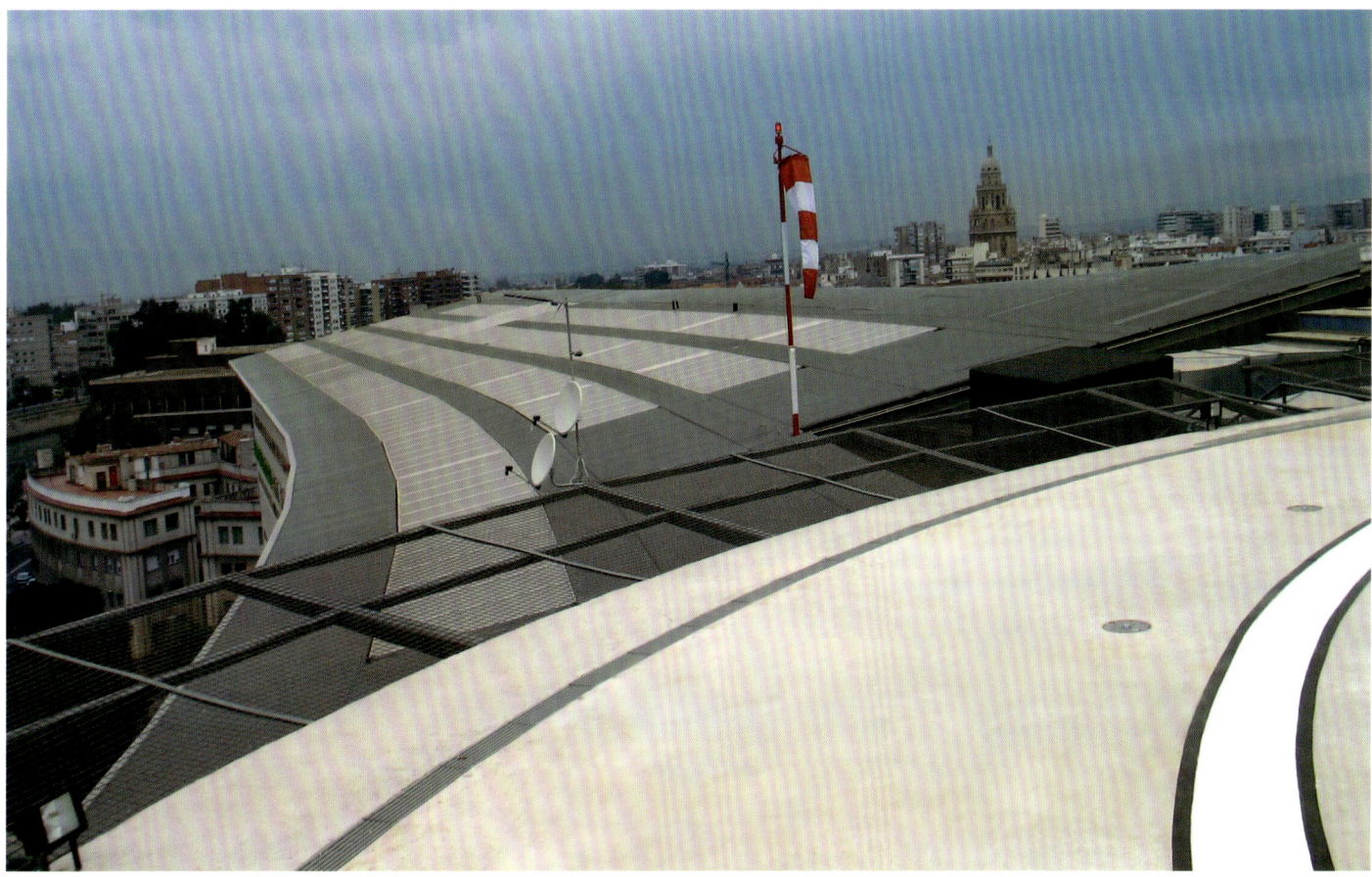

153

KMD Architects

CHA Women and Children's Hospital

Bundang, South Korea

Photographs: Jong O Kim

Designed to comply with strict height and bulk limitations, the CHA Women's Hospital brings to a dense, suburban Seoul neighborhood a sleek, gleaming, modernist building catering to avant-garde Korean women comfortable with the aesthetic of haut-couture shops, spas, hair salons and restaurants sweeping Asian capitals today. This new hospital is among the first in Korea to offer a full array of advances from the United States such as LDR (labor, delivery, recovery), water birthing and participation by family members in the birthing process that are taken for granted stateside. In addition, to meet Korean expectations, one entire floor of the hospital is given over to an extended stay spa, where those who can afford it may remain up to one month after giving birth.

CHA celebrates high technology but tempers it through the inclusion of elements from traditional Korean architecture, such as wood, plants, water features and organic forms contrasting with the glass, aluminum and stainless steel. Both inside and out, the design focus is on creating sleek, uncluttered surfaces to offer patients and visitors a respite from the surrounding neighborhood's visual noise. Organic, flowing interior surfaces offer warmth with a central, curved vertical wood slat wall flowing from top to bottom, connecting various functional areas and natural gathering spaces for patients, families and friends. Natural light flows through vast windows and a central atrium. A variety of open-air areas foster natural interaction and relaxation. The rooftop features an enjoyable and restful sky garden. Patient room windows rely on a dot pattern of changing densities to filter light and provide privacy while keeping interiors bright. The glass curtain wall serves as a veil of comfort, providing a sense of shelter without separating patients from the outdoors.

Because of the site's reduced dimensions the building program required four levels above grade and four below (for parking and support services). The primary design goal was to enhance the hospital experience through the maximization of daylight for greater patient and visitor satisfaction, as well as improved inpatient conditions through unique approaches for introducing and controlling daylight and creating a sense of privacy in patient bedrooms in a dense urban setting.

A second, equally important goal was the introduction of natural forms, plants, materials and water features throughout the hospital, forming a stark contrast to the harshness of the surrounding neighborhood. Nearly all floors of the building, from the basement to the rooftop garden, become accessible respite areas for patients, staff and visitors, either visually or through the experience of being outside in a peaceful environment.

Client:
CHA Health Care System, College of Medicine
Pochon CHA University
Surface area:
15,300 sqm (165,000 sqft)
Start date:
September 2005
Finish date:
June 2006
Associates:
Yo2 Architects
Contractor:
Doosan Construction & Engineering
Structural engineering:
ALT structure group
Cost:
$ 30,000,000
Awards:
AIA National Healthcare Design Award 2008

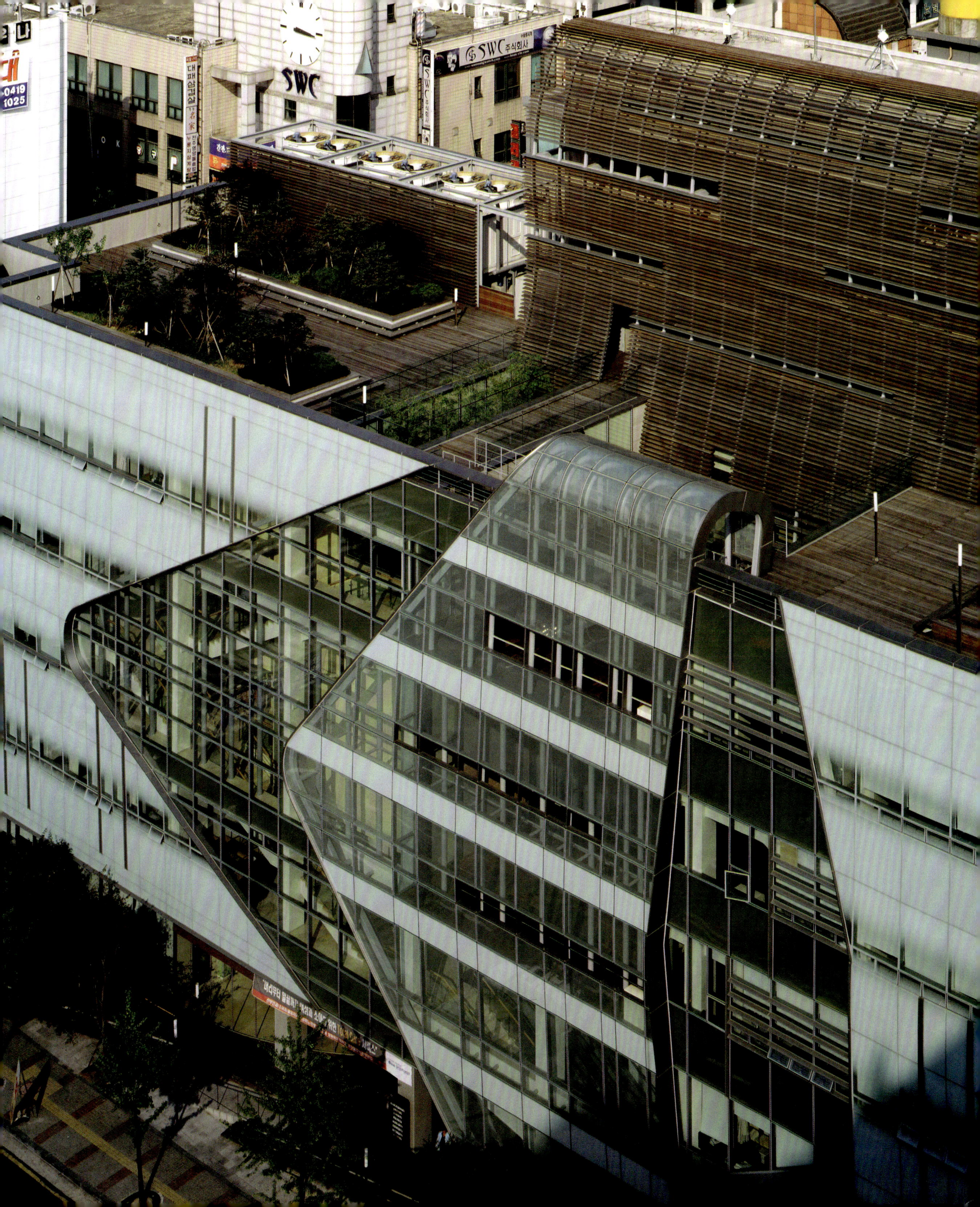
SWC
SWC 주식회사
0419
1025

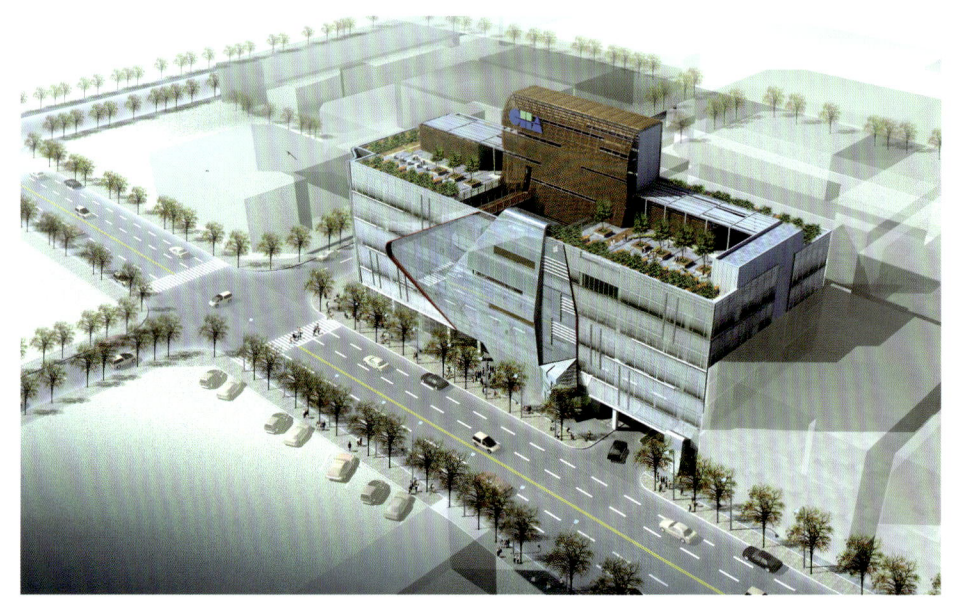

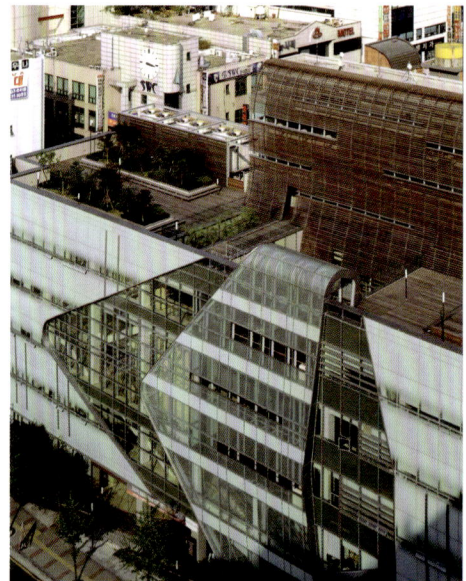

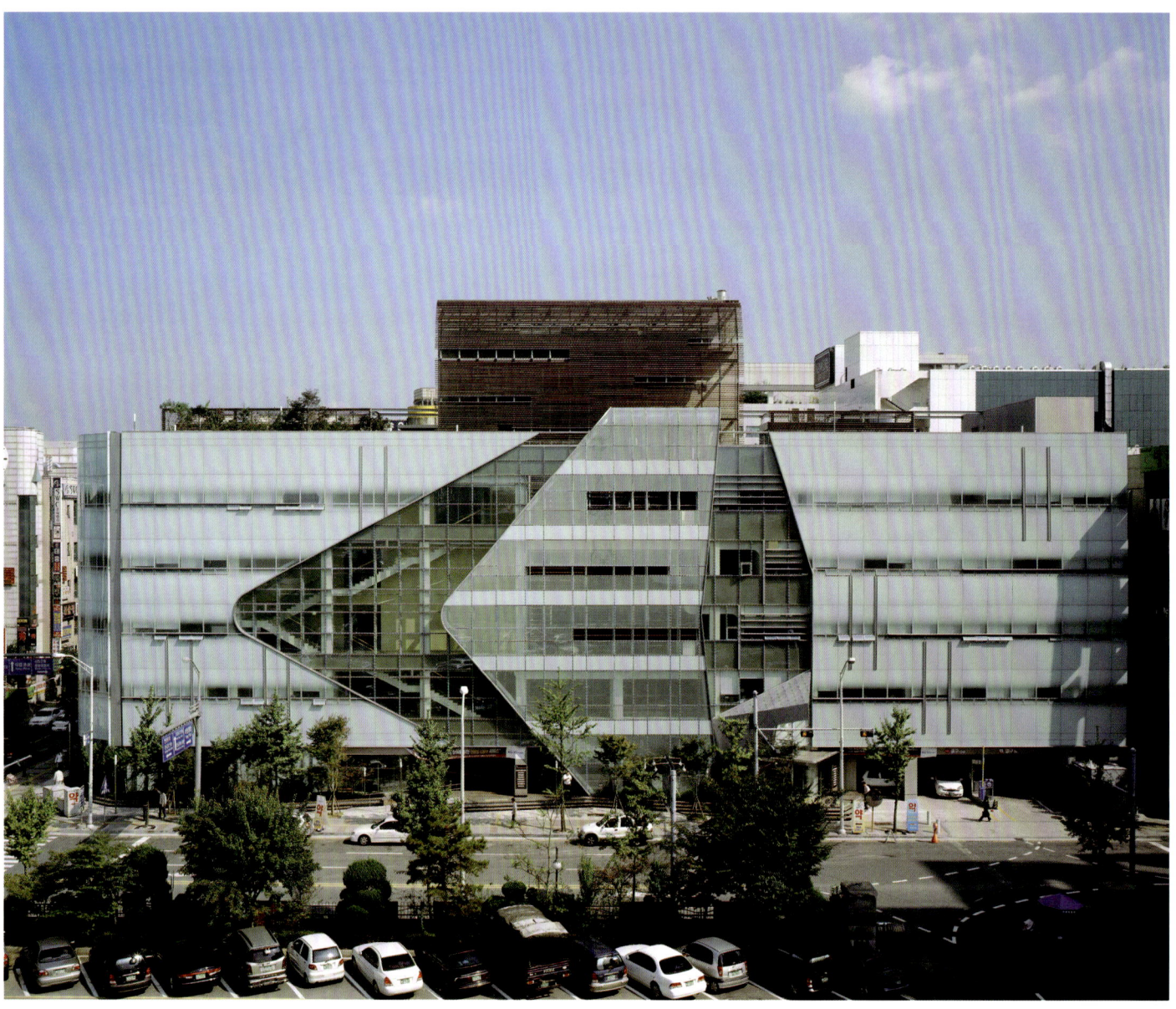

157

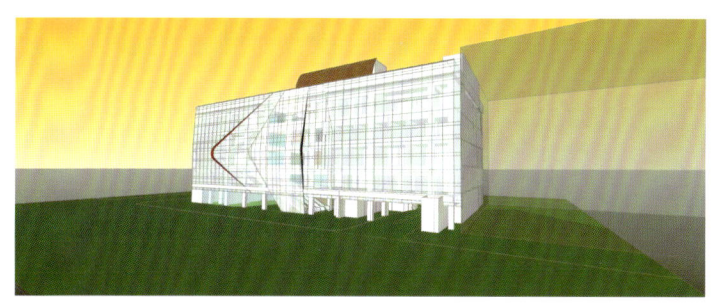

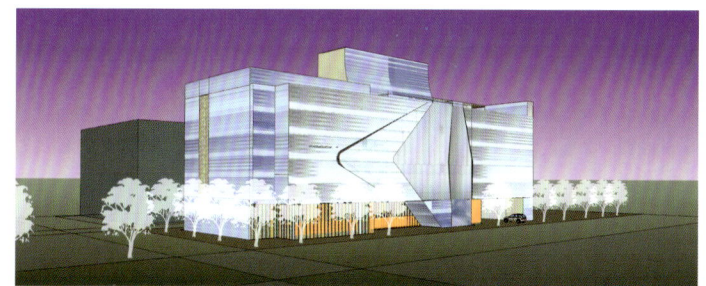

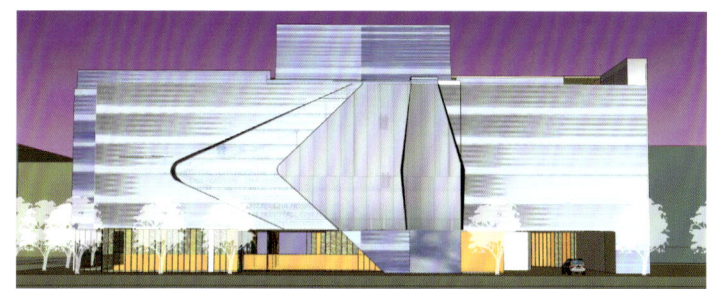

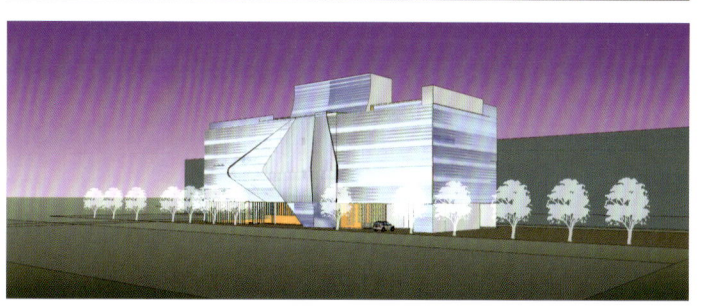

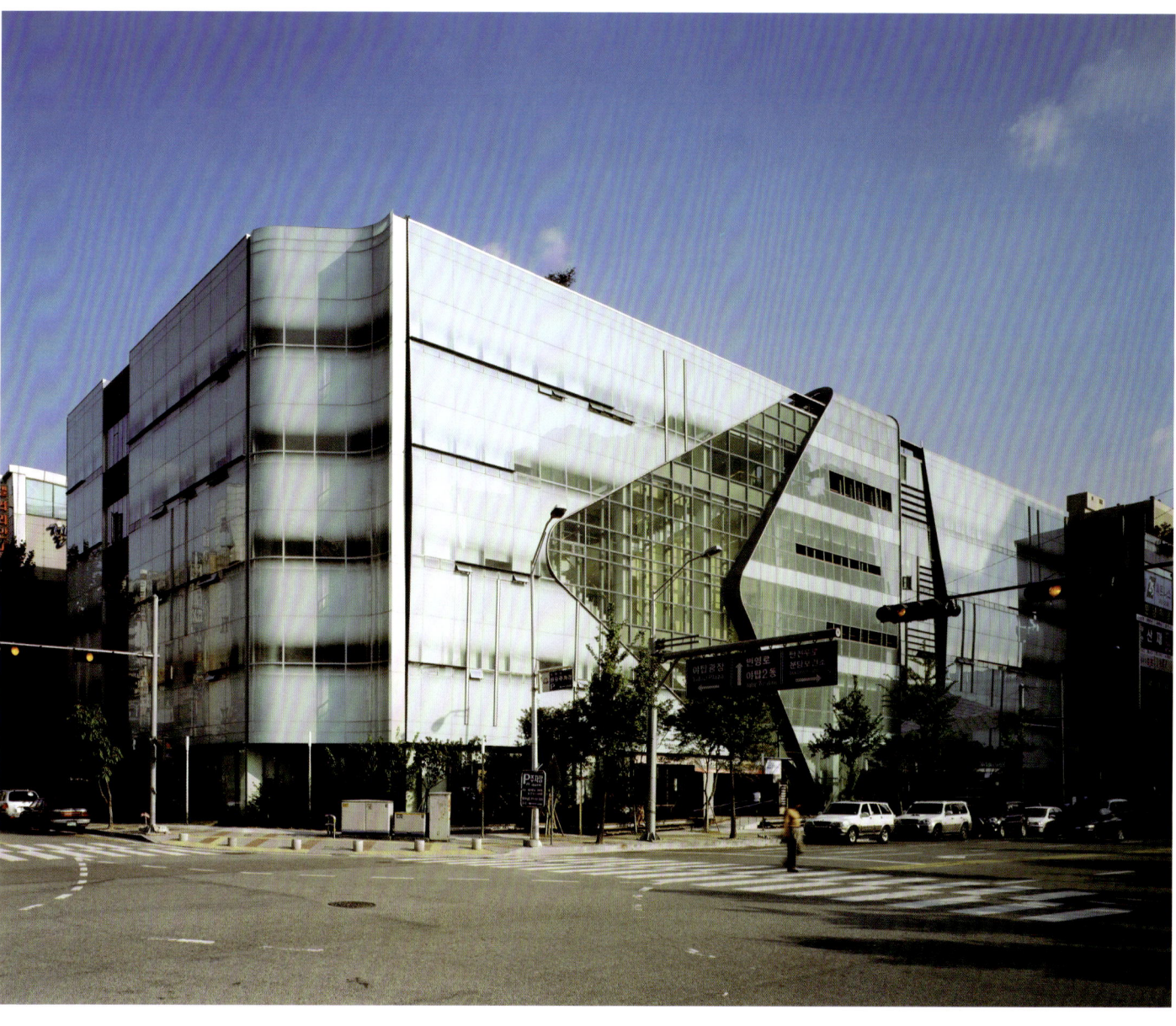

+1 floor plan

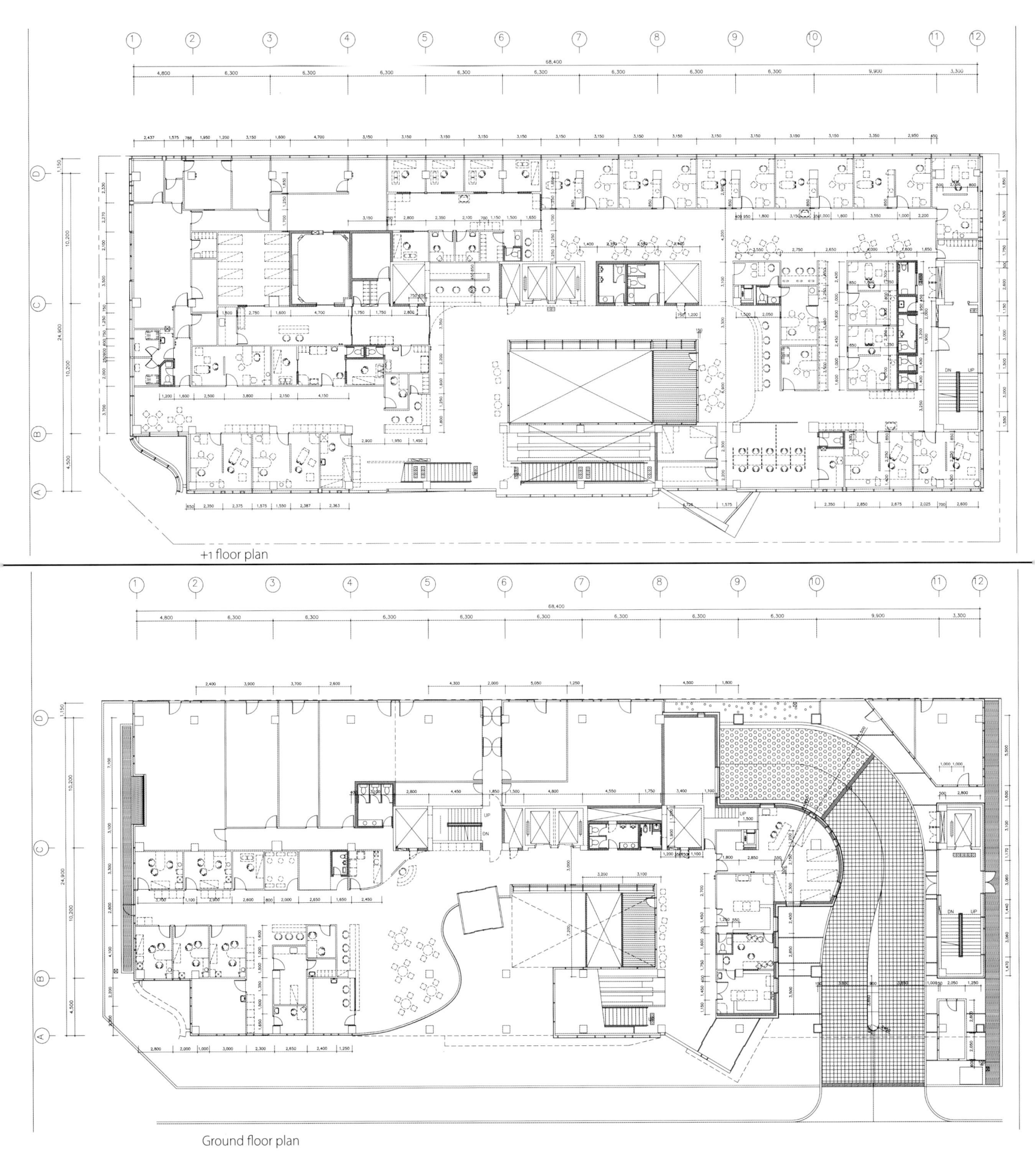

Ground floor plan

158

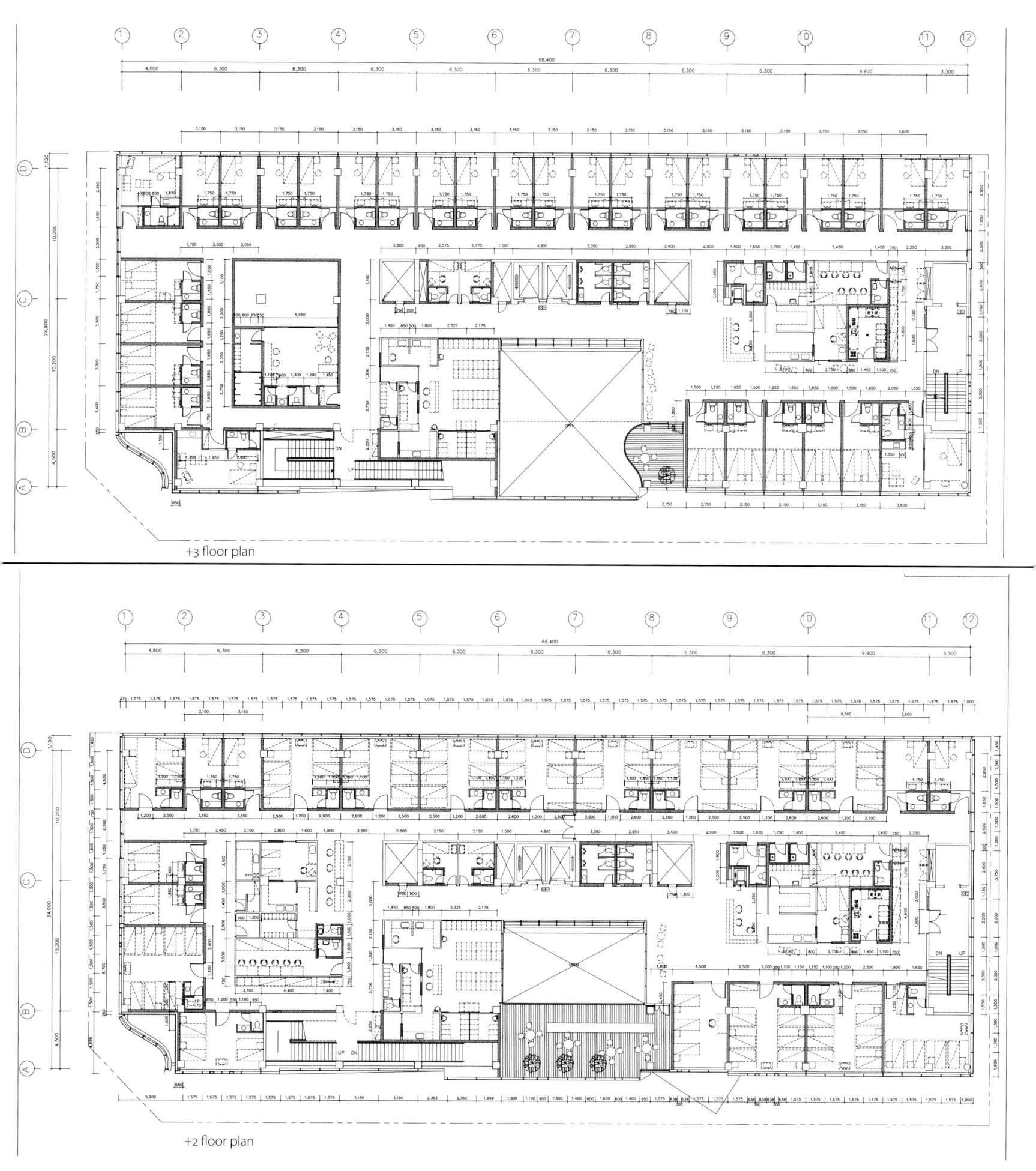

+3 floor plan

+2 floor plan

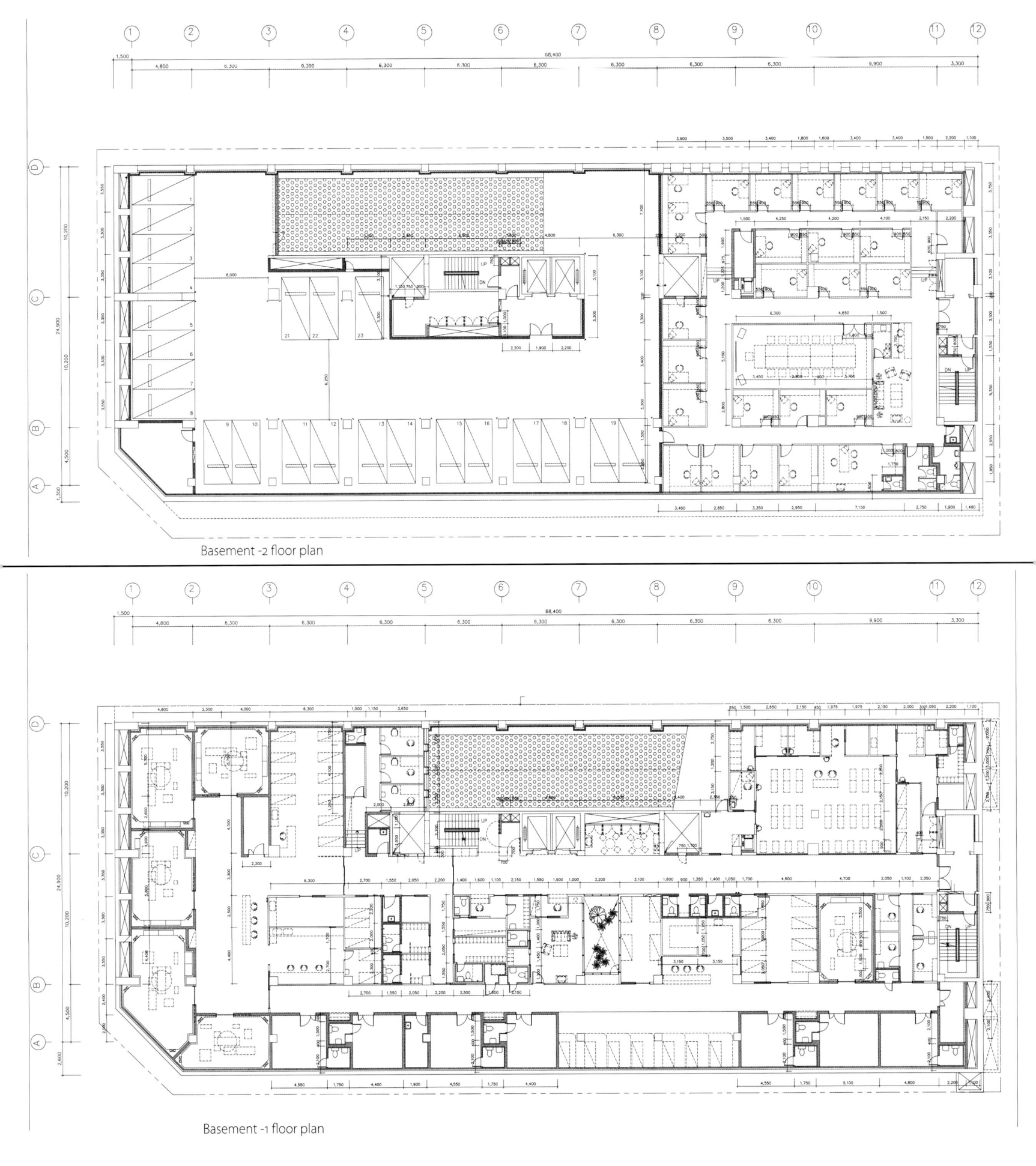

Basement -2 floor plan

Basement -1 floor plan

Basement -4 floor plan

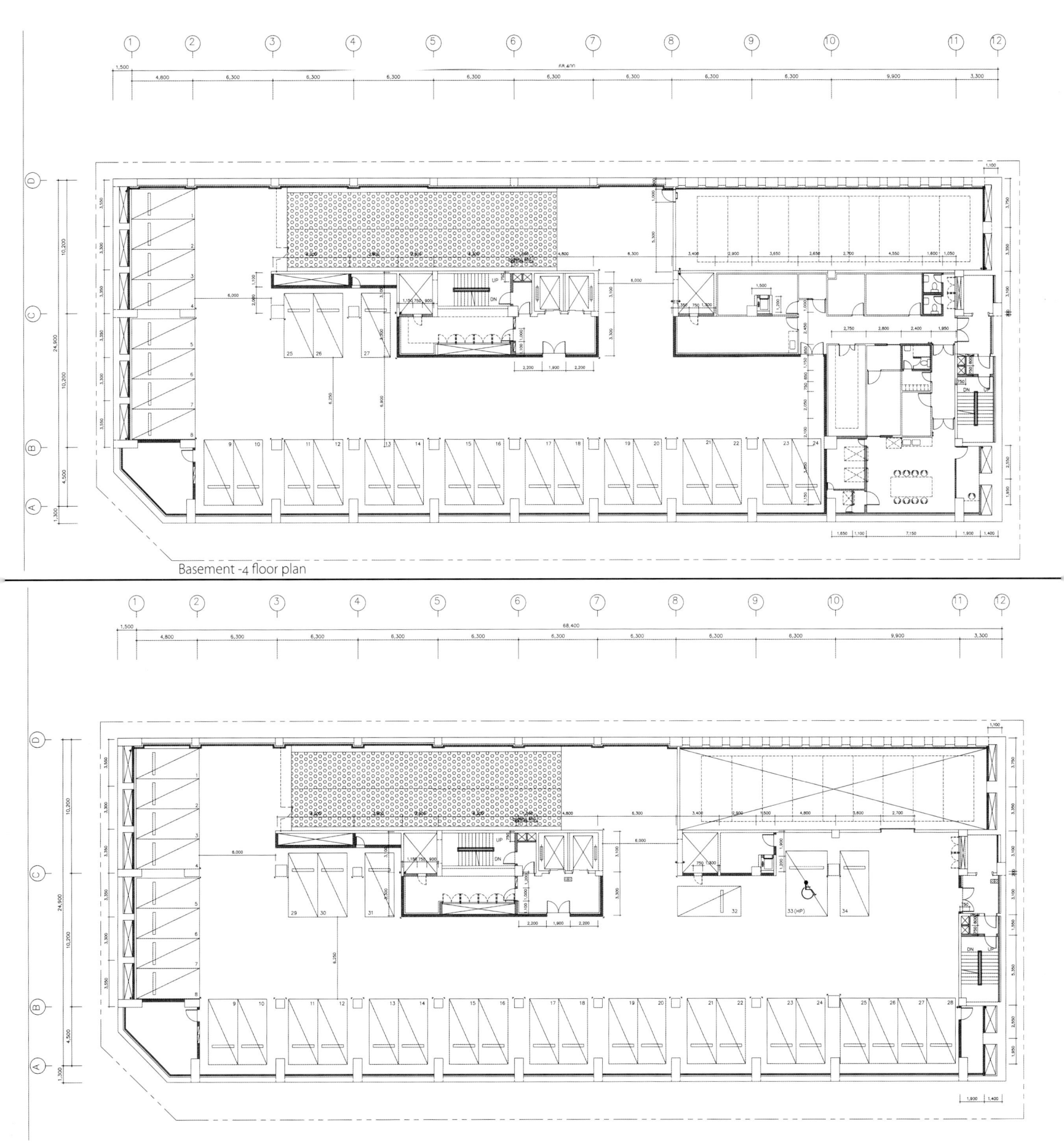

Basement -3 floor plan

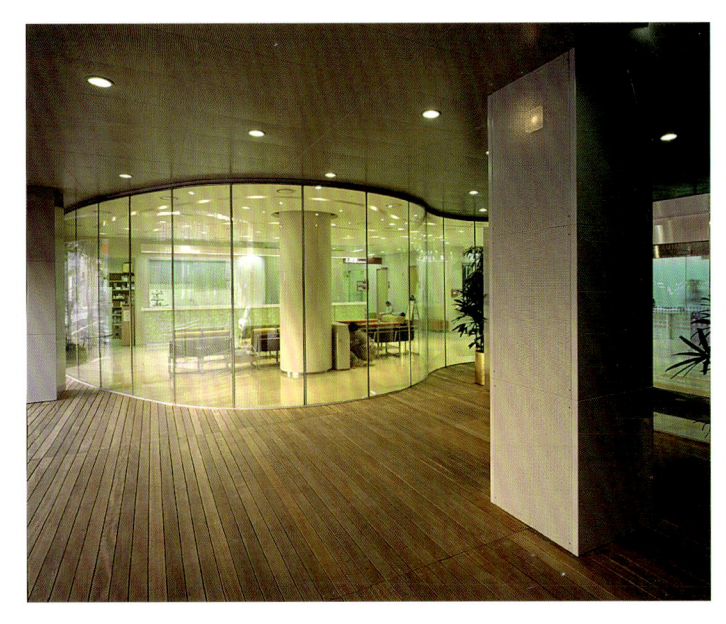

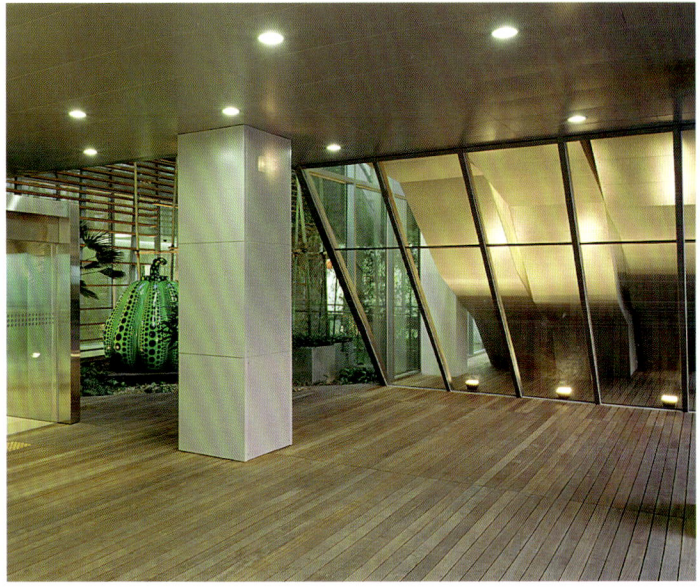

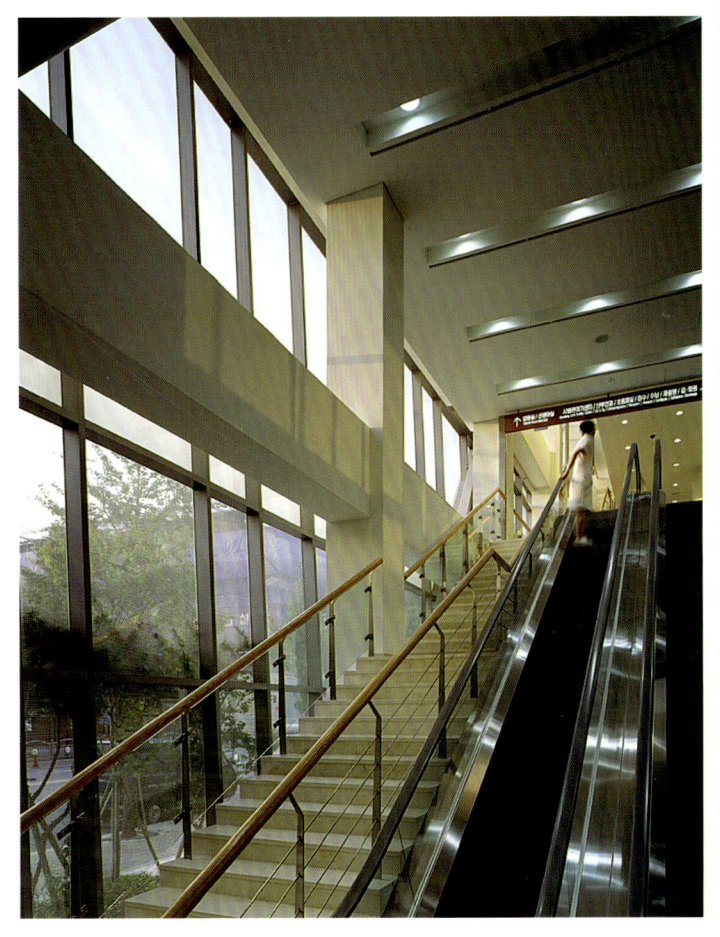

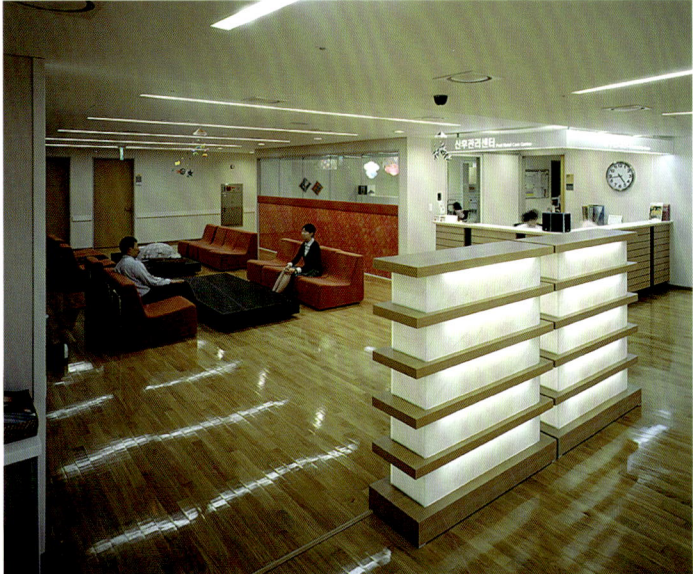

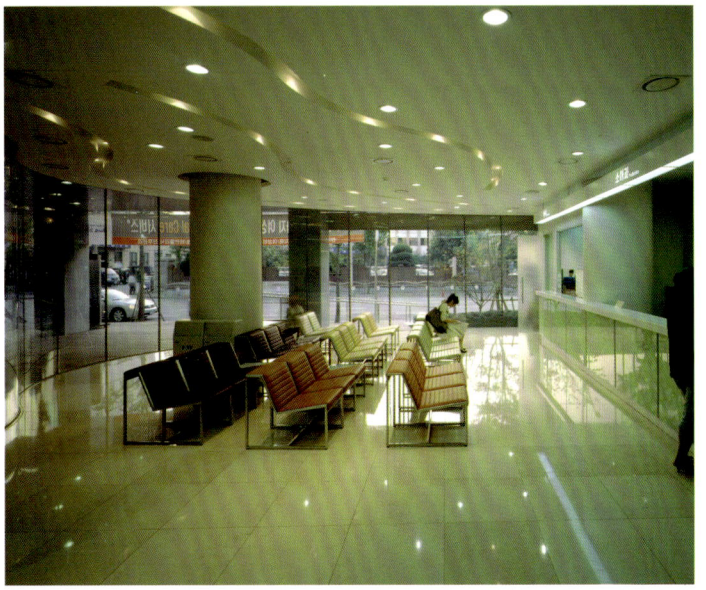

East-west section 1

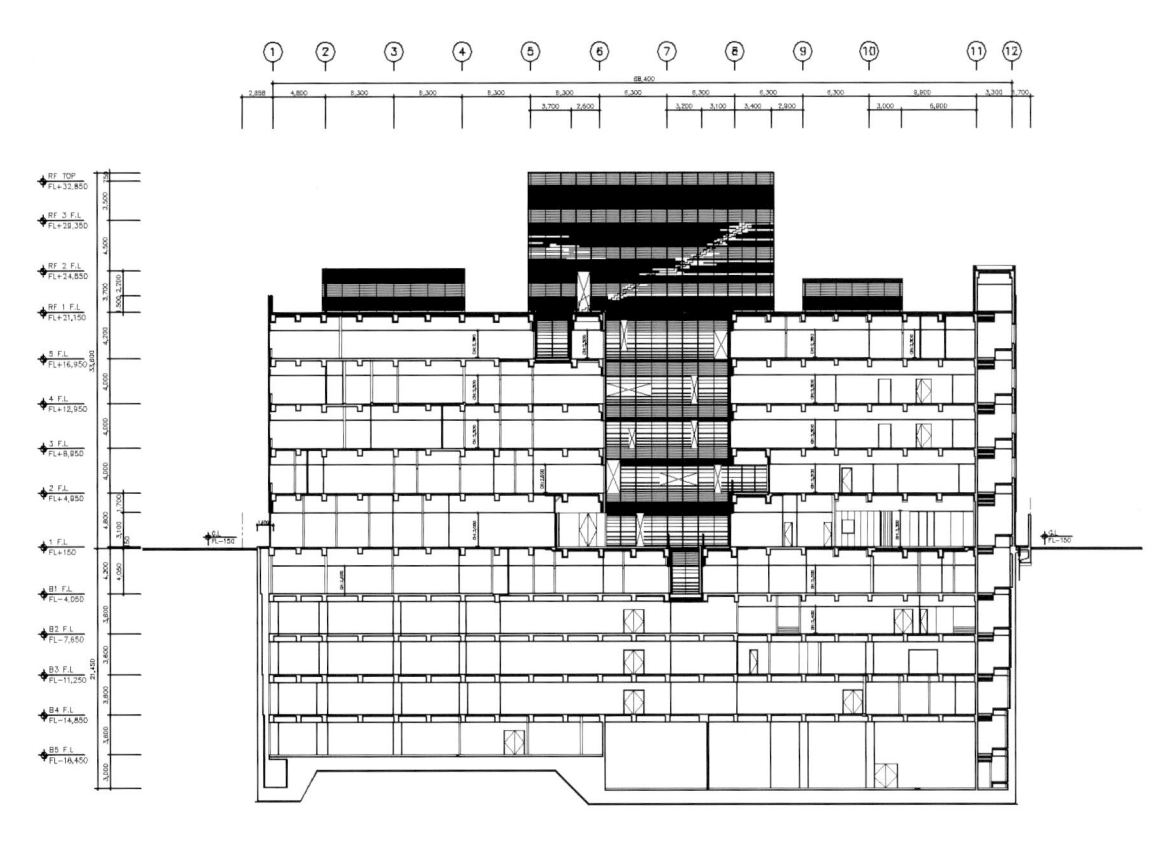

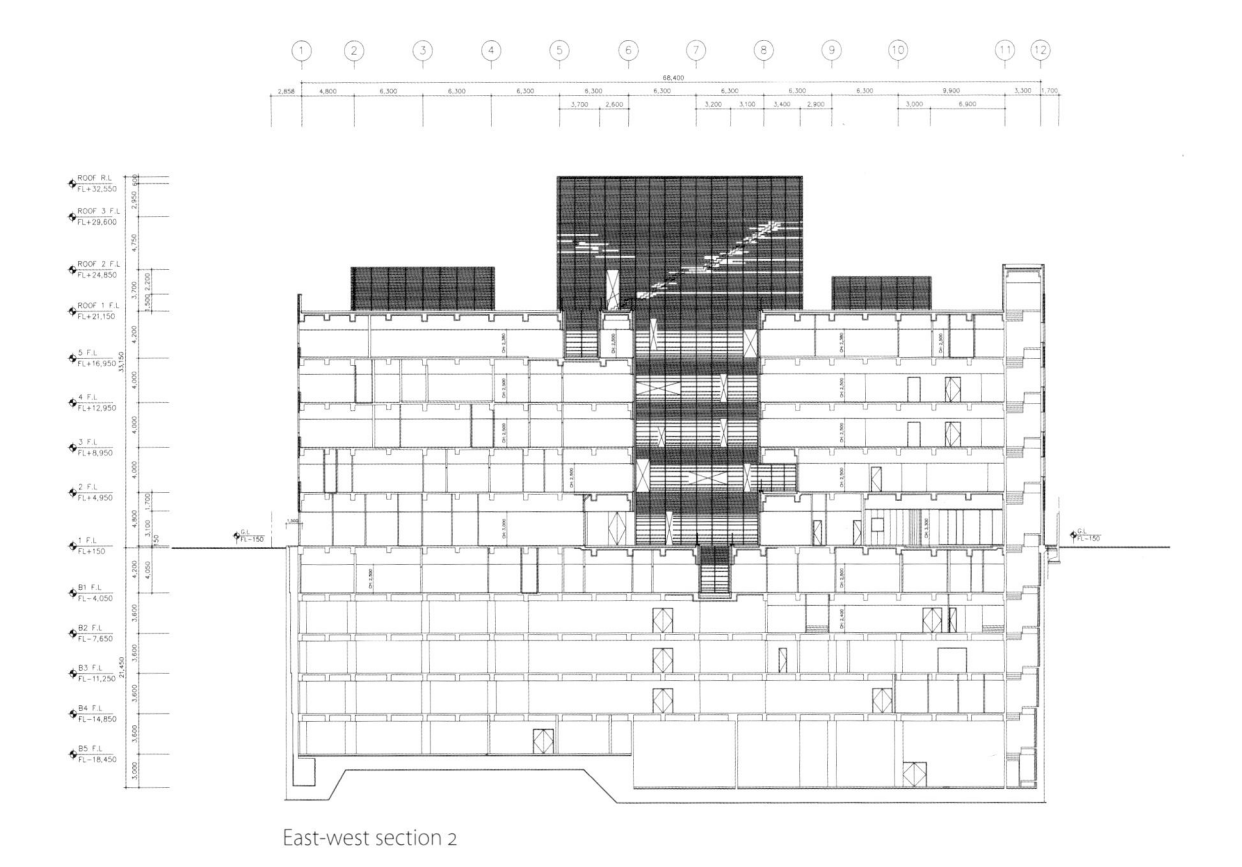

East-west section 2

North-south section 1

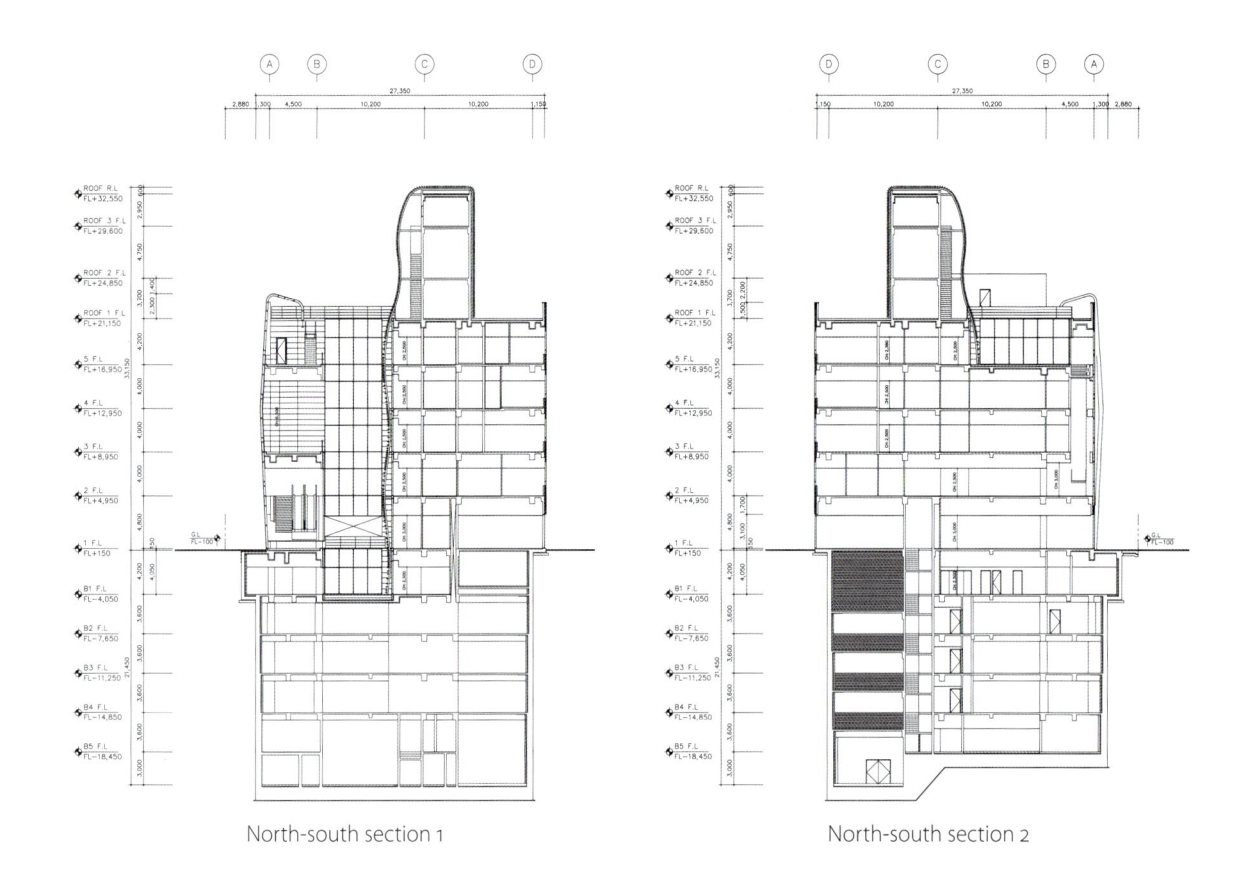

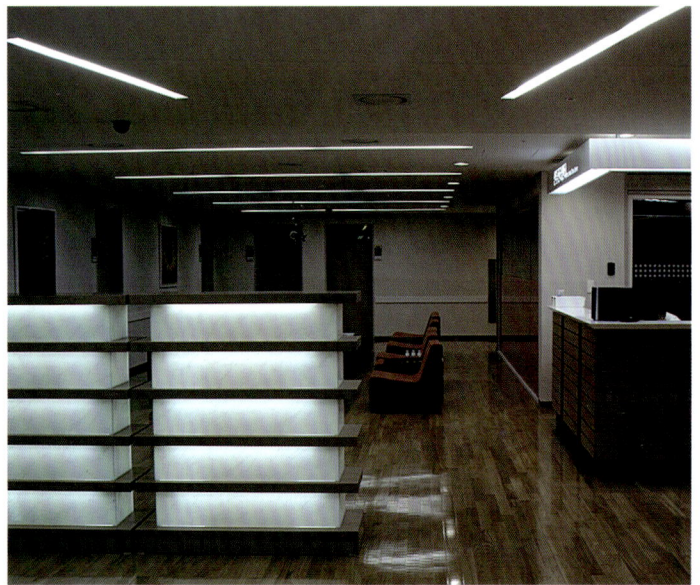

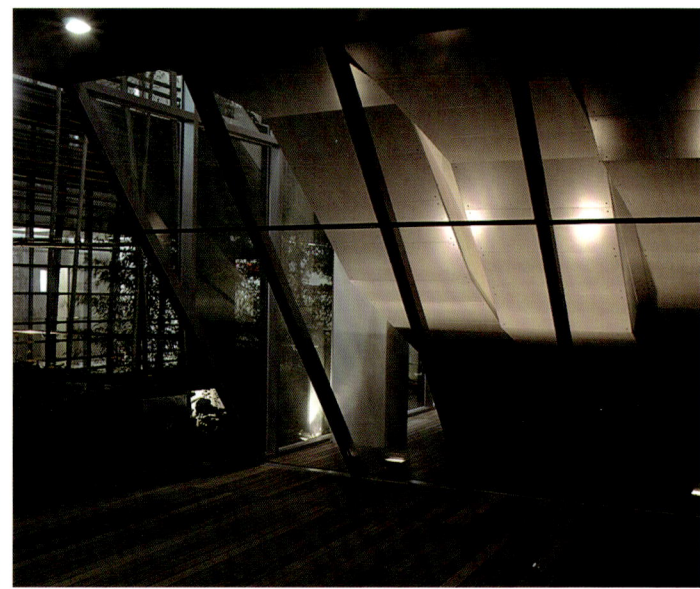

North-south section 2

165

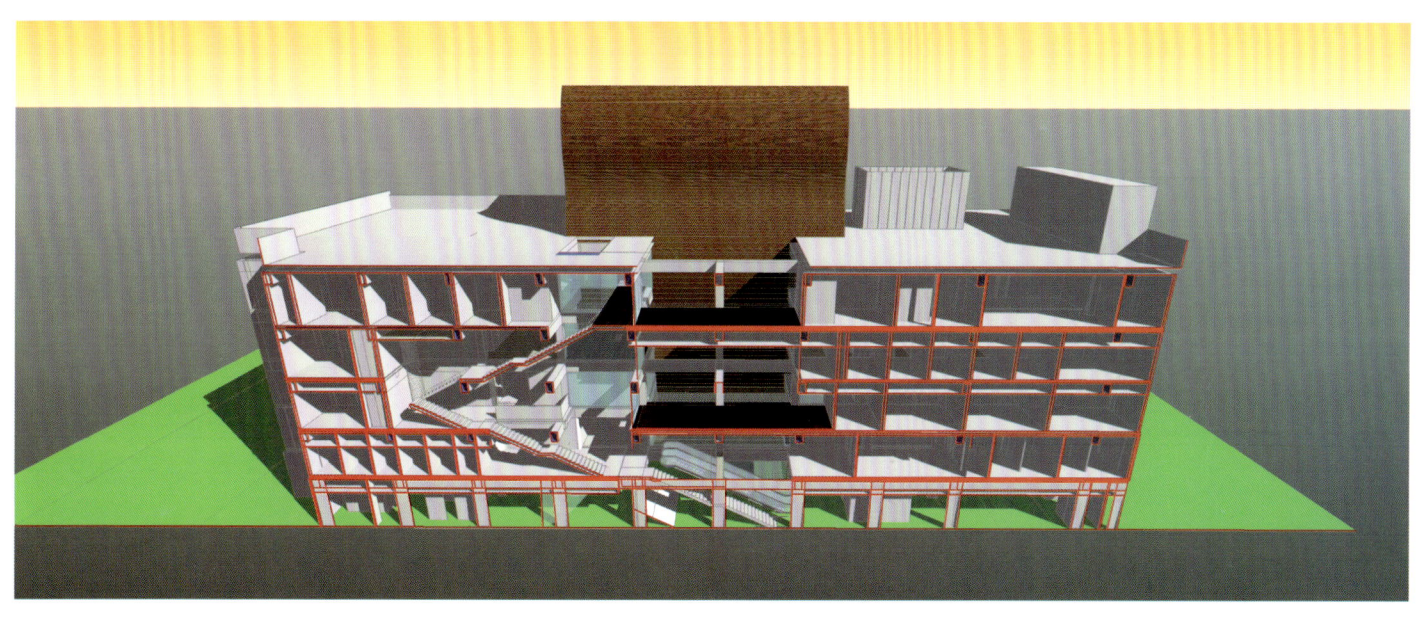

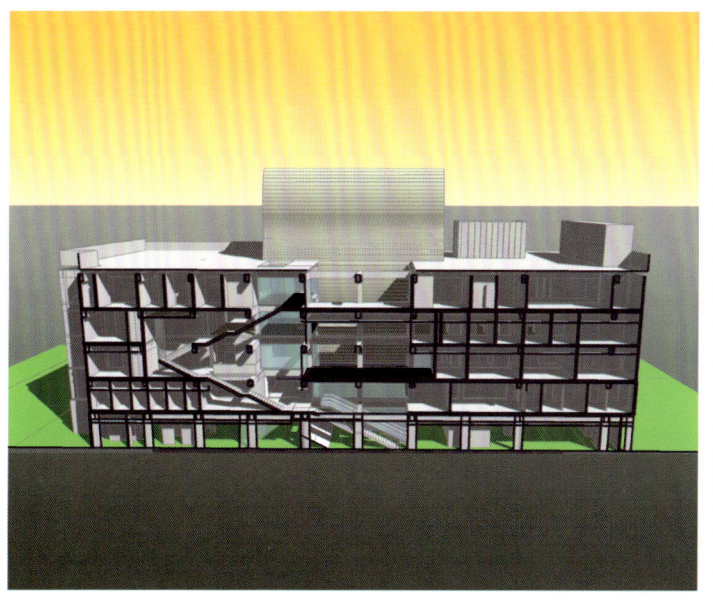

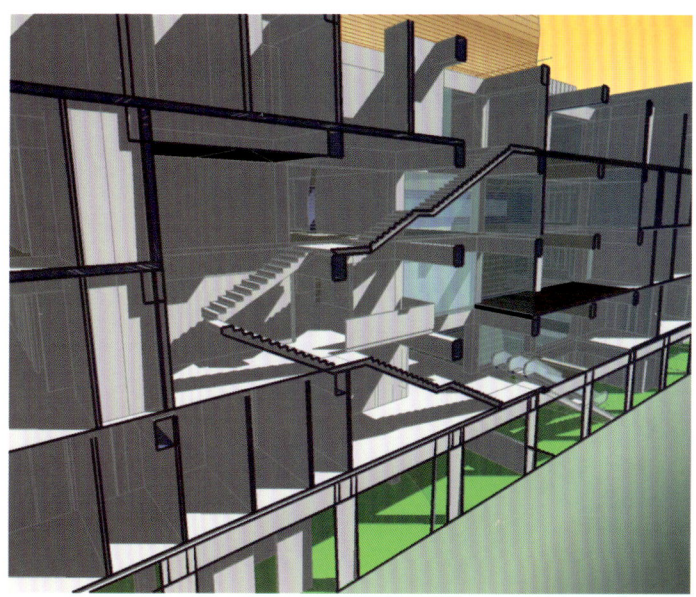

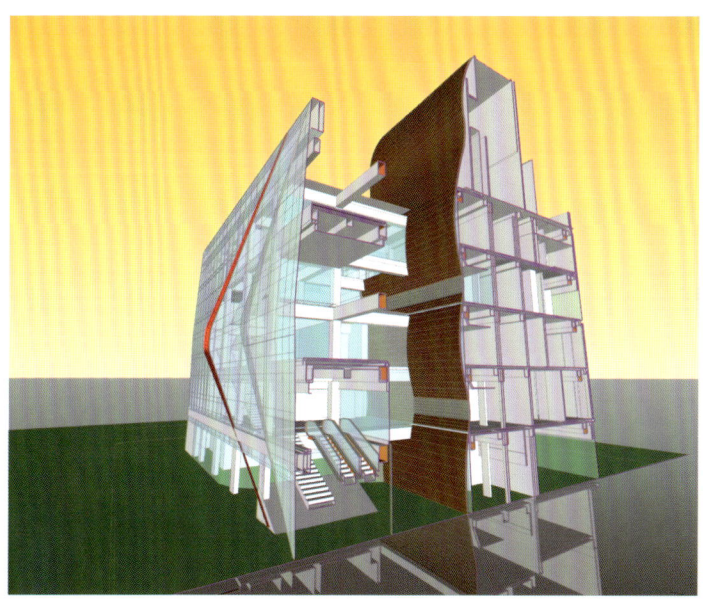

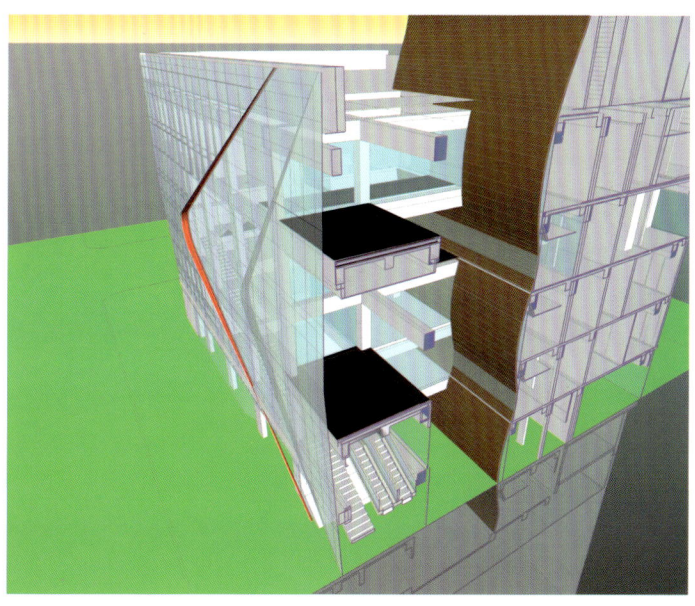

166

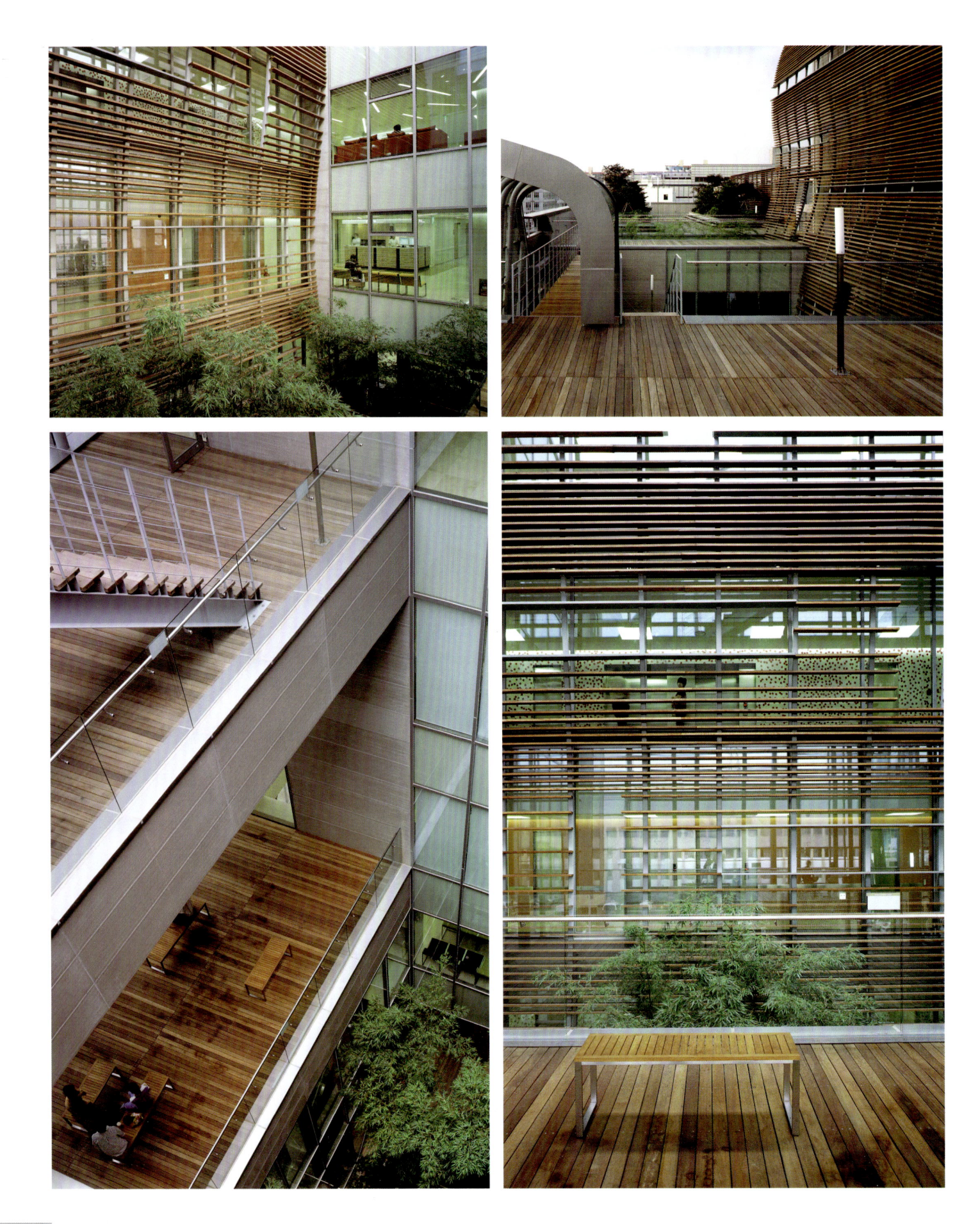

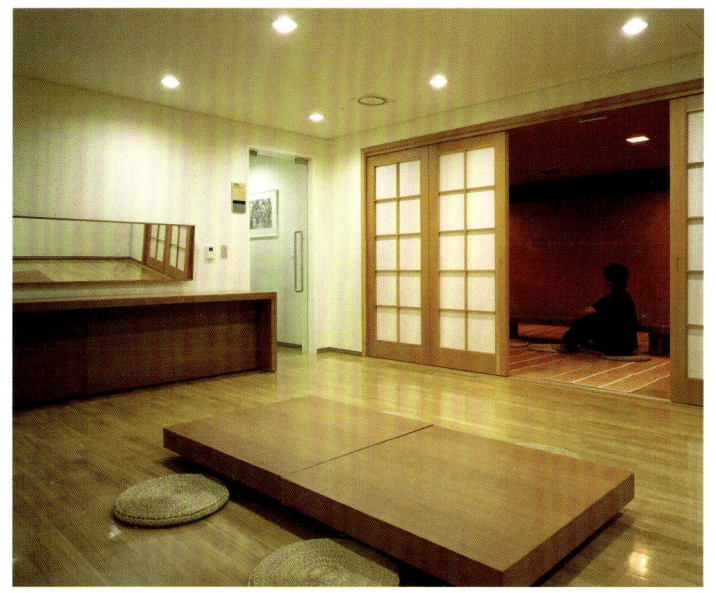

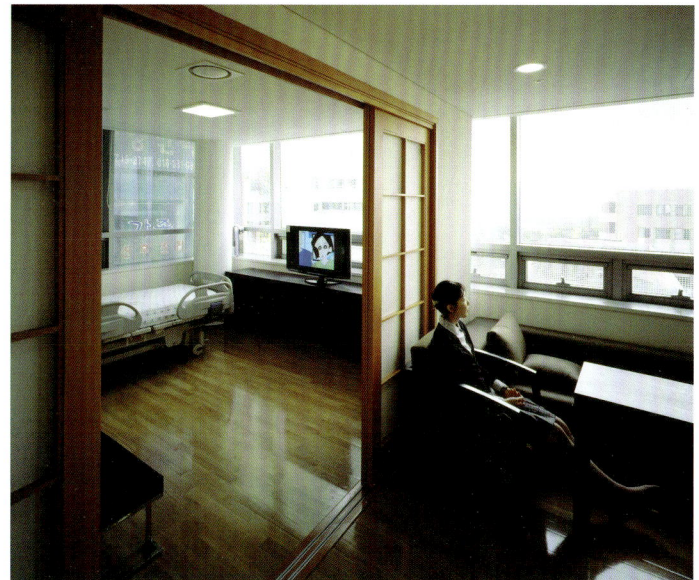

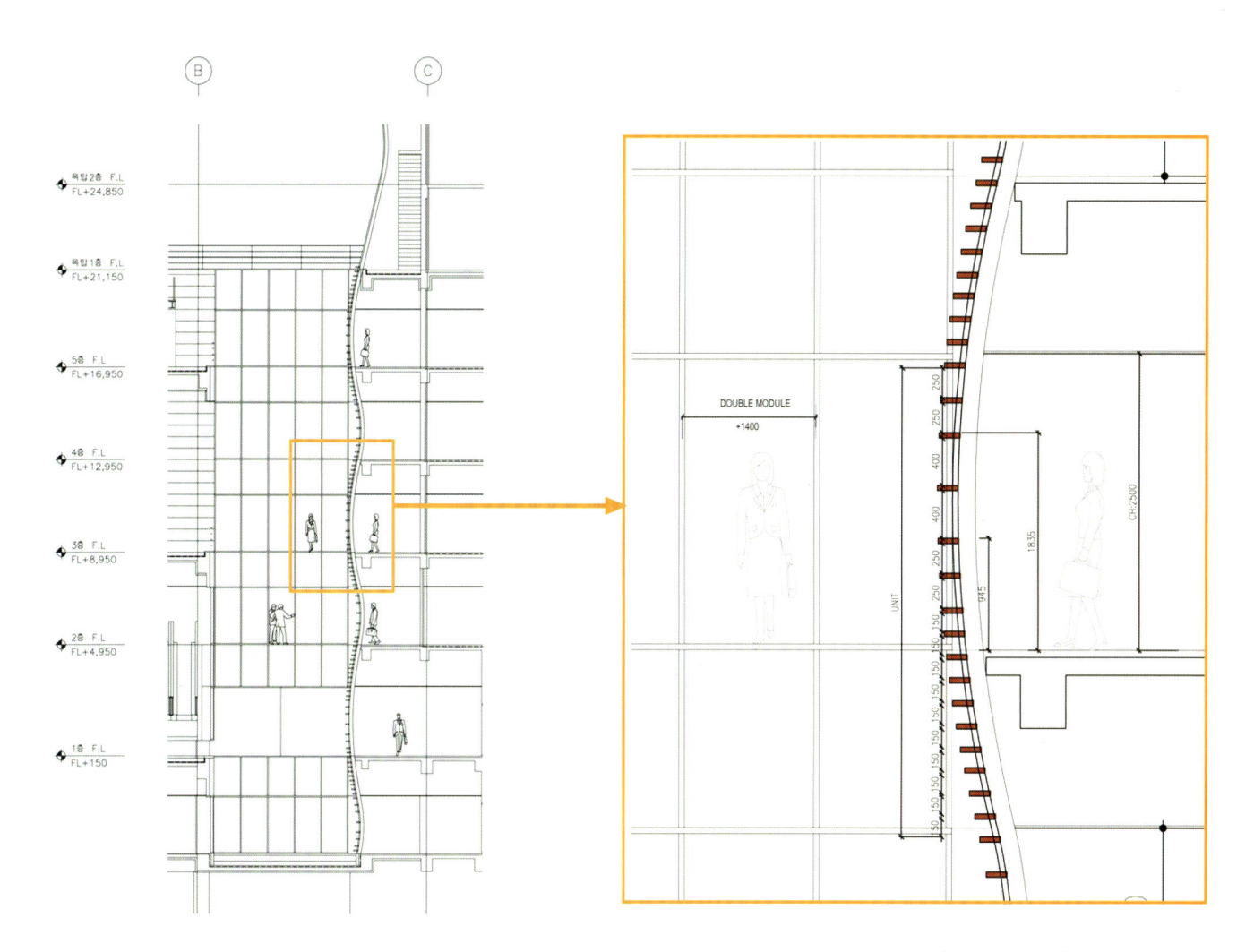

Glass curtain wall at atrium space
Wood screen profile

KMD

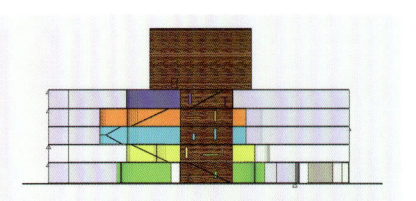

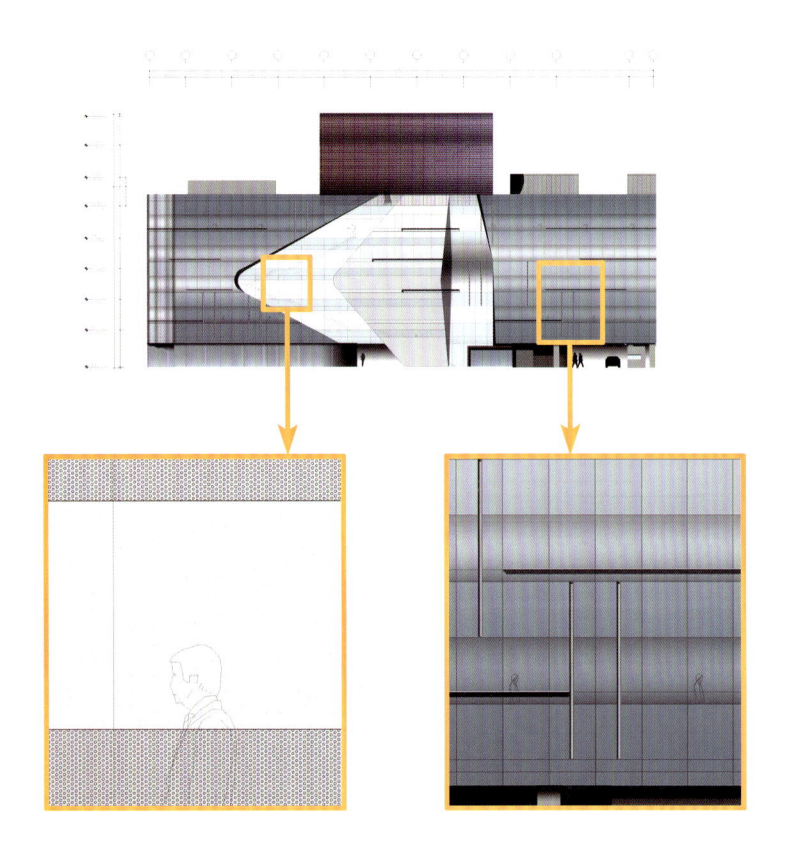

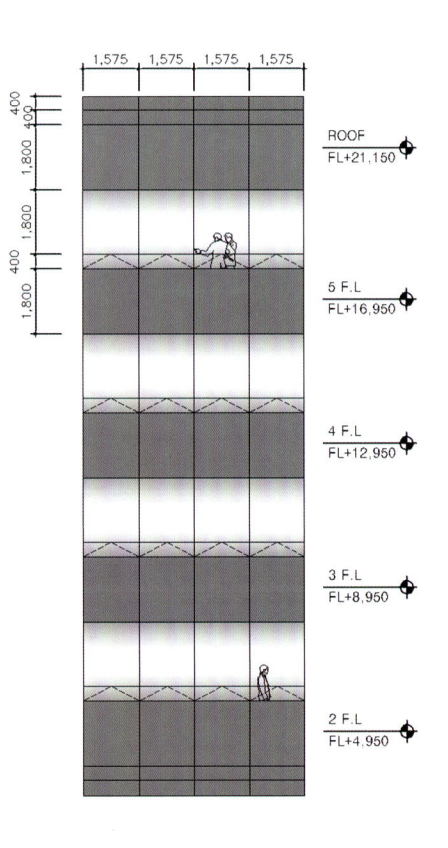

Enlarged glass pattern
at stair & corridor

Enlarged glass curtain wall at patient room
& facility

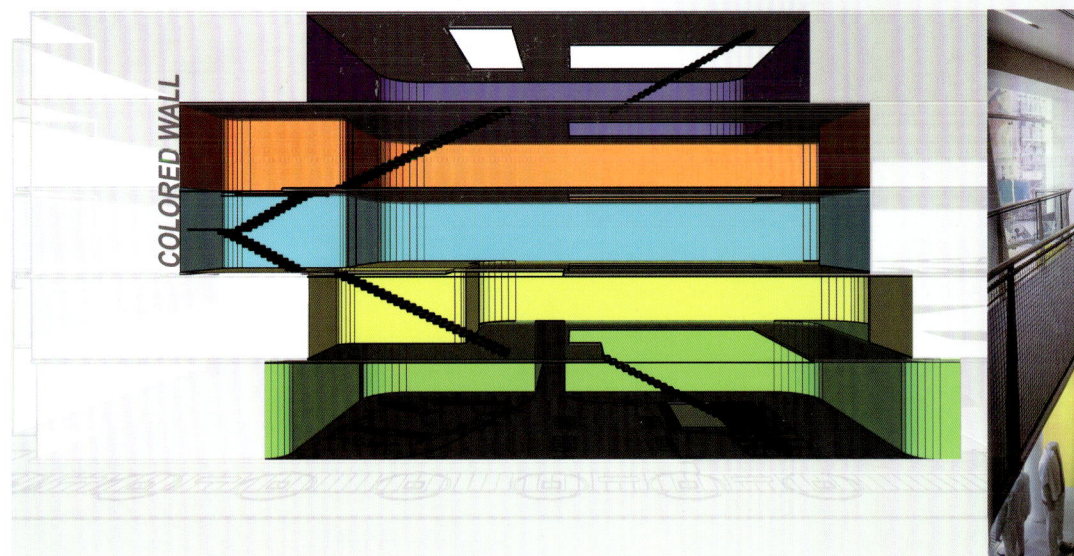

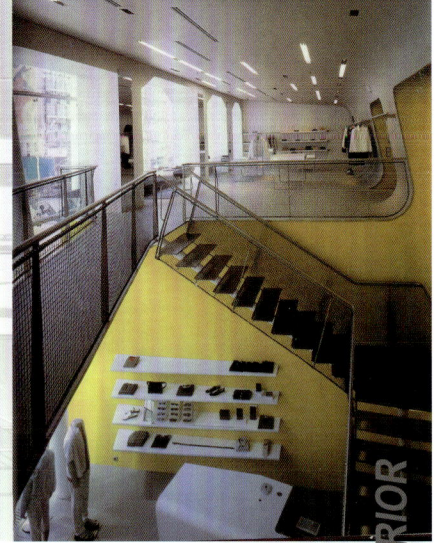

Typ. glass curtain wall

169

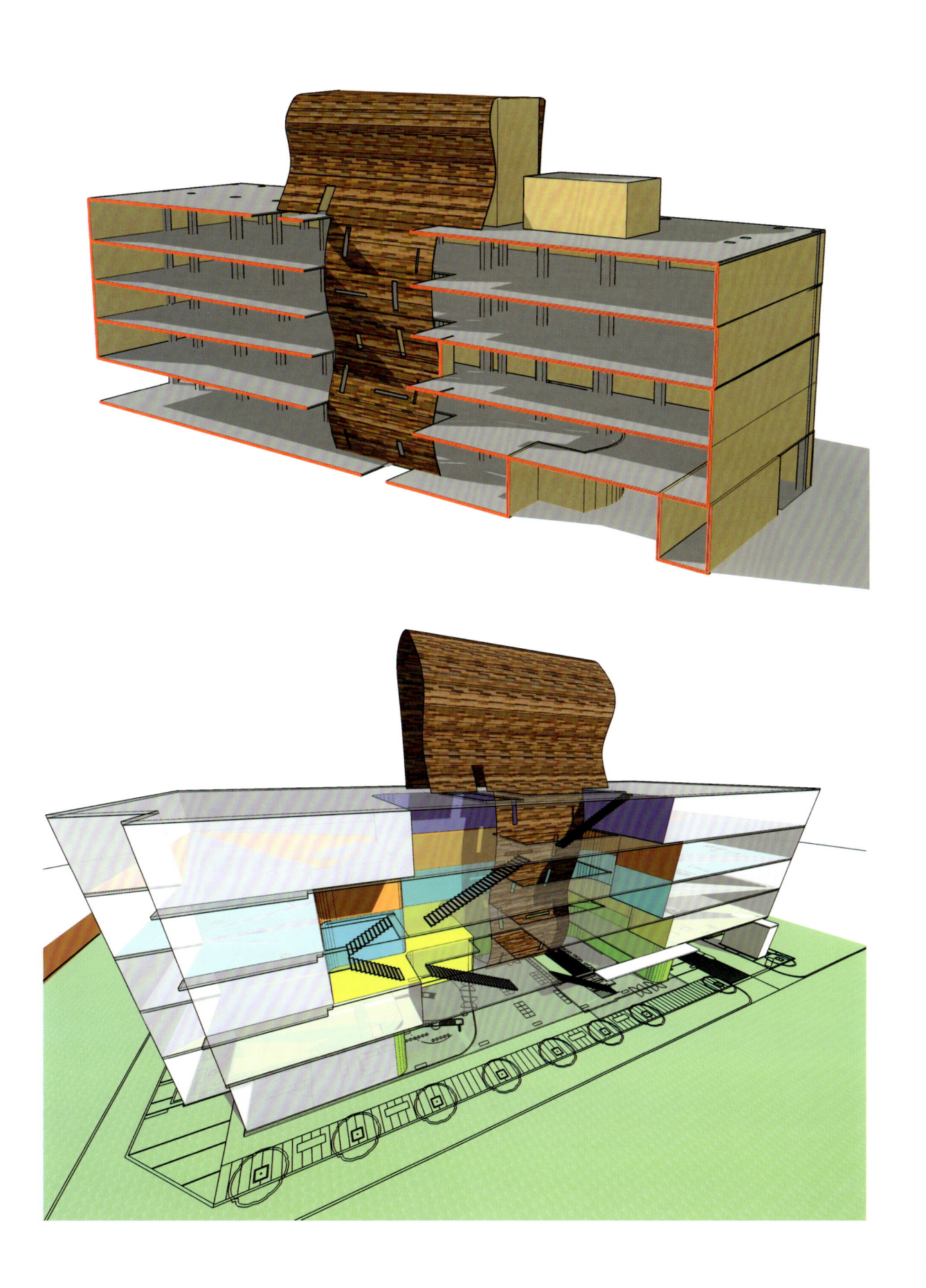

West elevation

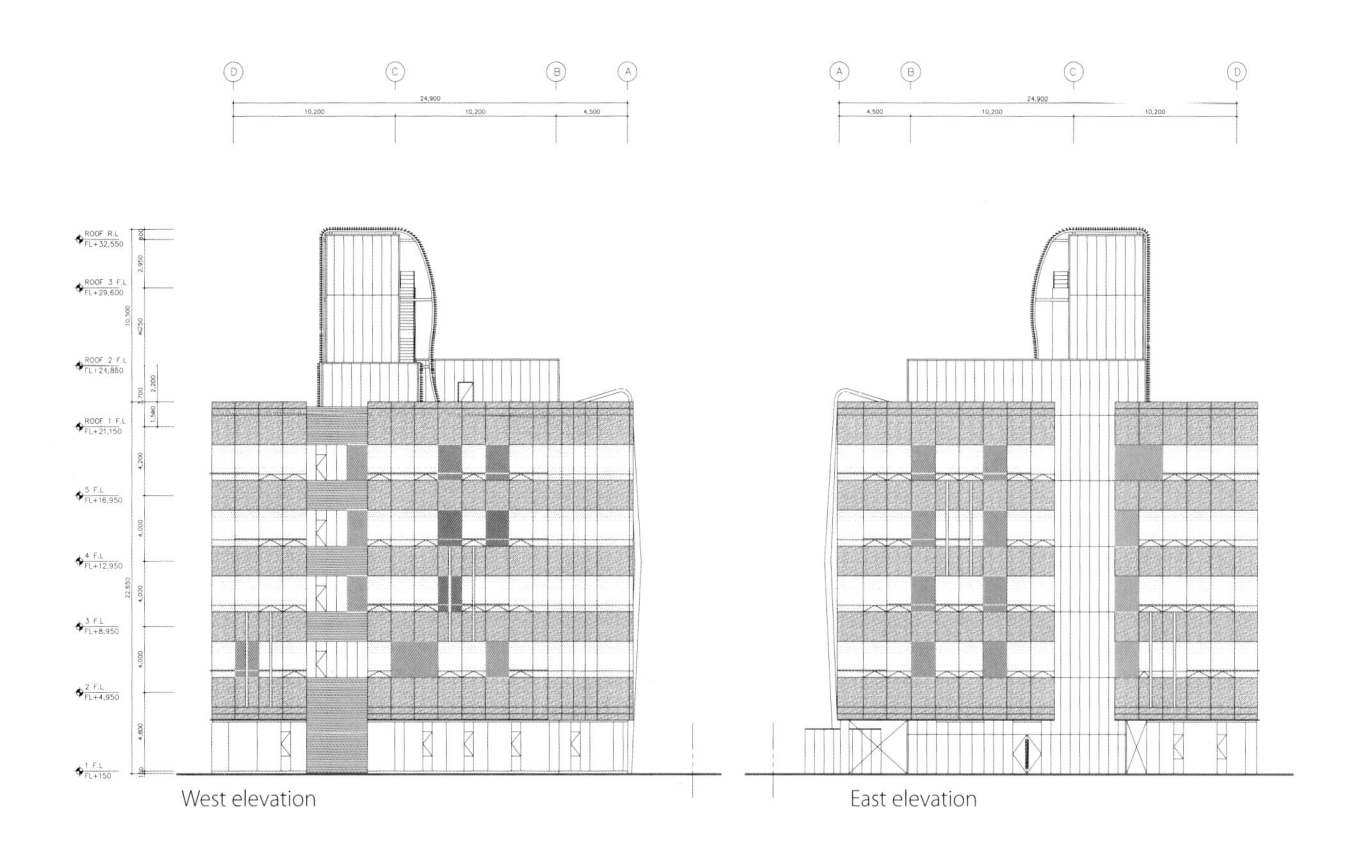

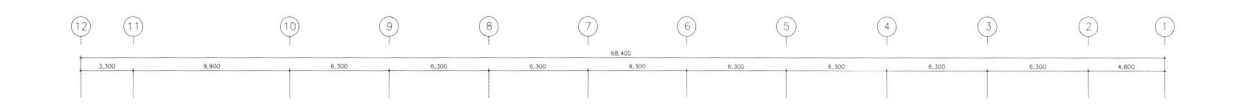

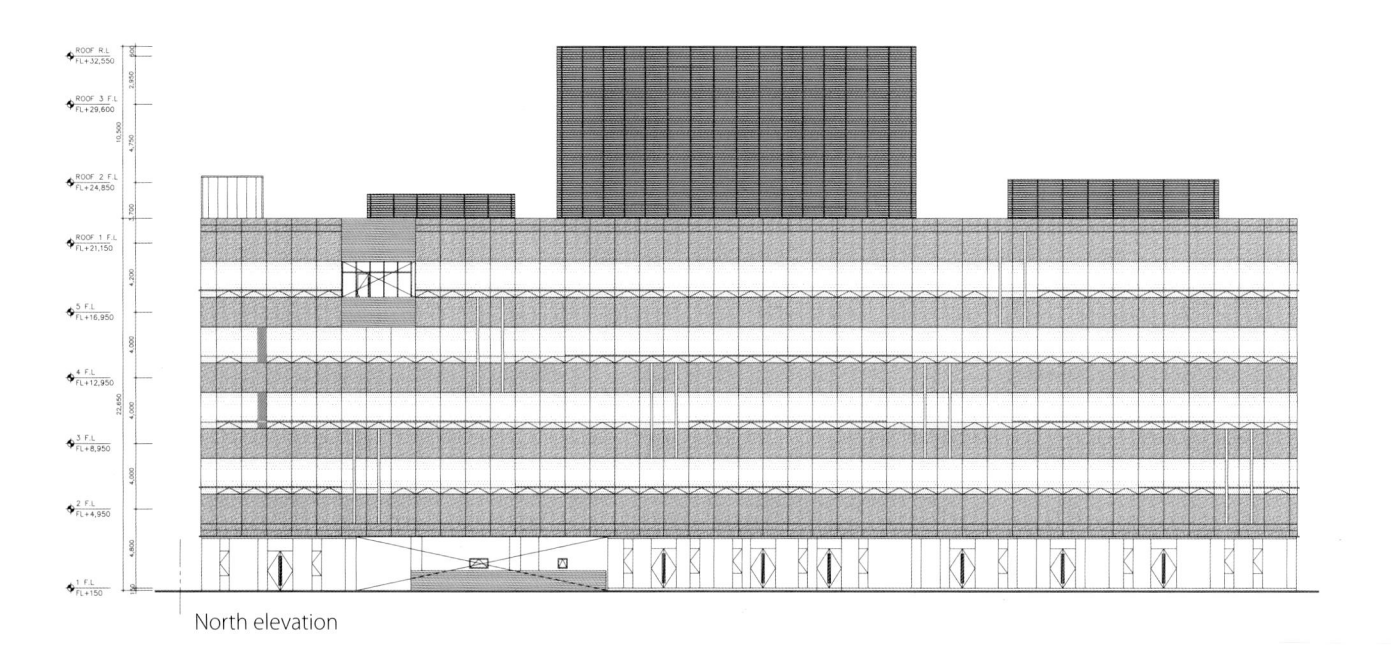

East elevation

North elevation

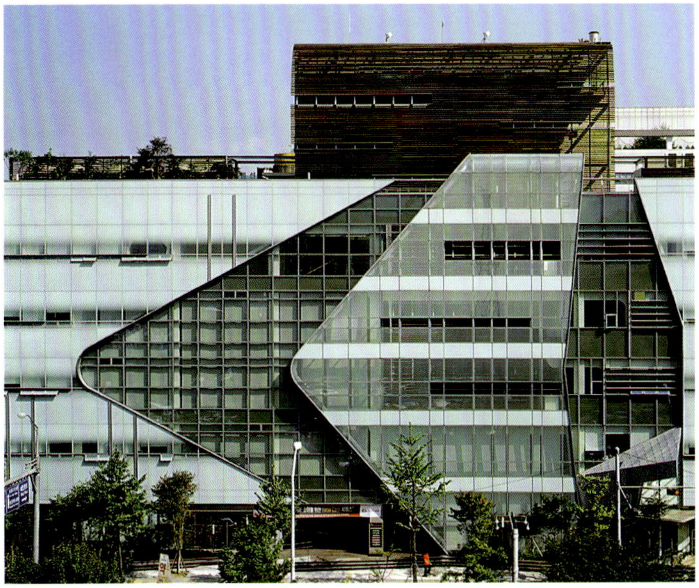

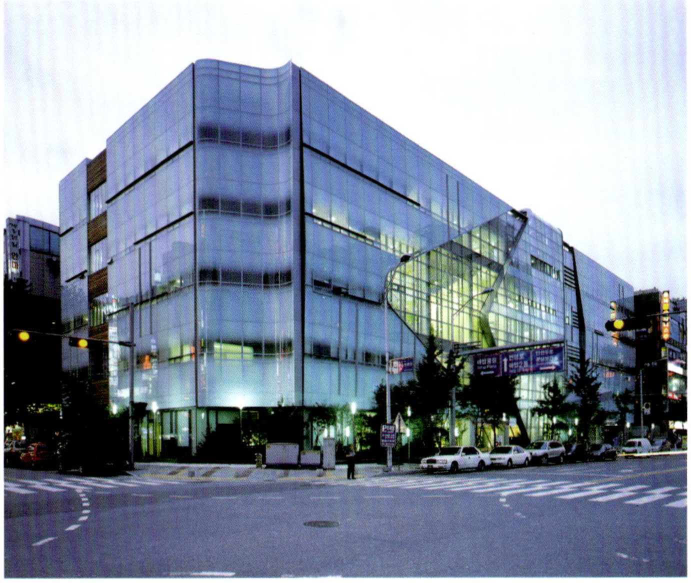

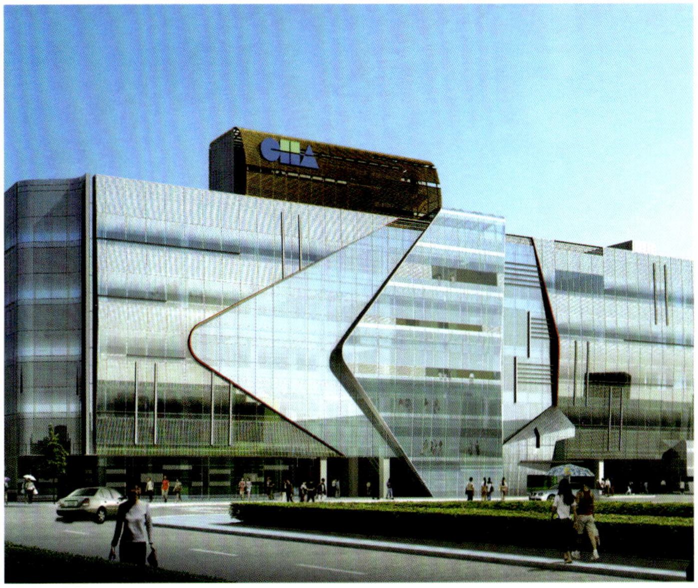
CHA

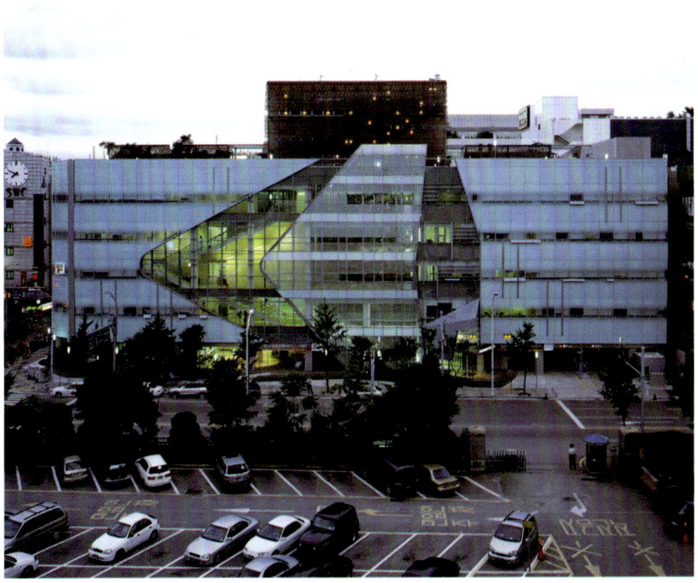

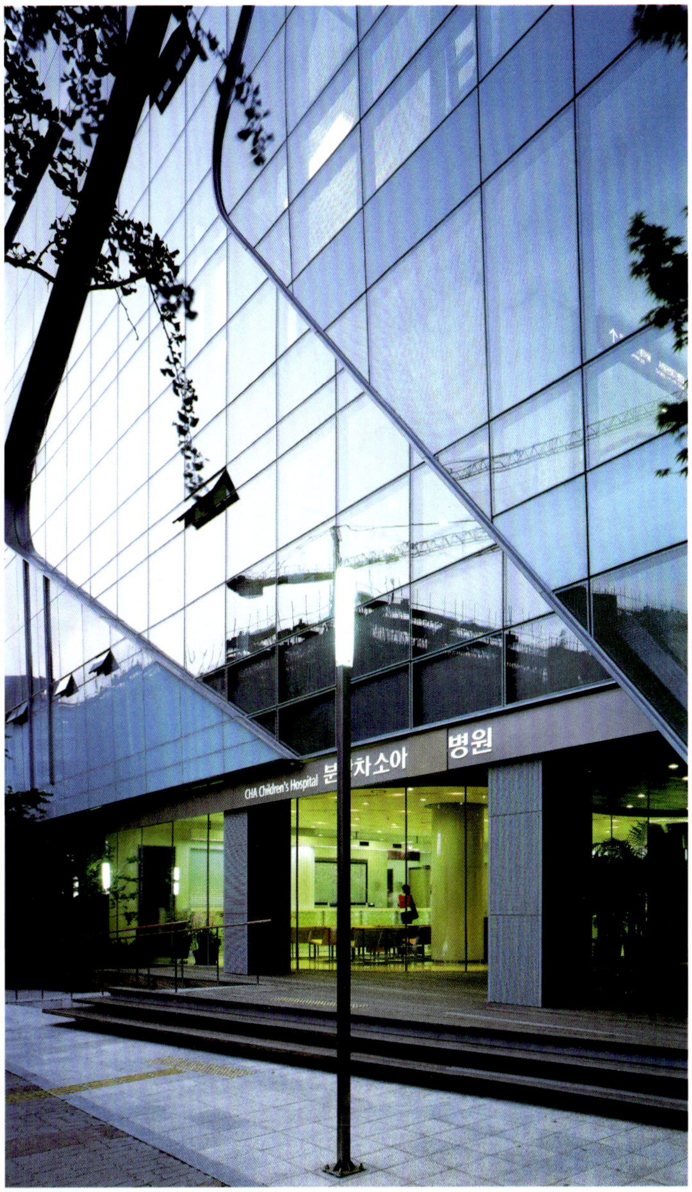
CHA Children's Hospital
분
차소아
병원

KMD

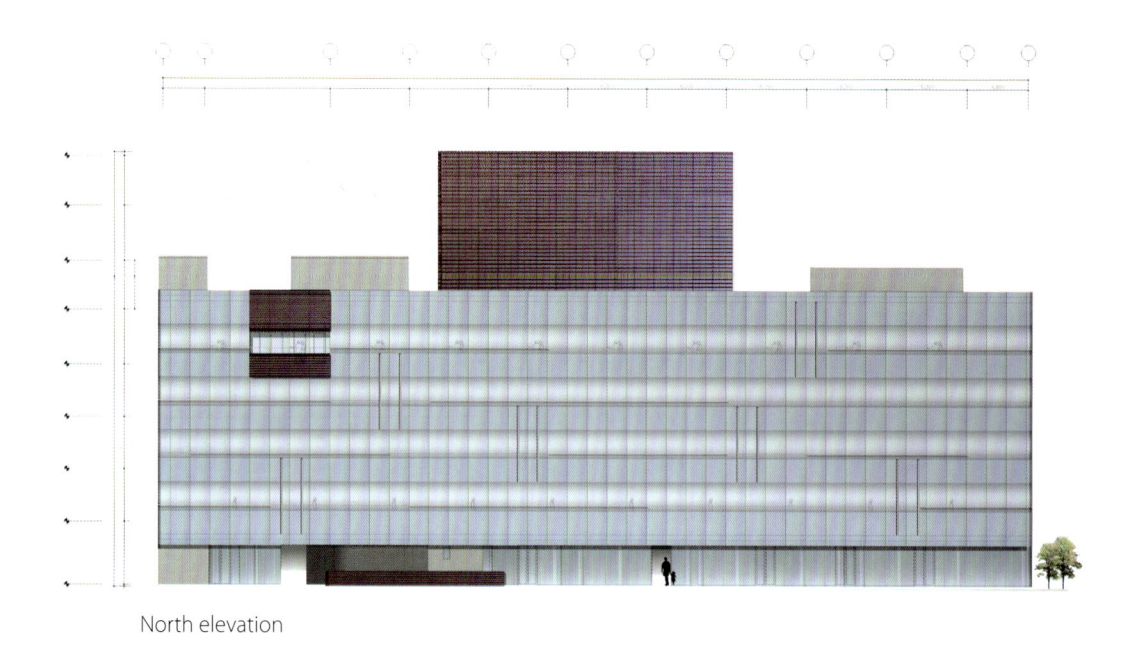

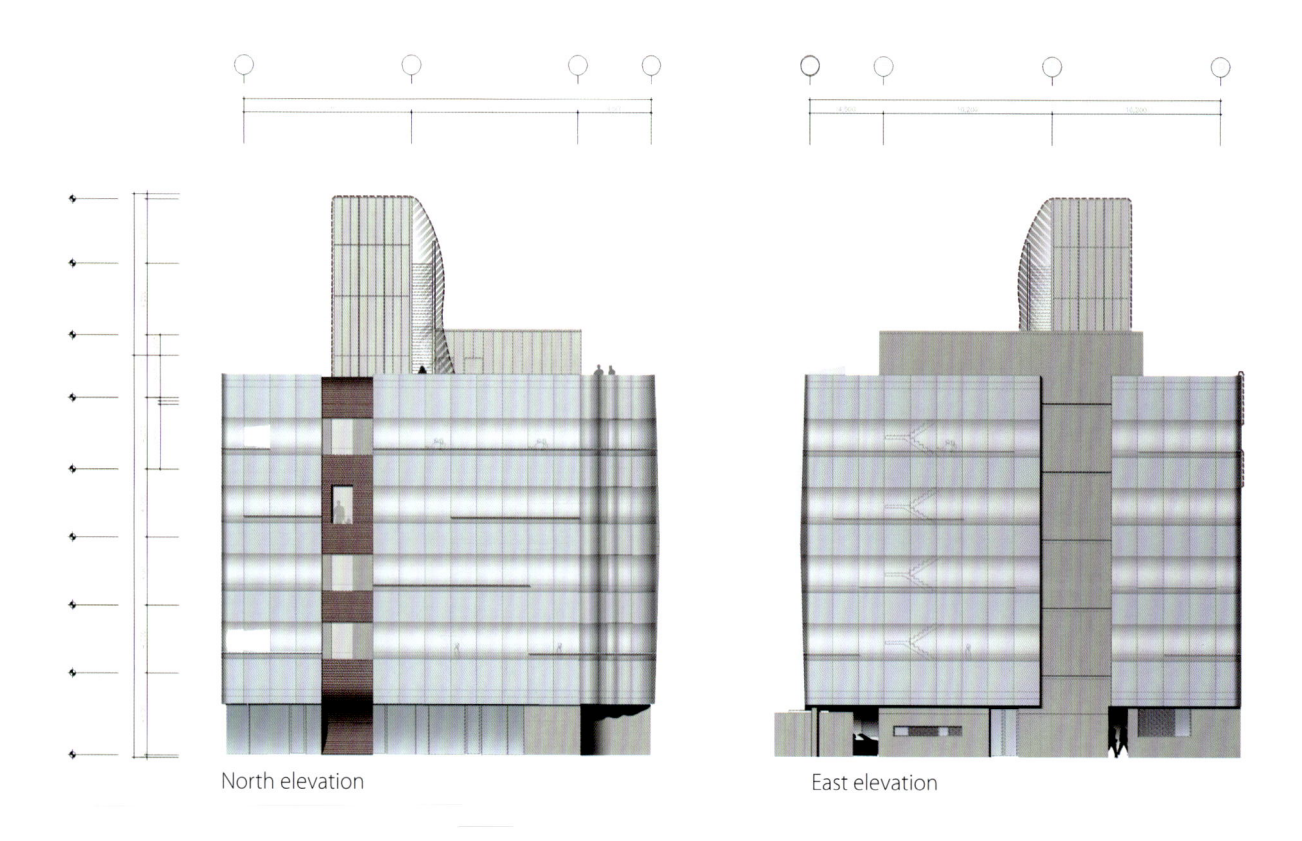

North elevation

North elevation

East elevation

West elevation

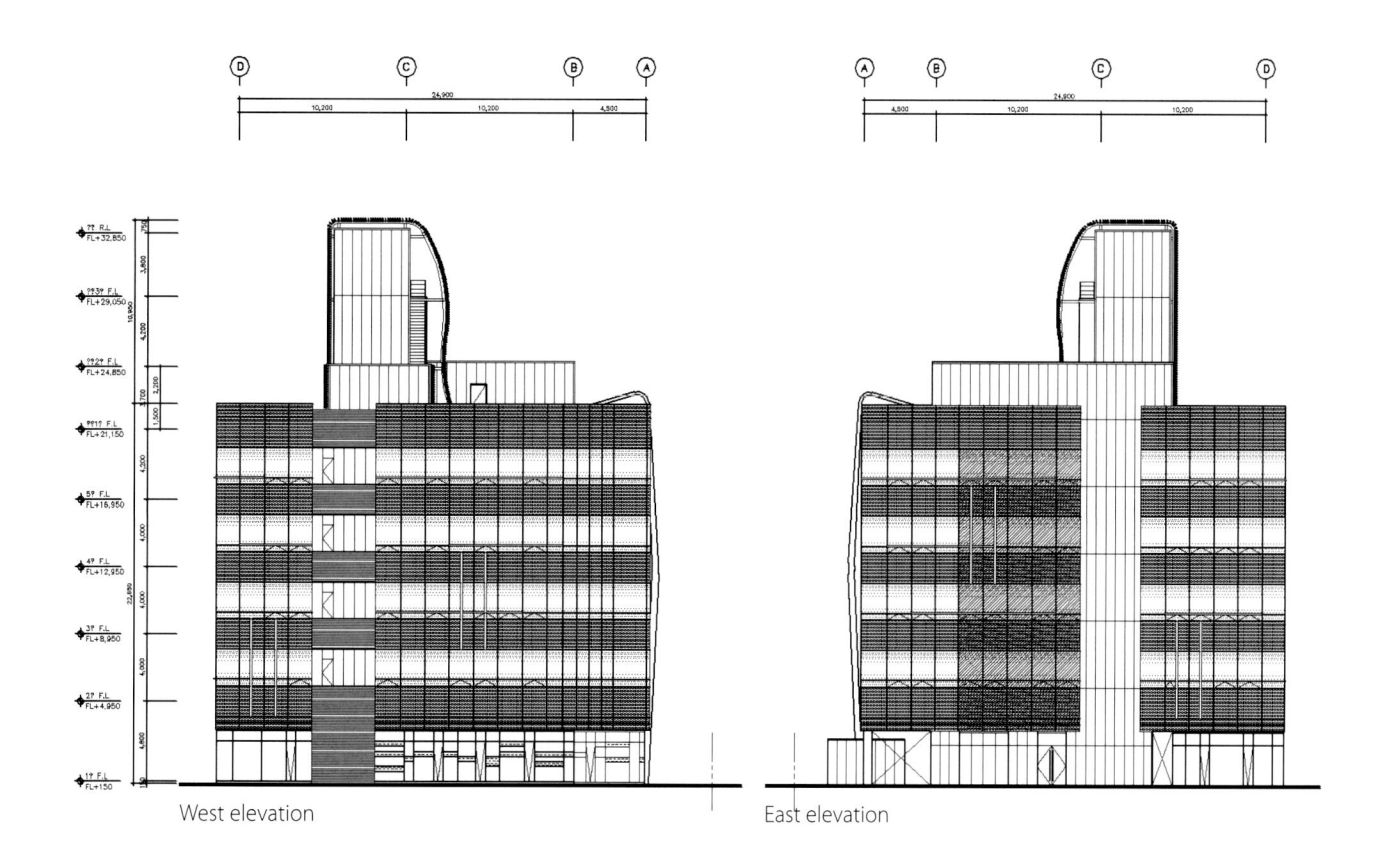

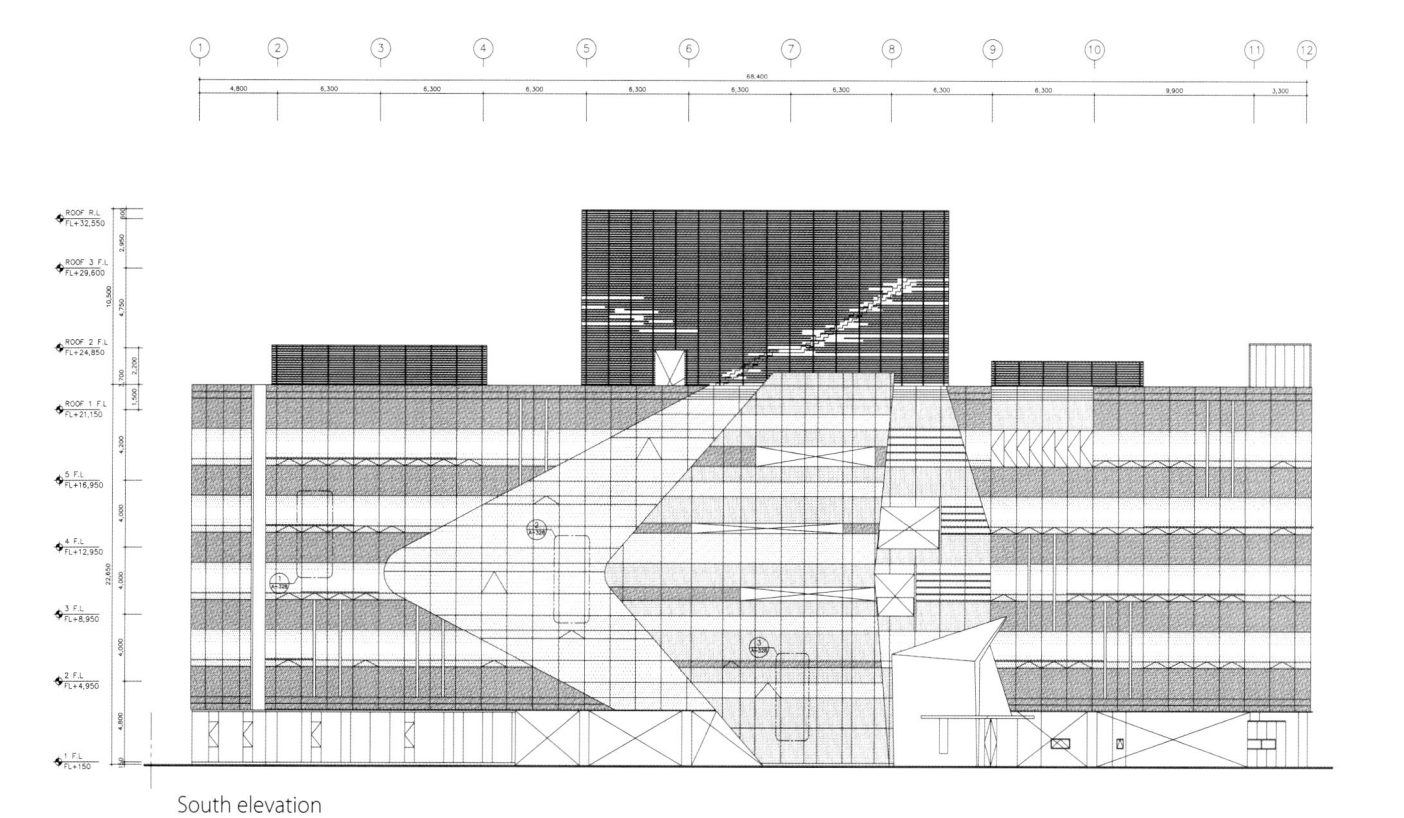

East elevation

South elevation

Corea & Moran Arquitectura

Mahón Hospital

Menorca, Spain

Photographs: *Pepo Segura*

The site proposed for the new Menorca General Hospital, in the city of Mahon consists of a vast flat surface area with a rectangular geometry. The ground floor plan covers approximately 35,000 sqm (375,000 sqft) and can be easily accessed by the front and one side of the building where there are service roads for vehicles. Ample parking space is provided next to the hospital.

The project for the hospital took advantage of the generous surface area offered by the site and developed primarily on a horizontal plane, rising to just two levels. The horizontal solution is actually much more effective than a vertical one, as the latter relies upon mechanical means of circulation, or endless flights of stairs. The building in itself is a system that organizes sub-systems of services. The areas for the public, medical staff and technicians are organized through and connected by circulation routes that form a sequence defining boundaries and access possibilities. This feature, however, does not hinder the exit possibilities in case of an emergency. The organizational layout generates clarity in the circuits, avoids patients and visitors obstructing movement and facilitates the control over hygiene standards. The system is capable of being adapted to changes in use, services, equipment, medical technologies and techniques, etc. Essentially, the hospital has been designed as a support architecture which is capable of accommodating the proposed program of 27,826 sqm (300,000 sqft) and 140 beds, and of being compatible with future needs and requirements.

The hospital has been designed as a massive volume on the ground floor penetrated by light courtyards, upon which float the four in-patient volumes forming the first floor. The project is organized about three circulation routes: a public circulation with escalators and double-height spaces, a circulation for use by medical staff only and a technical circulation located in a linear building housing the installations, services and supplies. The functional program is distributed across the ground floor, with the out-patients area at one end and intensive treatment at the other. The main roof extends beyond the limits of the building and folds to reach down to the floor providing a spacious courtyard for ambulances that is protected from the elements

Client:
IB-Salut
Surface area:
27,826 sqm (300,000 sqft)
Start date:
2002
Finish date:
2006
Project team:
Mario Corea, Lluis Moran, Emiliano Lopez
Collaborators:
Diego Nakamatsu
Cost:
€ 34,910,362

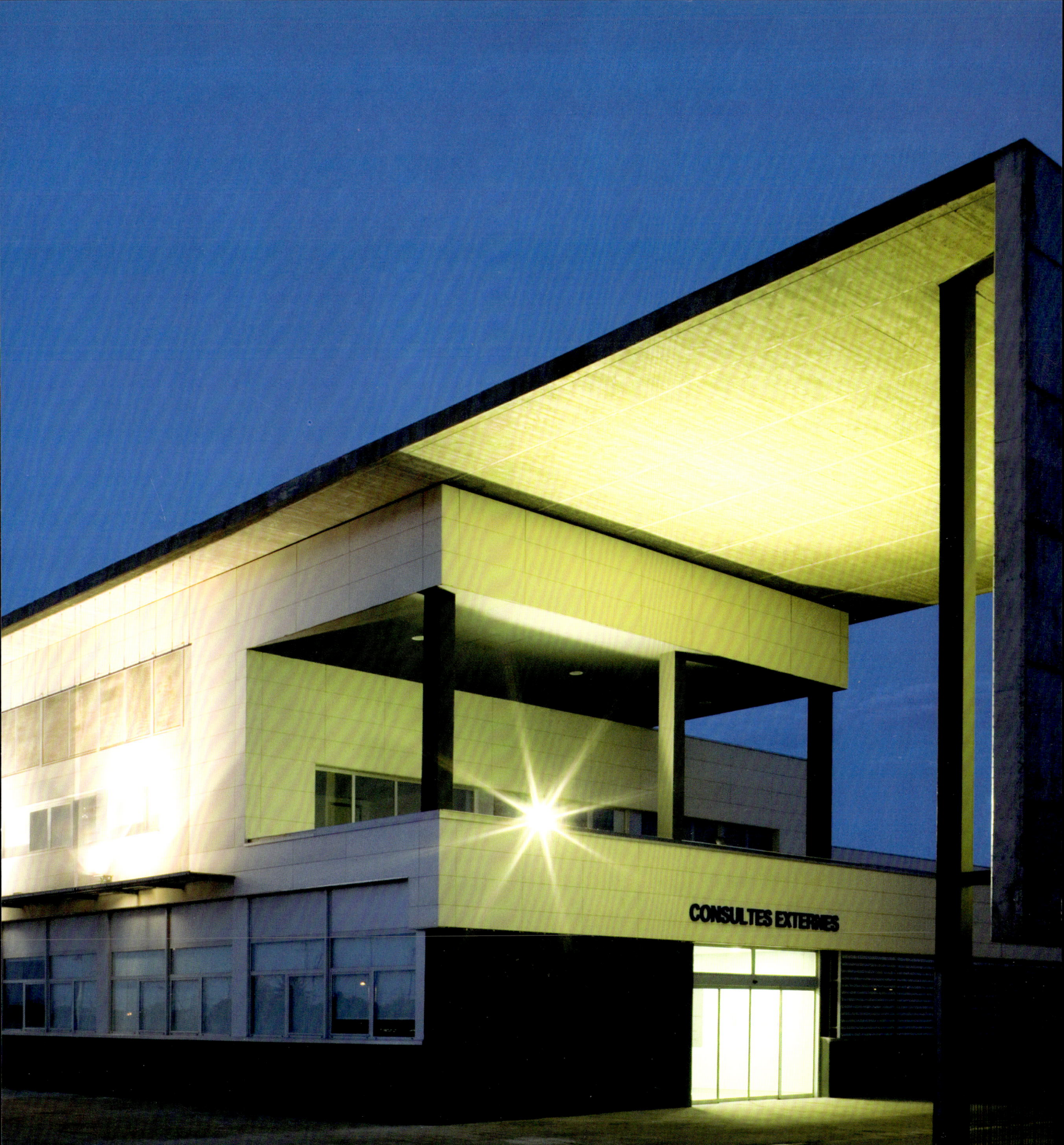

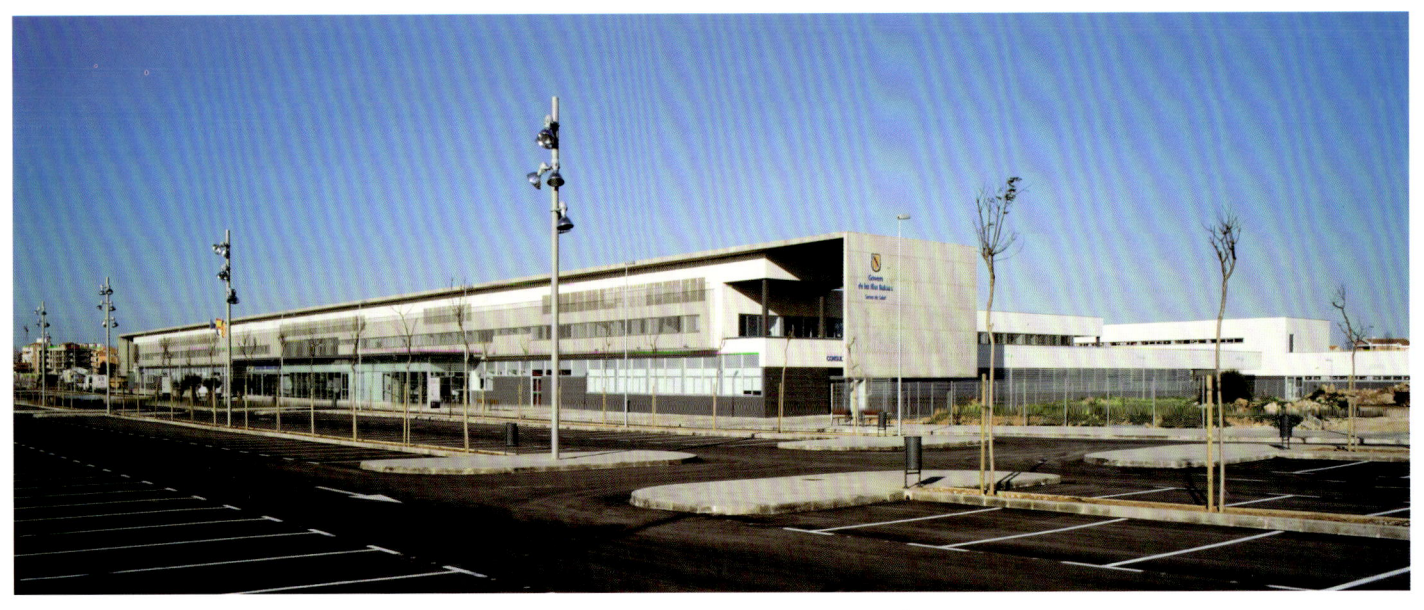

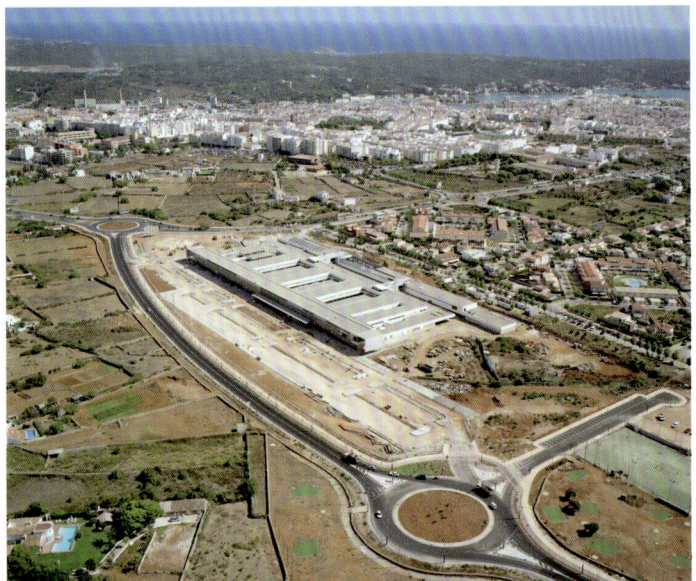

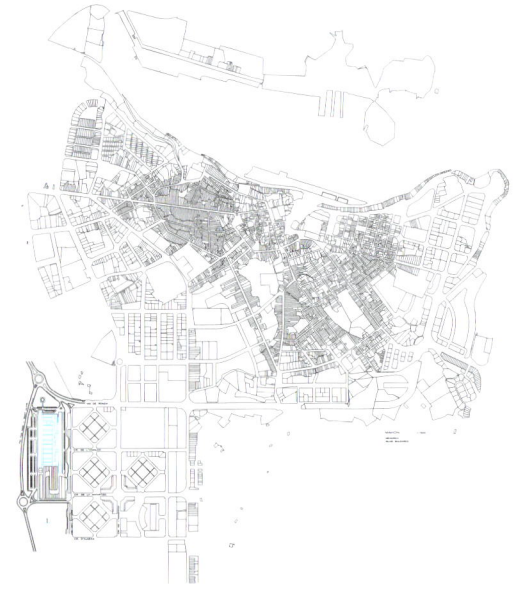

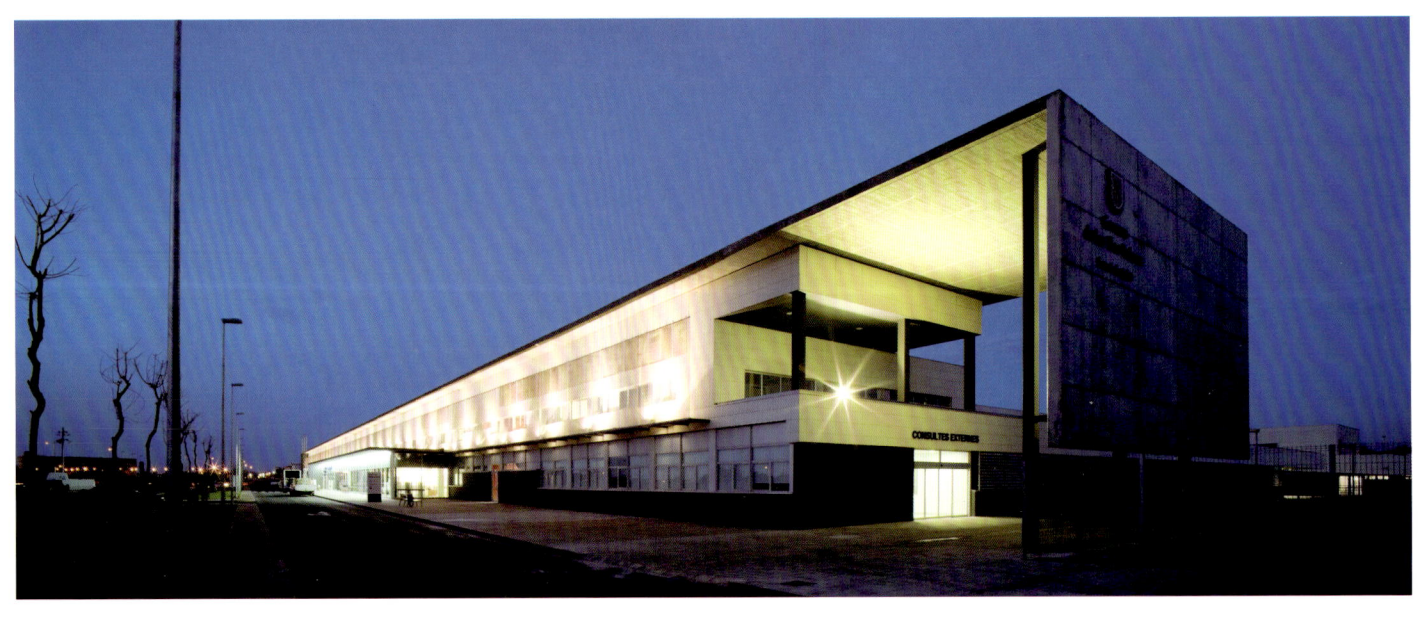

177

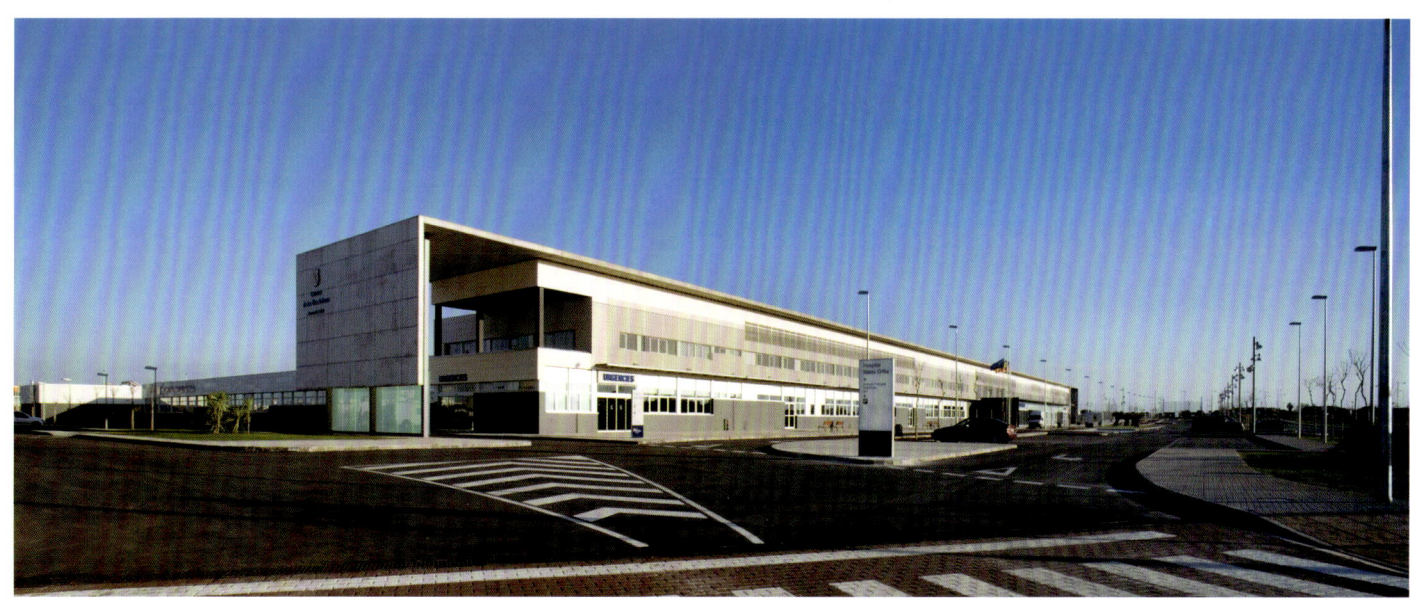

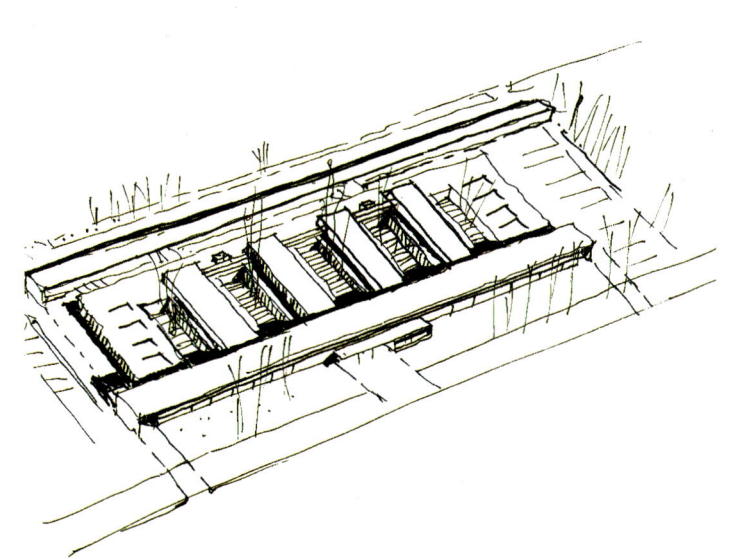

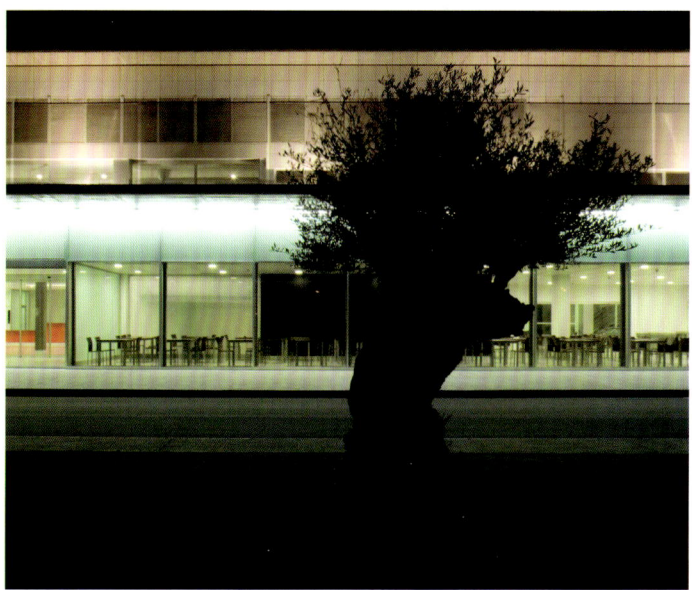

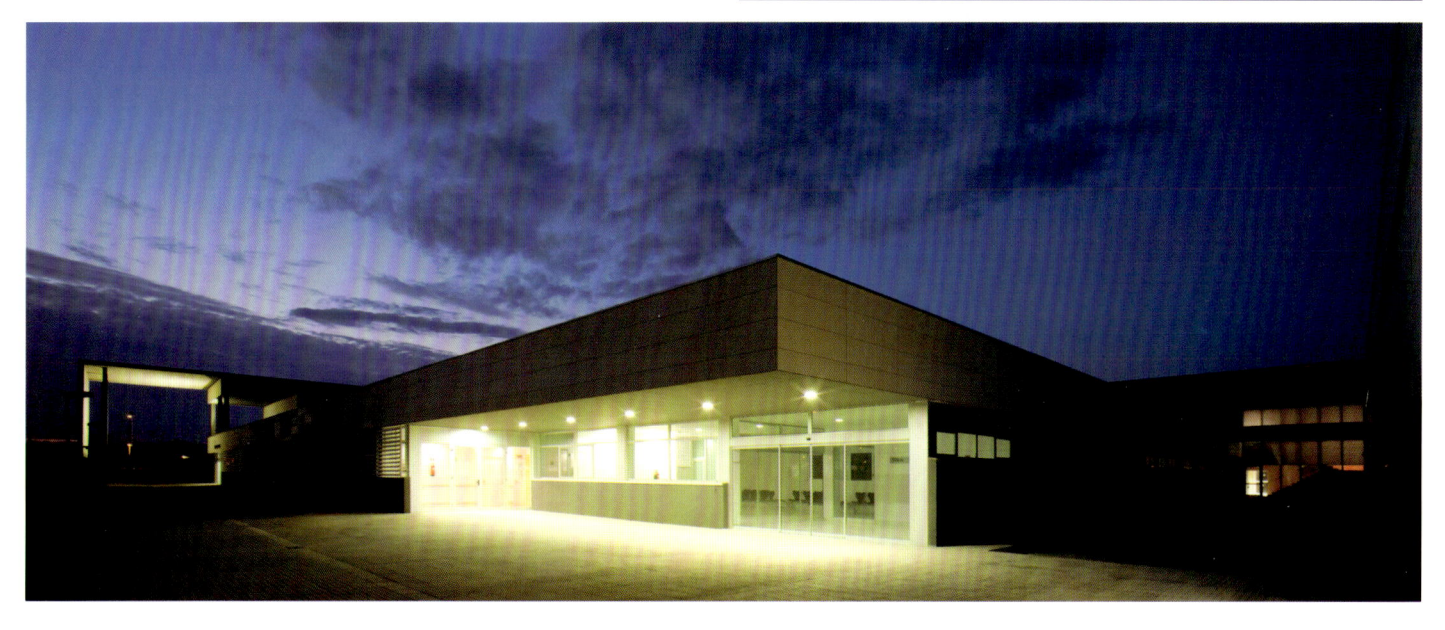

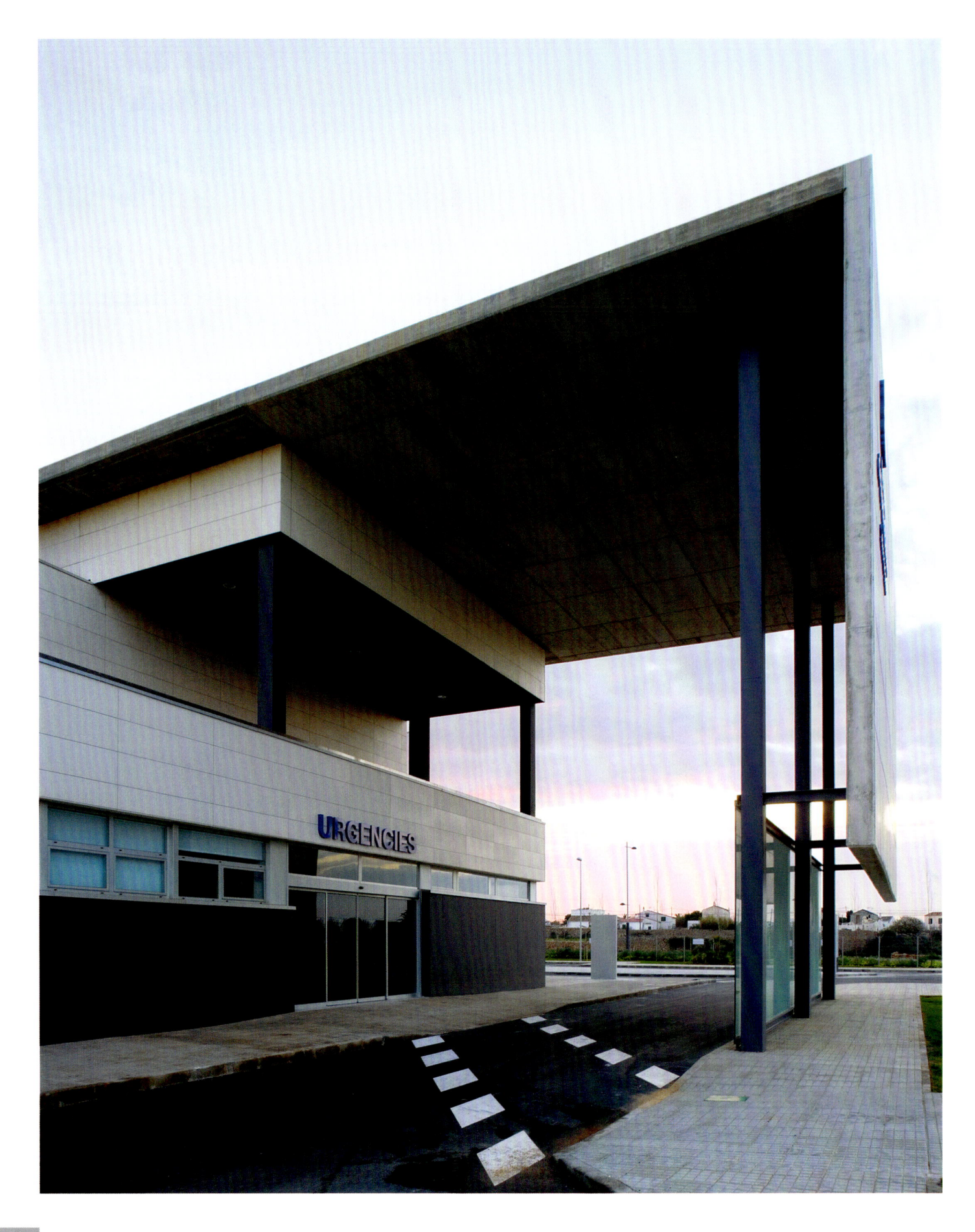

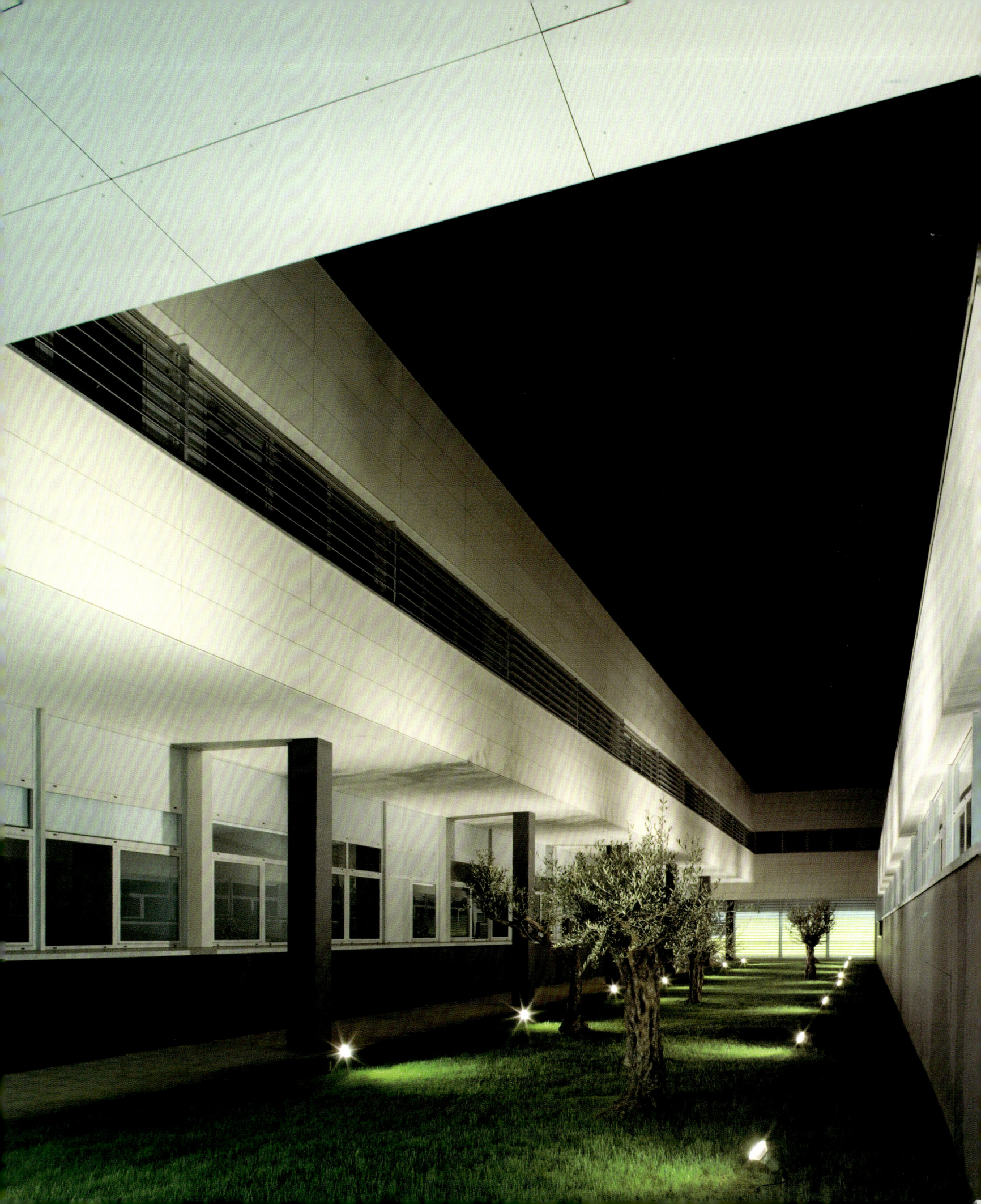

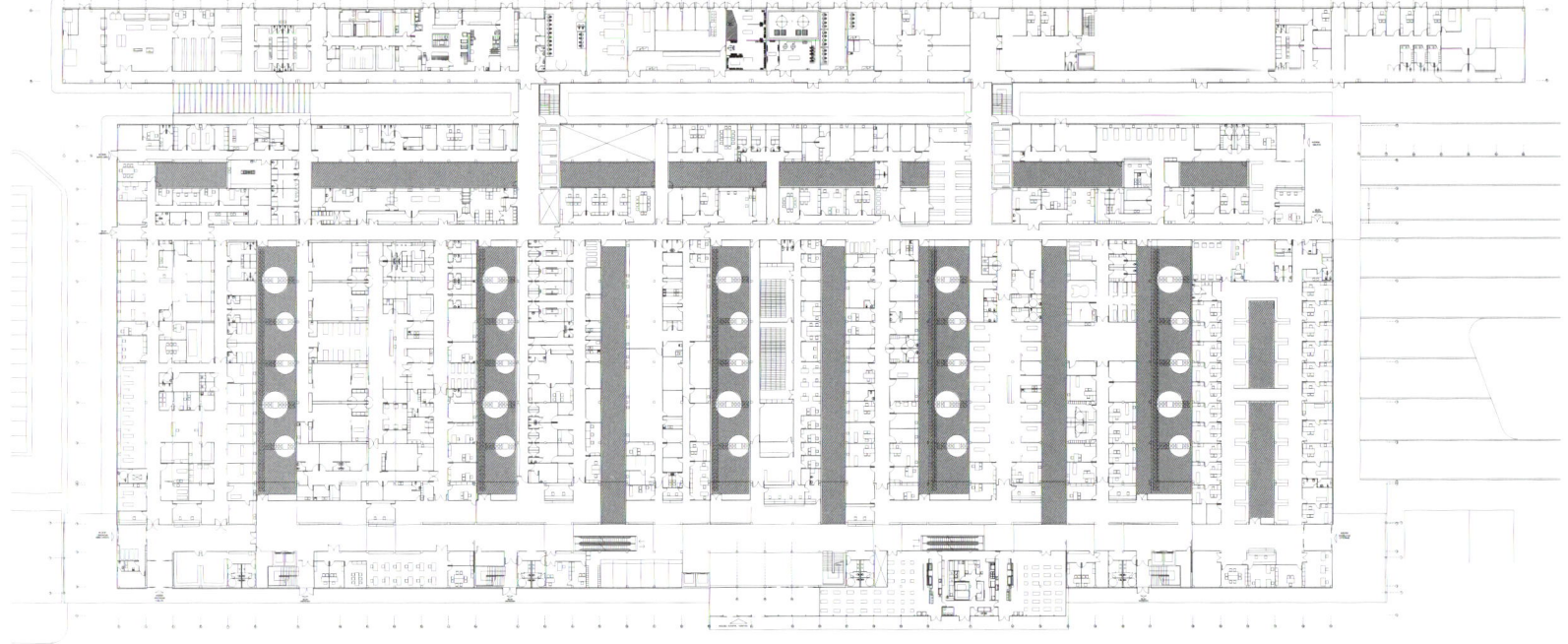

Ground floor plan

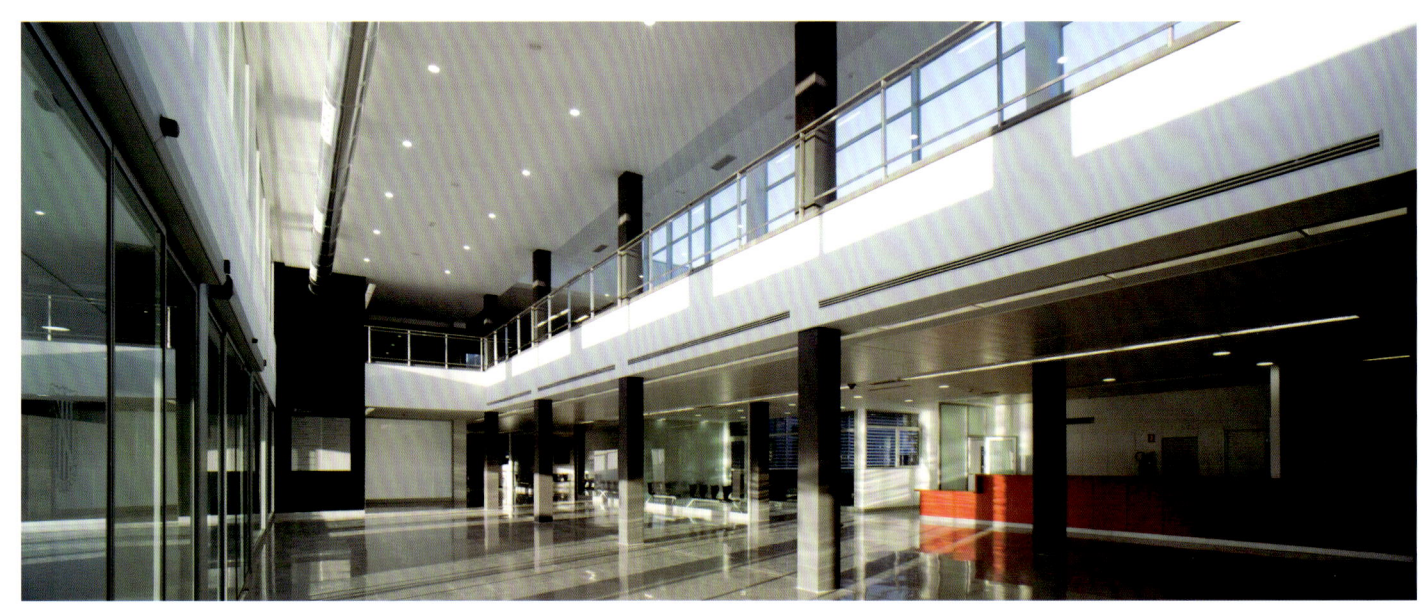

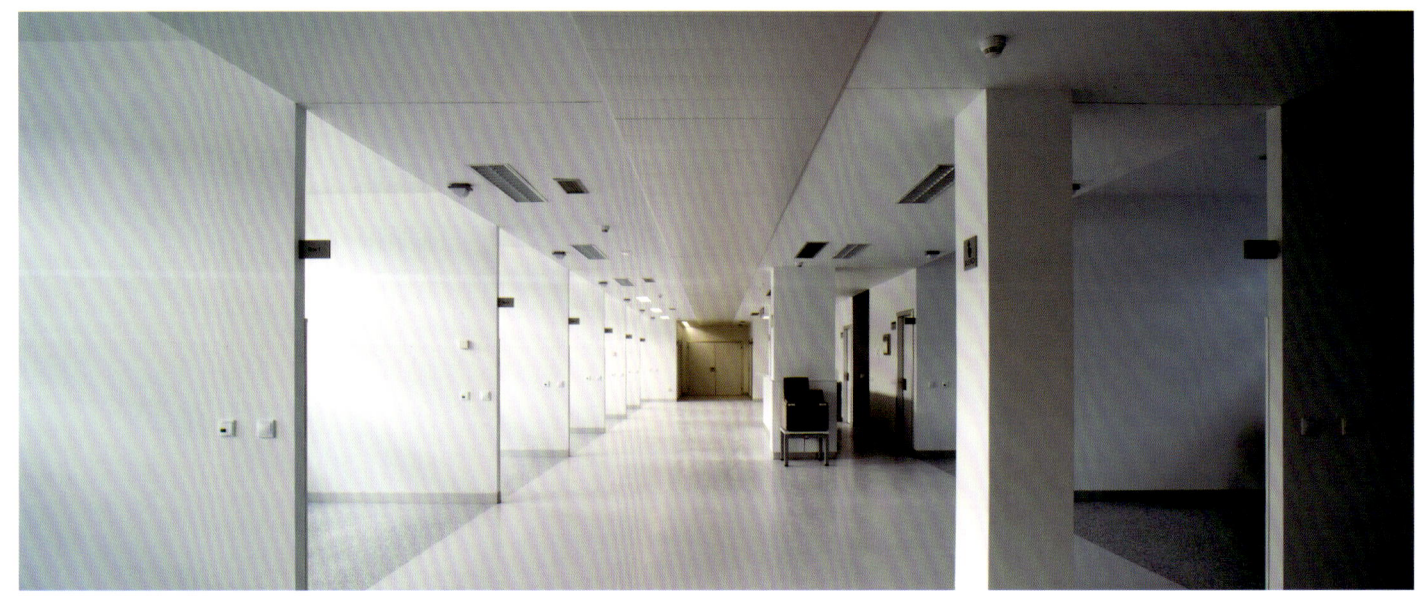

First floor plan

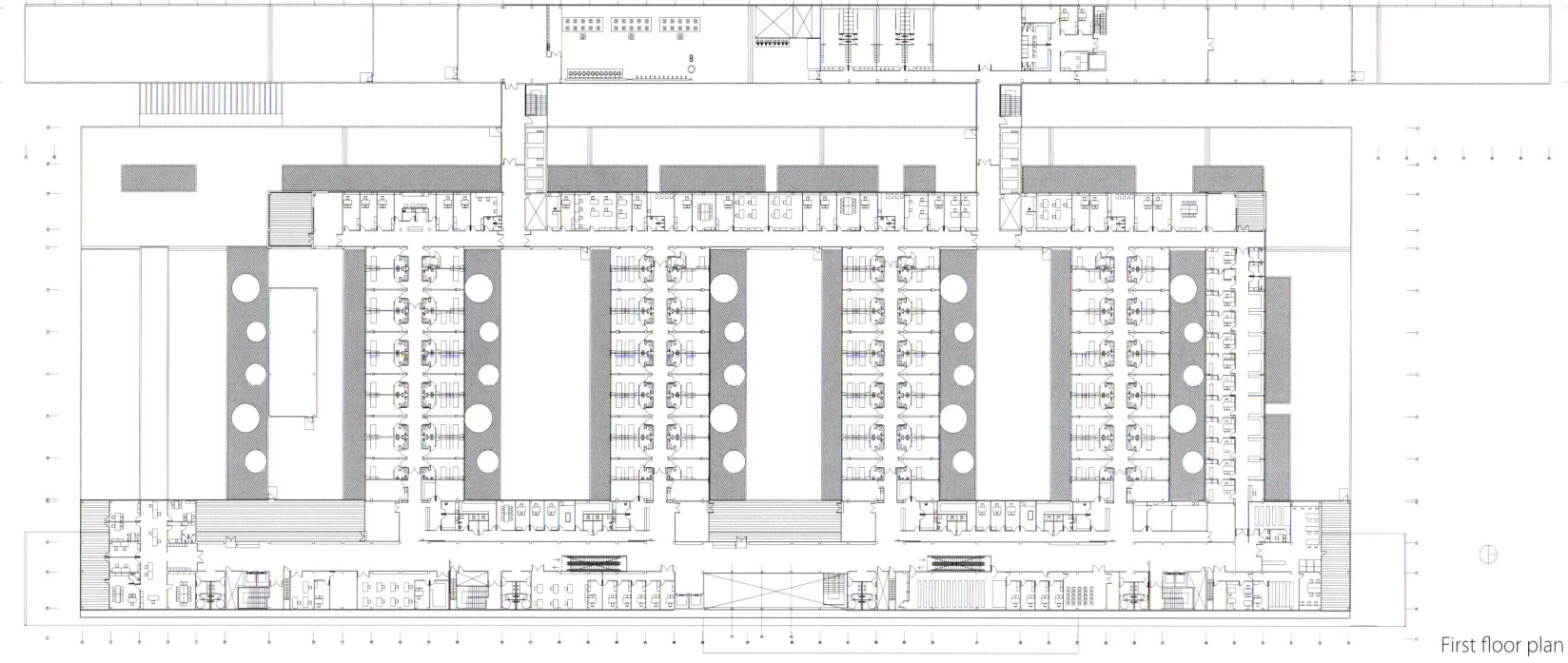

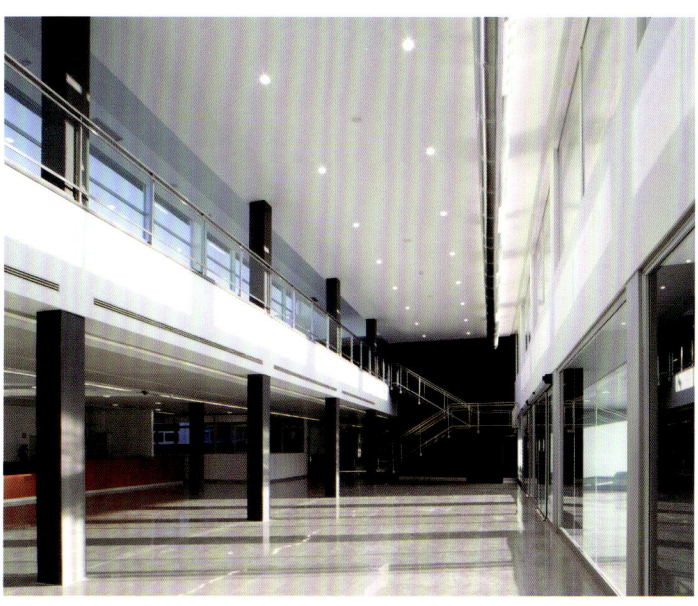

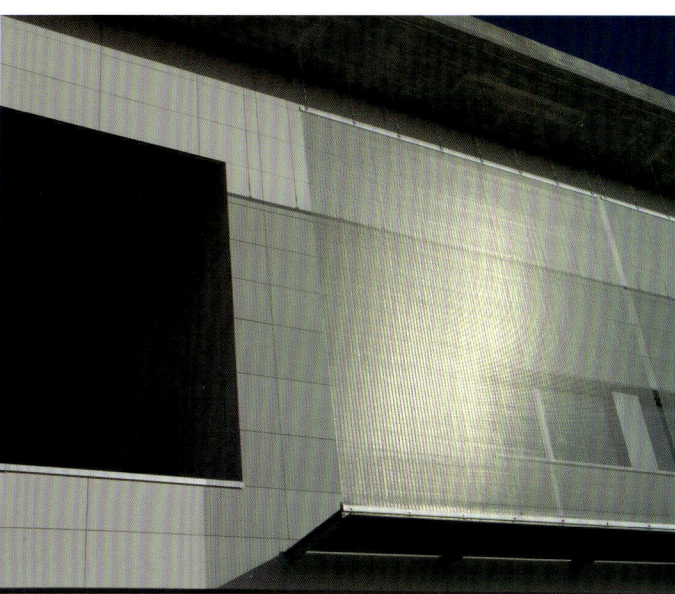

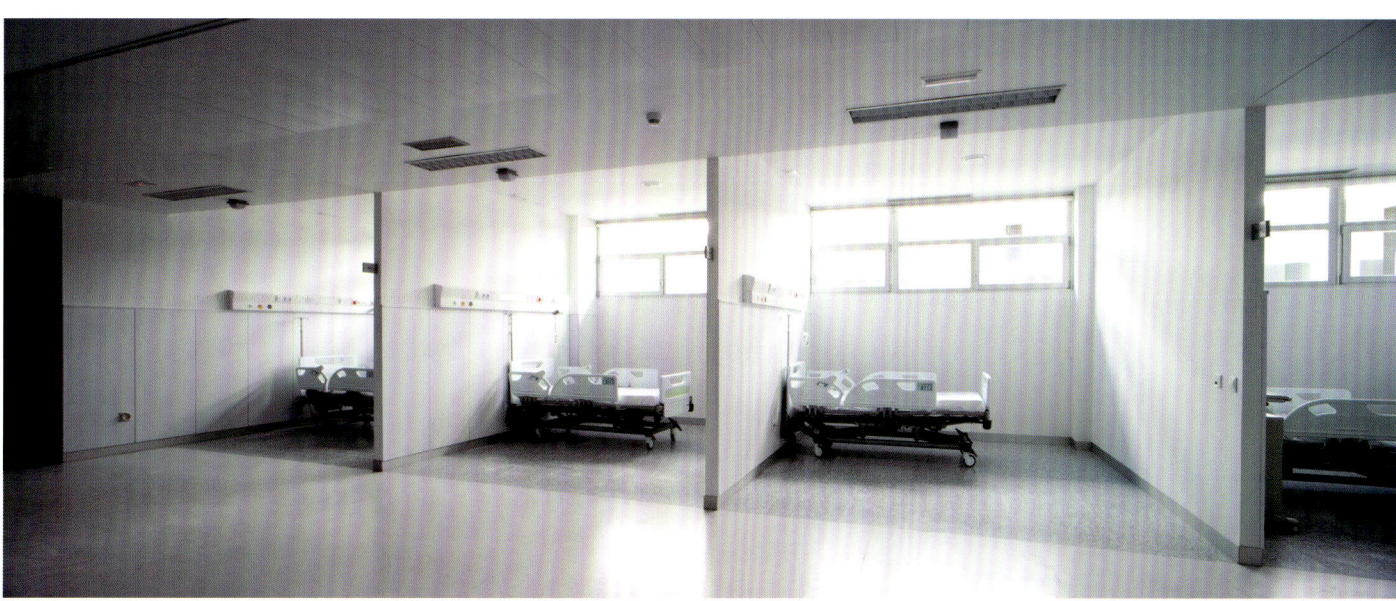

Section 1

Section 2

Section 3

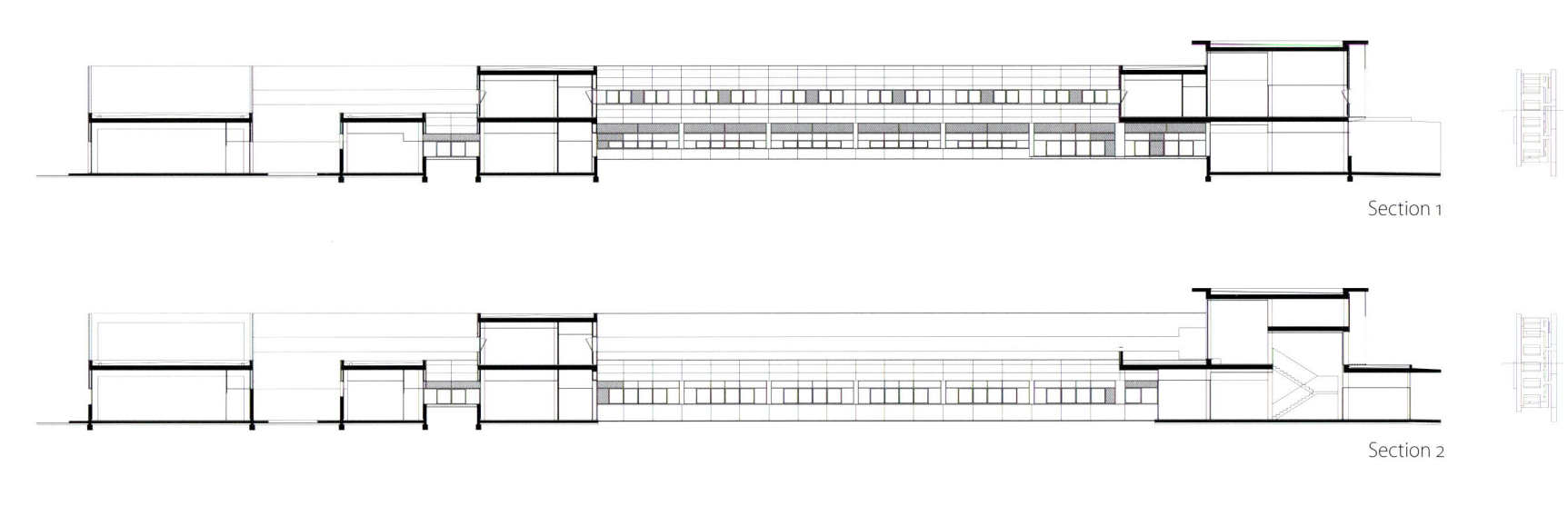

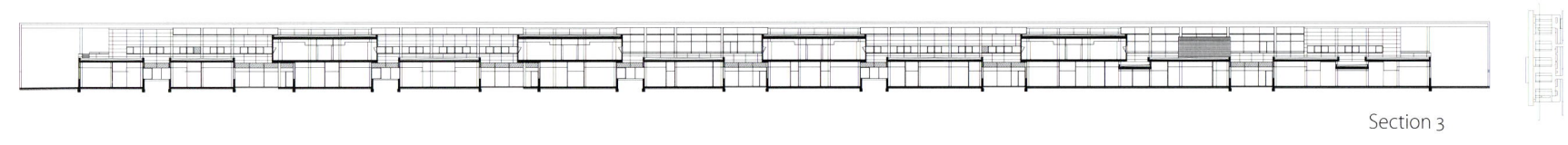

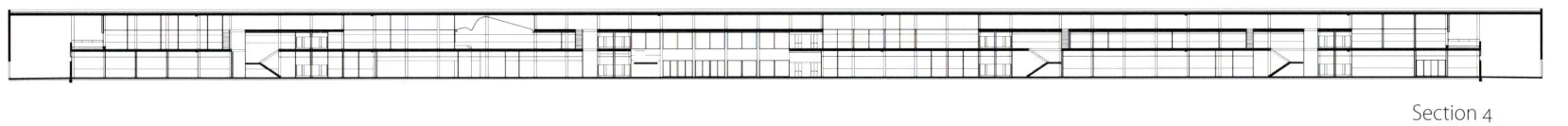

Section 4

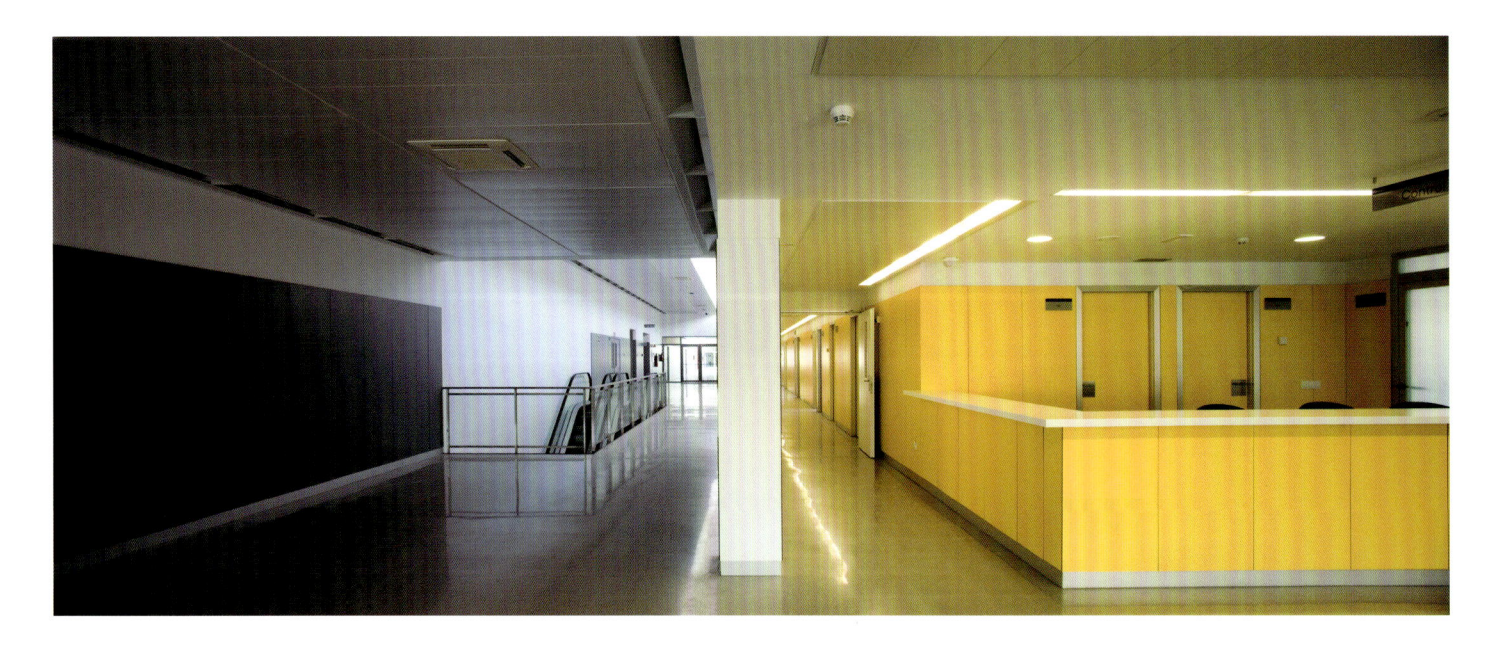

182

1. Corner finish of anodized aluminum sheet
2. "L" galvanized steel angle iron, with naturvex cap
3. "L" galvanized steel angle iron, with omega fixture
4. Omega fixture for fermacell type wall-panels
5. Sheet-rock paneling, fermacell type, 15mm
6. Sheet-rock paneling, fermacell type, 12.5mm
7. Acoustic membrane 4mm
8. Sheet-rock paneling, fermacell type, 12.5mm
9. Suspended ceiling, plaster, fermacell type 10mm
10. Joint cover of galvanized steel
11. Panel: naturvex 8x600x2025
12. Ventilation space
13. Panels of extruded polystyrene
14. Omega fixtures of galvanized steel to support naturvex
15. "L" galvanized steel angle iron, with omega fixture
16. Outer frame of galvanized steel 80x40mm
17. Carpentry, anodized aluminum, natural finish
18. Netting omega 1520 tensed stainless steel
19. Carpentry, anodized aluminum, natural finish
20. Paving: terrazzo
21. Tramex grid of galvanized steel 30x30mm
22. Sandwiched anodized aluminum sheet, natural finish
23. Anodized aluminum sheet, natural finish
24. Pre-frame of galvanized steel 80x40mm
25. Carpentry, anodized aluminum, natural finish
26. Sheet metal, anodized aluminum, natural finish
27. "L" of galvanized steel 80x80 fixed to the outer frame
28. Panel of sheet-rock, fermacell or similar 15mm
29. Panels of extruded polystyrene
30. In situ concrete, painted
31. Baseboard, anodized aluminum 10cm
32. Pavement, hydraulic floor tiles

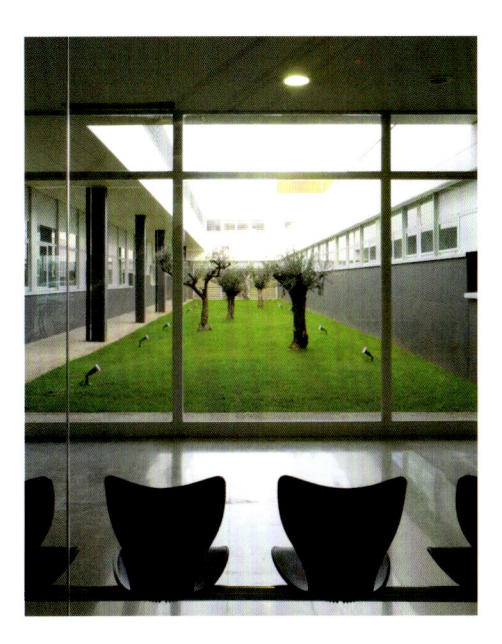

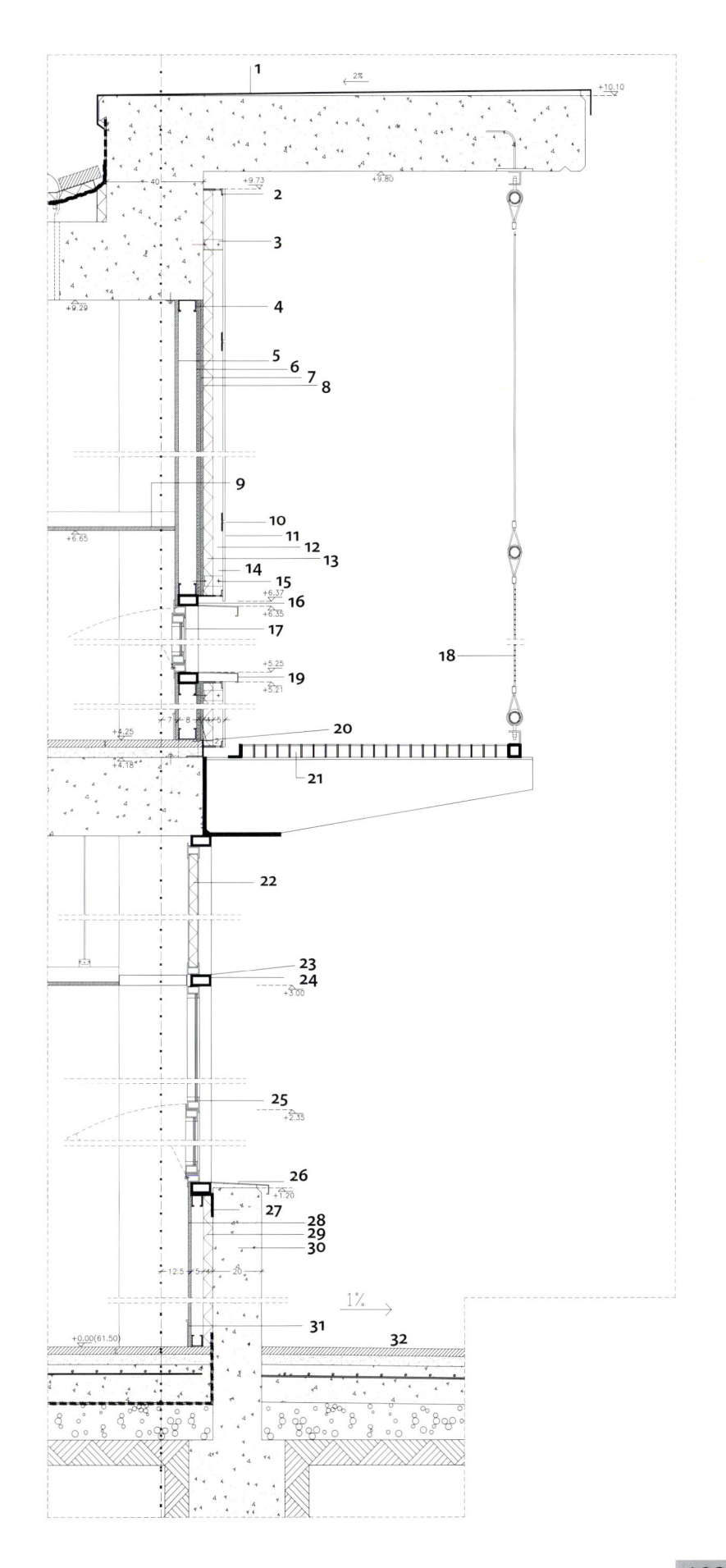

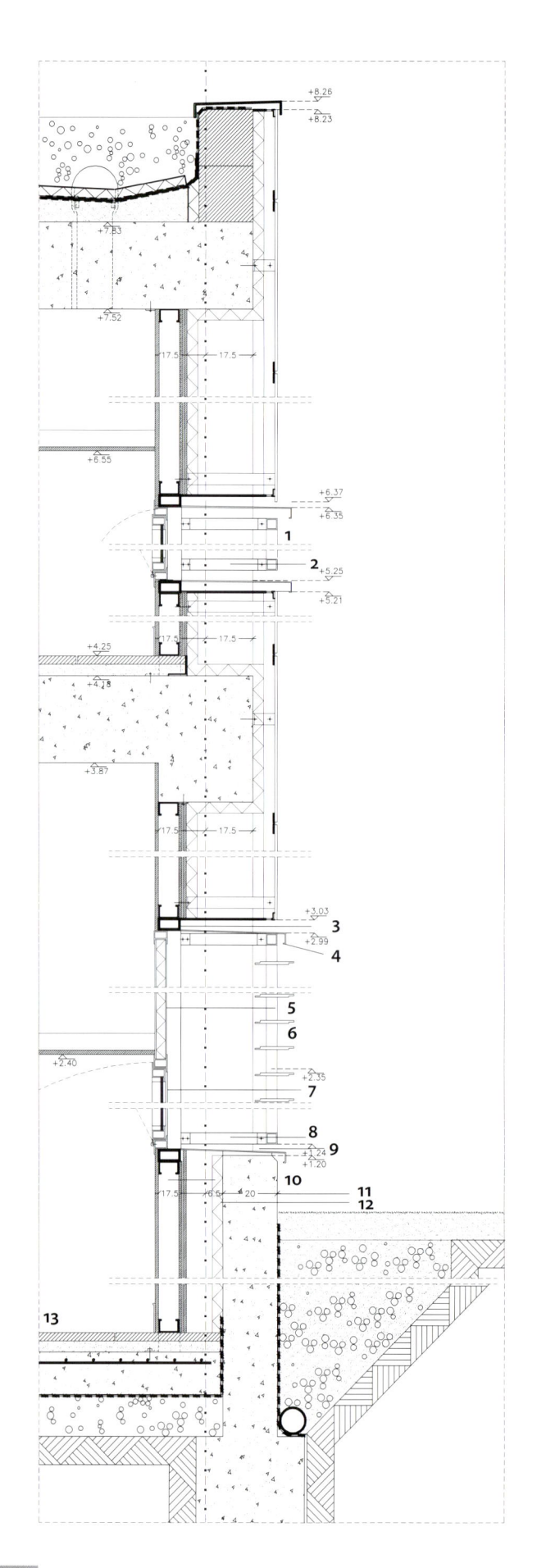

1. Mobile lamellae of anodized aluminum. Type: gradermetic 120
2. Structure to hold the lamellae, galvanized steel
3. Outer frame of galvanized steel 80x40mm
4. Sheet metal, anodized aluminum, natural finish
5. Sandwich sheet of anodized aluminum, natural finish
6. Mobile lamellae of anodized aluminum. Type: gradermetic 120
7. Carpentry of anodized aluminum, natural finish
8. Structure to hold the lamellae, galvanized steel
9. Sheet metal, anodized aluminum, natural finish
10. Substructure of galvanized steel 80x80 anchoring frame
11. In situ concrete, fairfaced, painted.
12. Panels of extruded polystyrene
13. Paving, smooth terrazzo

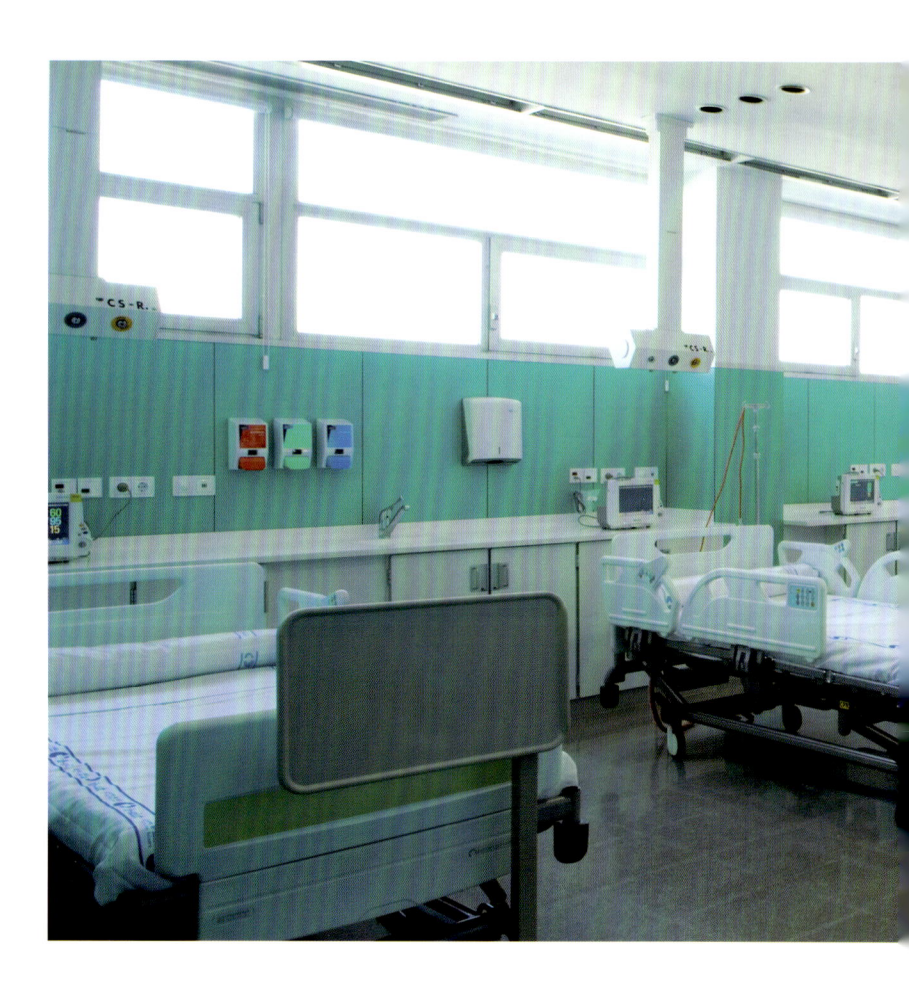

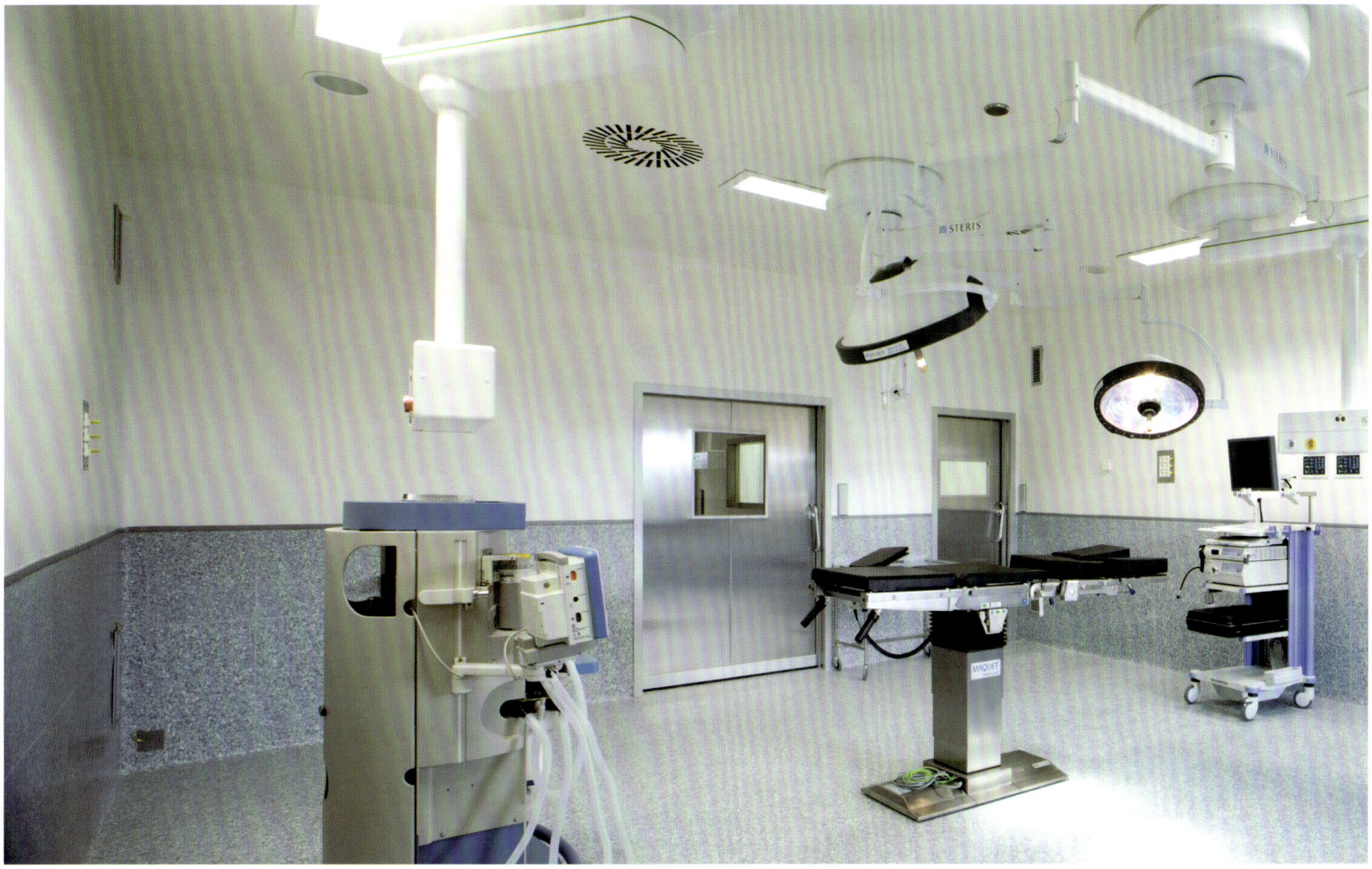

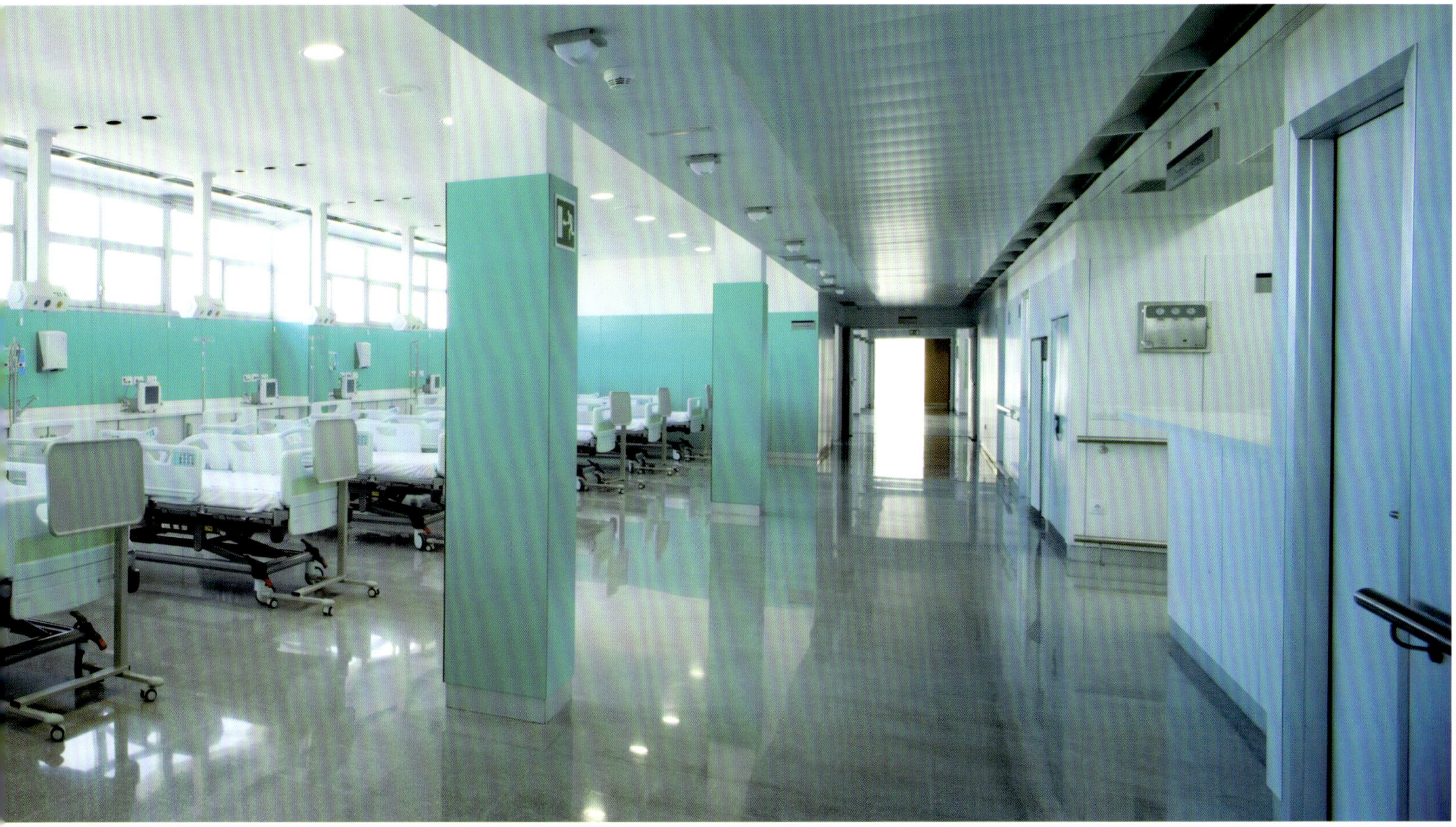

Estudio Lamela

Center For Alzheimer Patients

Madrid, Spain

Photographs: *contributed by the architects*

The Alzheimer Project of the Reina Sofía Foundation adopts a medical-social approach which attempts to reduce the effects of Alzheimer's disease, both for those affected and their families. The project comprises the construction of the Center for Alzheimer Patients, designed by Estudio Lamela.

There are four sections to the project: an inpatient facility for 156 Alzheimer patients; an outpatient day center for 40 Alzheimer patients; a research center and a training center for healthcare personnel, family members and volunteers. Functionality and aesthetics were priorities throughout in order to create spaces that are easy to use, accessible and visibly identifiable by patients, as well as being warm and homely. To this end all architectural barriers have been avoided where possible and spacious corridors resembling pedestrian motorways have been designed for heavy traffic. Color has been used throughout to aid orientation, afford warmth, and to benefit from the light, and bright murals decorate the main passageways.

The medical-social area includes a day center and shared spaces. The former has a large multi-purpose hall which opens to an outdoor area where the residents can carry out activities such as gardening therapy, physiotherapeutic exercises in the open air, etc. The majority of the rooms in the day center are multifunctional, with movable partition walls allowing the rooms to be used for dining, recreation or occupational therapy. Patients spend most of their time in the shared spaces, located on the ground and upper floors. These spaces are grouped around accessible courtyards. The spaces contain the bedrooms, the dining rooms, the lounge, etc. There is also a shared intensive care space, dedicated to patients in a more advanced stage of the disease, as well as a training area for caretakers and family members.

The concept of the outdoor spaces was to recreate traditional village squares with trees and benches to sit on, and few green spaces. Each garden is the center of each unit, and is quite distinct so that patients may orientate themselves. A recreational area has been designed for visiting children and is located in front of the cafeteria.

The research building consists of four floors above a ground level with offices and one underground floor where magnetic resonance (used to detect the disease) will be concentrated. An independent entrance allows the research area to function autonomously from the residence.

The project stands out for its great respect for the environment, expressed through the bioclimatic measures it incorporates. An orientation adapted to its location, measures against excessive heat gain, natural ventilation, water treatment, the use of ecological roofing and thermal and photovoltaic solar panels make the center a model for bioclimatic measures.

Client:
Reina Sofía Foundation
Surface area:
12,910 sqm (139,000 sqft)
Start date:
December 2002
Finish Date:
March 2007
Structural engineer:
Ingeniería Valladares
Contractor:
Grupo Rayet
Cost:
€ 17,115,510

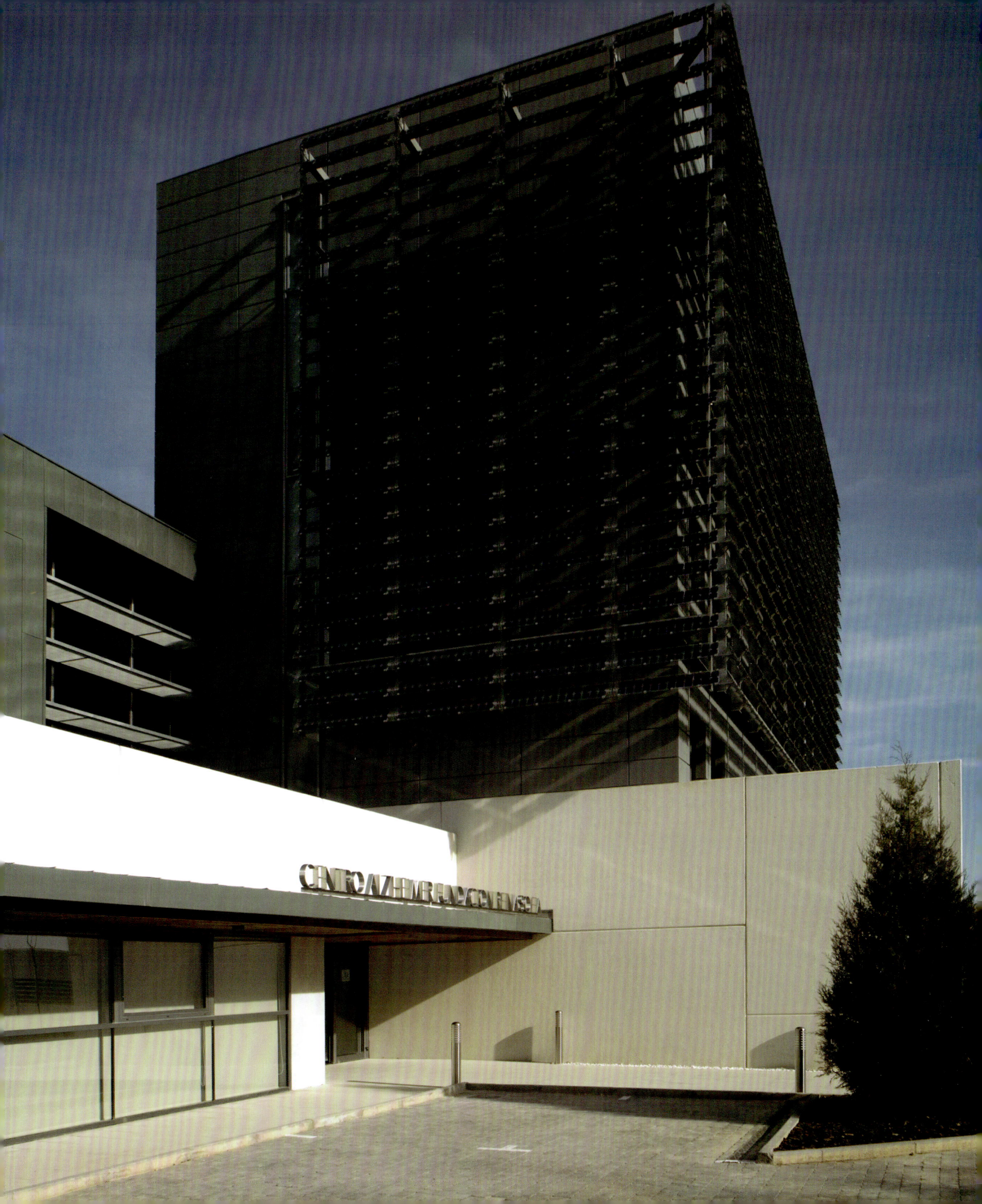

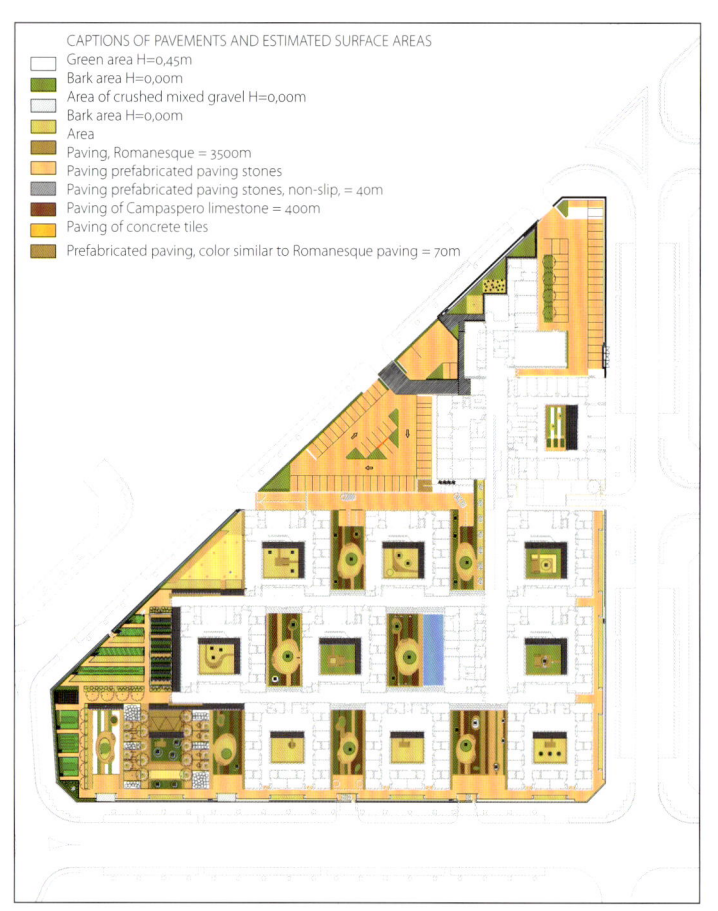

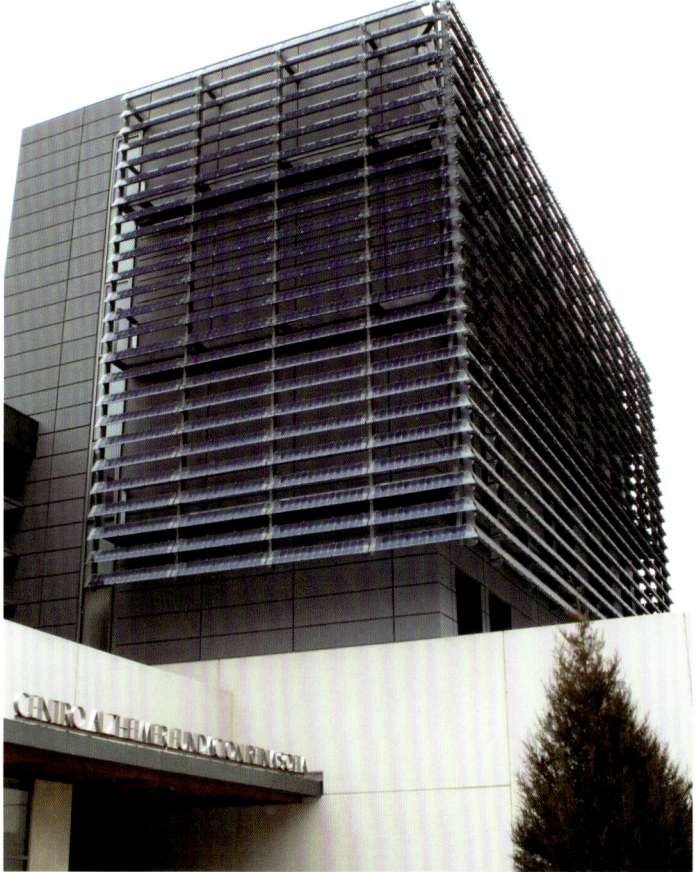

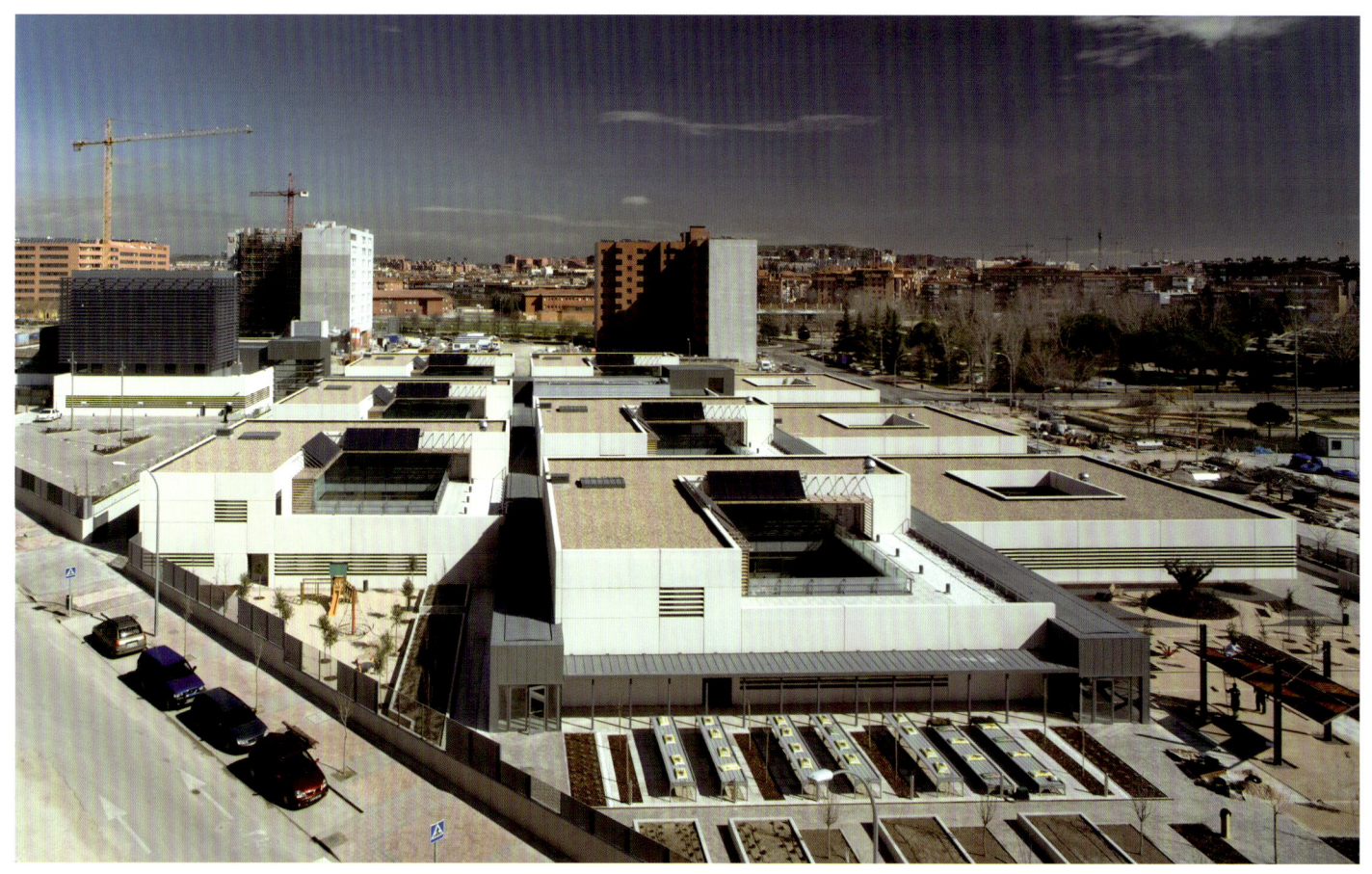

CAPTIONS OF PAVEMENTS AND ESTIMATED SURFACE AREAS
- Green area H=0,45m
- Bark area H=0,00m
- Area of crushed mixed gravel H=0,00m
- Bark area H=0,00m
- Area
- Paving, Romanesque = 3500m
- Paving prefabricated paving stones
- Paving prefabricated paving stones, non-slip, = 40m
- Paving of Campaspero limestone = 400m
- Paving of concrete tiles
- Prefabricated paving, color similar to Romanesque paving = 70m

189

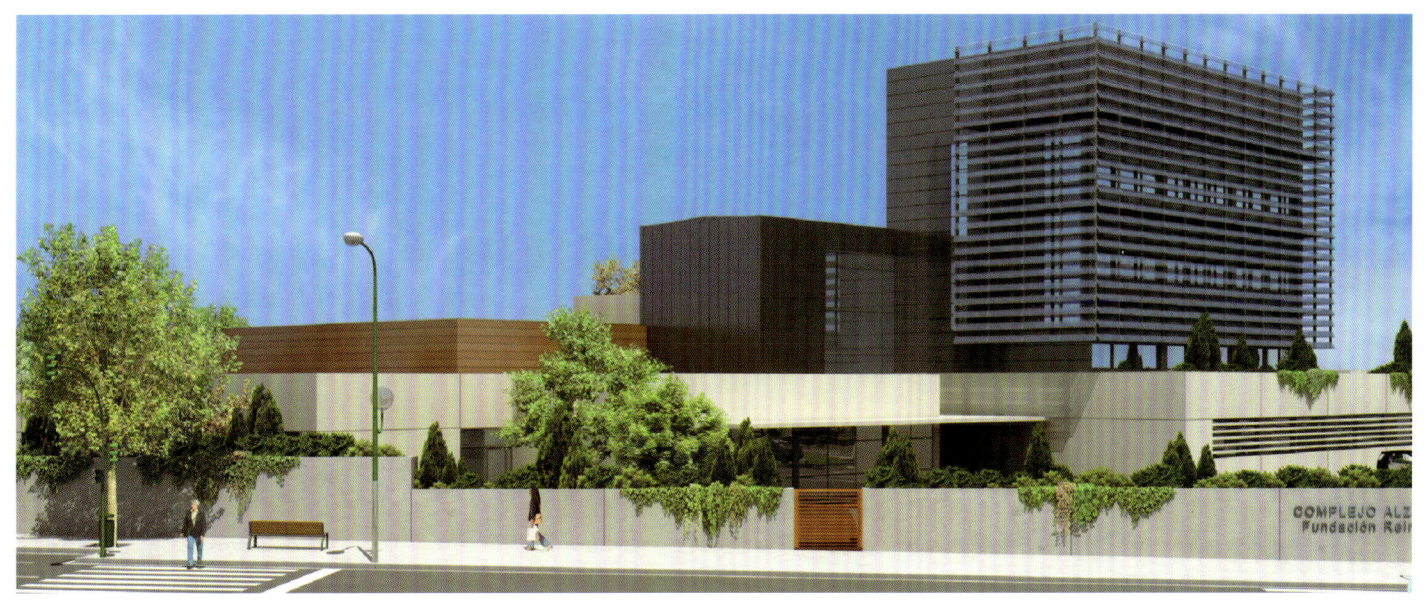

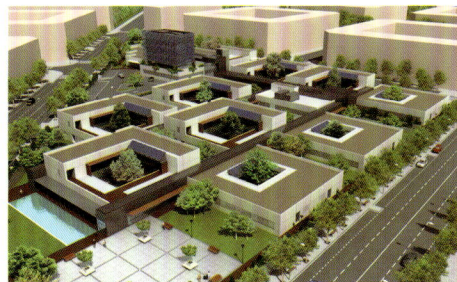

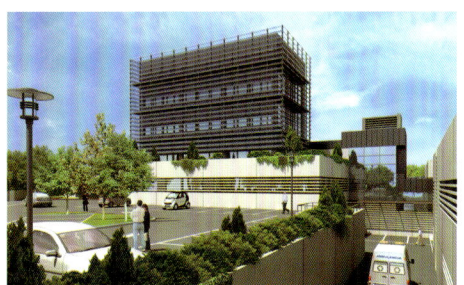

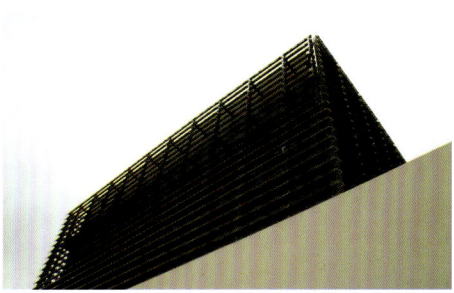

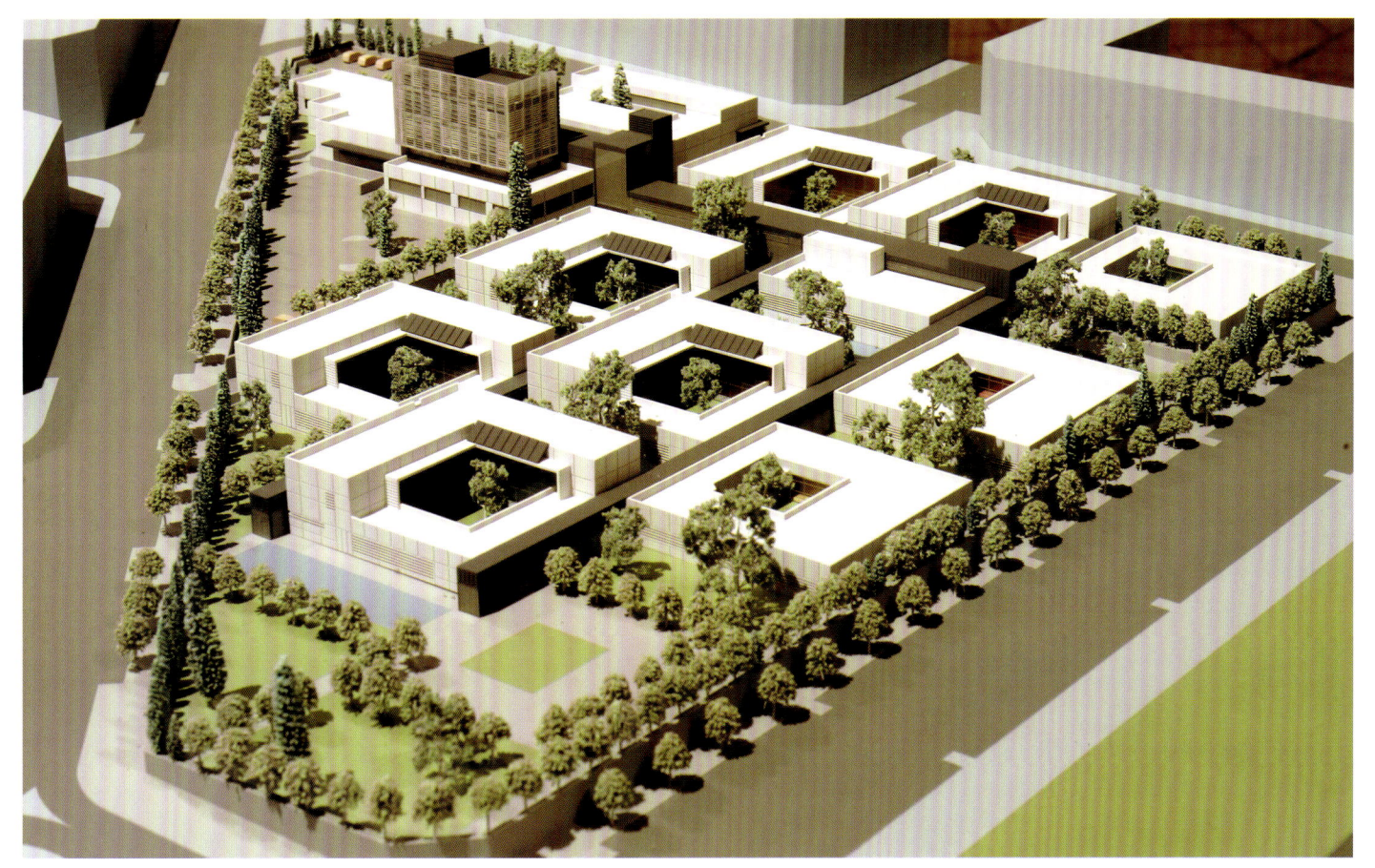

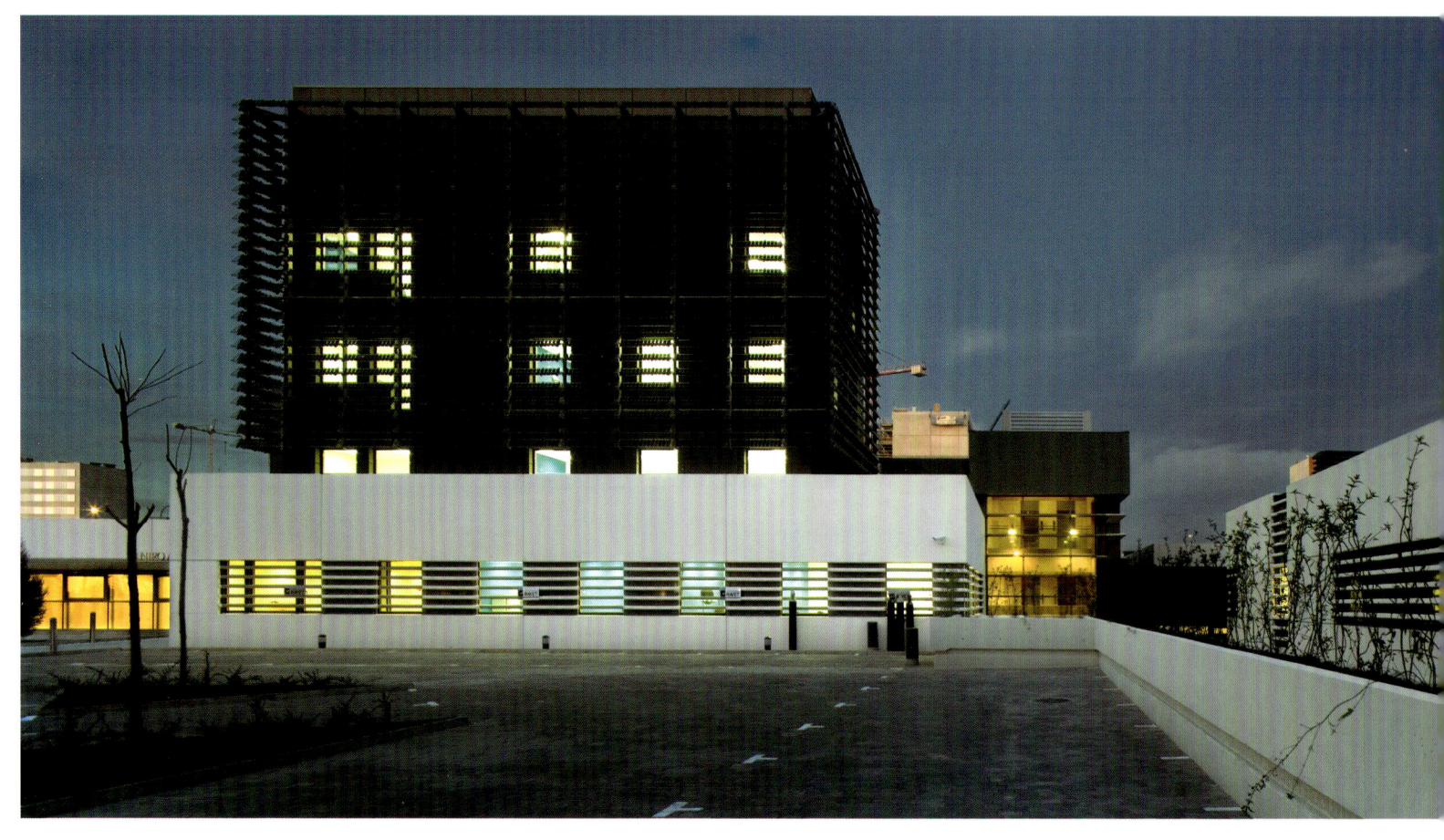

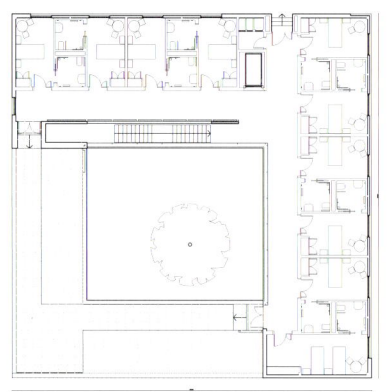

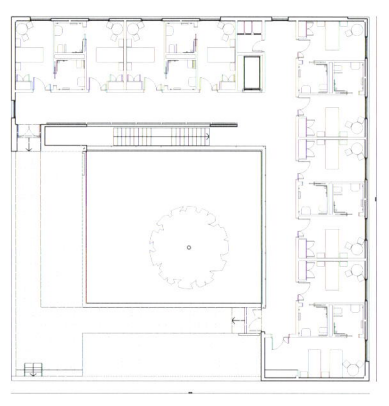

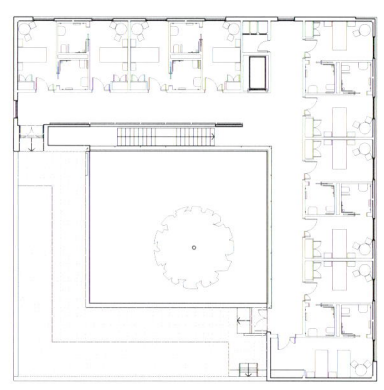

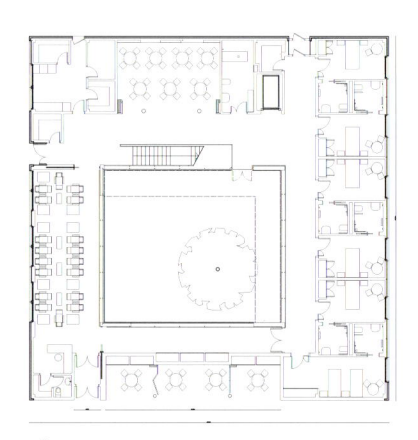

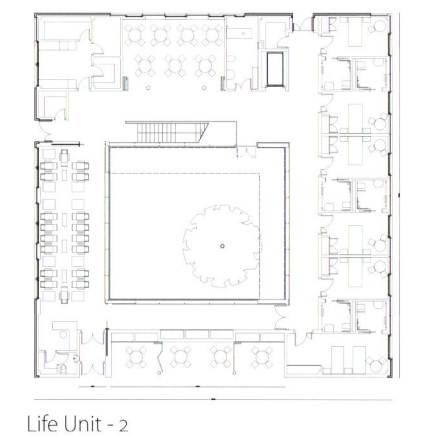

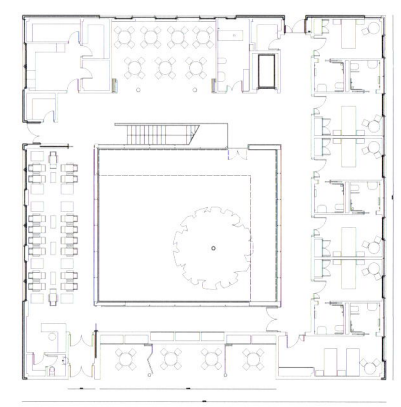

Life Unit - 1

Life Unit - 2

Life Unit - 3

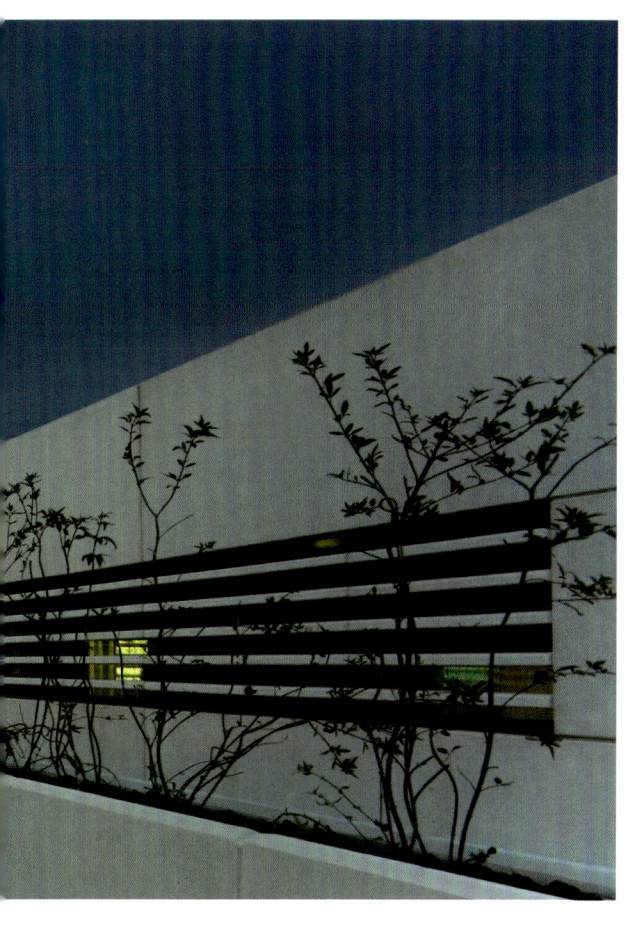

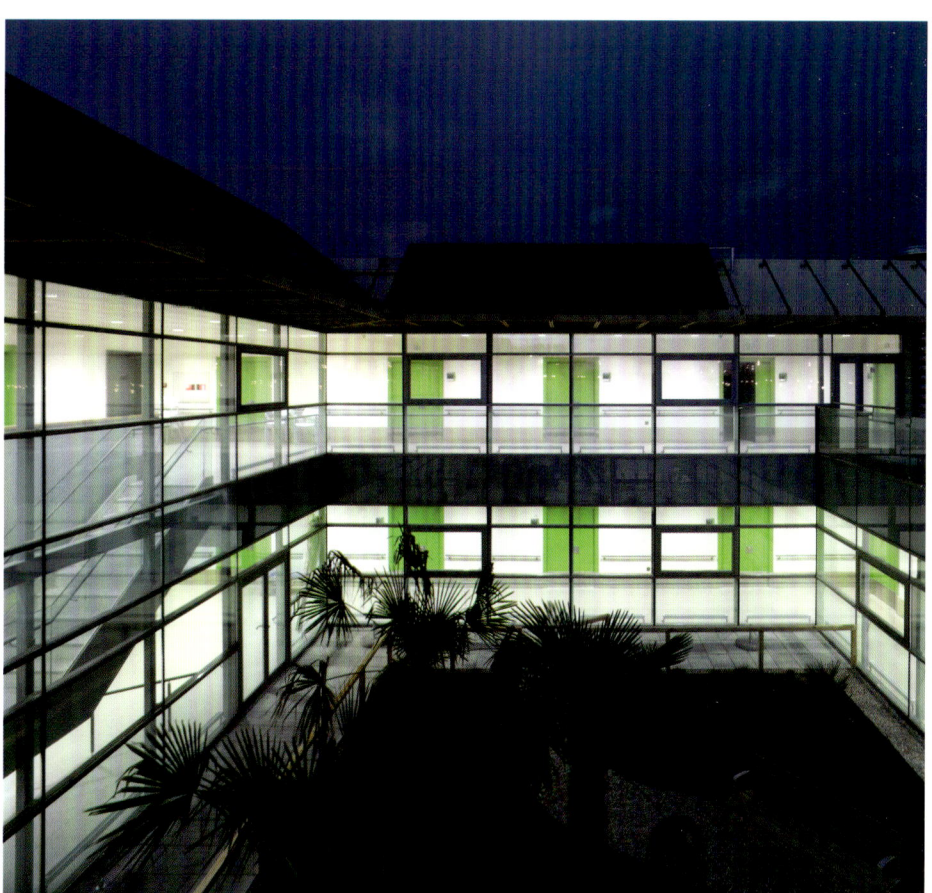

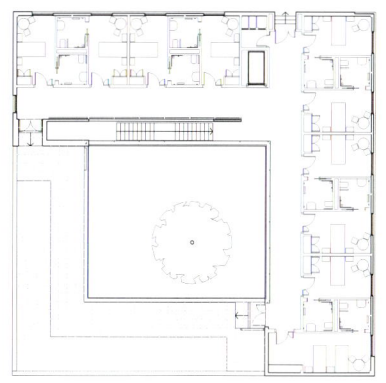

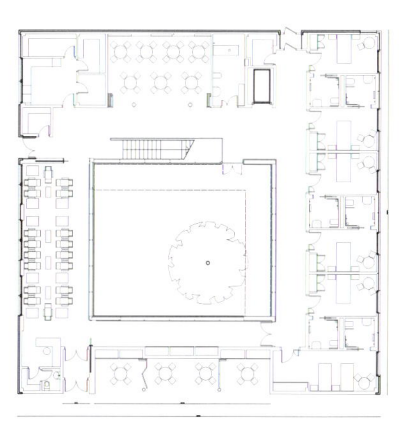

Life Unit - 4

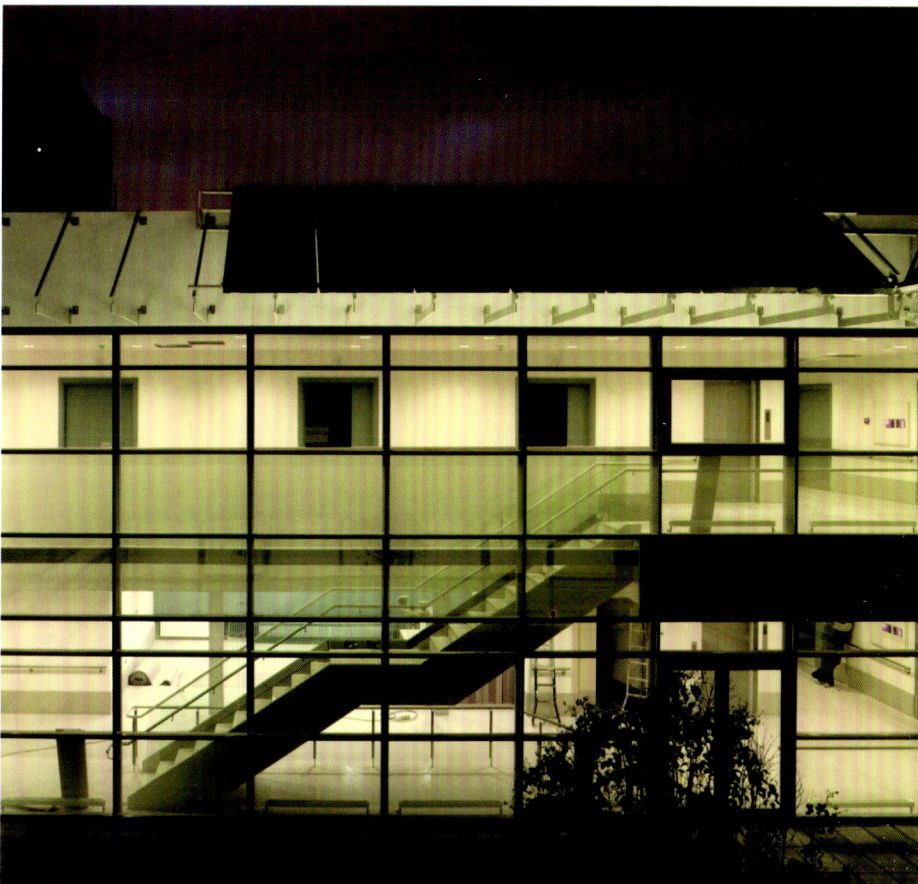

191

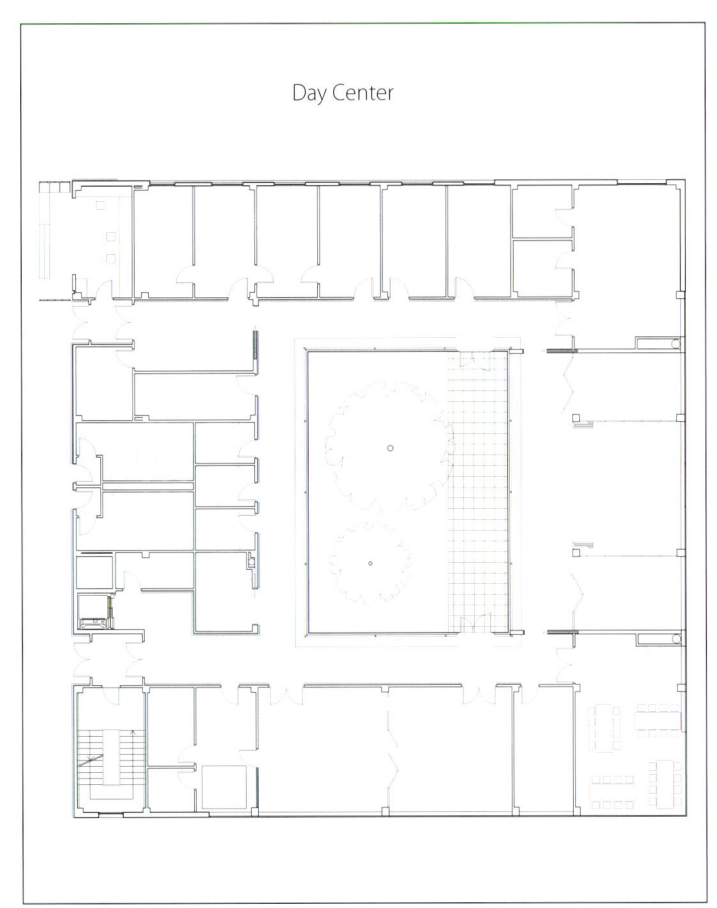

Day Center

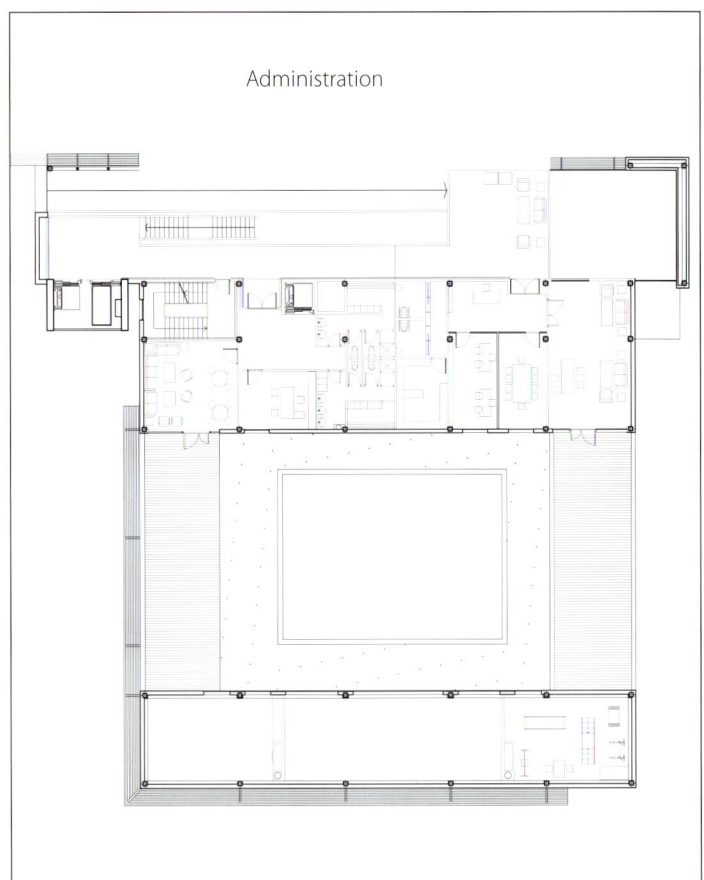

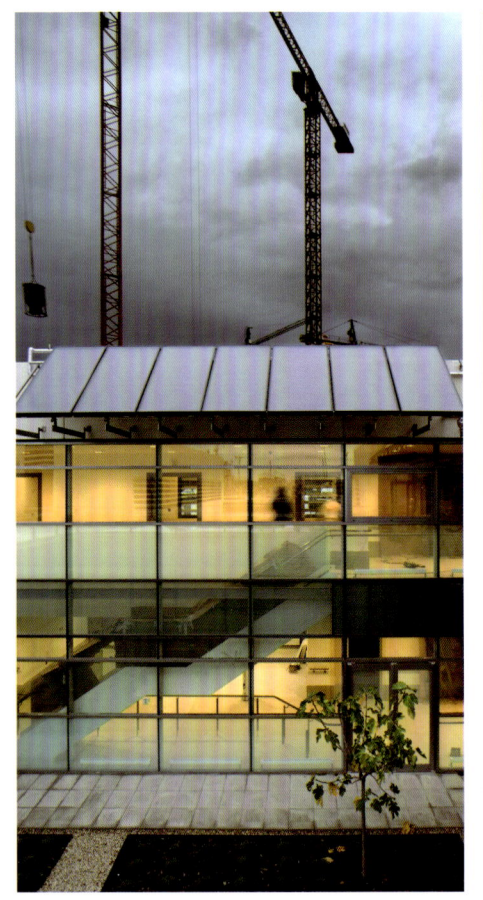

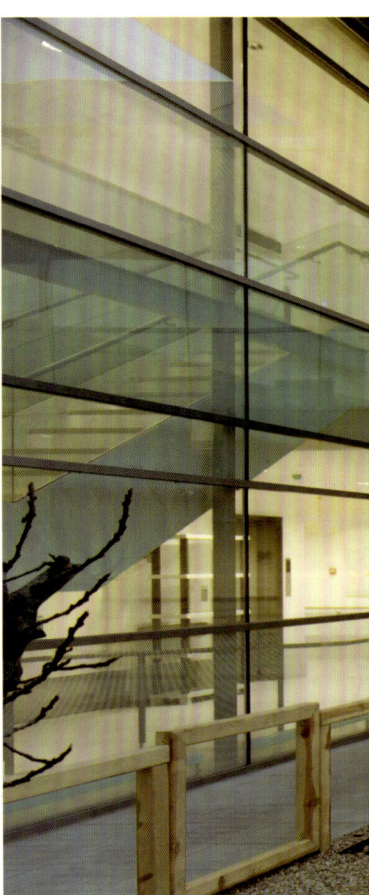

Administration

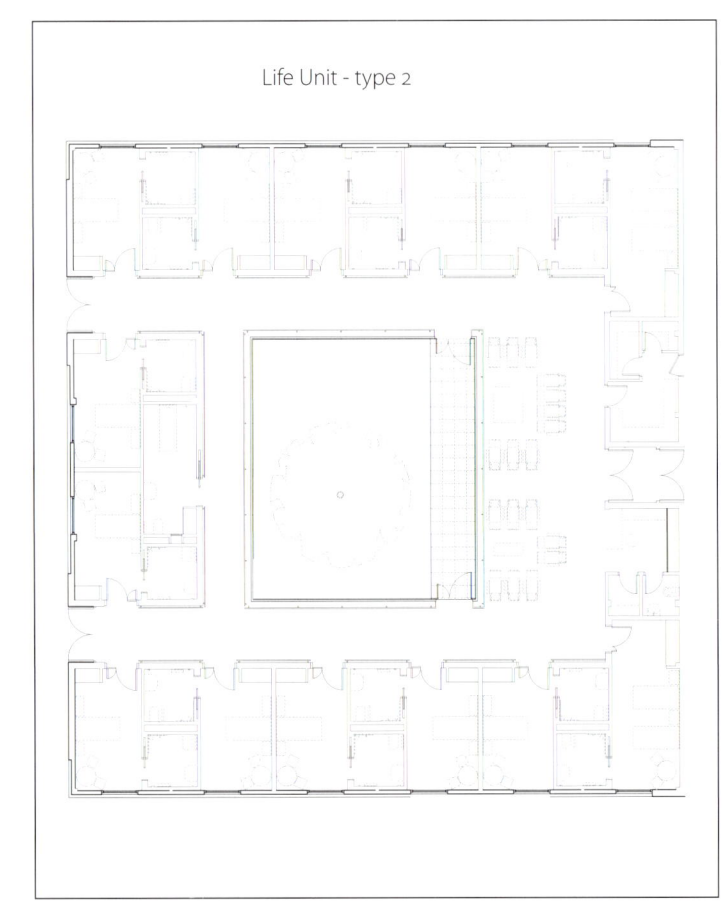

Life Unit - type 2

192

Ground Floor Plan - Specialized Attention

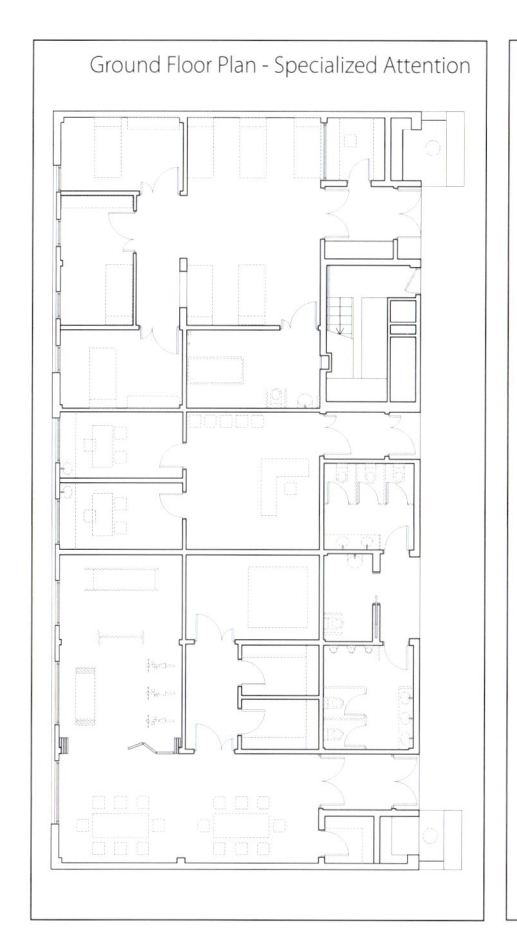

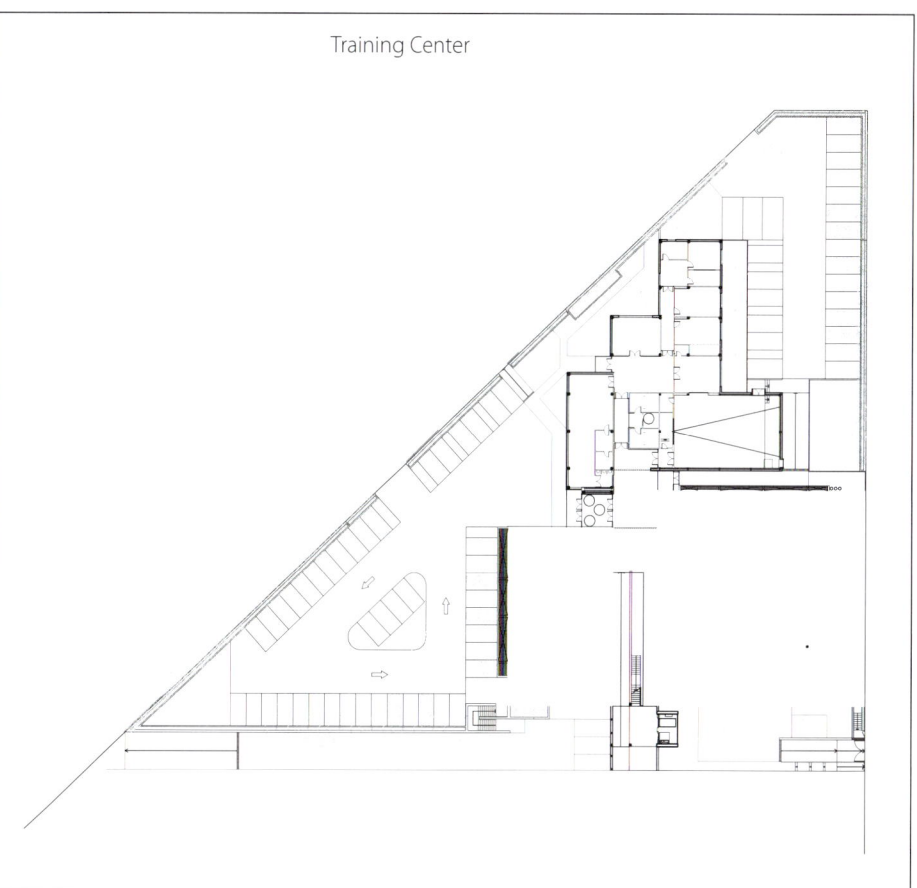

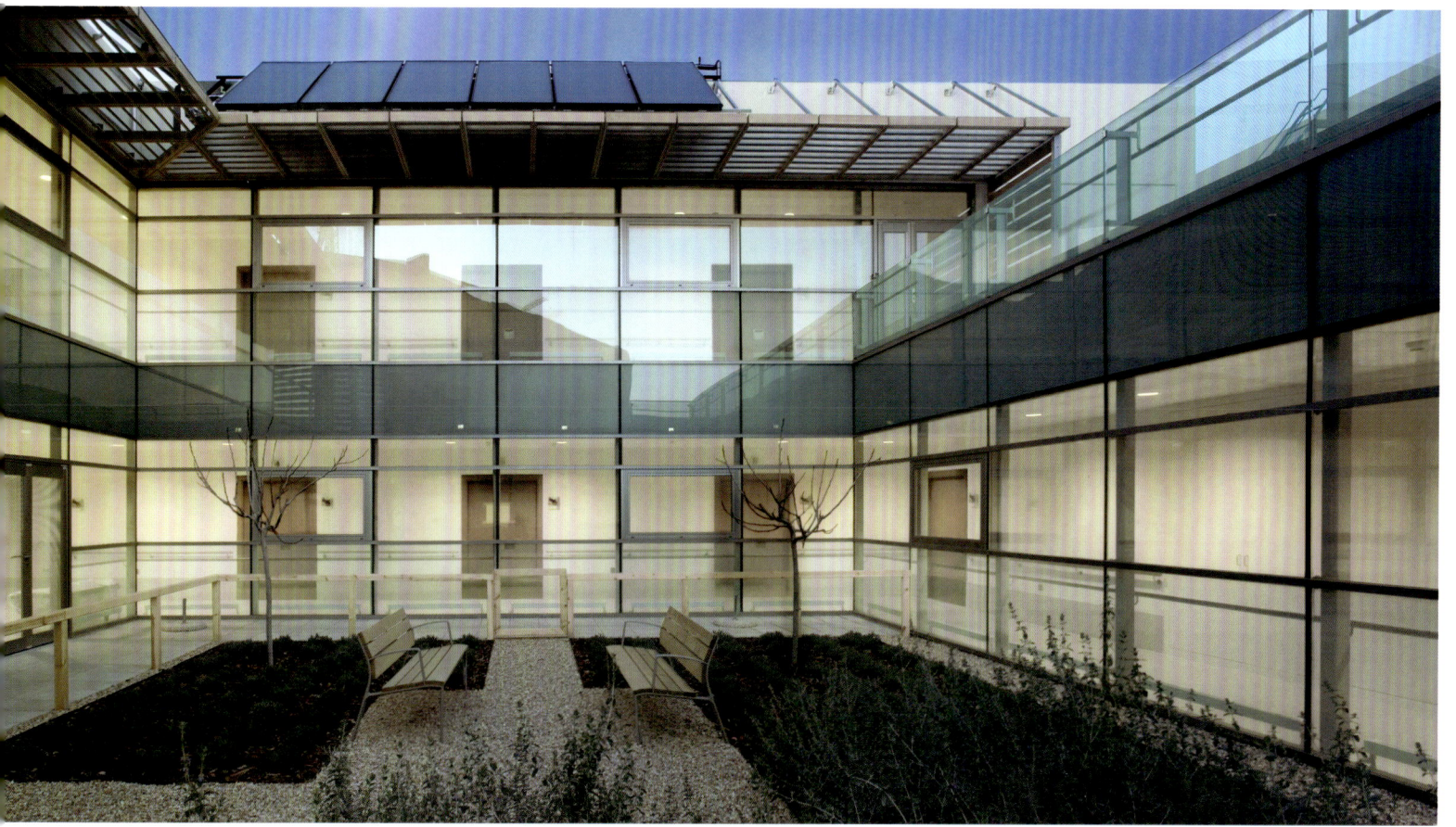

Training Center

193

194

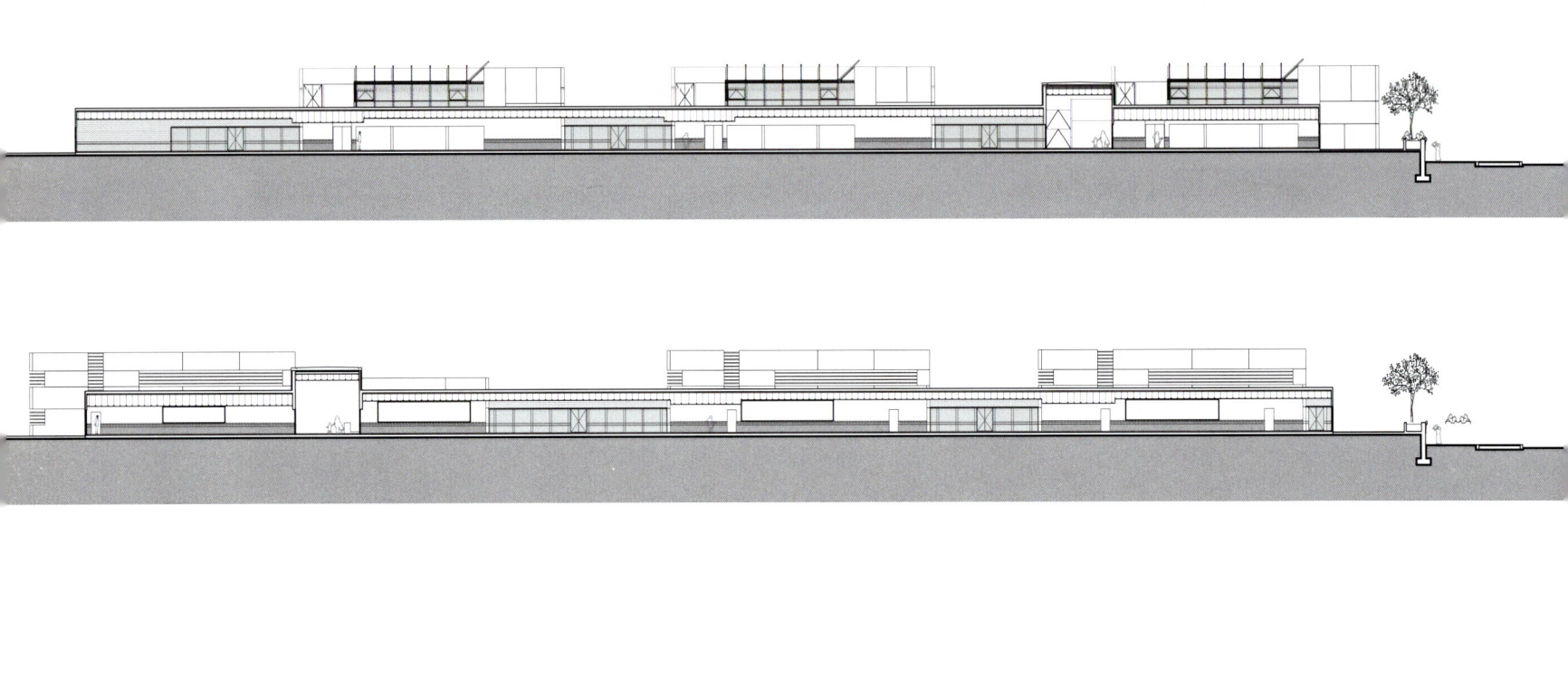

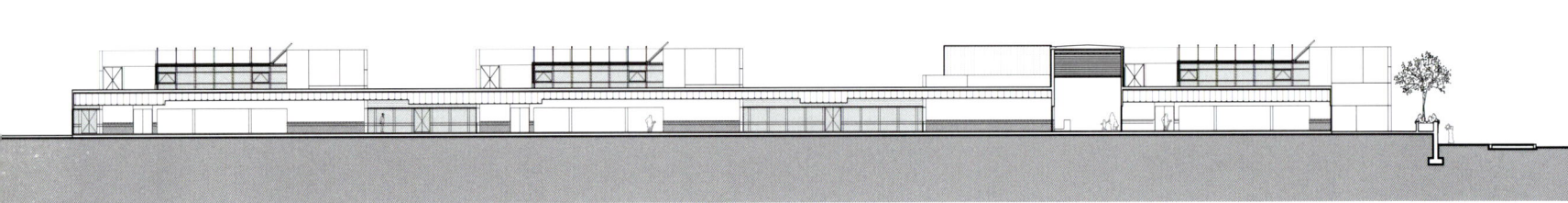

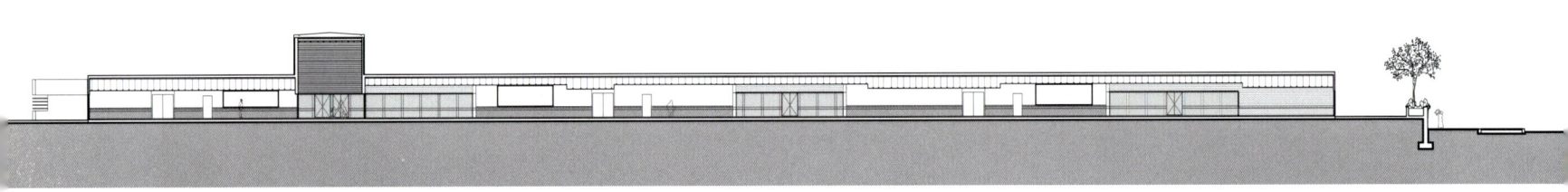

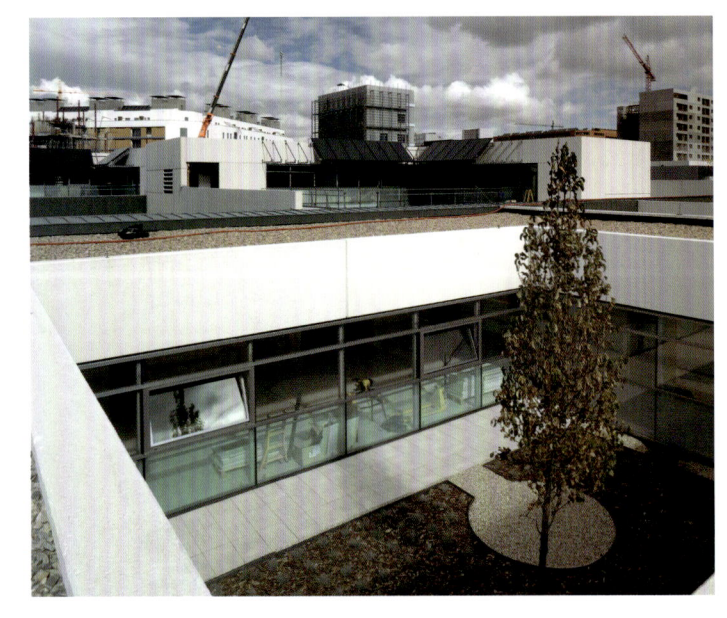

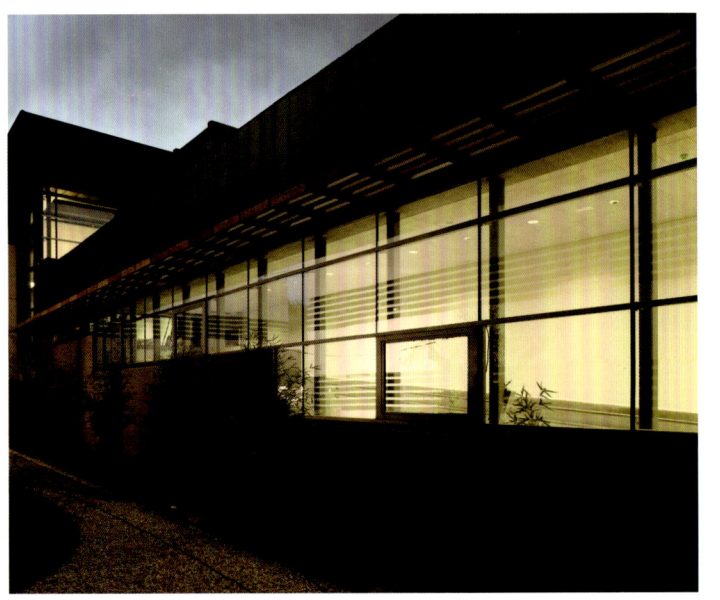

195

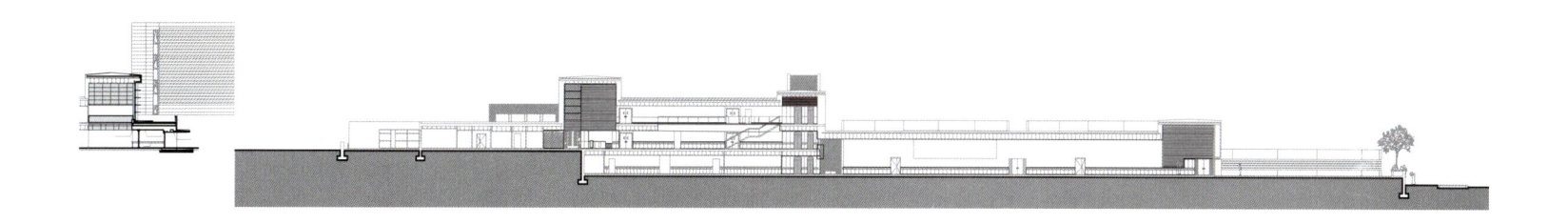

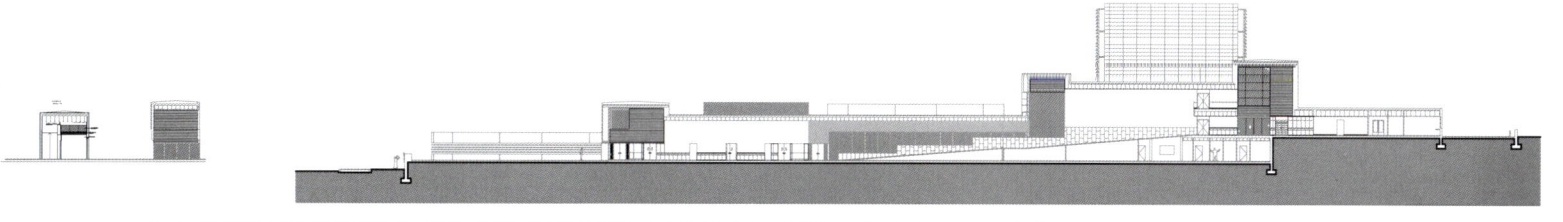

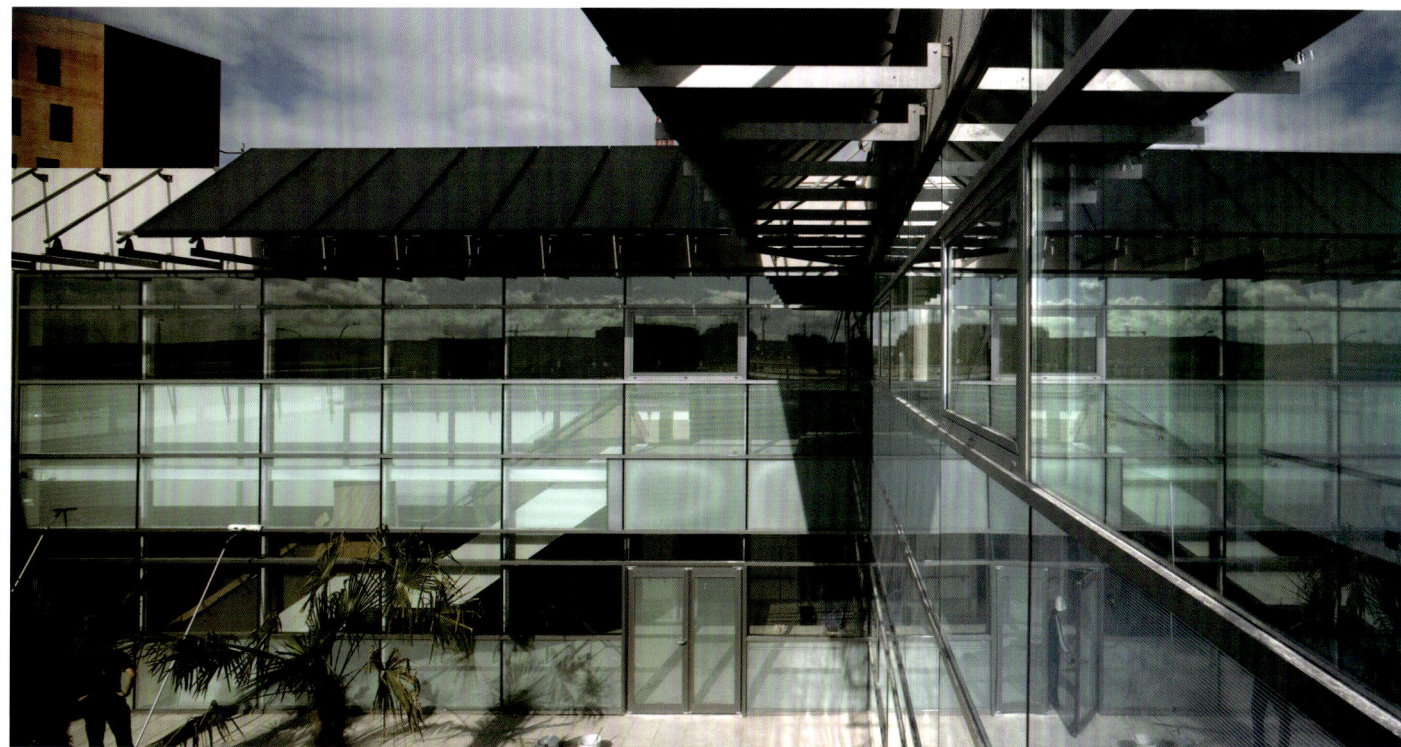

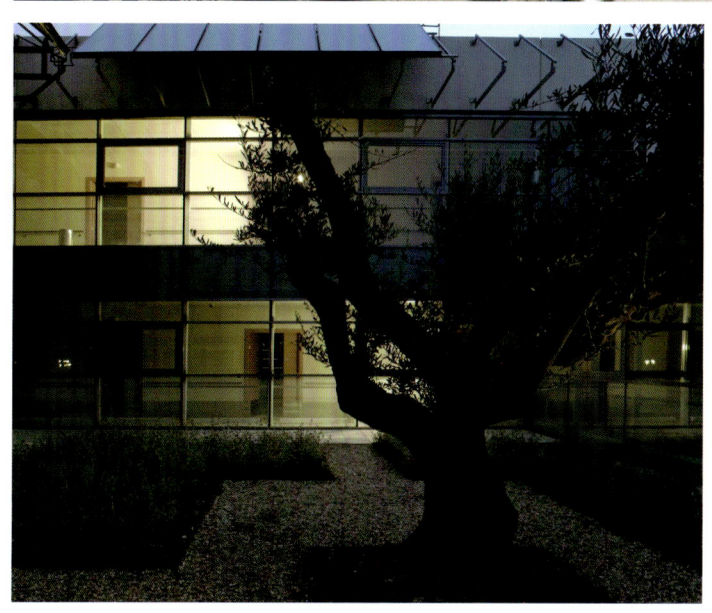

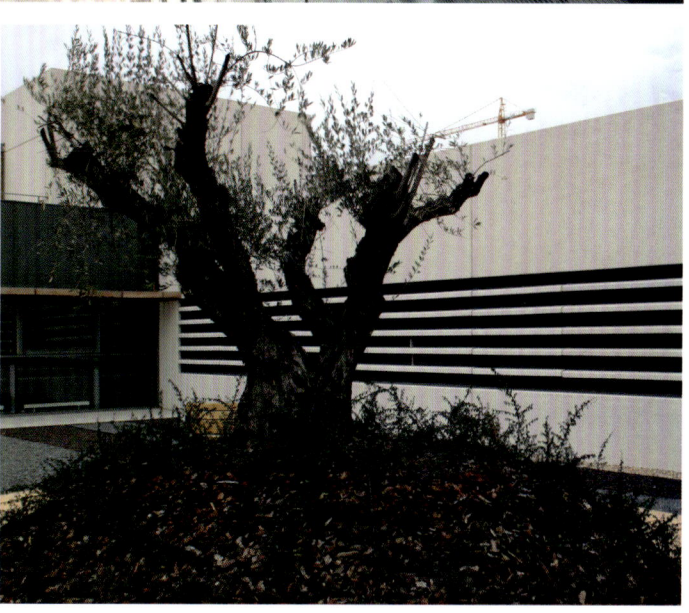

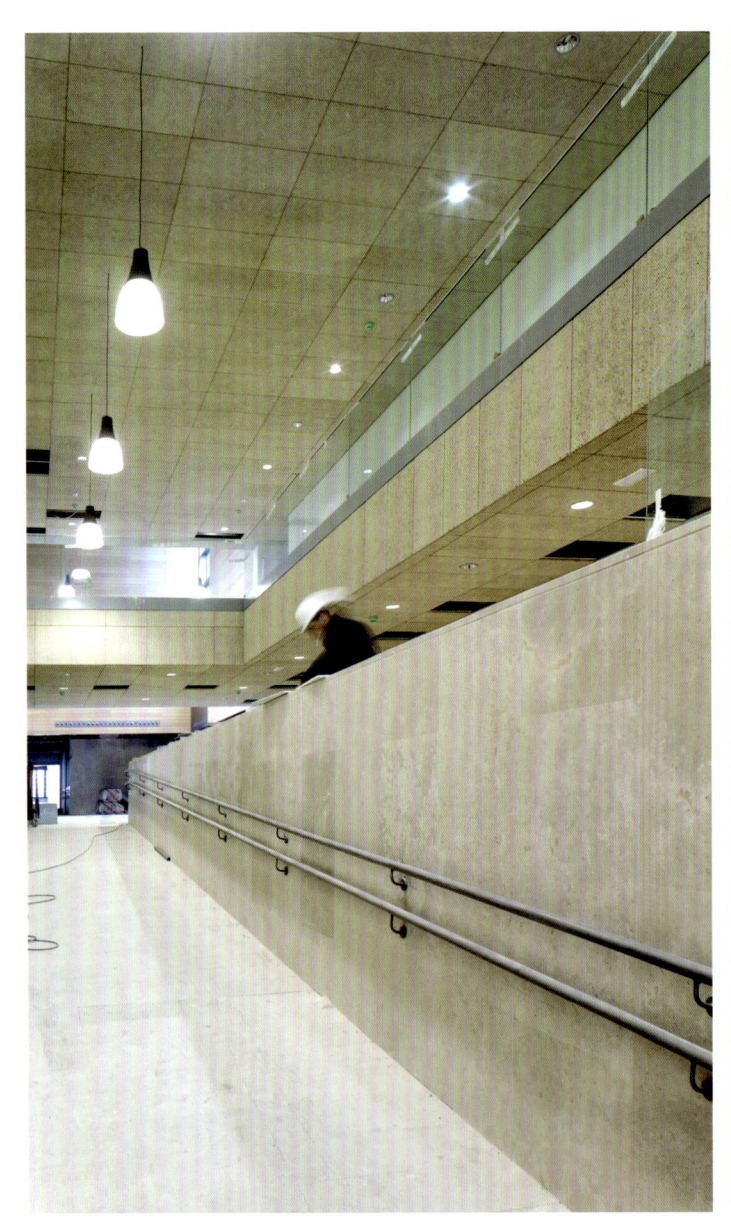

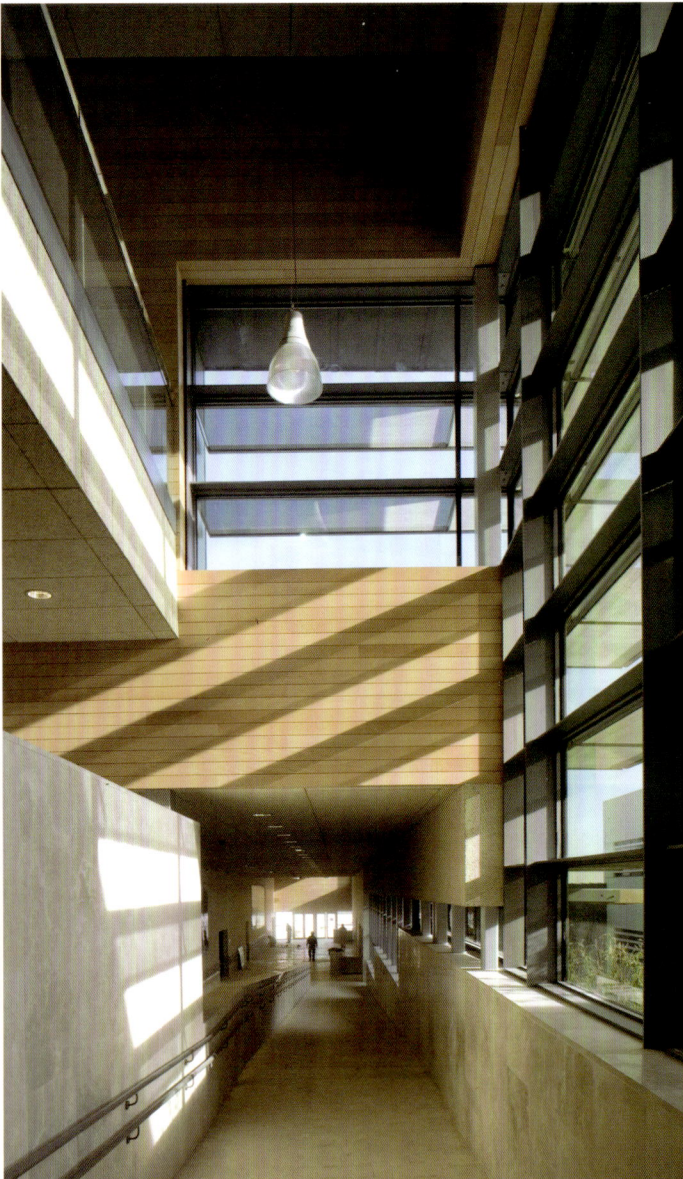

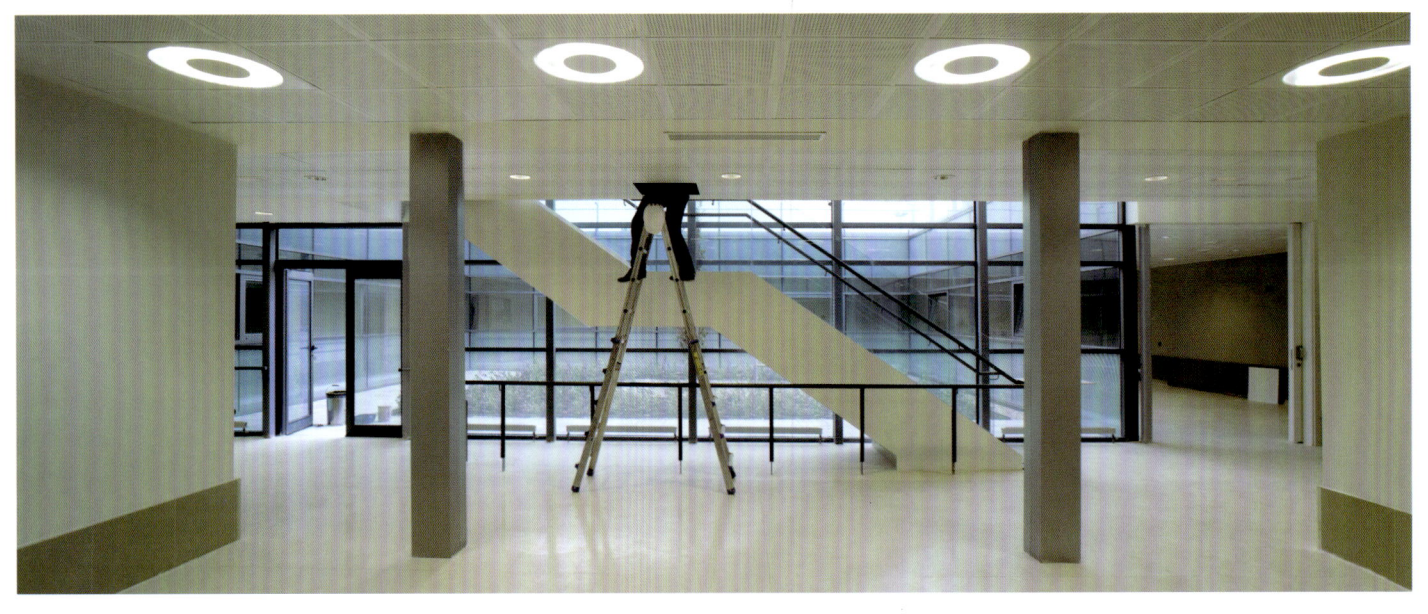

197

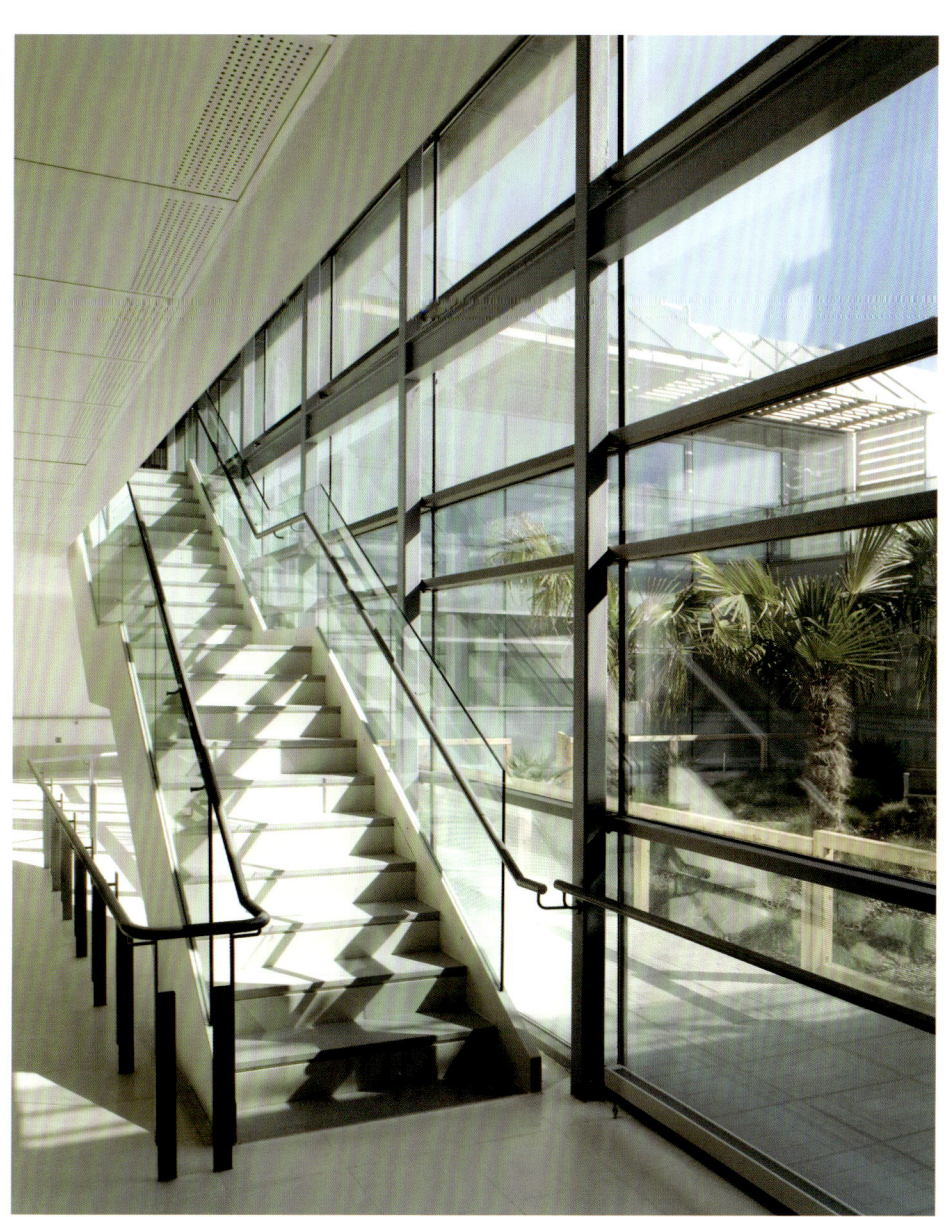

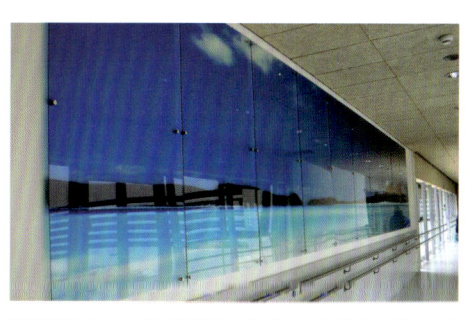

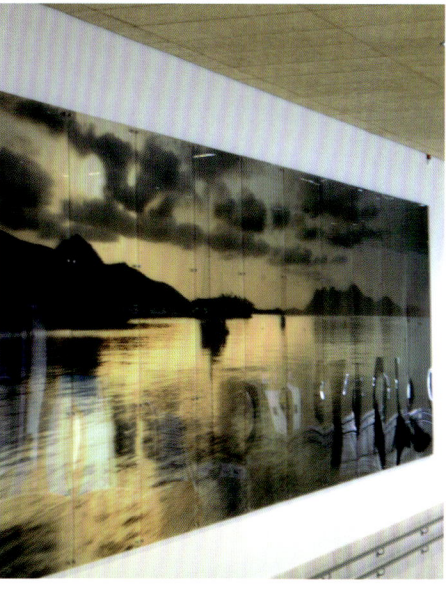

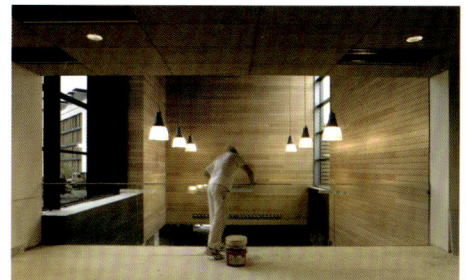

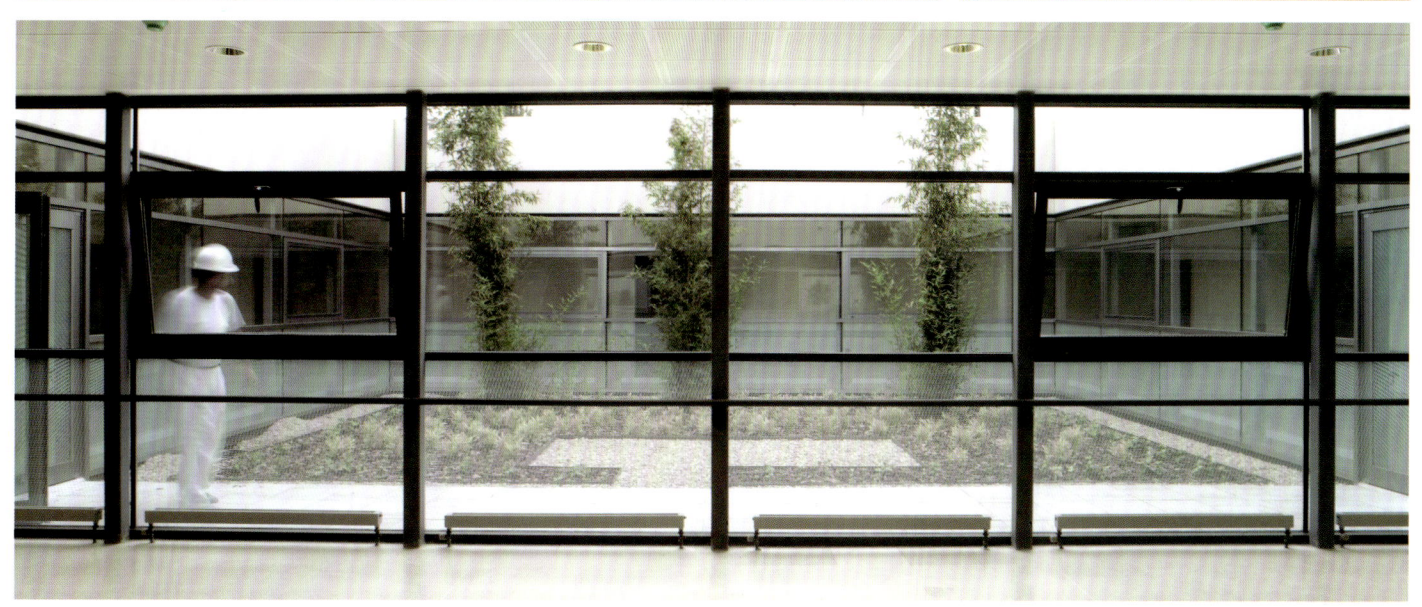

198

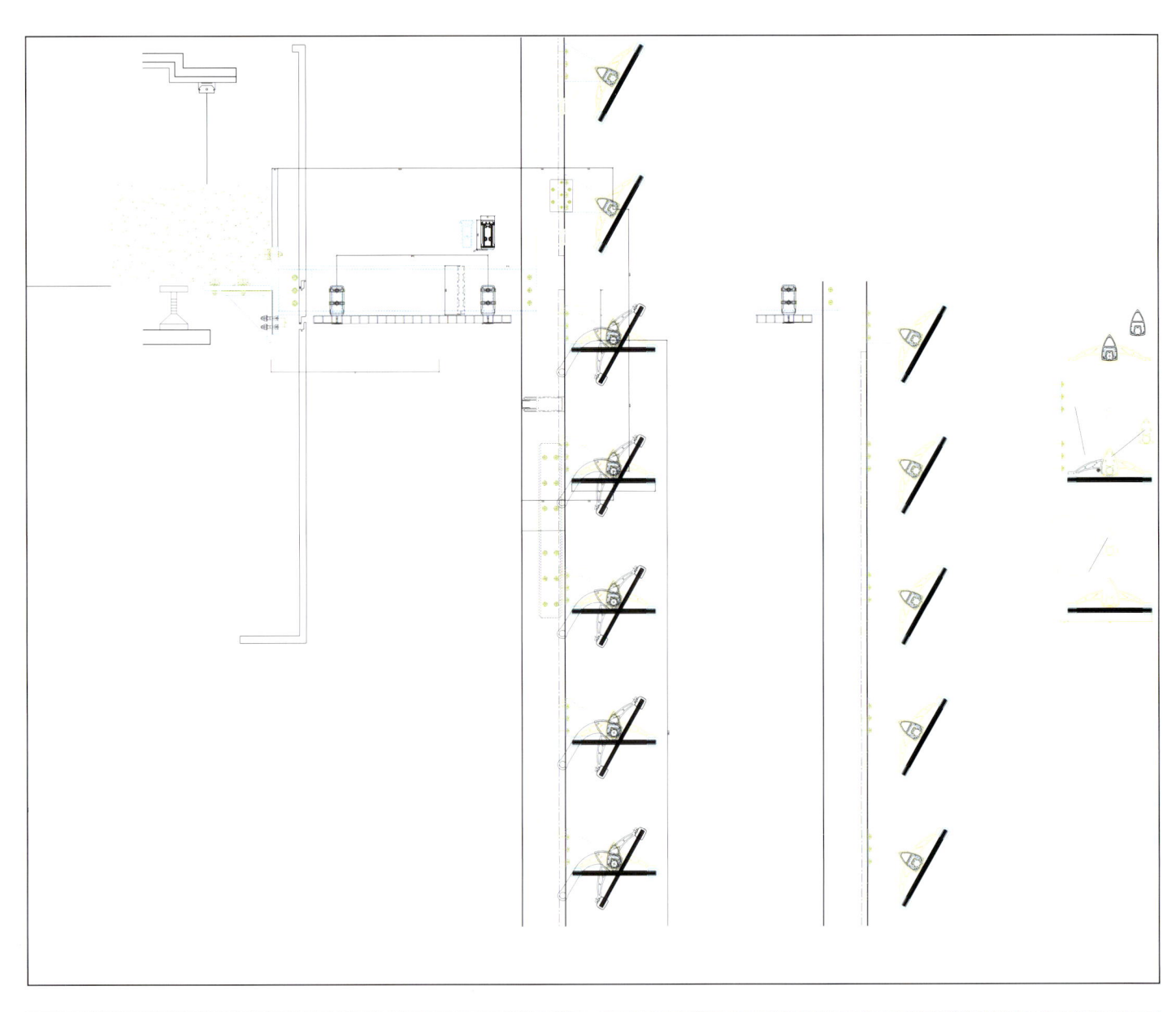

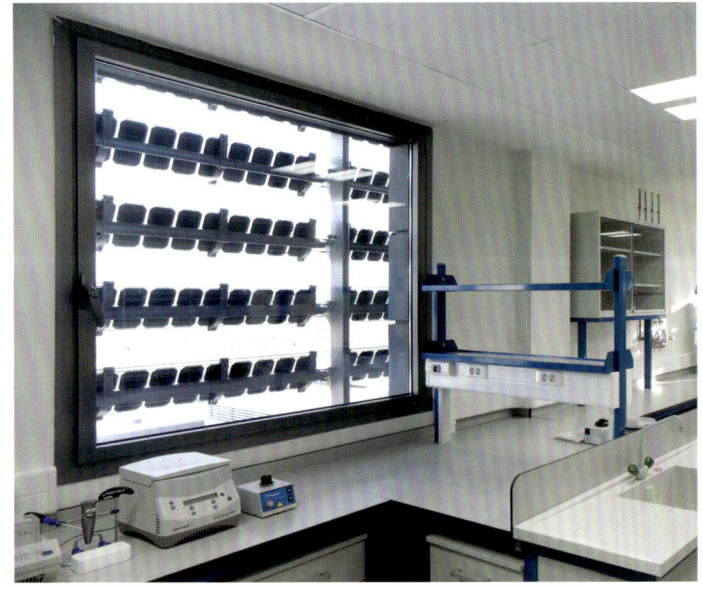

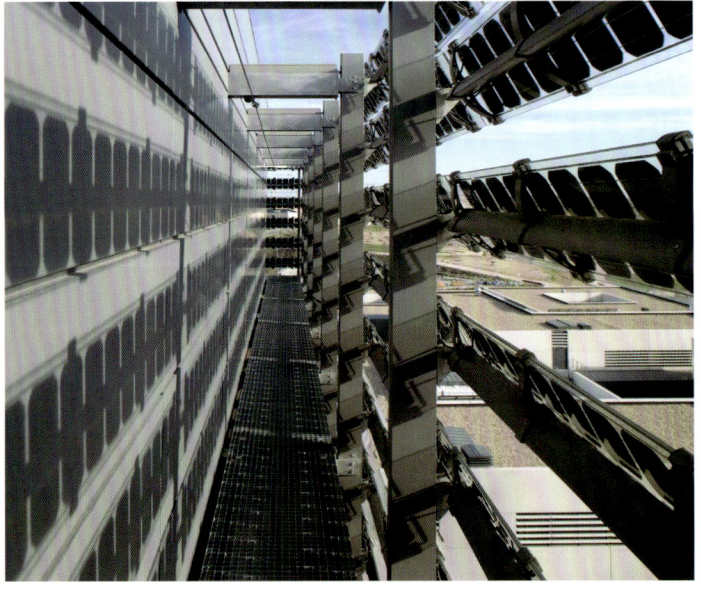

199

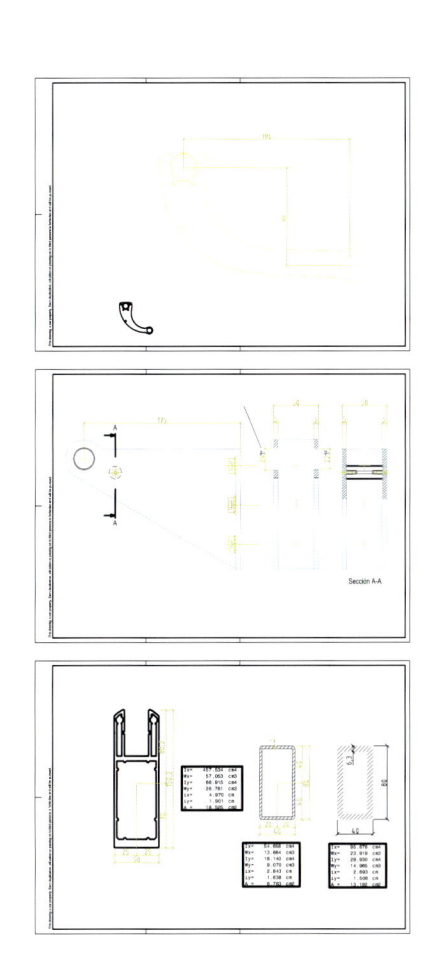

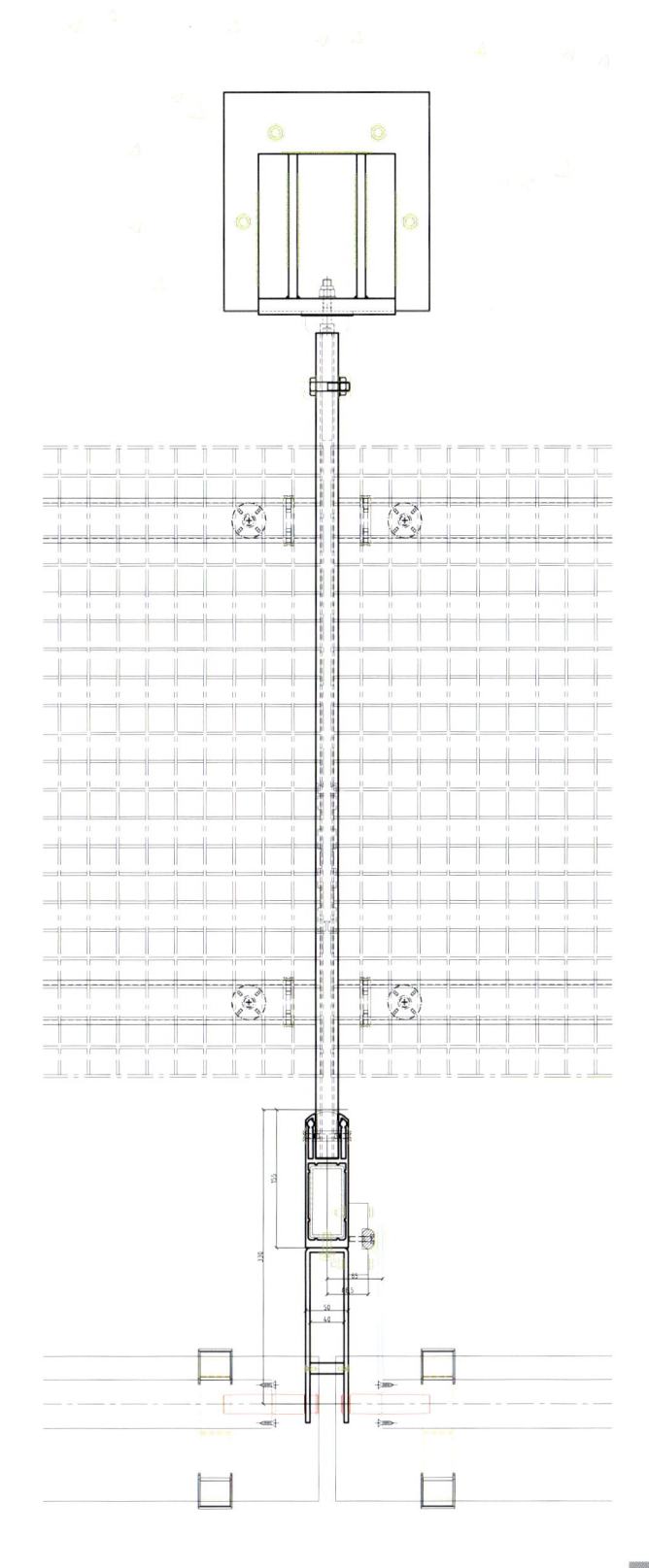

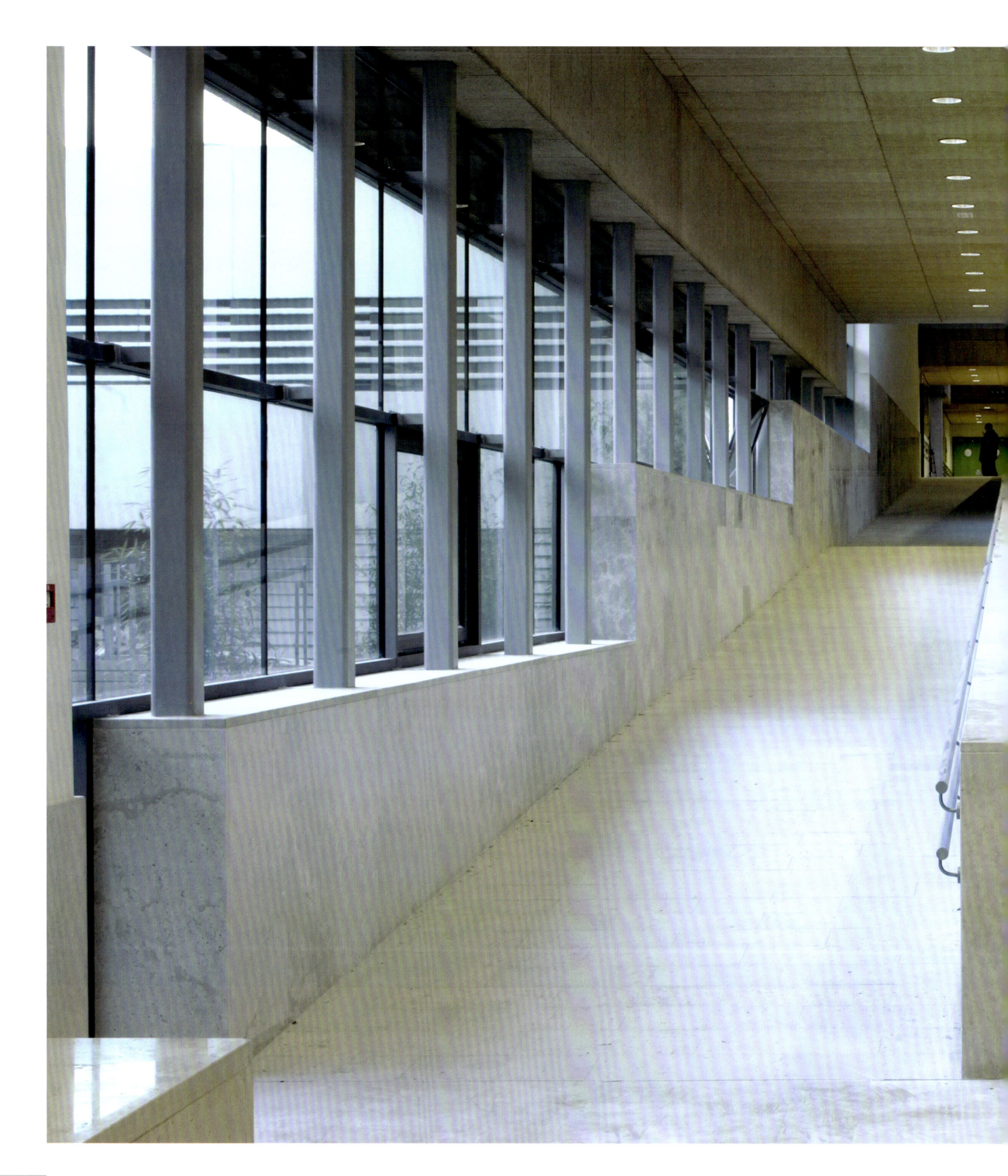

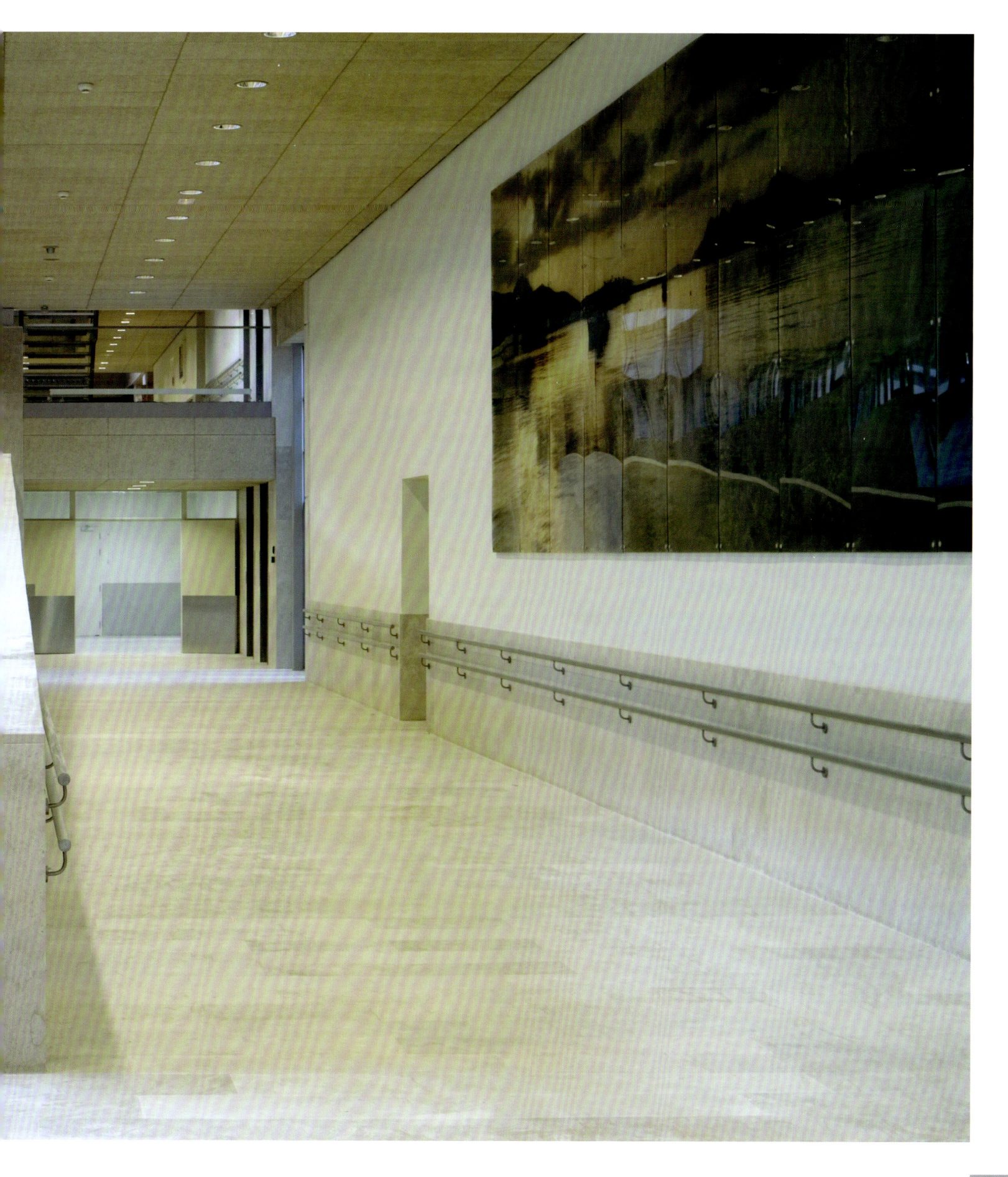

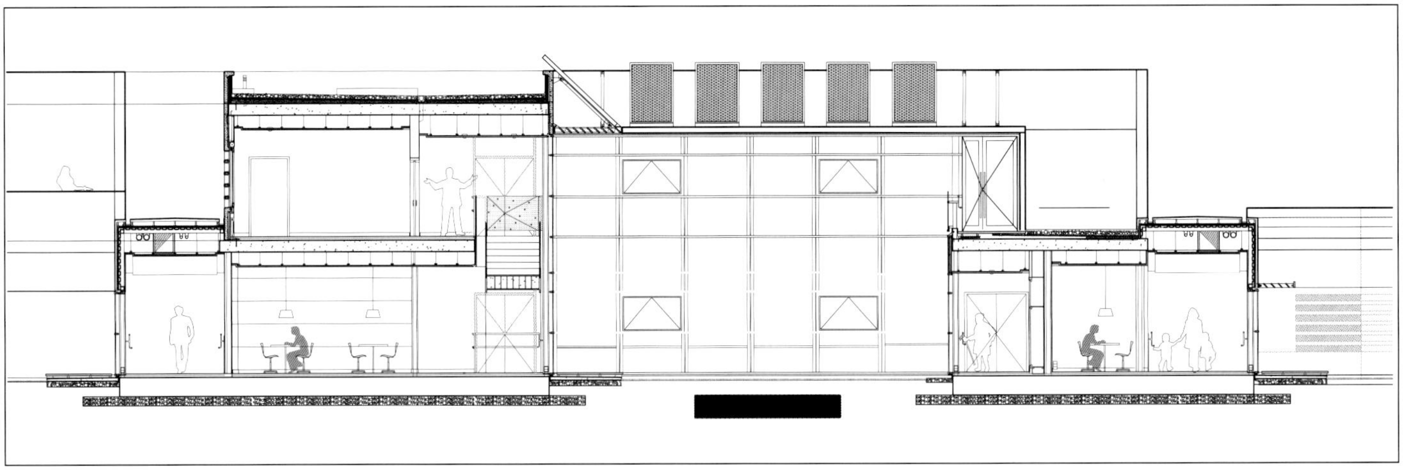

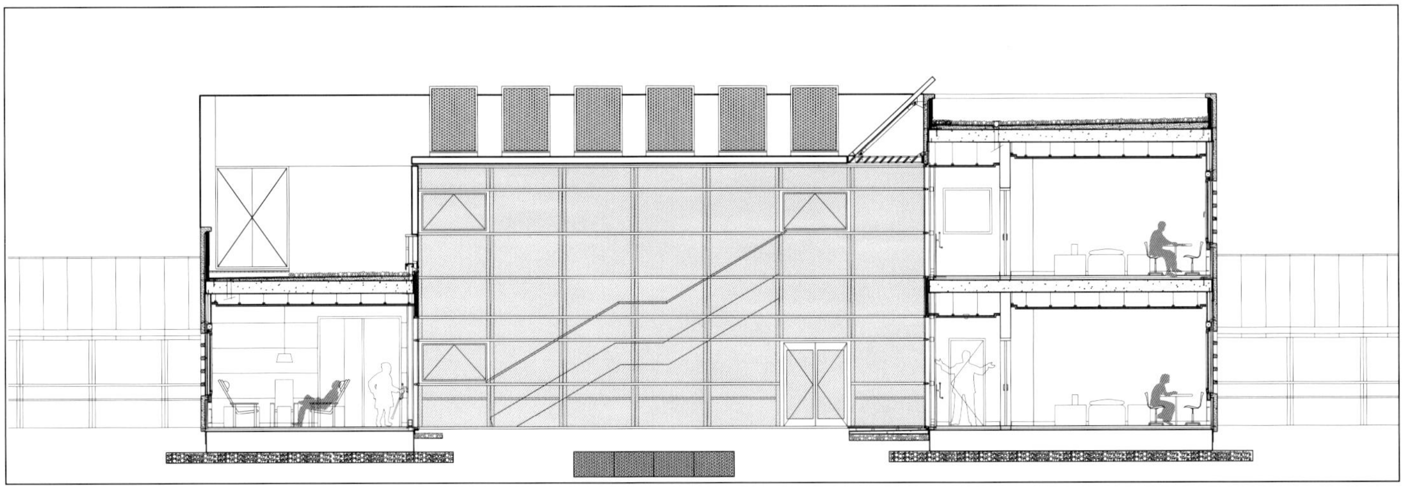

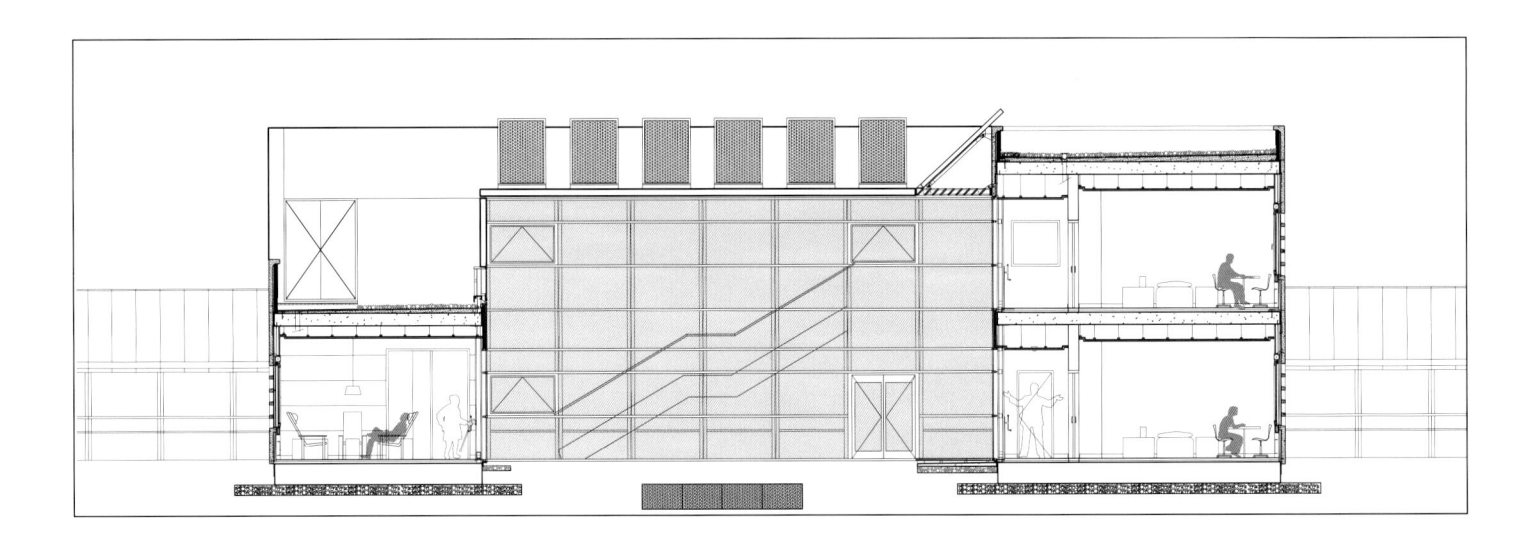

203

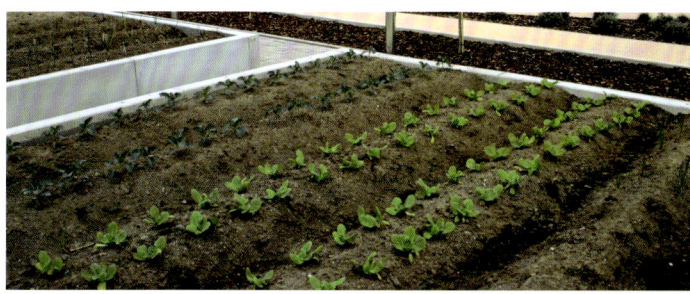

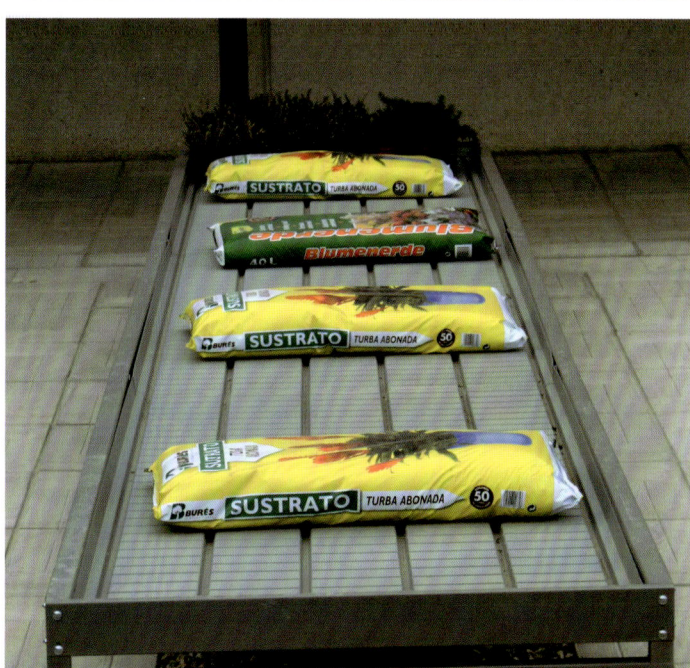

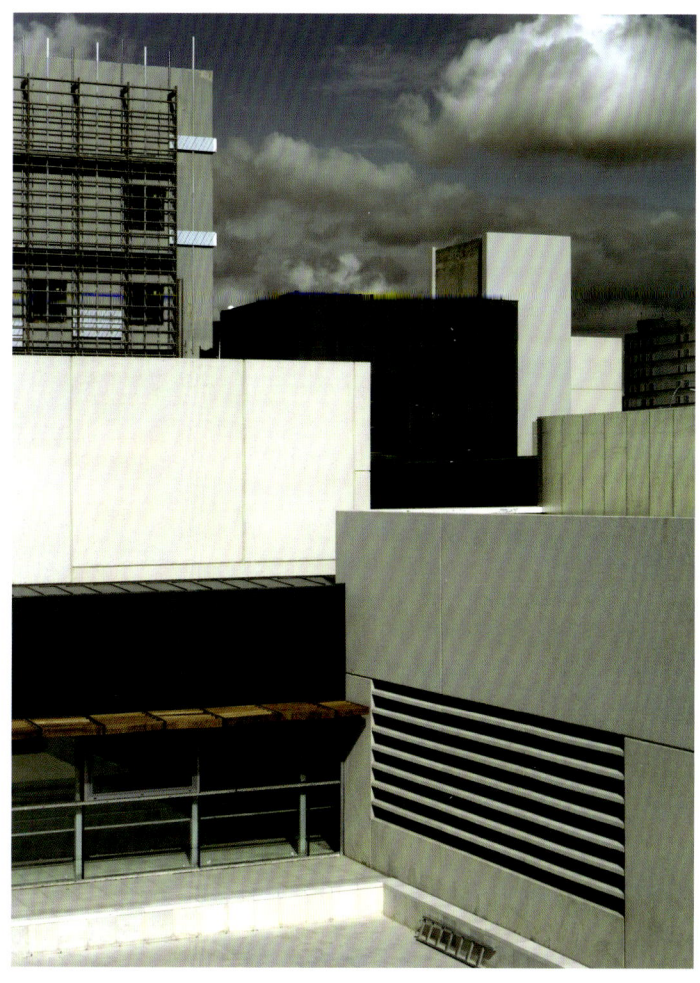

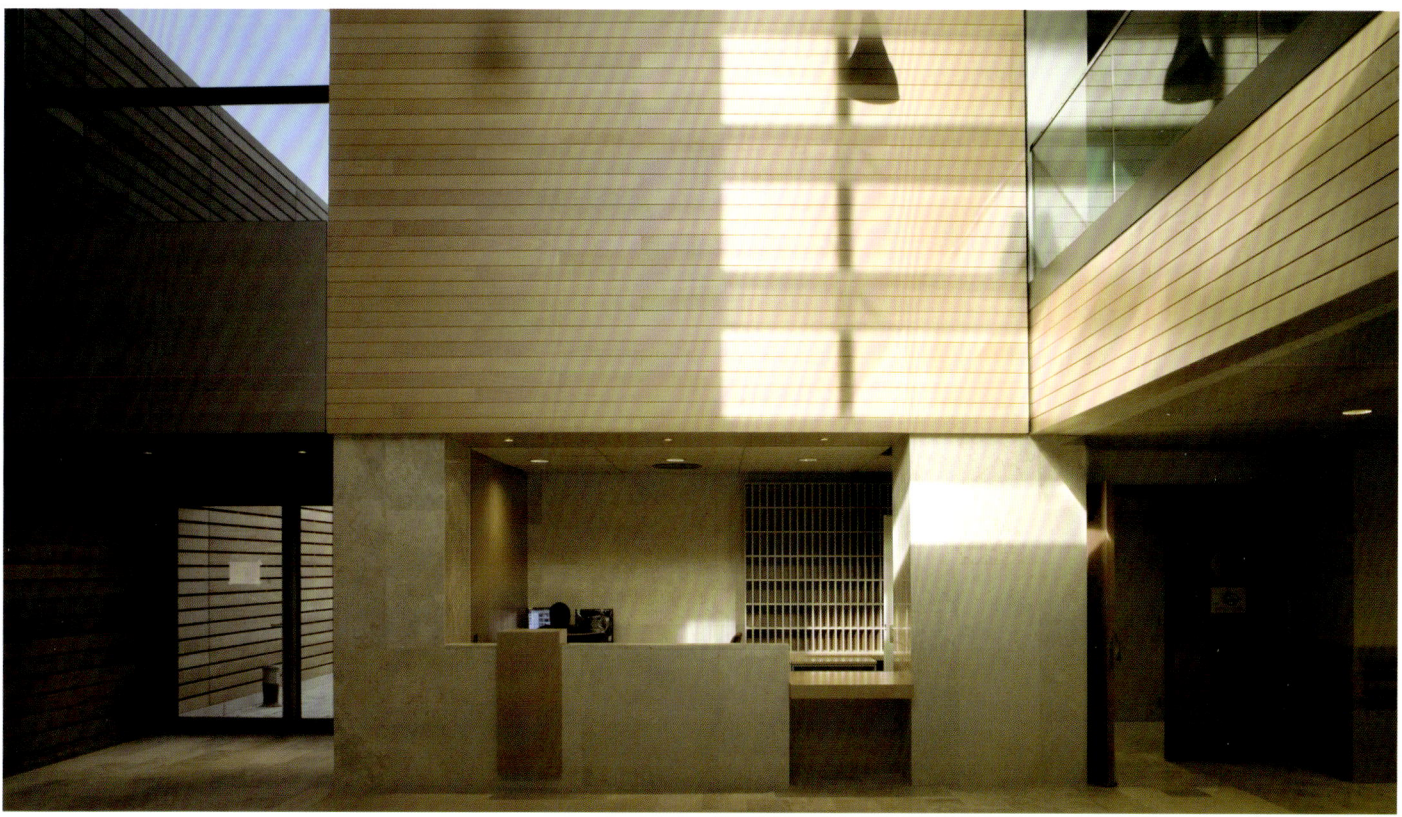

Tonet Sunyer Arquitecte - LKS Estudio

Villablino Hospital

León, Spain

Photographs: Eugeni Pons

The building is situated at the highest point of a site with a pronounced north-south inclination, which generates a 40 m (130 ft) change in floor level, and forms a long and narrow volume running from east to west. Like the base of a comb this building connects the volumes that extend southwards which contain the different areas of the program. These elements with their connecting "vertebra" are built into the land and rise above it as they develop, resolving the level differences. Their different geometries, heights and rhythms generate a dynamic and lightweight architecture that integrates smoothly with the surroundings.

The longitudinal spine is closed to the north with an opaque, hermetic wall that resolves the access points and accommodates the central circulation and installations. On its south façade a long corridor opens with glazed viewing points, interspaced between the different wings. The backbone resolves and links with all the functional areas, affording them independence but at the same time functional fluidity.

The architecture adapts to the uneven topography without staggering the building and allowing for a strong linear component. The projecting bodies arise from the need for functional and operative differentiations without sacrificing simple orientation and visual connections. The usual problems of continuity associated with the compact nature of this building typology are thus avoided. The building envelope is conceived in a similar way distinguishing externally the concrete and glass longitudinal axis from the more compact brickwork of the projecting bodies, which echoes the vernacular architecture.

All spaces are treated with a precise and equivalent geometry. As stated in the brief, the modules can be easily modified allowing for possible changes regarding technologies, regulations and uses. The uniform geometry is altered in just one of the central wings, where the cafeteria, dining area and main hall are located, since this section should not undergo significant changes during the life of the center. On the north façade a concrete wall contains and closes the access platform and conceals the installations, ending in a glazed wall that encloses the rehabilitation unit, which is open to the south.

Two volumes either side of the center stand out thanks to their unusual and attractive aesthetics. A large glazed body with louvers projects from the second floor at one end of the main volume, while at the other end a vertical wooden landmark houses the funeral building and the multi-use chapel. The latter rises above the main building like a translucent wooden box creating a secluded and quiet interior space which lights up like a beacon at night.

Client:
Villablino Town Council
Surface area:
8,523 sqm (91,740 sqft)
Start date:
1998
Finish date:
2002
Collaborators:
Rute Carlos, Eva Moral, Alberto Pérez, Cristina Soler, Diana Garay, María Antonia Mir, Alfonso Días Prats, Philip Esperanza
Structure:
Eduardo Doce
Quantity surveyors:
Francisco Varela y Jose Manuel Lafuente
Contractor:
Martínez Núñez
Cost:
€ 7,550,000

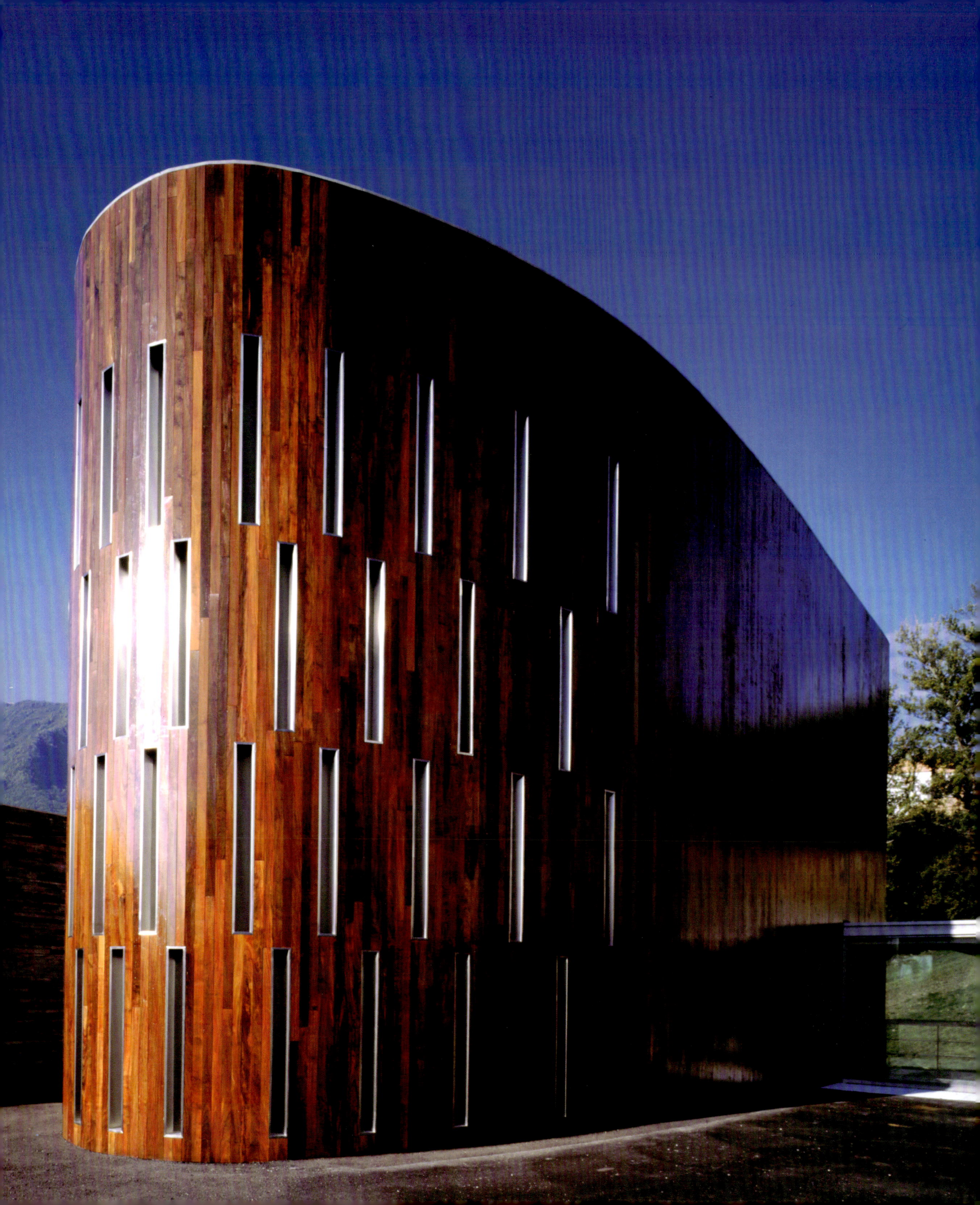

206

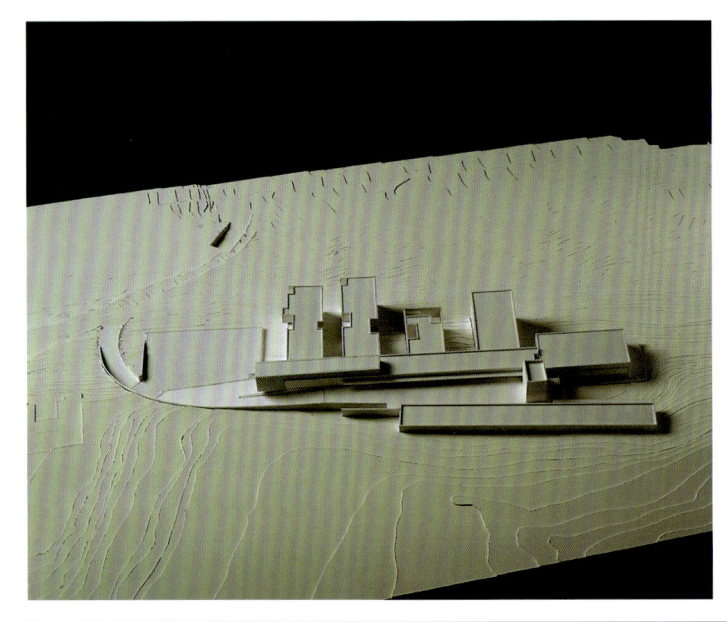

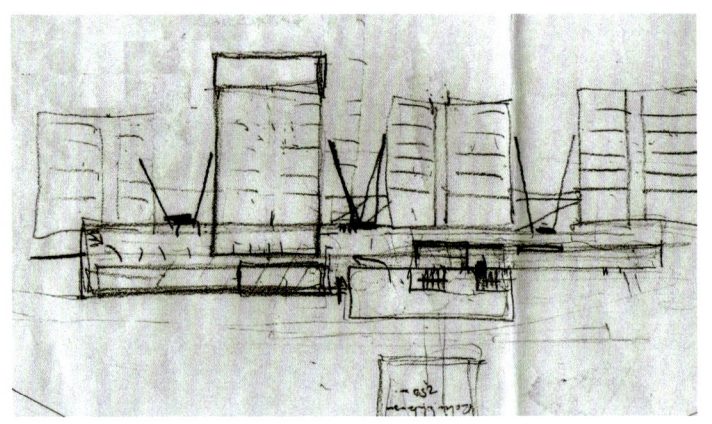

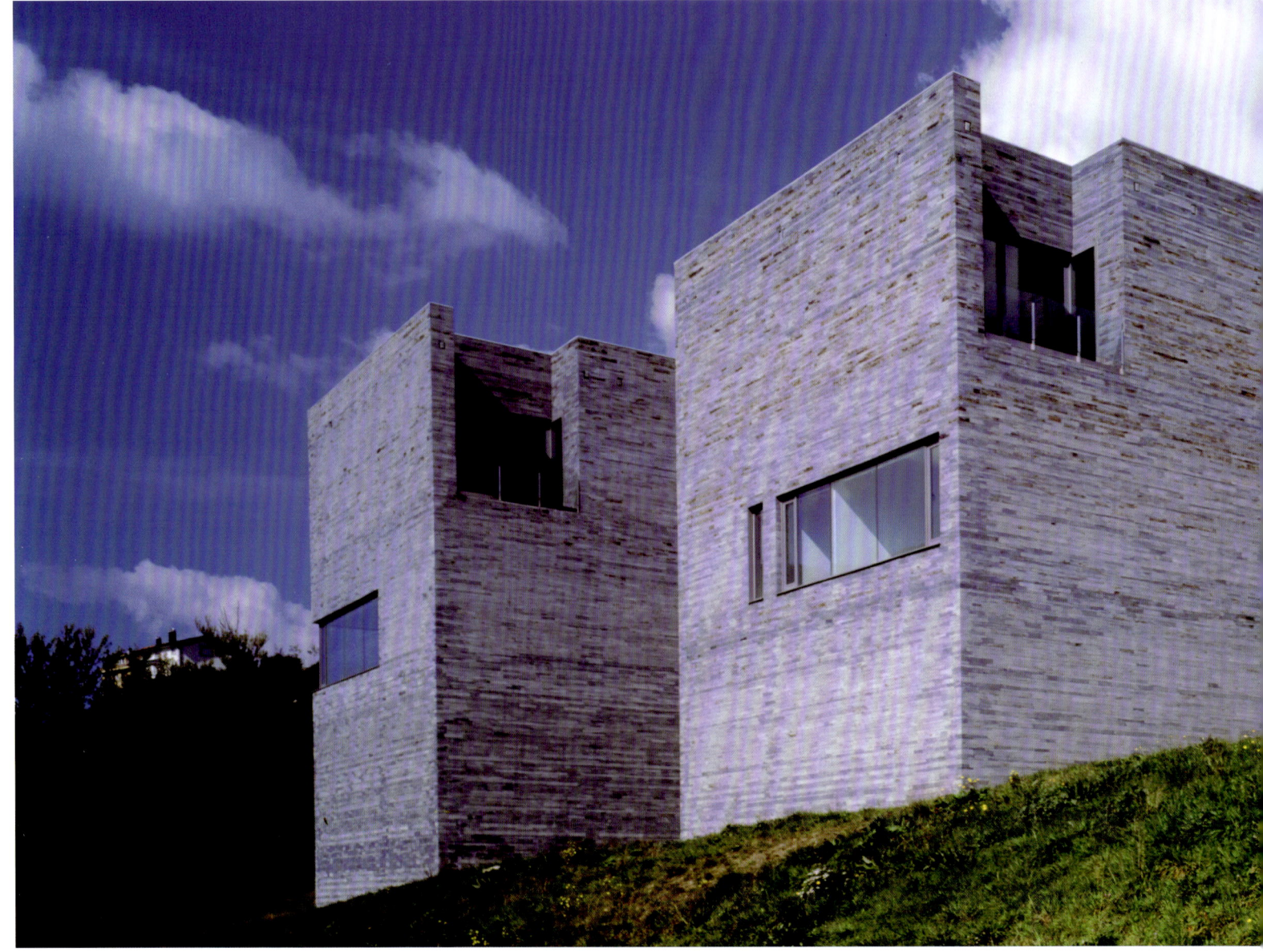

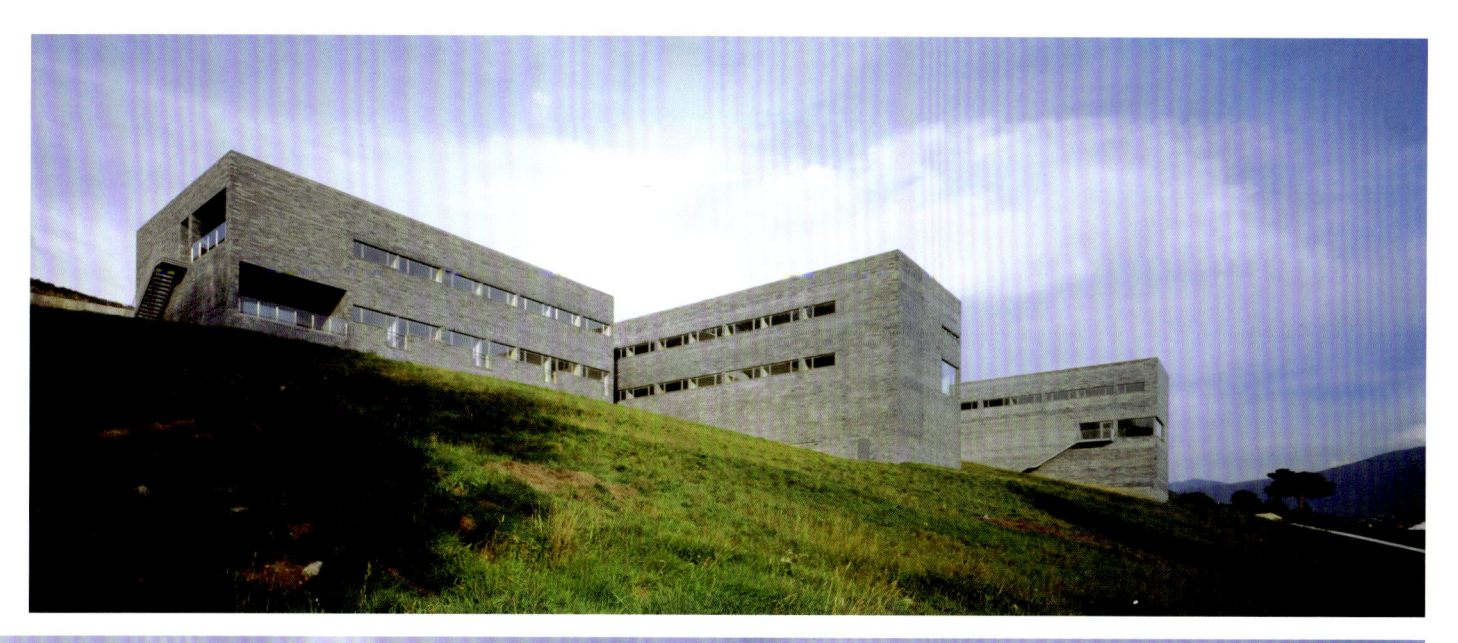

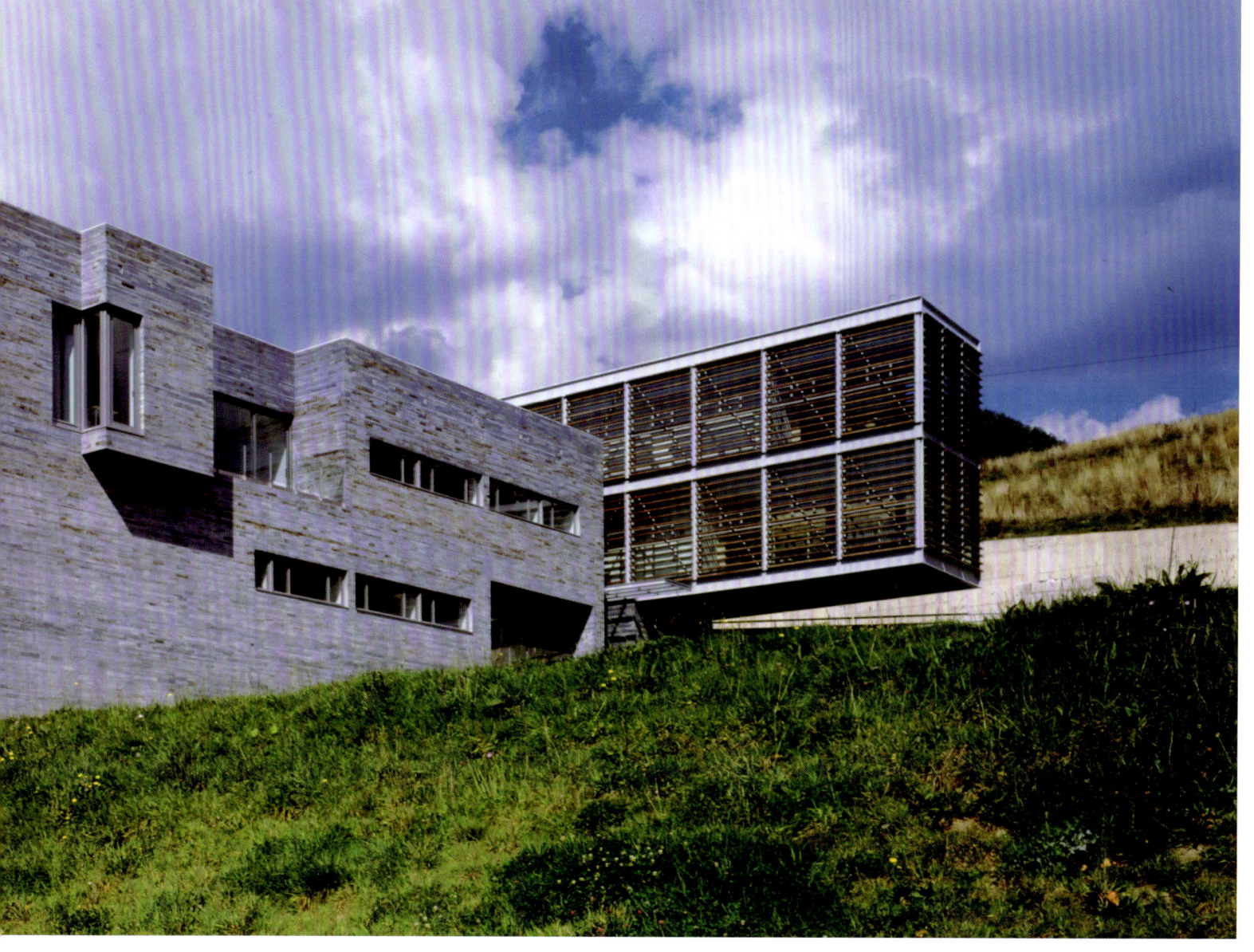

Ground floor plan

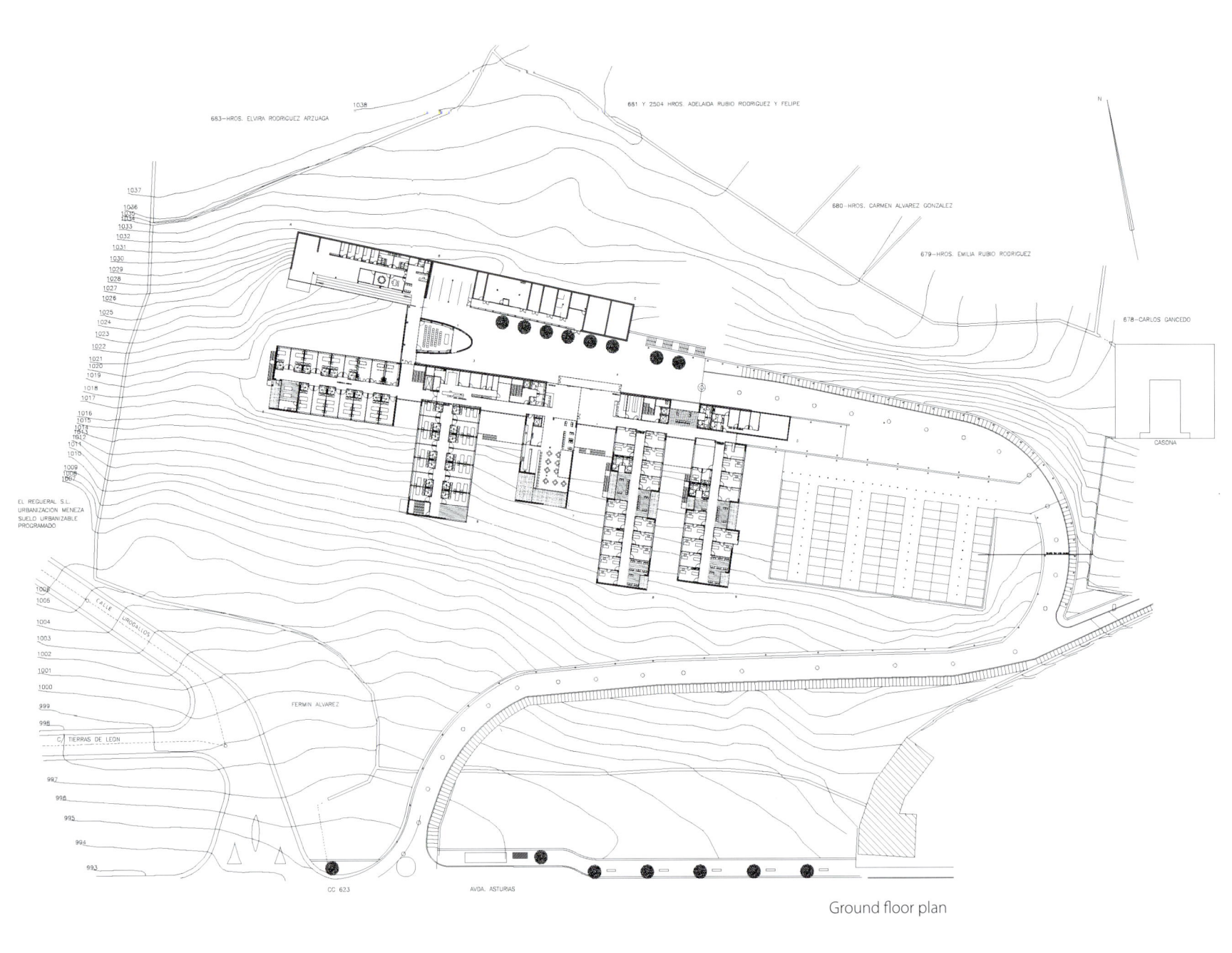

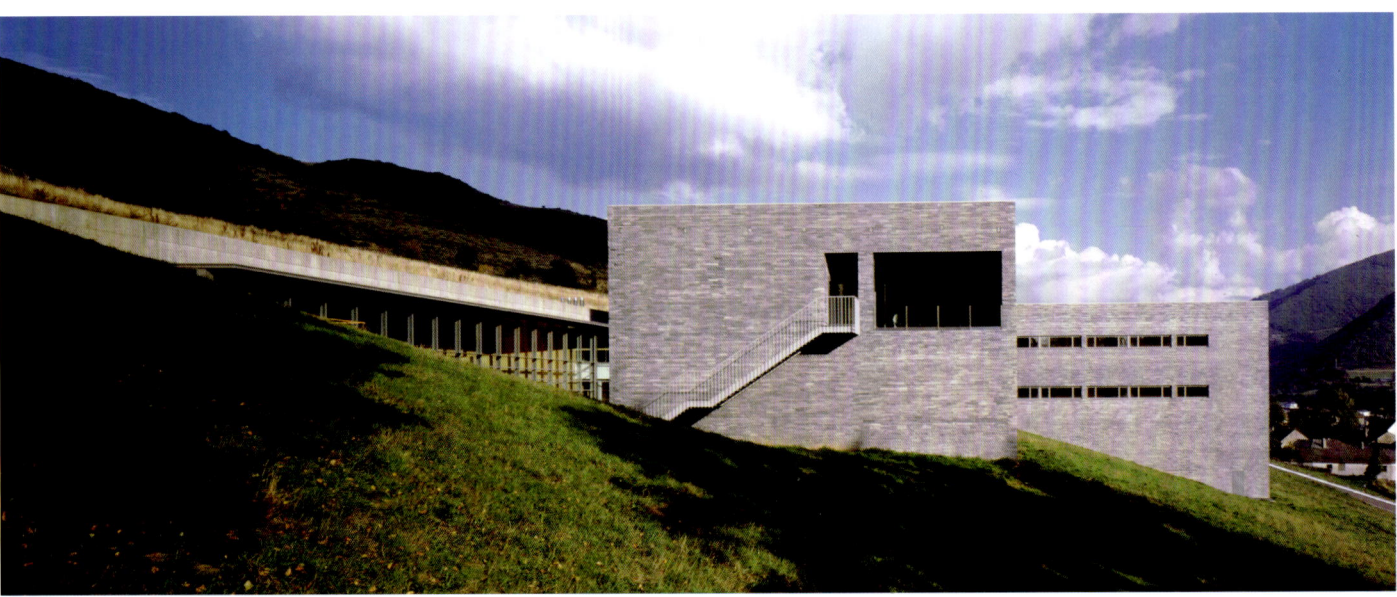

208

The architecture adapts to the uneven topography without staggering the building and allowing for a strong linear component. The projecting bodies arise from the need for functional and operative differentiations without sacrificing simple orientation and visual connections.

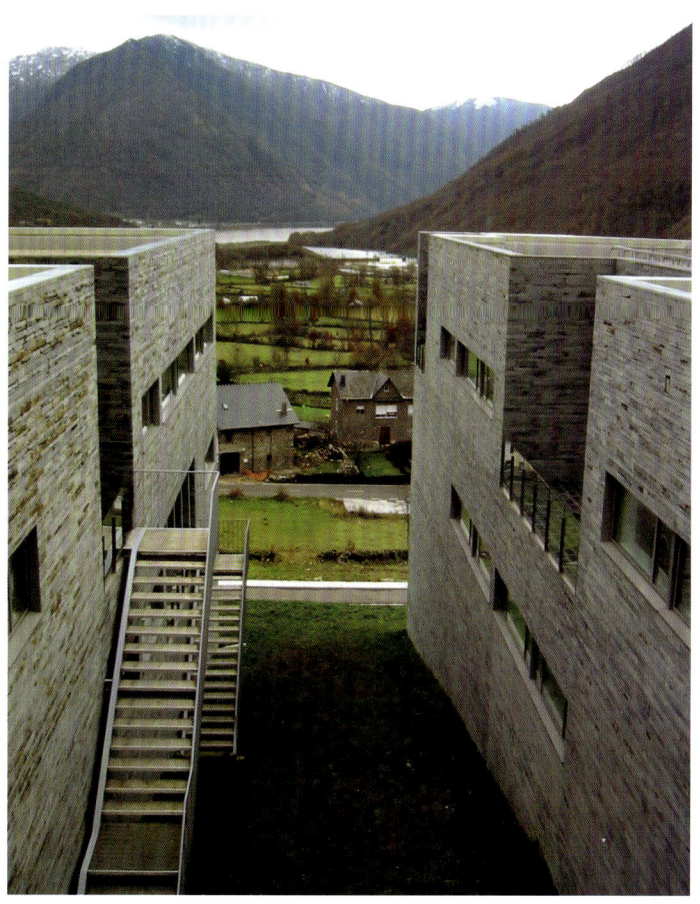

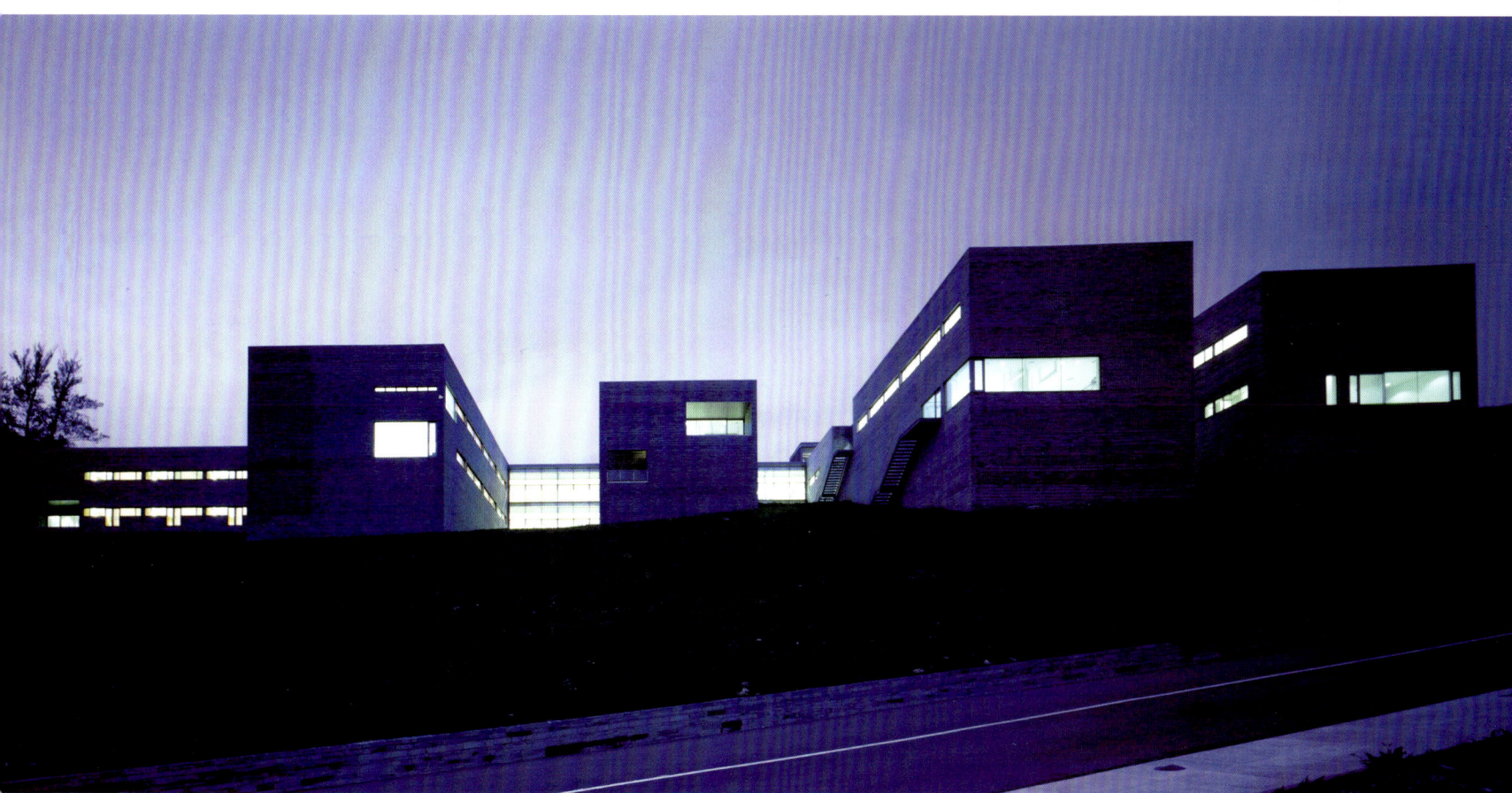

First floor plan

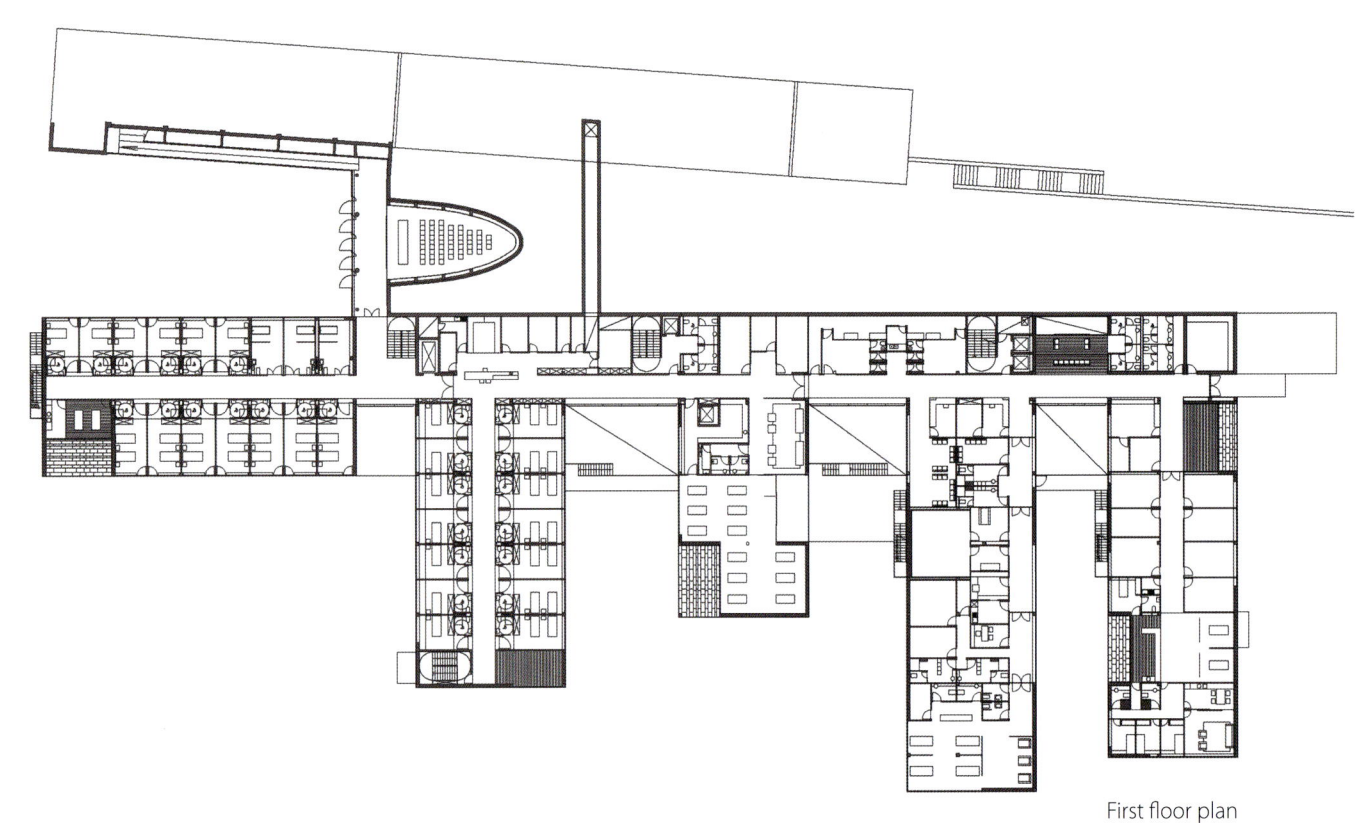

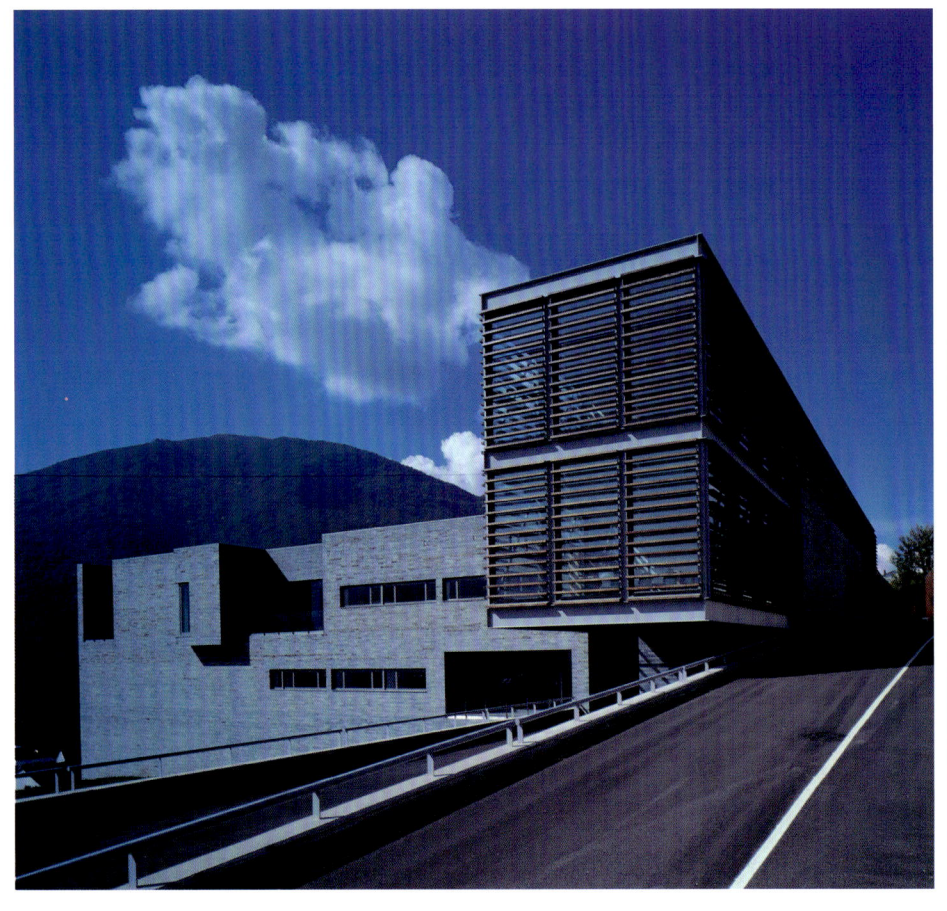

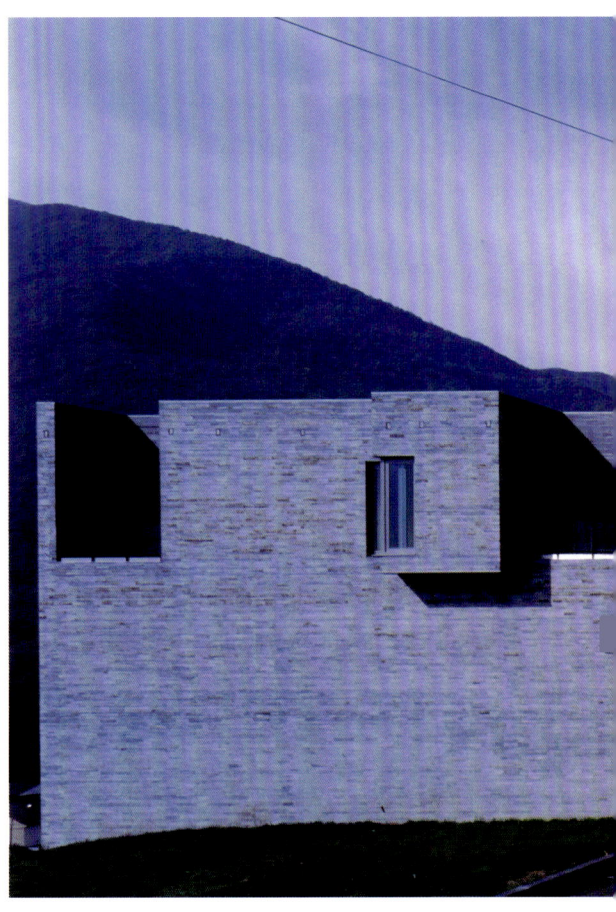

Second floor plan

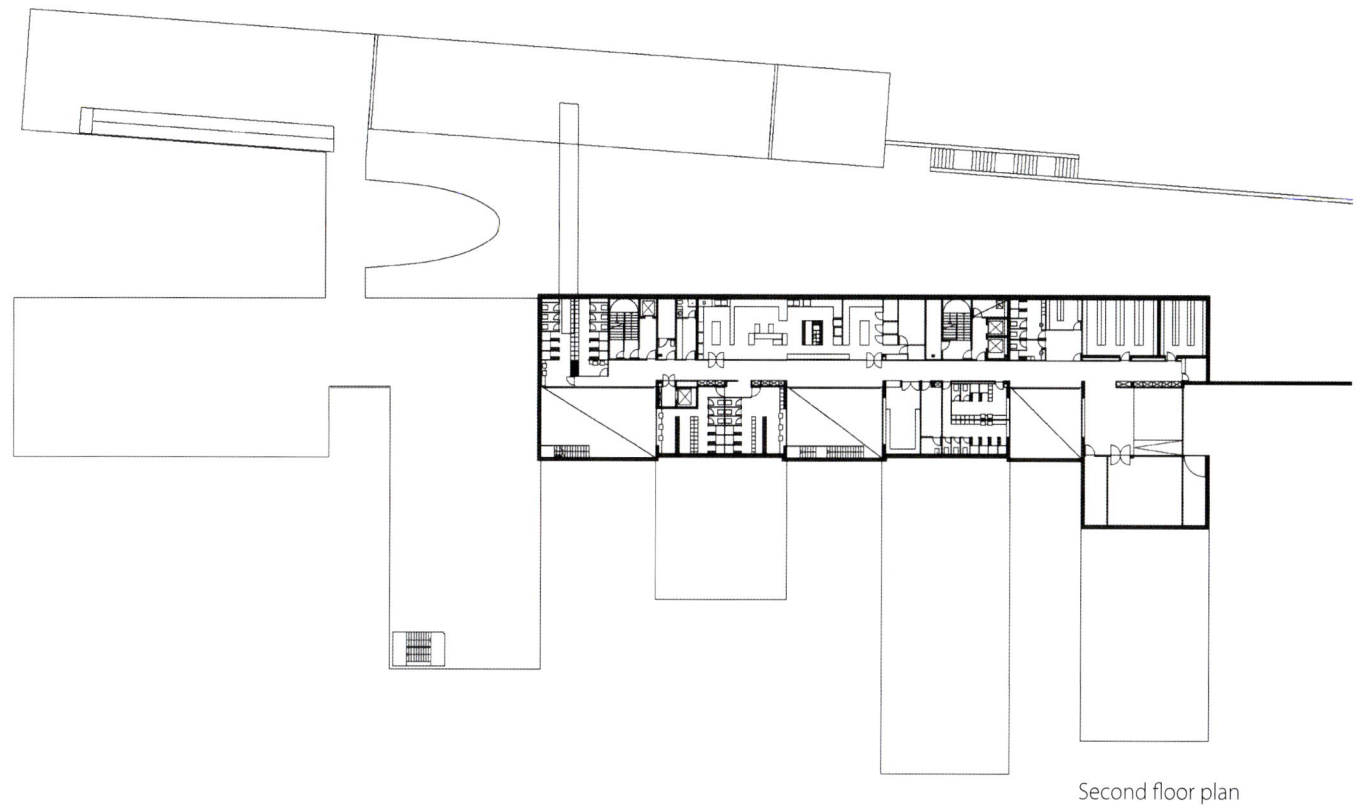

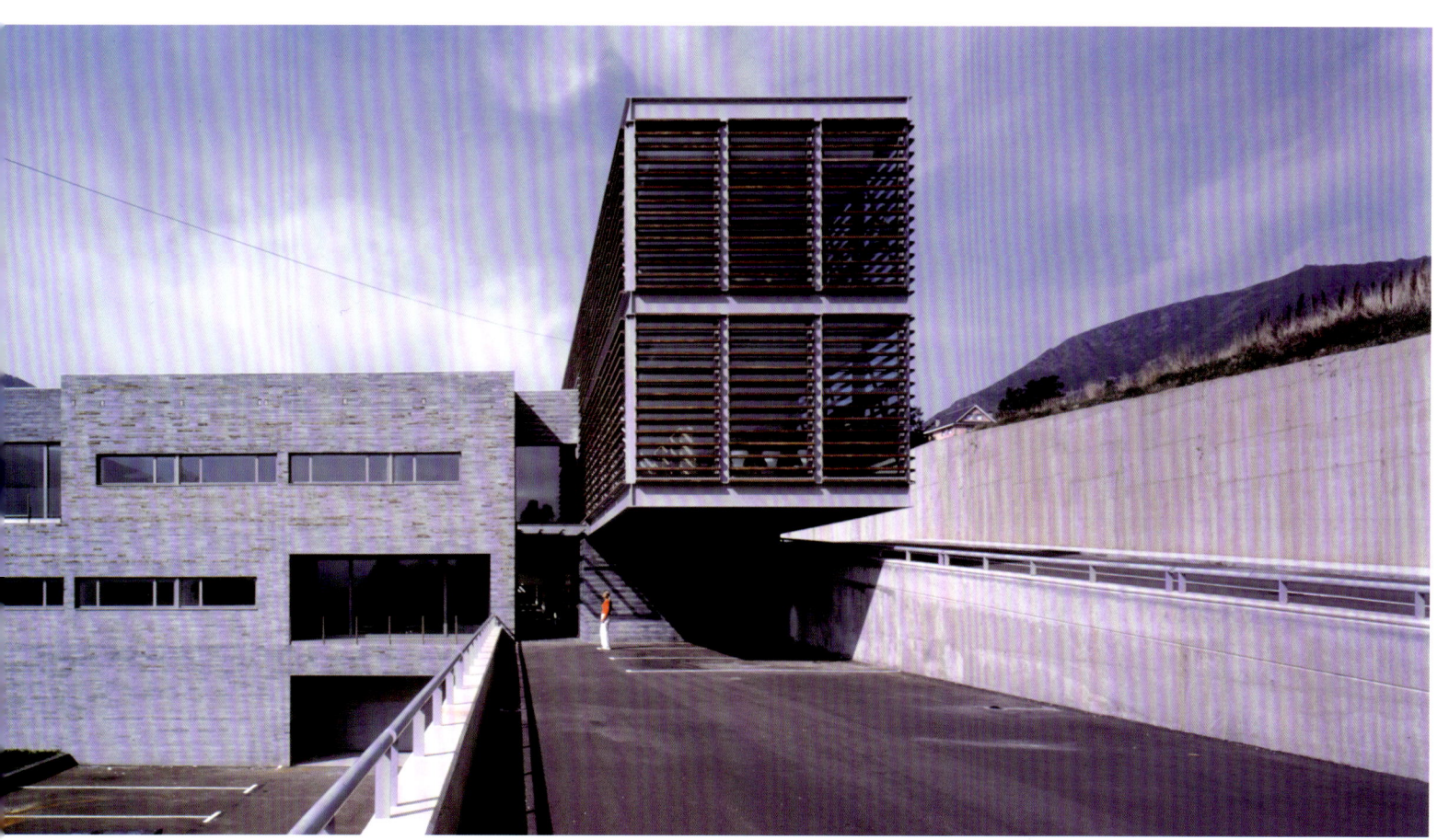

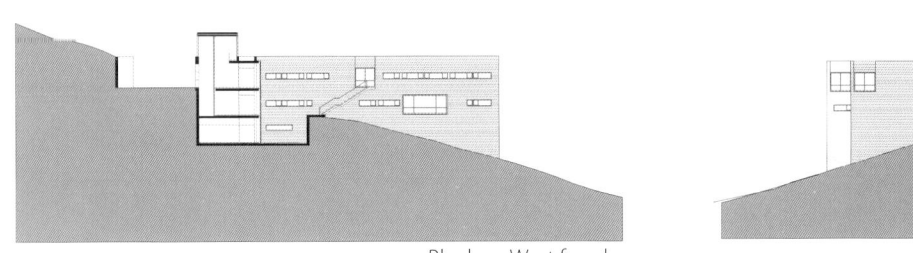

Block 9 - West façade

Block 9 - East façade

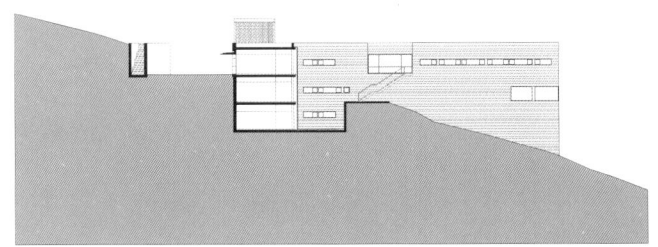

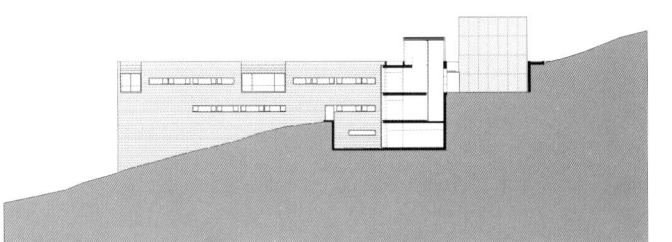

Block 8 - West façade

Block 8 - East façade

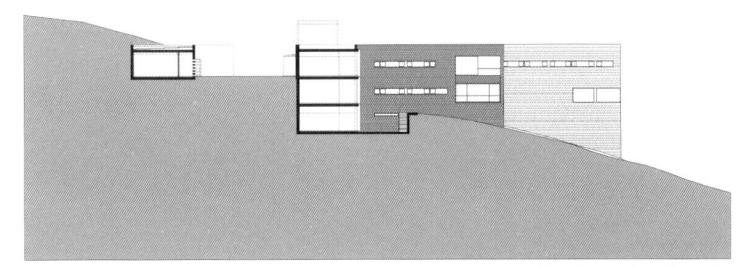

Block 7 - West façade

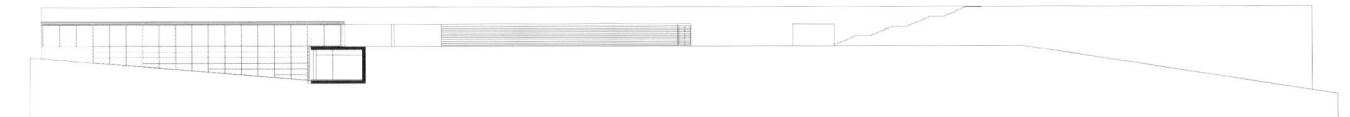

Rehabilitation block - South façade

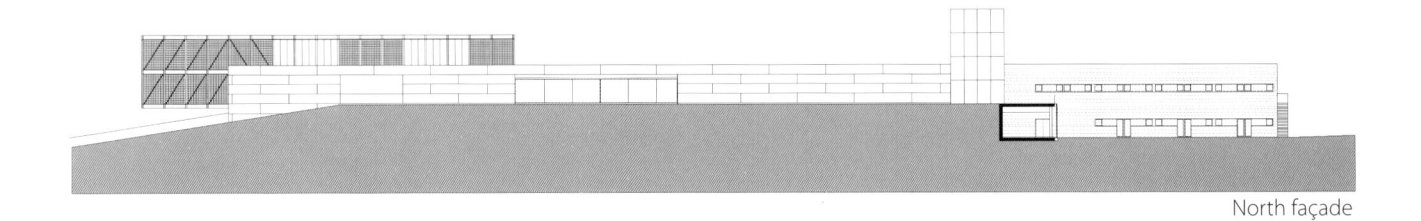

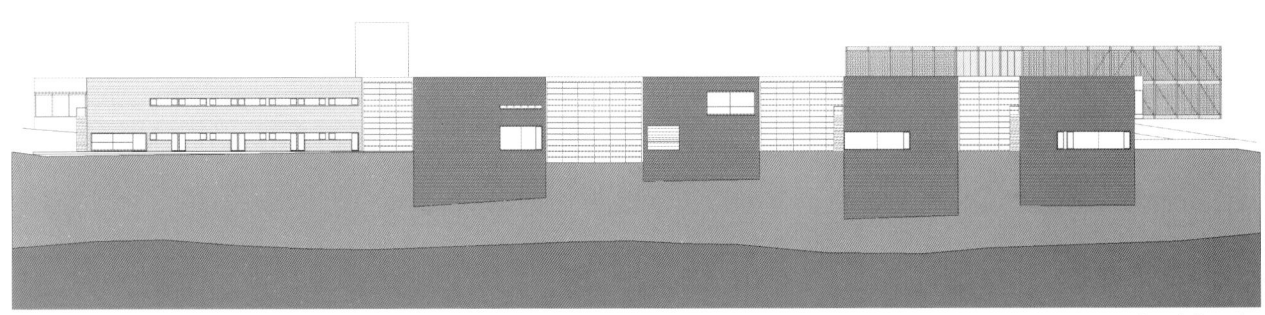

North façade

South façade

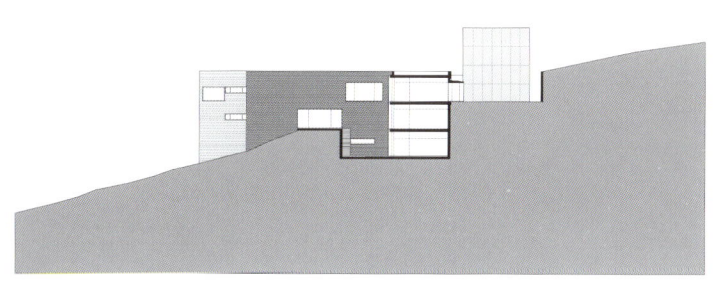

Block 7 - East façade

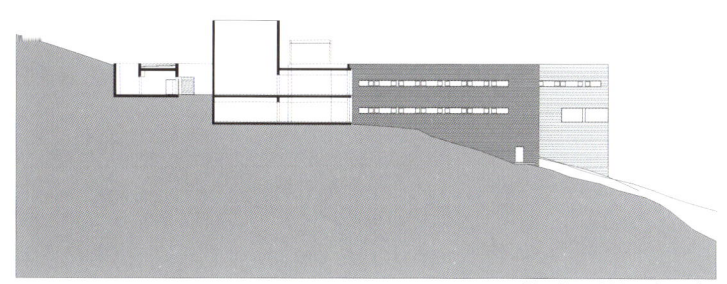

Block 6 - West façade

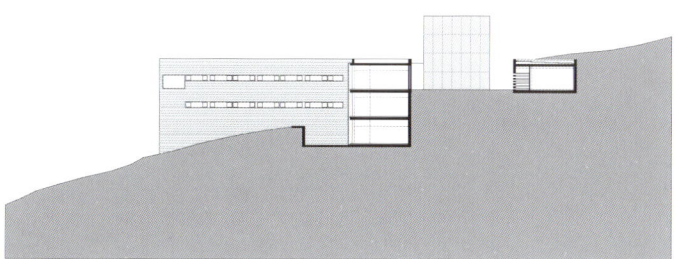

Block 6 - East façade

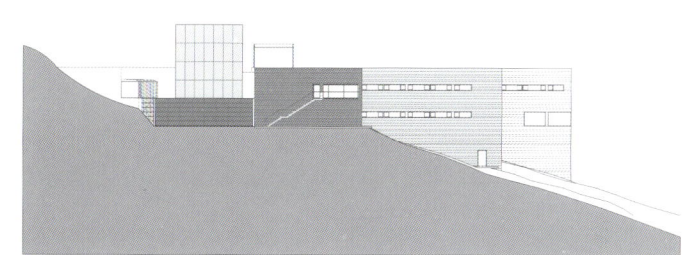

Block 2 - West façade

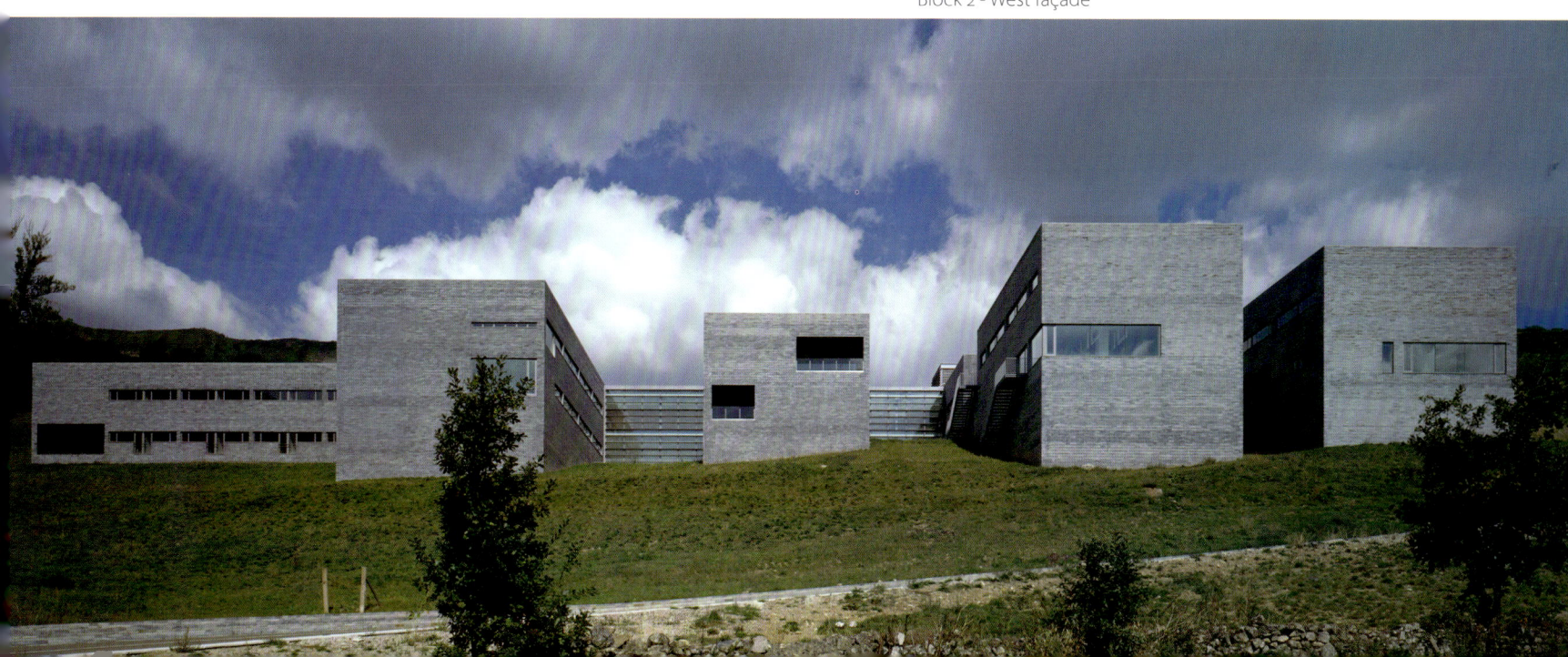

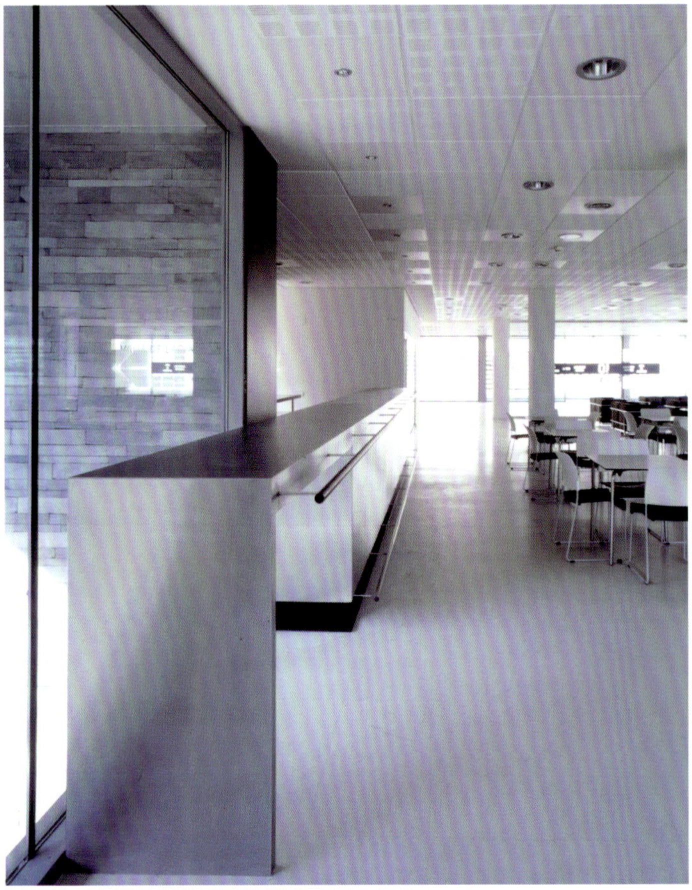

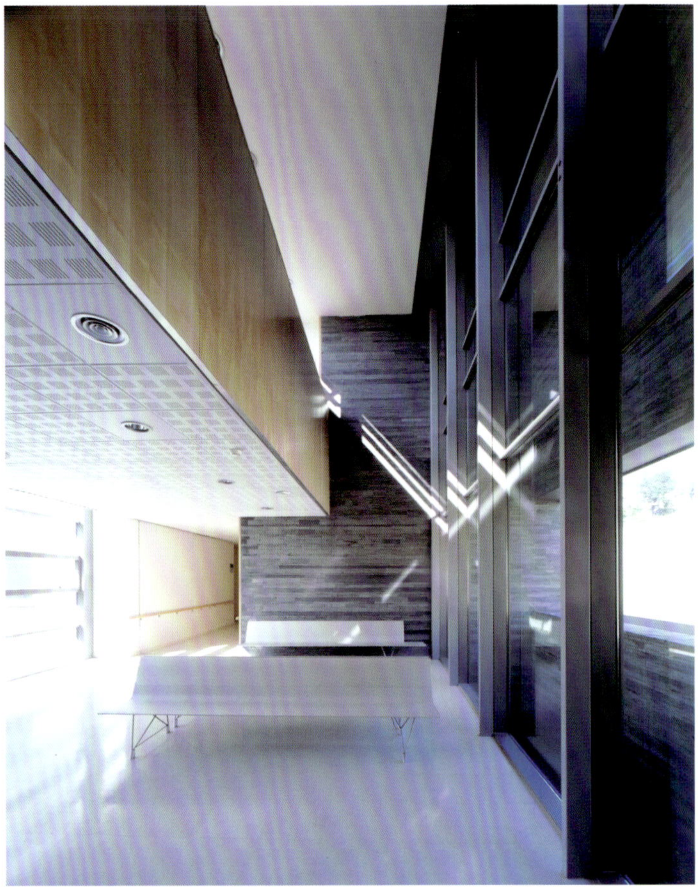

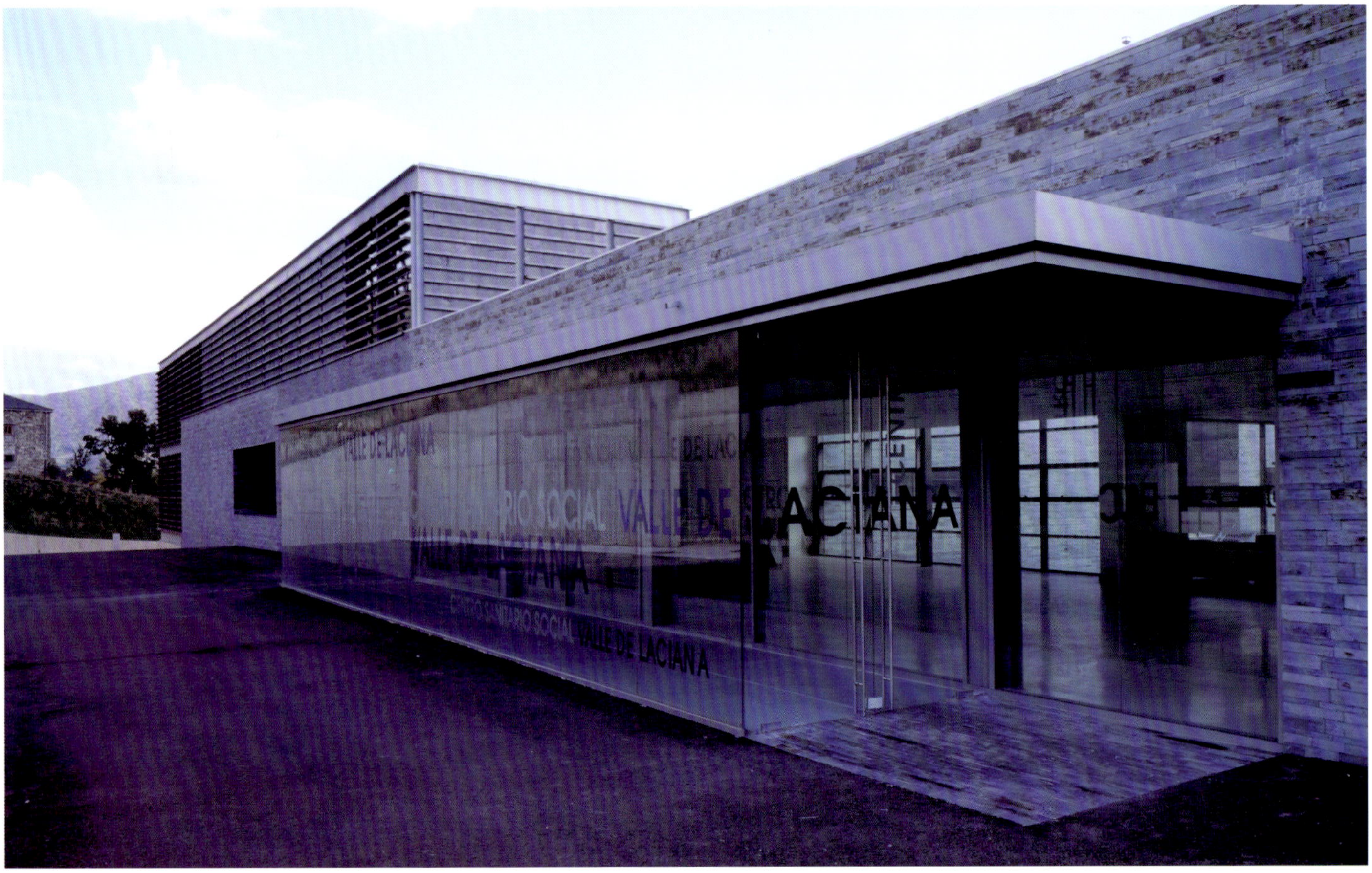
VALLE DE LACIANA
CENTRO SANITARIO SOCIAL VALLE DE LACIANA

A - LIST OF MATERIALS
1. Terrazzo tiles, micro-aggregate, white, 60x60cm
2. Parquet floor, maple
3. Gres tiles 10x10cm
4. Linoleum

CLADDING
5. Fair-faced concrete
6. Stratified panel
7. Maple wood
8. Tongue-and-groove maple
9. Phenolic resin panels
10. Gres tiles 10x10cm
11. Stainless steel
12. Transparent glass
13. Mirror

CEILINGS
14. Suspended Pladur ceiling
15. Suspended maple wood ceiling
16. Suspended maple wood ceiling
17. Suspended ceiling of stratified panels

ENCLOSURES
18. Fixed espalu carpentry
19. Sliding espalu carpentry
20. Pivoting espalu carpentry
21. Pivoting espalu carpentry
22. Hinged espalu carpentry

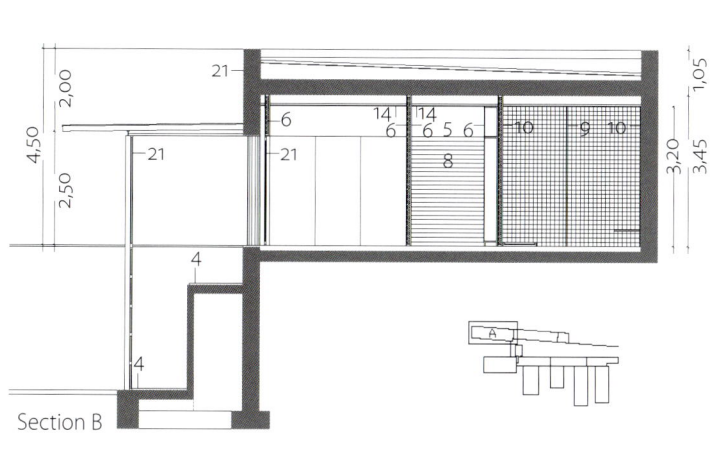

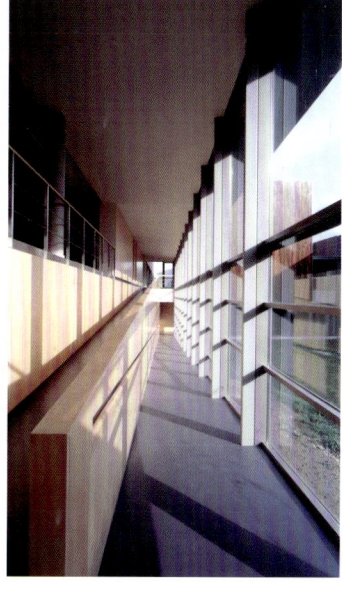

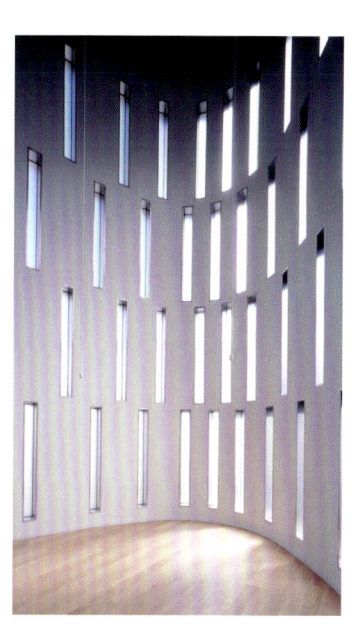

Section B

Rehabilitation block - Detail

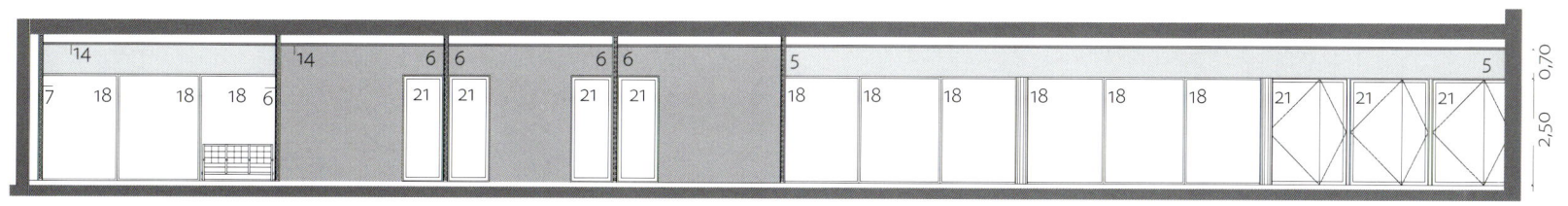

Section C

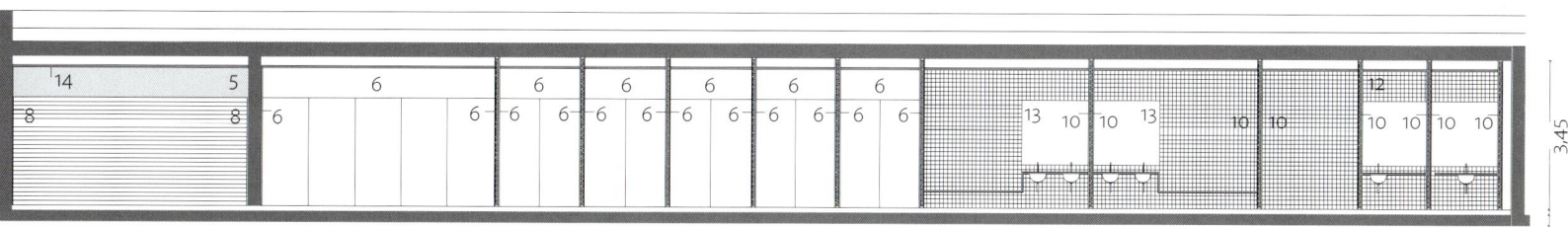

Section D

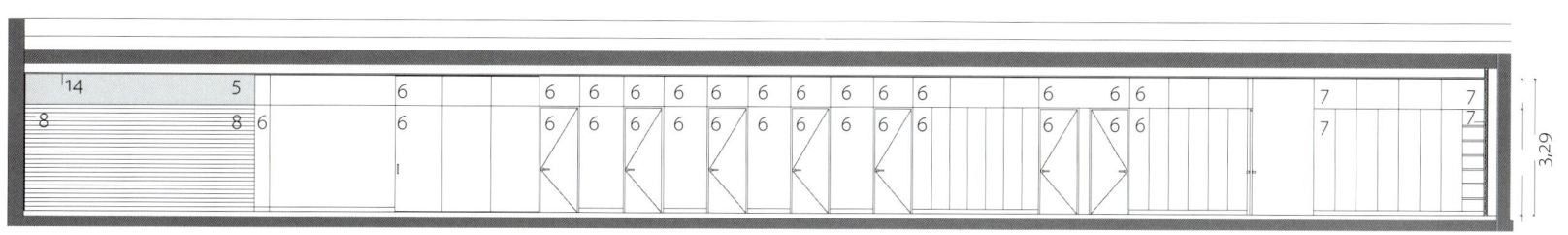

Section E

215

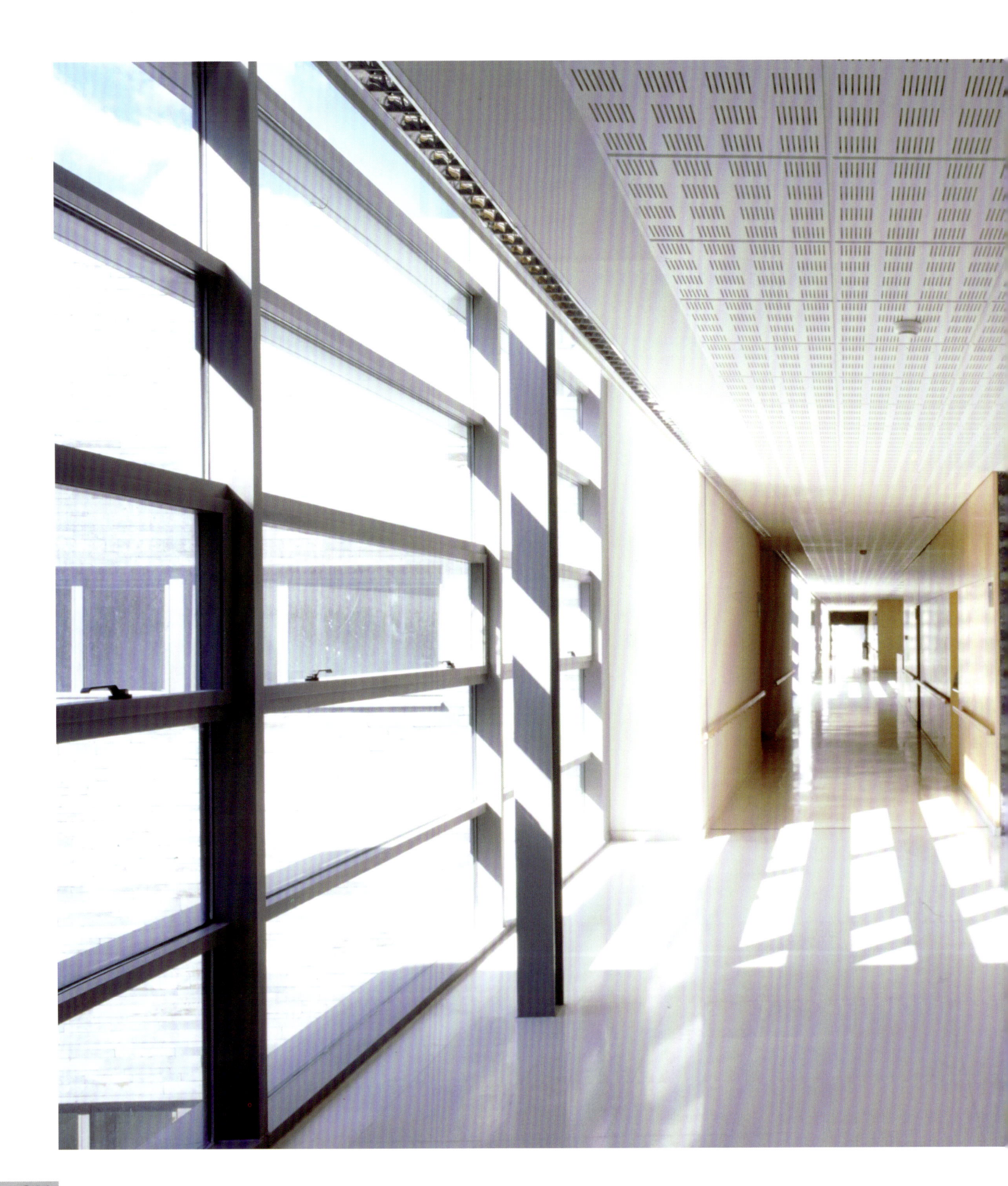

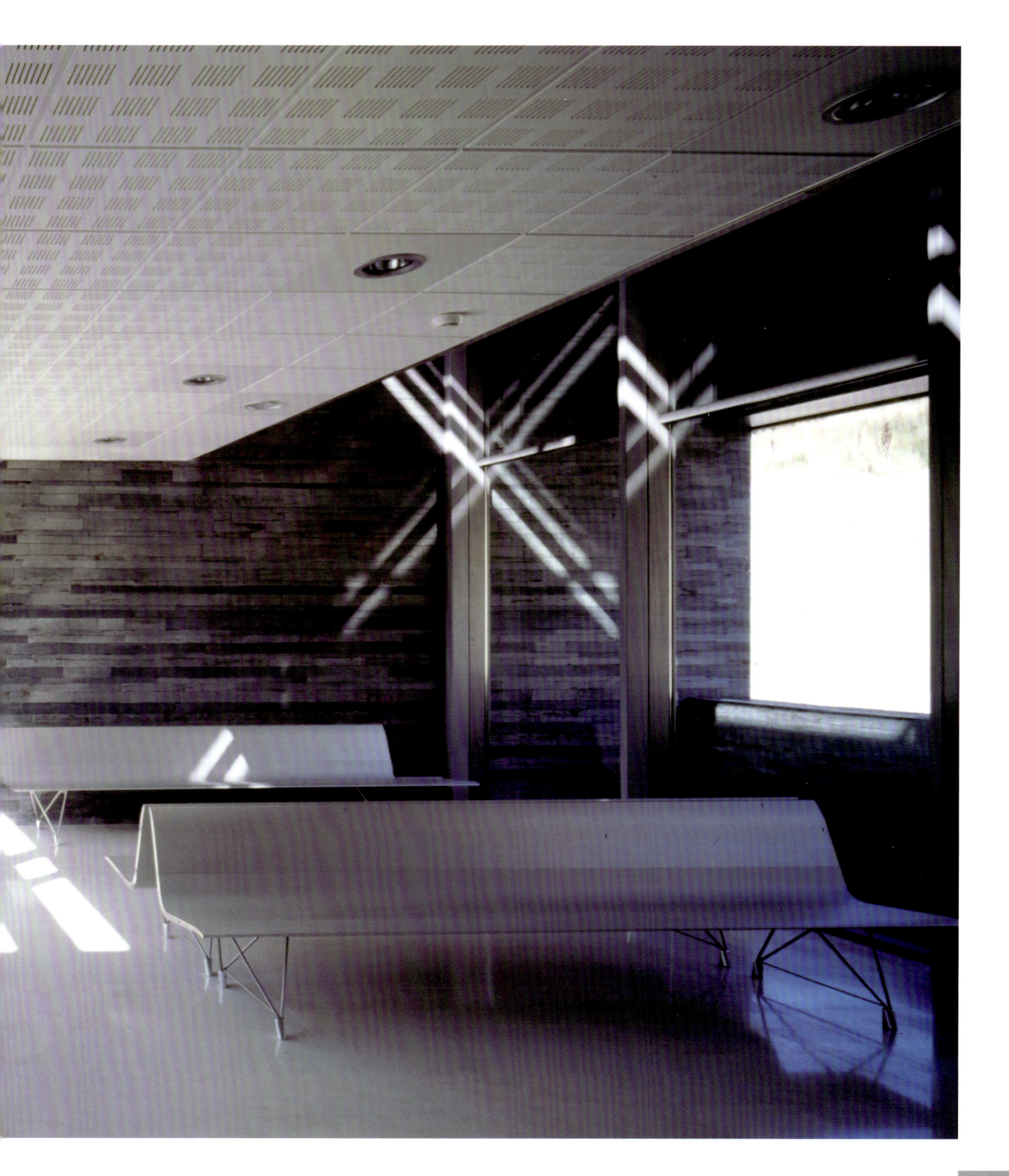

Rehabilitation block - Detail

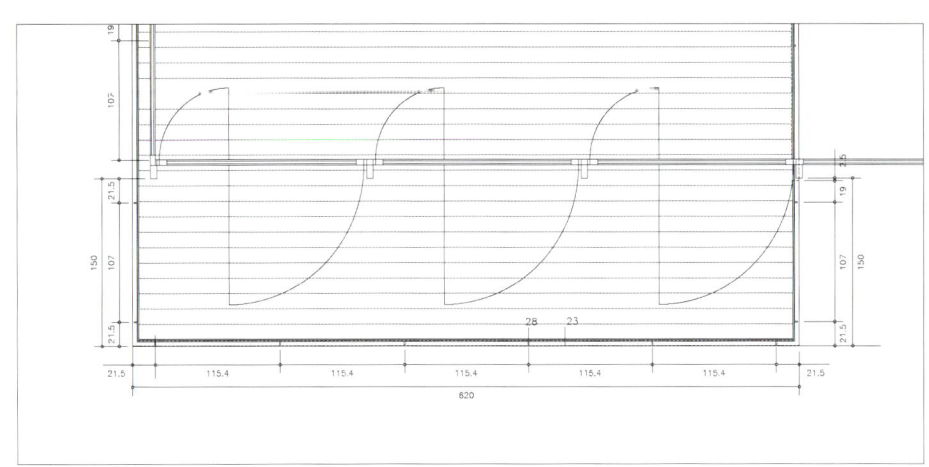

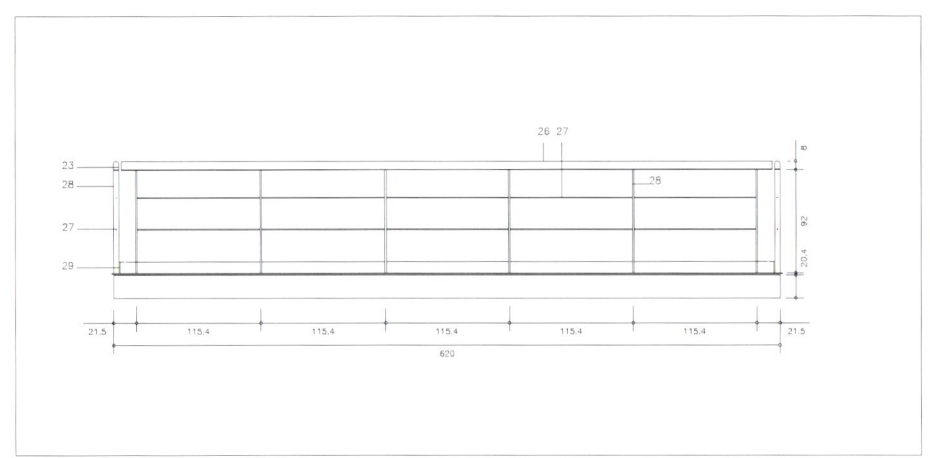

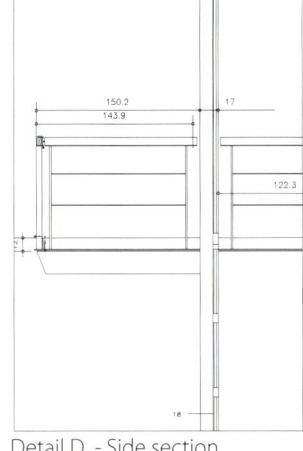

Detail D - Balcony

Detail D - Frontal facade

Detail D - Side section

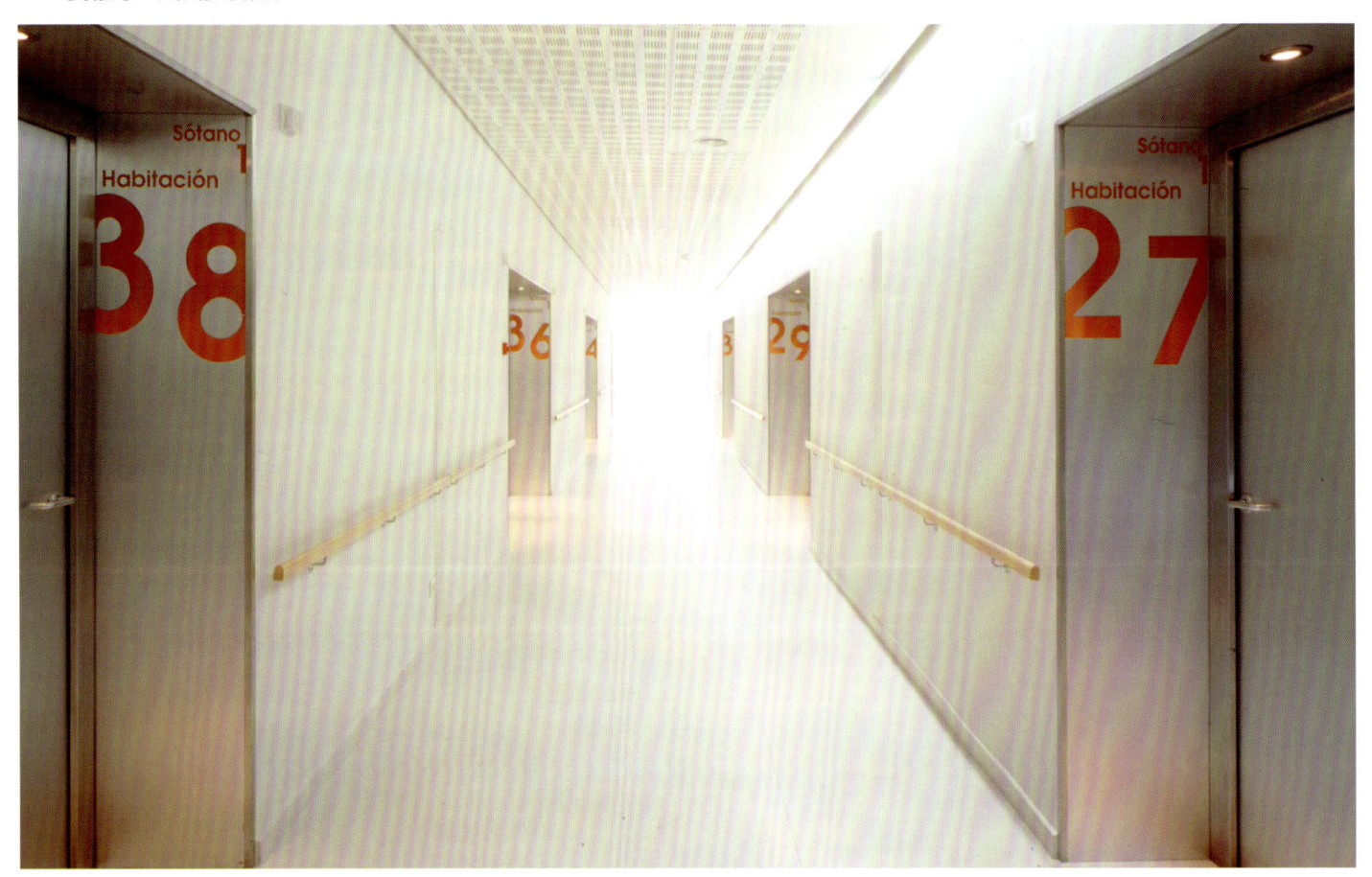

LIST OF MATERIALS

FLOORS
1. Terrazzo, micro-aggregate, white, 60x60 cm
1.2 Marble, white Tasso, 40 cm wide
   (=private bedroom bathroom)
2. Parquet, Listone Giordano
3. Gres tiles 10x10 cm.
4. Linoleum DL

CLADDING
5. Fairfaced concrete
6. Stratified panelling
7. Maple-wood
8. Tongue-and-groove maple-wood
9. Phenol-resin panelling
10. Gres tiles 10x10 cm
11. Stainless steel
12. Transparent glass
13. Mirror

CEILINGS
14. Suspended ceiling of Pladur
15a. Suspended ceiling of Luxalon 300c
15b. Suspended ceiling of maple-wood
16. Suspended ceiling of maple-wood
17. Suspended ceiling of stratified panelling

WINDOWS AND ENCLOSURES
18. Fixed Espalu carpentry
19. Sliding Espalu carpentry
20. Vertical and horizontal hinged Espalu carpentry
21. Pivoting Espalu carpentry
22. Hinged Espalu carpentry
23. Custom made railing of stainless steel and solid maple-wood
24. Fluorescent light
25. Maple-wood held by 10 mm clips
26. Skirting-board - turned linoleum from paved ramp
27. Turn-shackle tensor, stainless steel, diameter 7.5 mm
28. Vertical member, stainless steel, rectangular, 15x30x920 m
29. Trim, angle iron, stainless steel, 110x7 mm

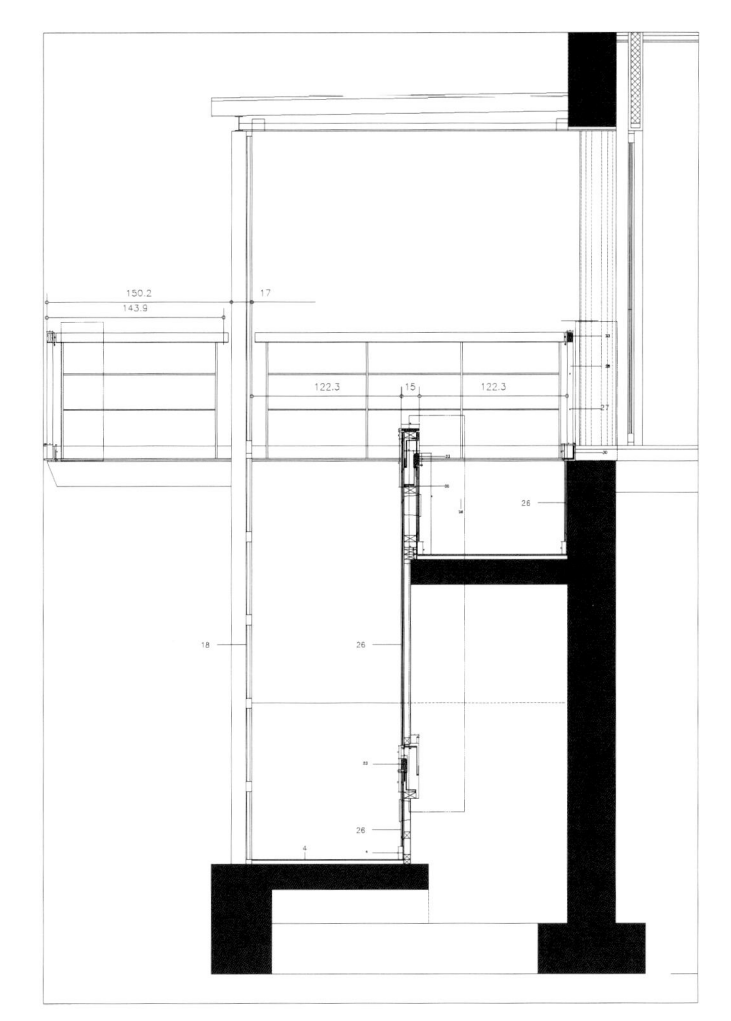

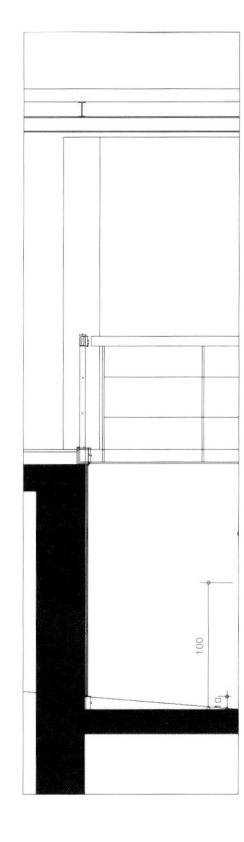

Section through ramp

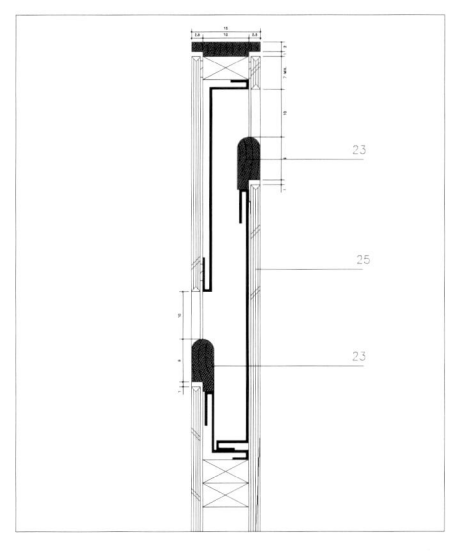

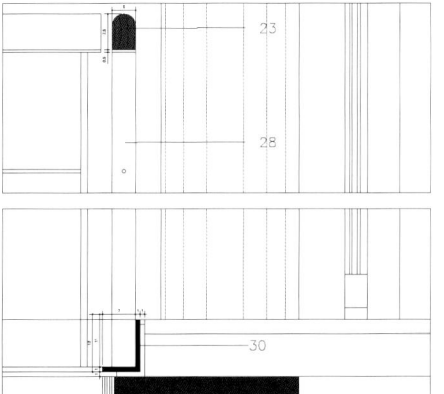

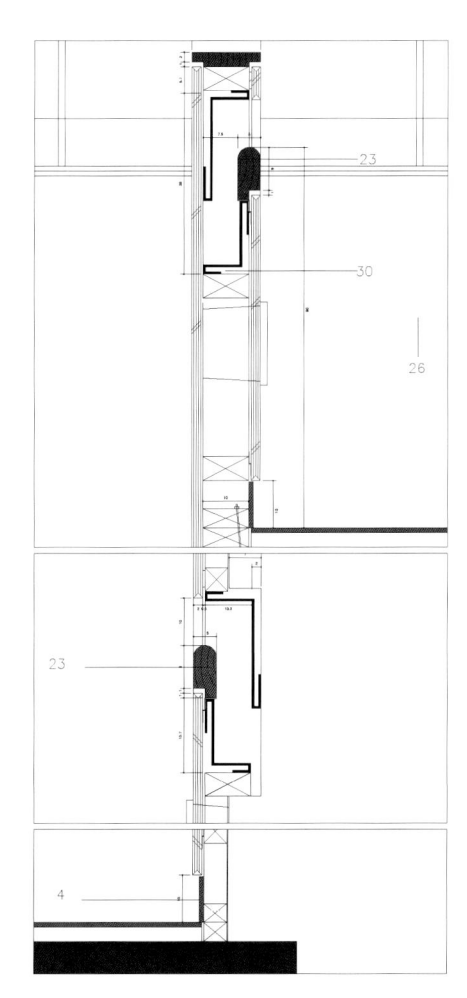

Rehabilitation block - Detail

Estudio Entresitio

CEDT Daimiel

Daimiel, Spain

Photographs: *Roland Halbe*

For an architect, a health program represents highly demanding work in terms of precision and organization of floorplans. The circulation of staff and patients alike needs to be very carefully considered to avoid crossovers and minimize movement. In order to be able to achieve this, the architect needs to have a keen understanding of the processes that take place there. This hospital carried out by Madrid-based studio estudio.entresitio demonstrates this understanding, creating an environment which is user-friendly for patients and staff, while at the same time generating an atmosphere of calm and tranquility, which is so important in buildings of this nature.

The CEDT in Daimiel resolves the program for outpatients and emergencies on the ground floor, since this is the area where the flow of people is at its densest. The same functional scheme of parallel corridors has been repeated on the top floor to house the specialist consulting rooms, residence for health workers and surgery block.

Externally the project attempts to resolve the image of a building destined to public use located on the perimeter of a residential area. This is done through a metallic cladding of galvanized microperforated sheets, which allows the building to be scaled down and presents a texturized volume. This finish is able to protect the interiors from being seen by nearby buildings and improves the insulating qualities, thereby lessening the need for energy consumption, through either air-conditioning in summer or heating in winter. Splashes of red enliven the façade and give the whole space a friendlier and more welcoming feel.

Inside, the building opens to five courtyards clad in corrugated sheet metal, around which on one side are the consulting rooms and on the other the circulation and waiting rooms. The use of glazed panes in these areas allows them to enjoy optimal conditions in terms of ventilation and lighting.

The building's profile seems to be interwoven like a patchwork quilt thanks to the incorporation of the volumes of the installation rooms, which align with the floorplan of the façade, and the spaces produced by the different accesses and the roof terrace. In the same way, the corner access points fold up allowing for the enlargement of the walkways, which become urban hallways in the areas where traffic is heaviest, blurring the building's perimeter.

The interiors are resolved with white materials, taking care to precisely adapt the finishes to the different uses. Thus the wall finishes are stone, phenolic panels, glass or plaster, and the ceilings absorb the acoustics, which together with the natural cork floor guarantee low sound levels in order to achieve greater interior comfort.

Architecture:
María Hurtado de Mendoza Wahrolén,
César Jiménez de Tejada Benavides,
José María Hurtado de Mendoza Wahrolén
Client:
SESCAM
Start Date:
2004
End Date:
2007
Team:
Carolina Leveroni, Jorge Martínez Martín, Verena Ruhm, Raquel, Fernández Antoñanzas, Vidal Fernández Díez, Cristina Fidalgo García, Vincent Rodriguez, Fabrice Quemeneur, Filipe Minderico, Laura Sánchez Carrasco, Irene de la Cruz García
Structural Engineer:
Geasyt
Quantity Surveyors:
Juan Carlos Corona Ruiz
Santiago Hernán Martín
Graphic Design:
Diego Hurtado de Mendoza

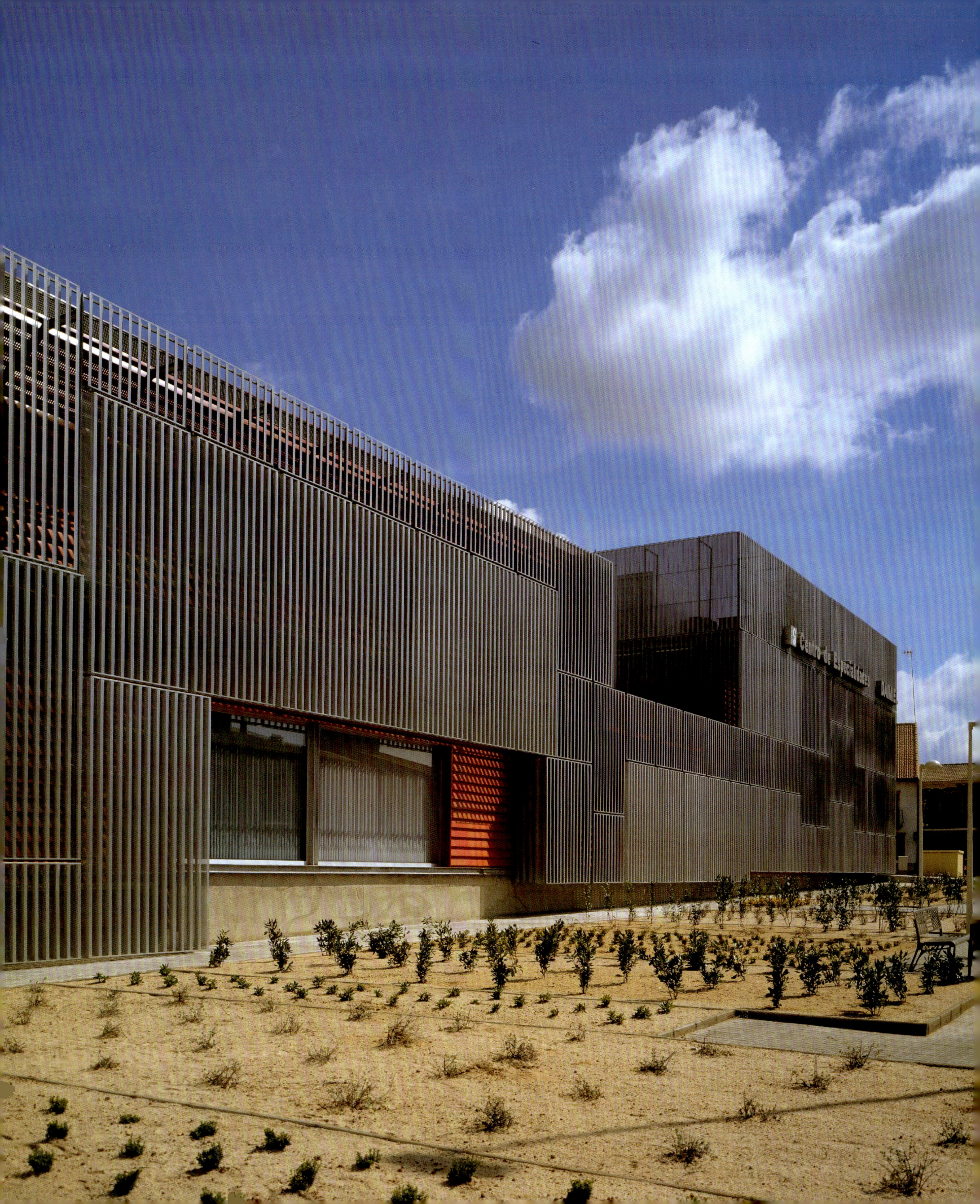
Centro de Especialidades

Site plan

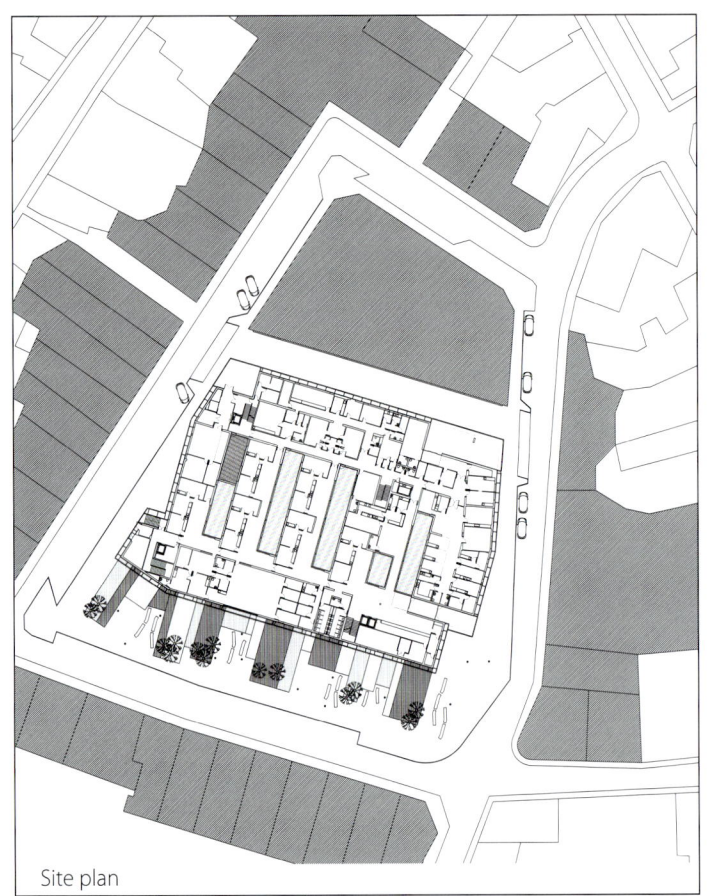

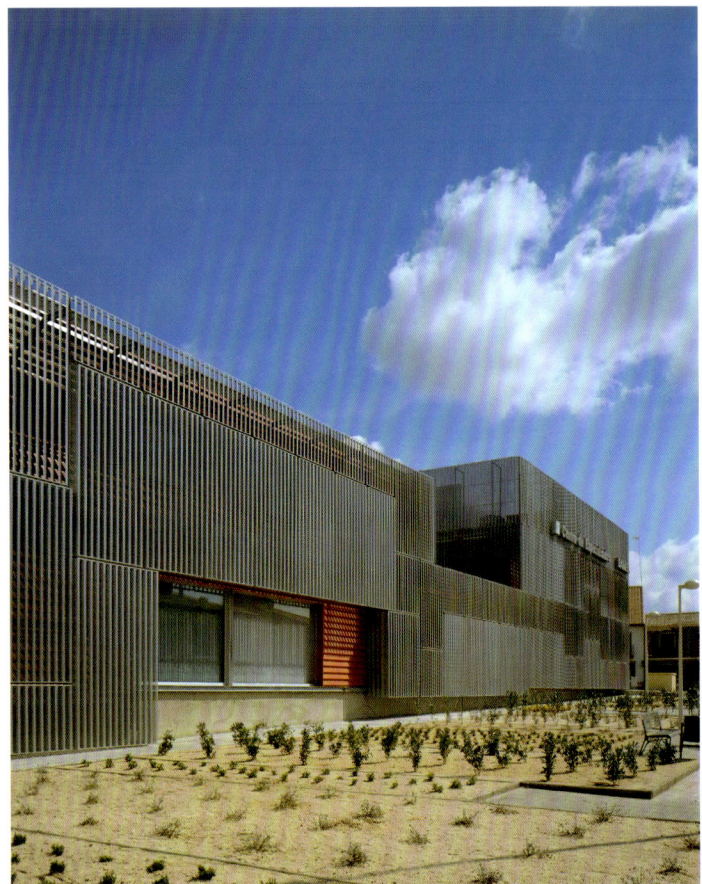

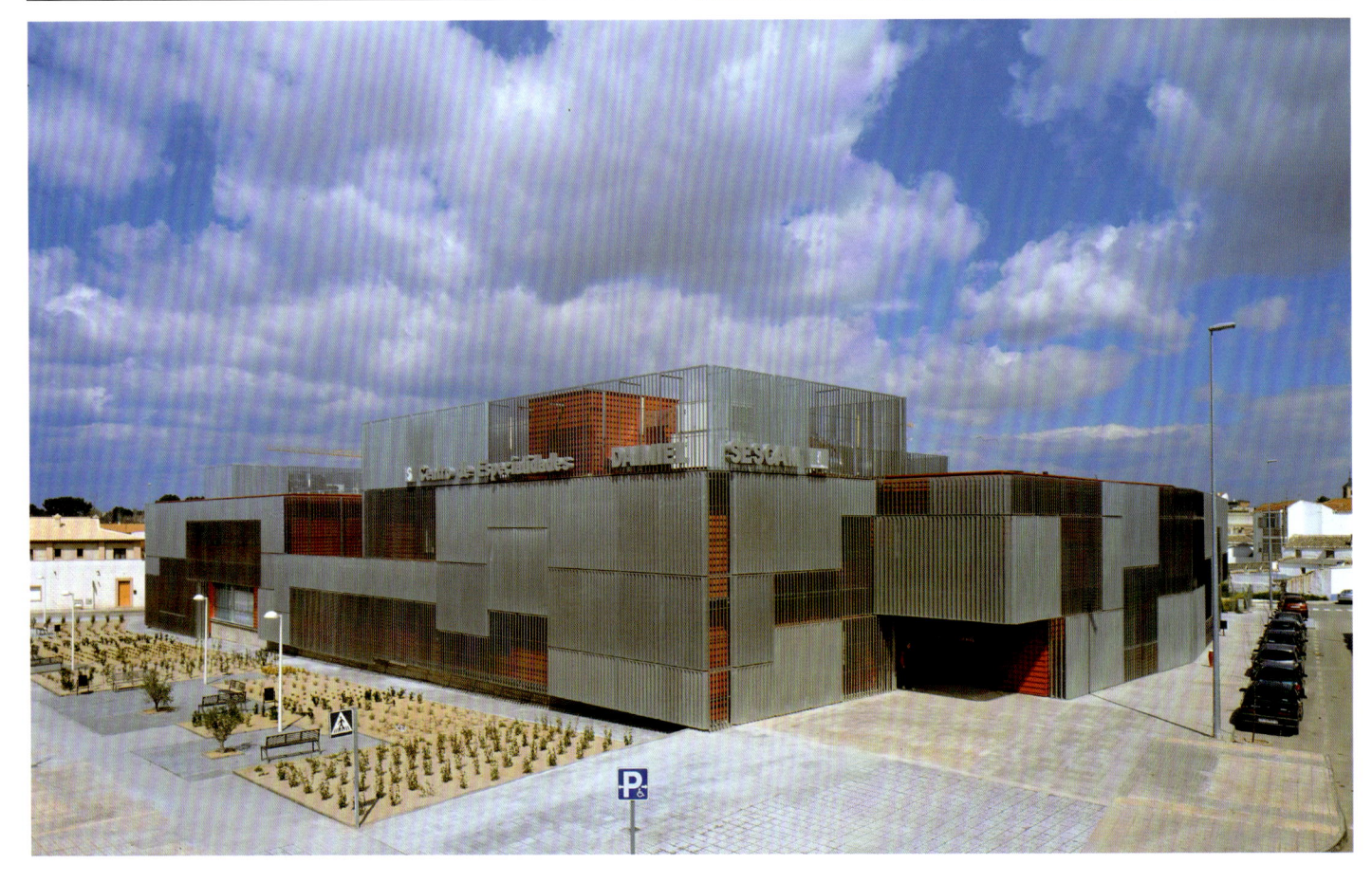

223

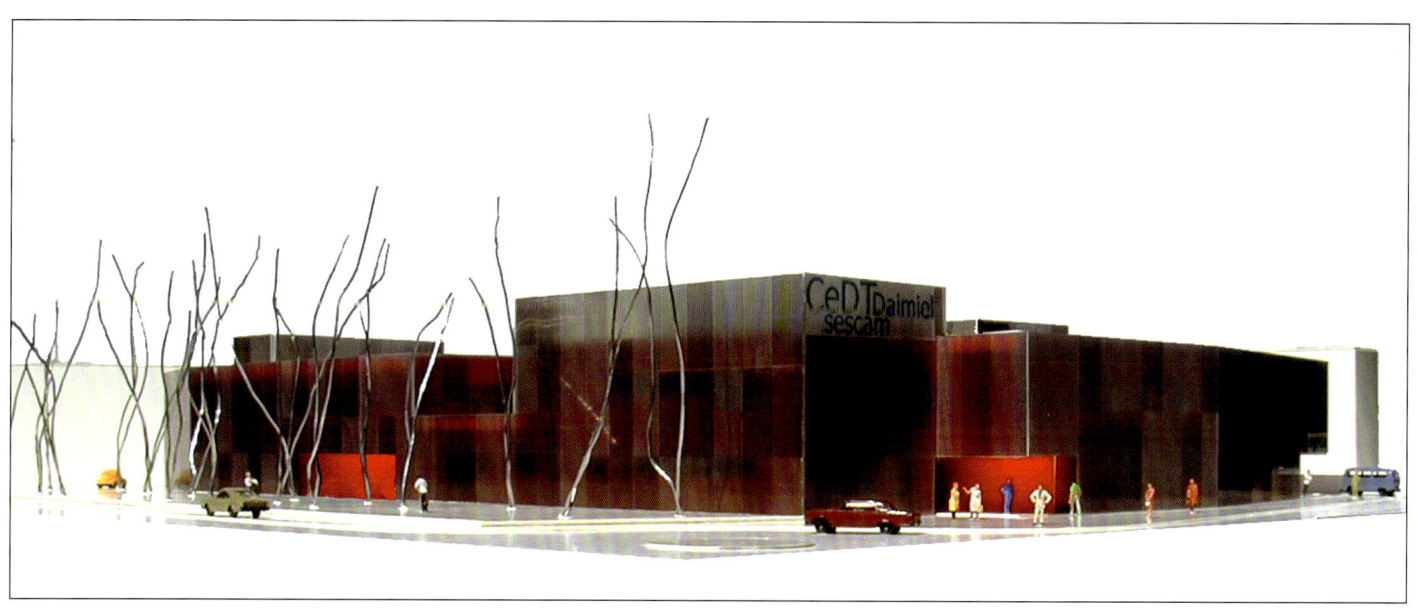

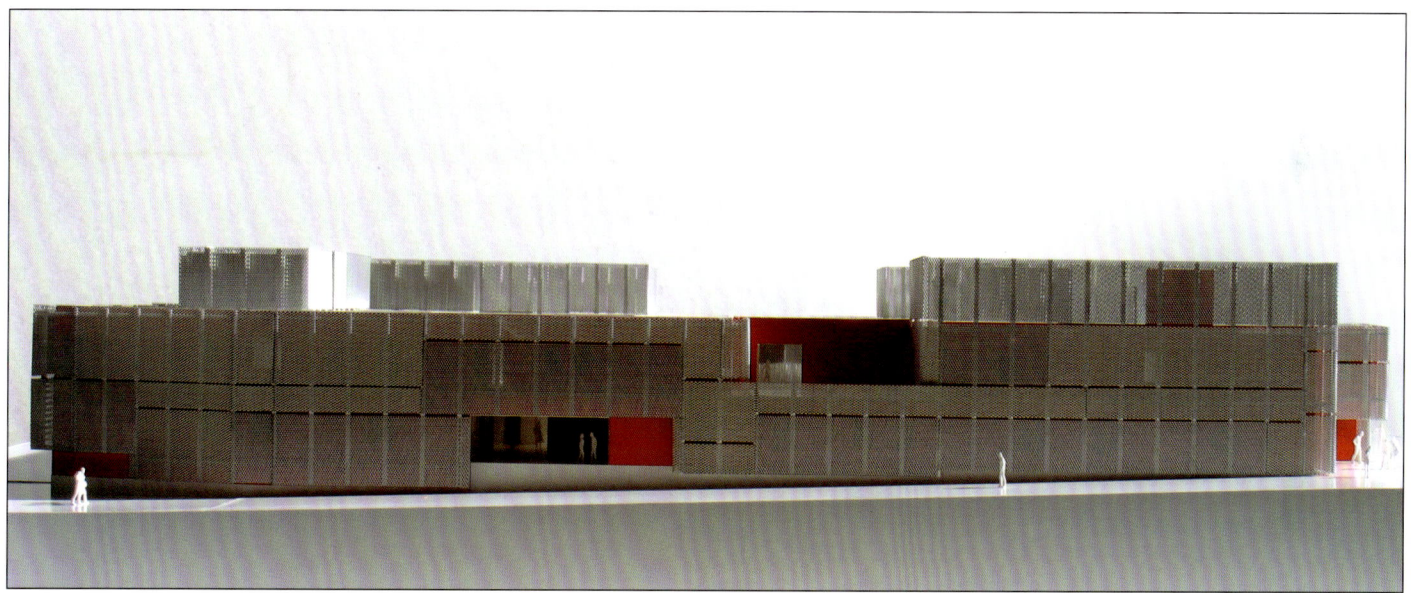

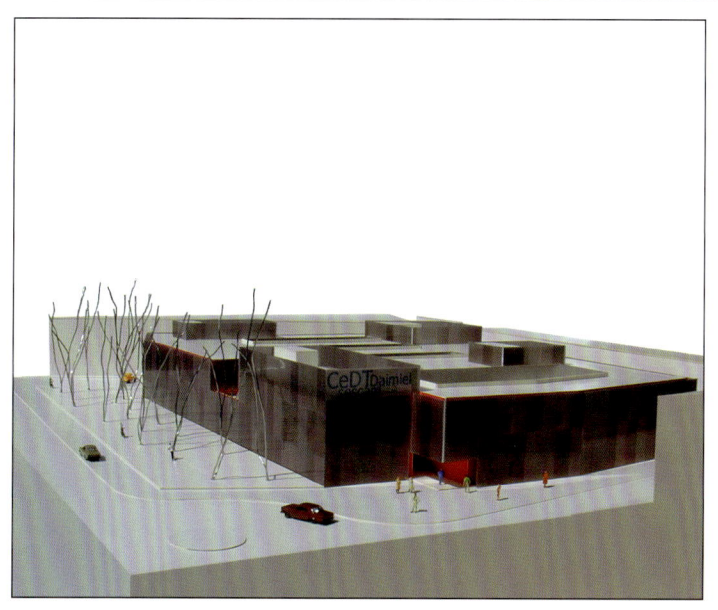

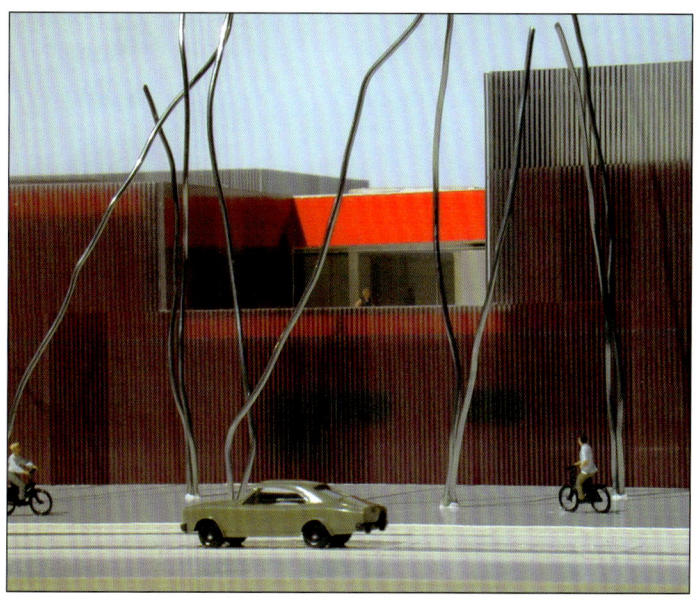

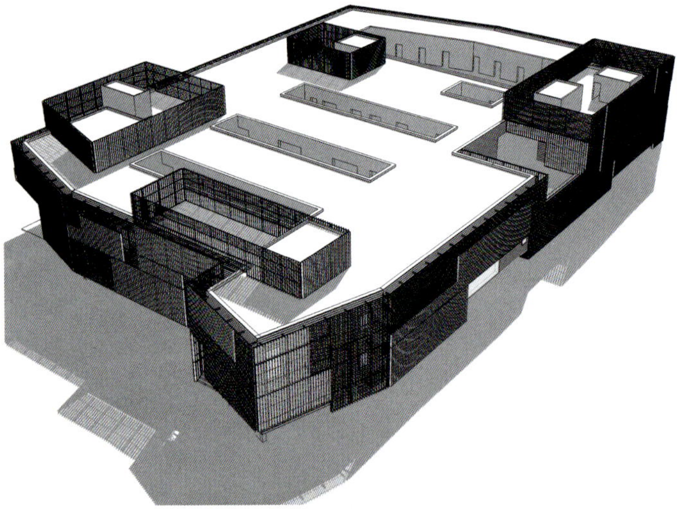

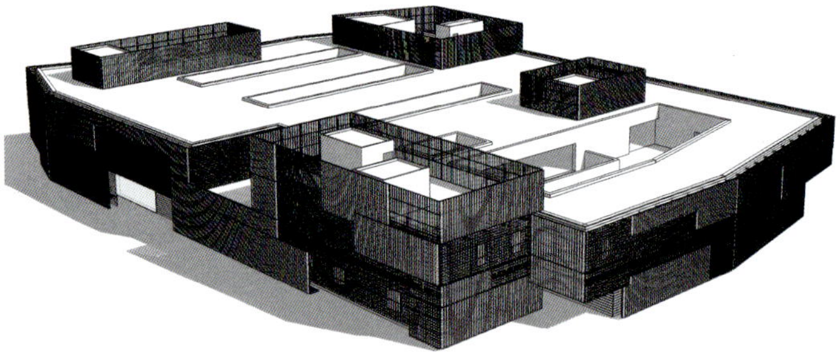

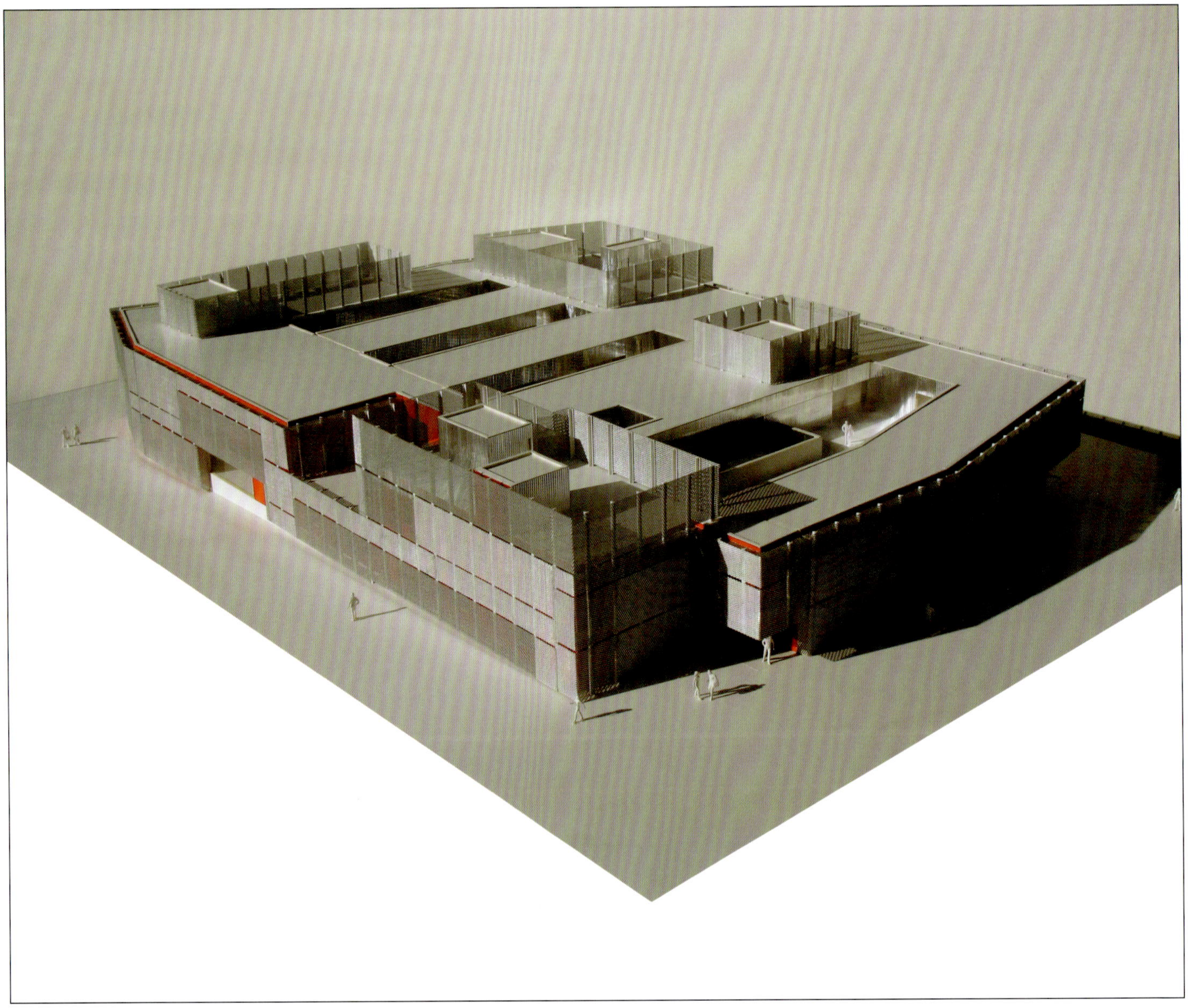

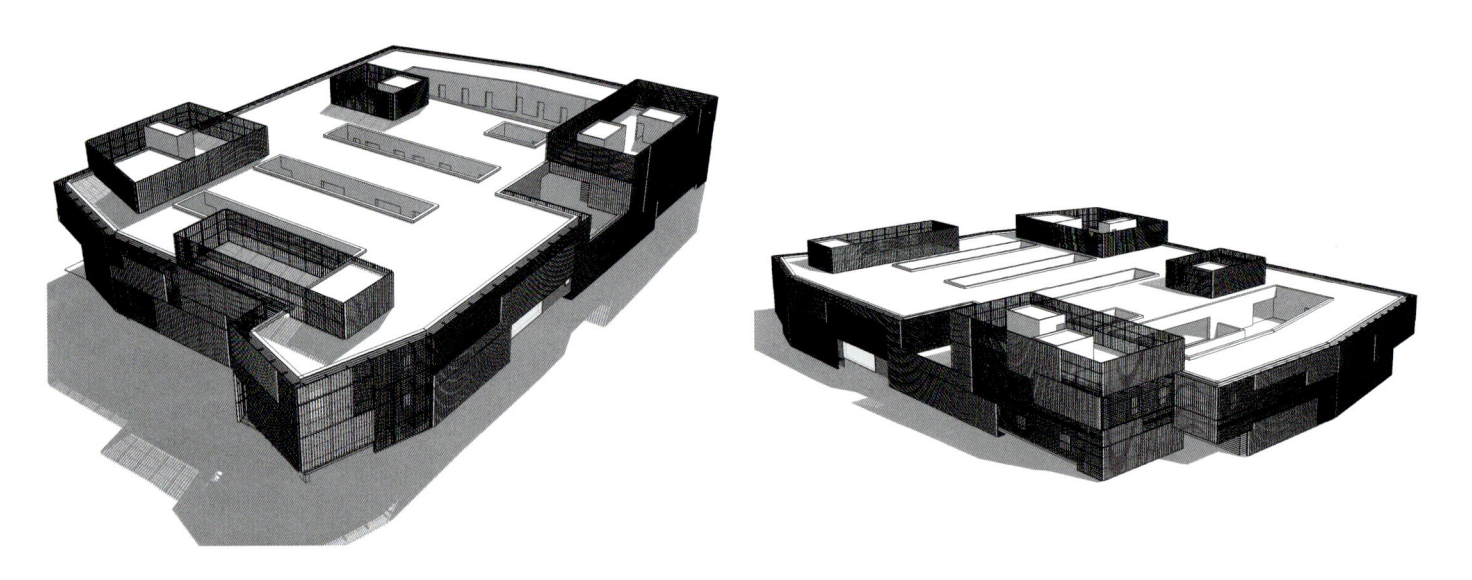

225

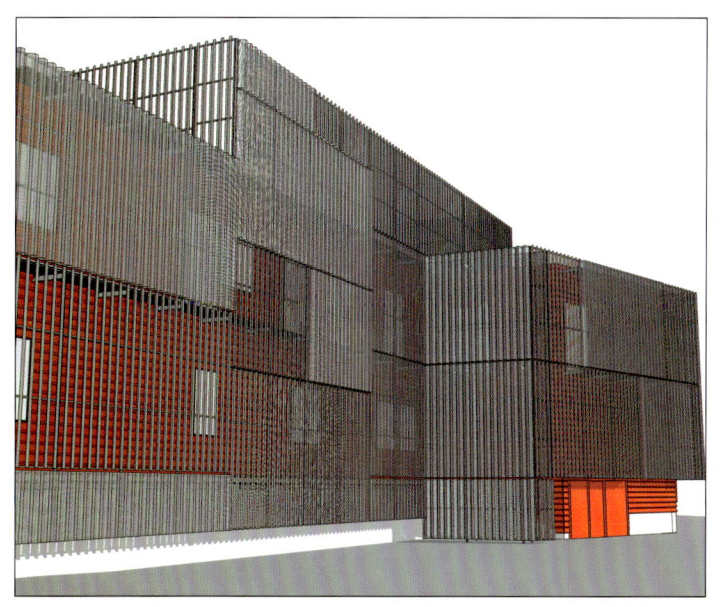

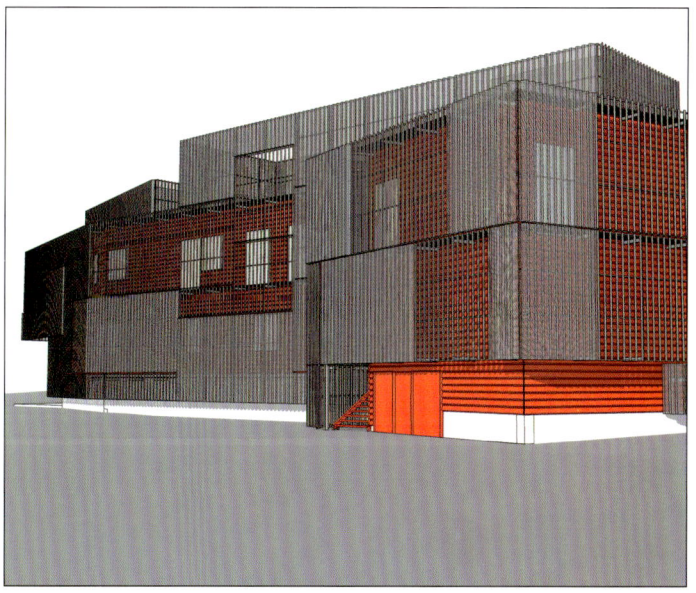

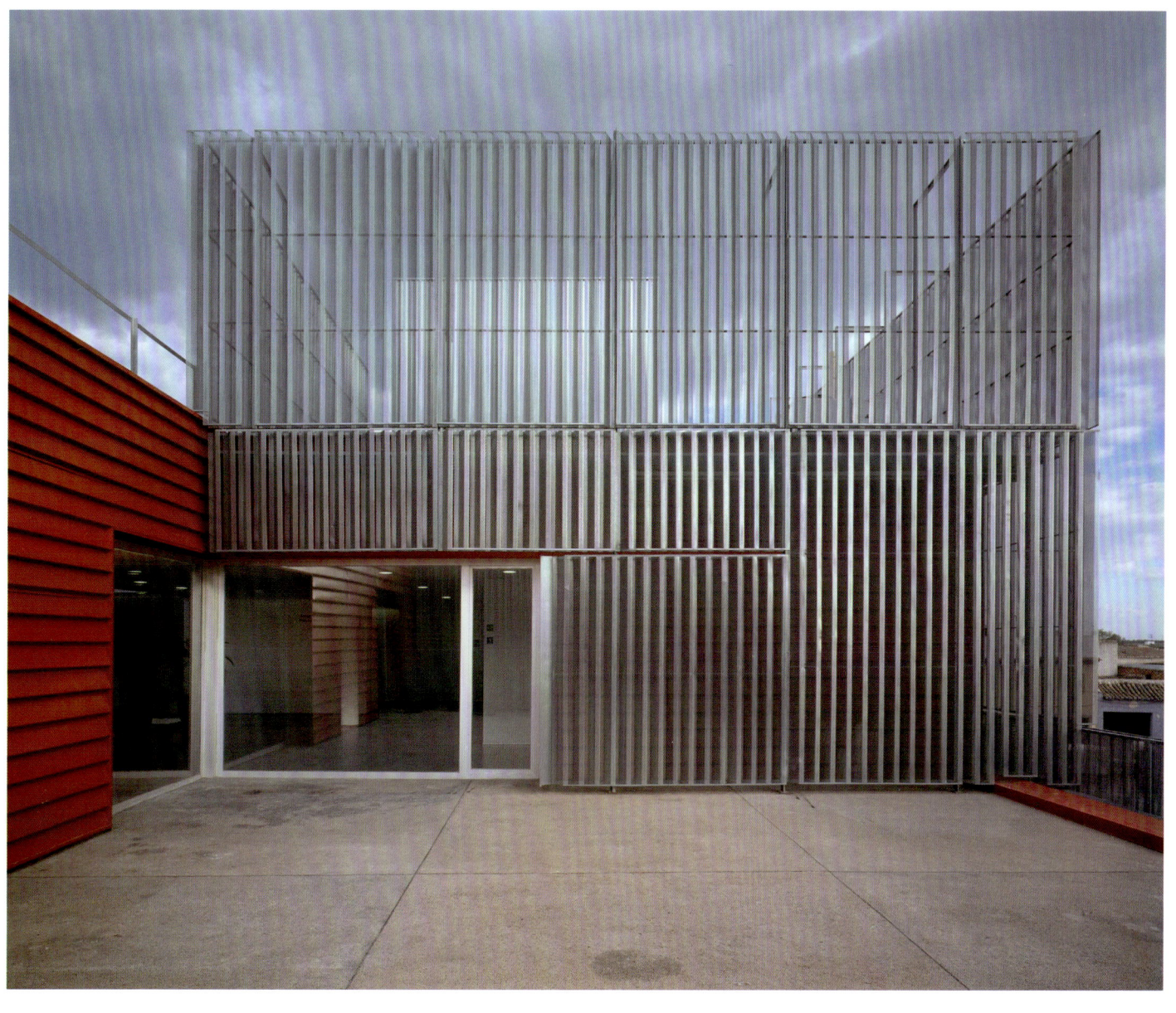

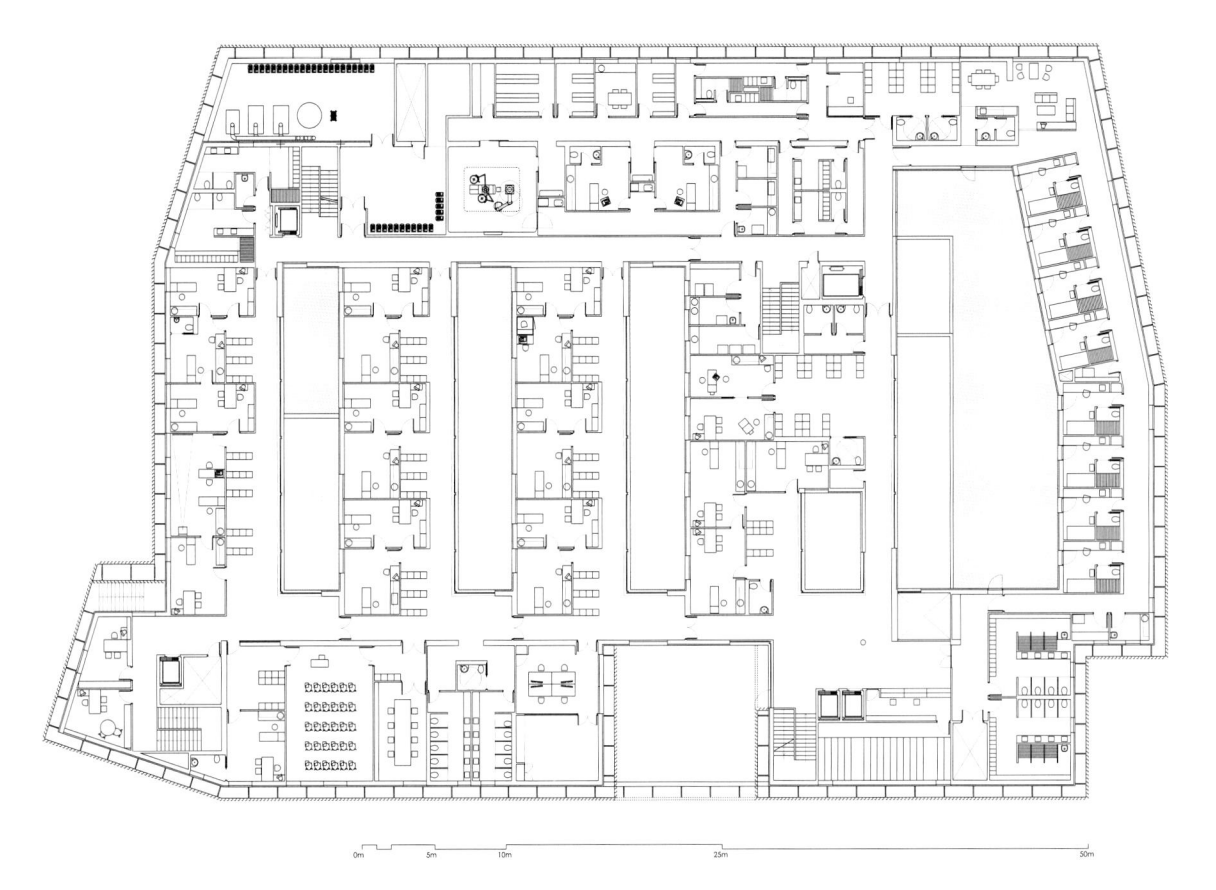

Second floor plan

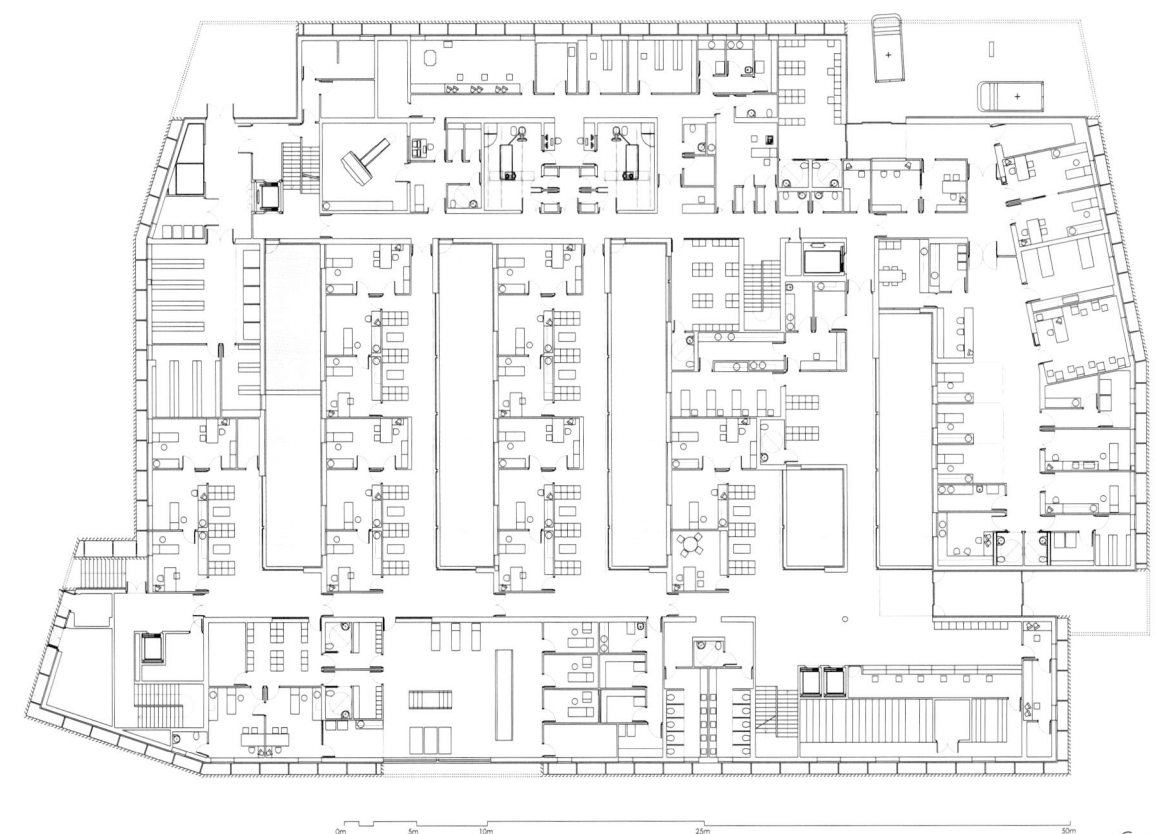

Ground Floor Plan

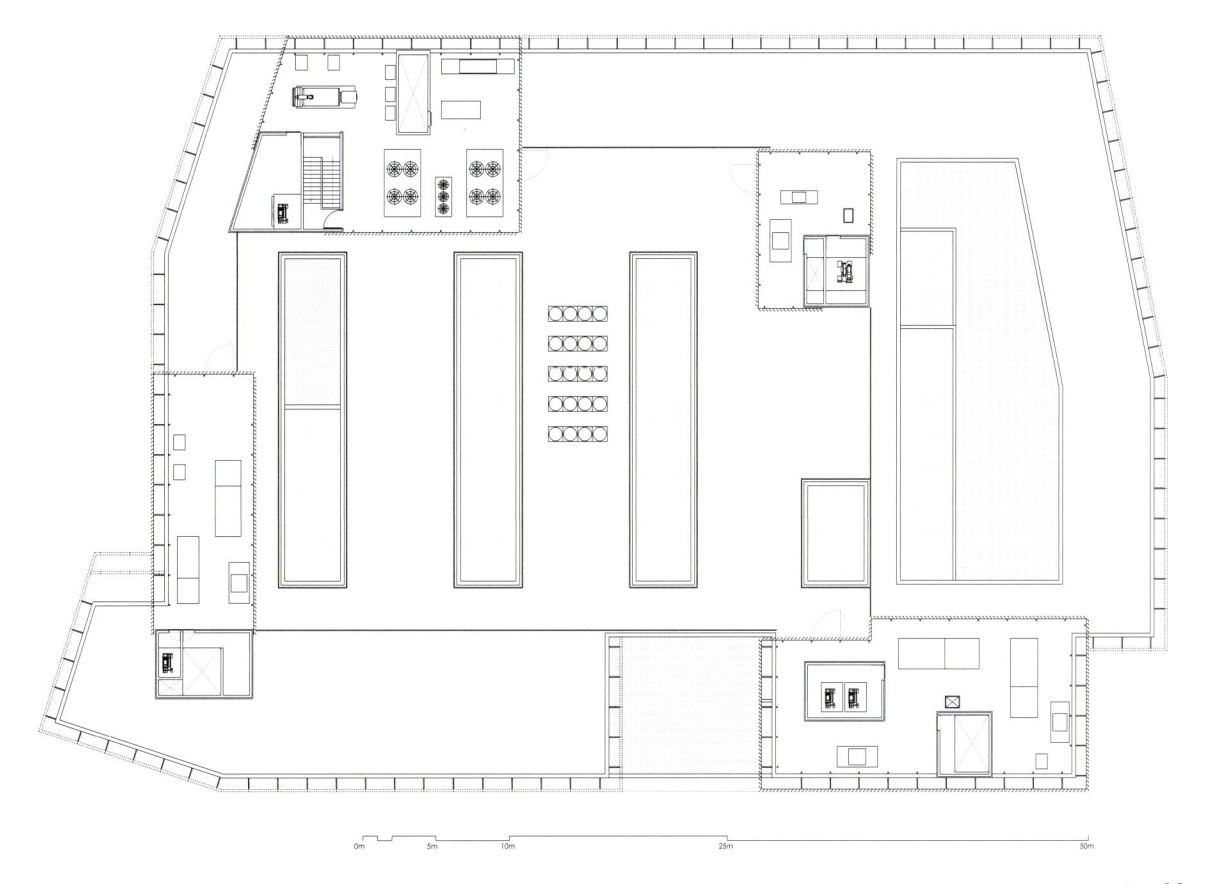

Roof floor plan

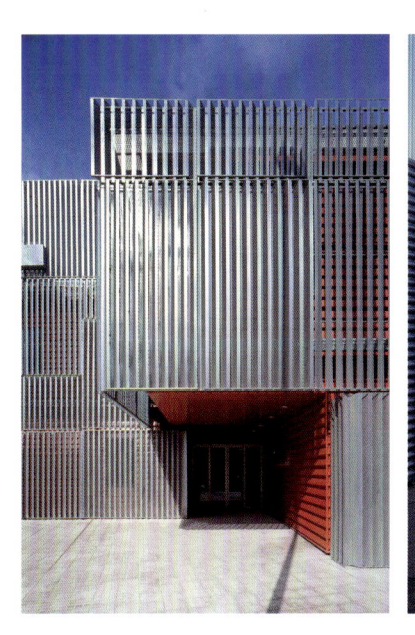

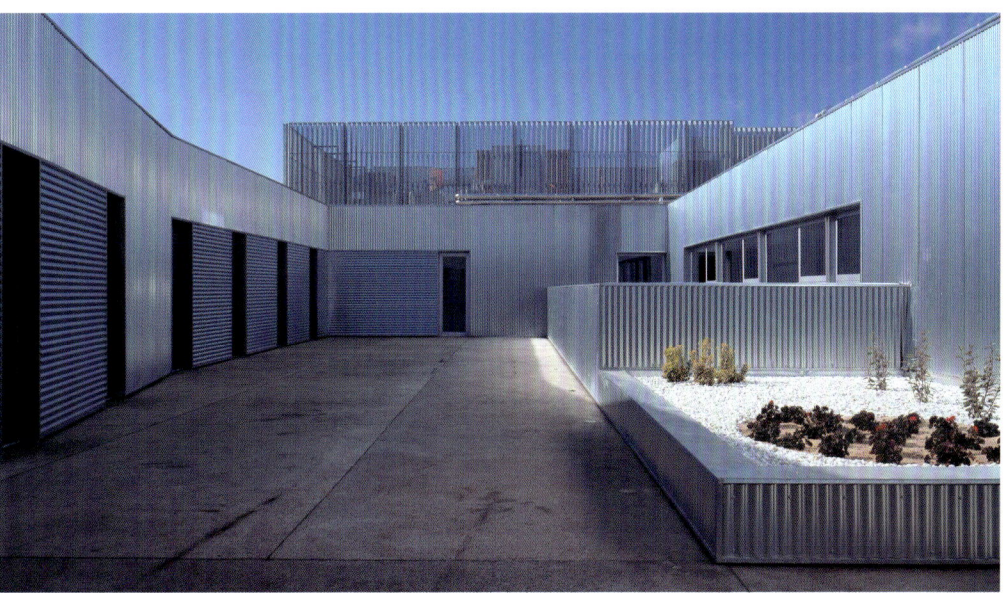

Longitudinal section 1

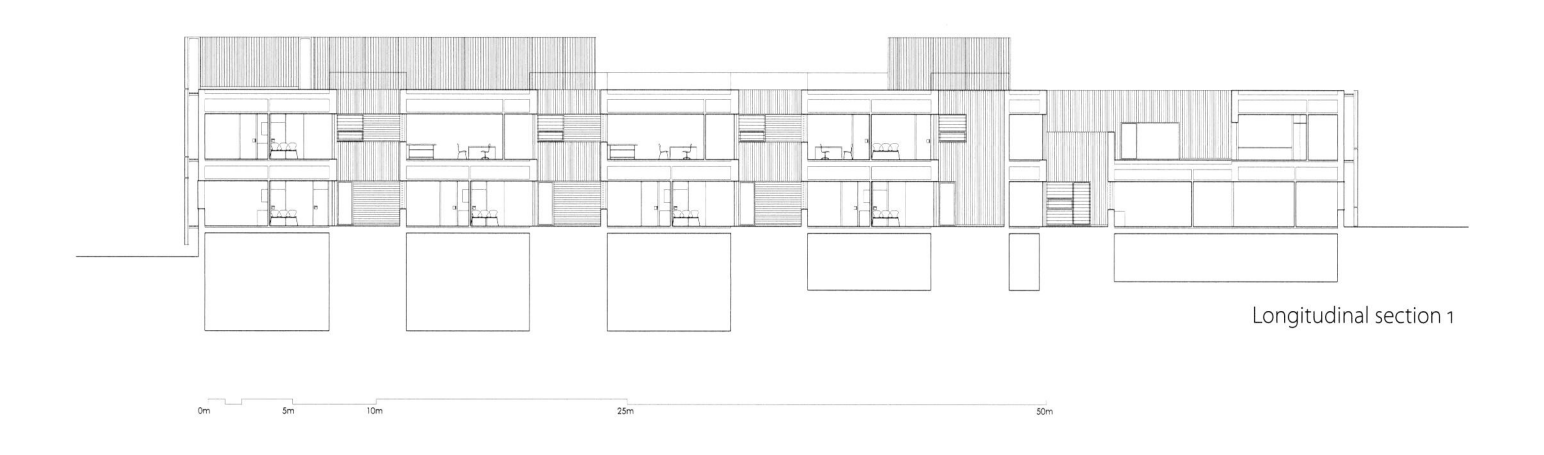

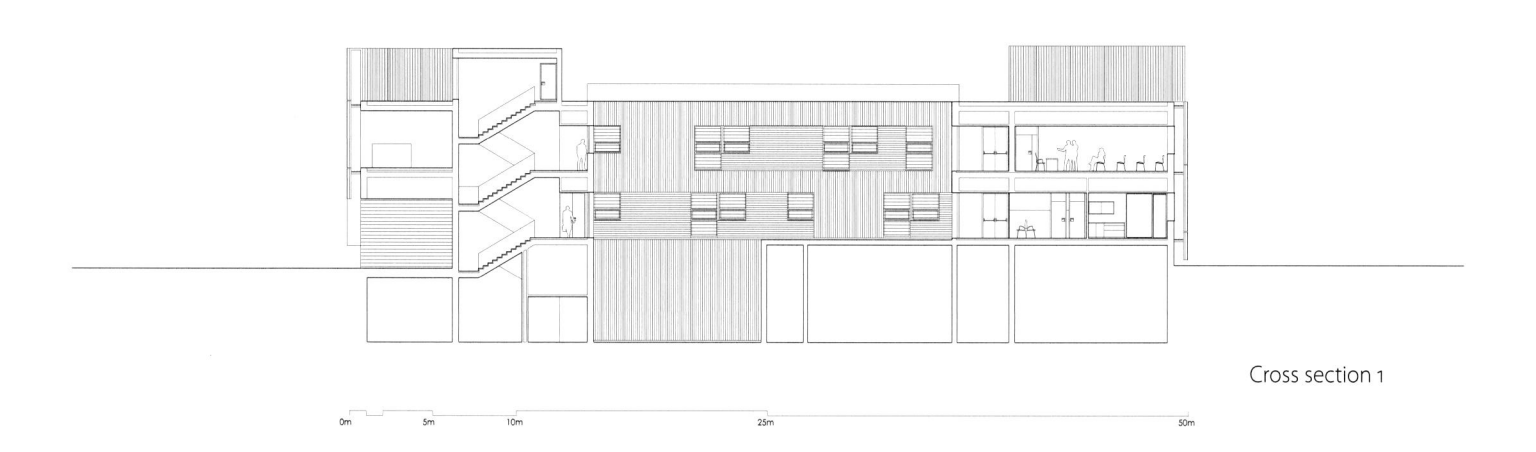

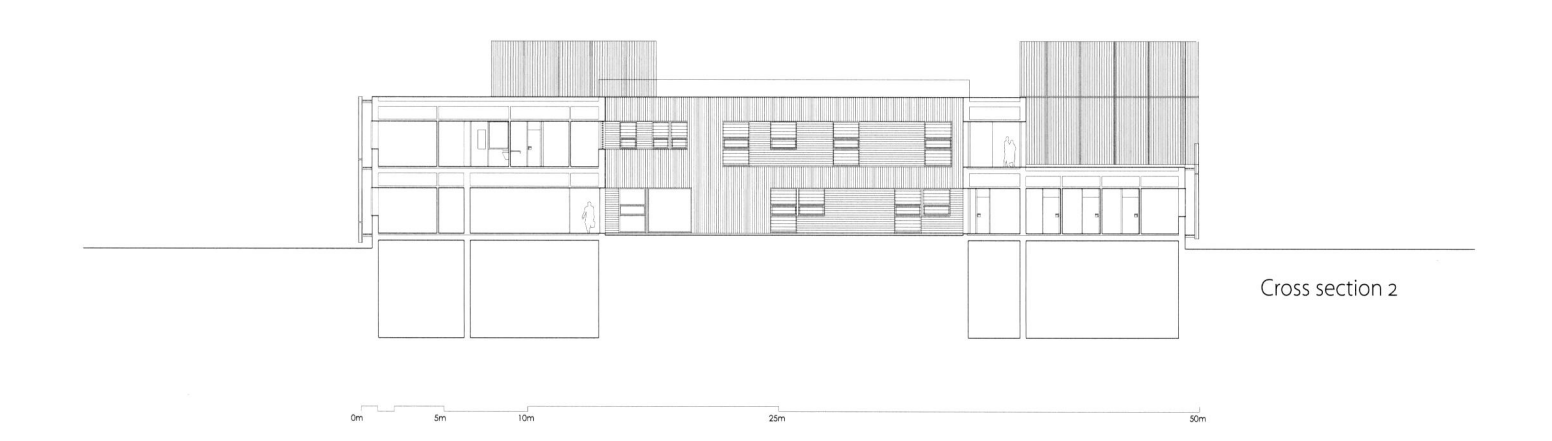

Cross section 1

Cross section 2

Longitudinal section 2

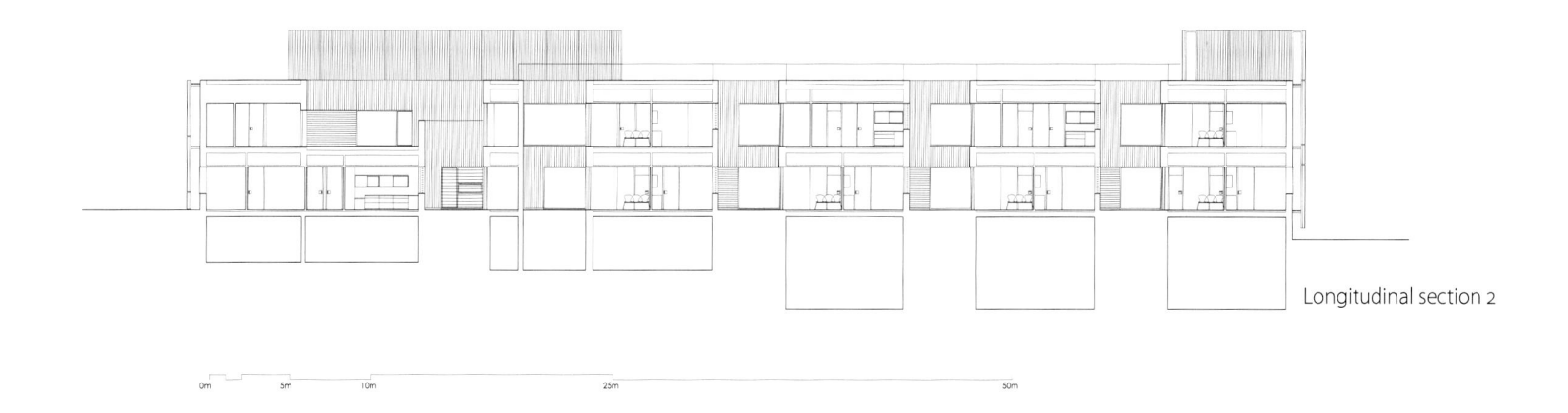

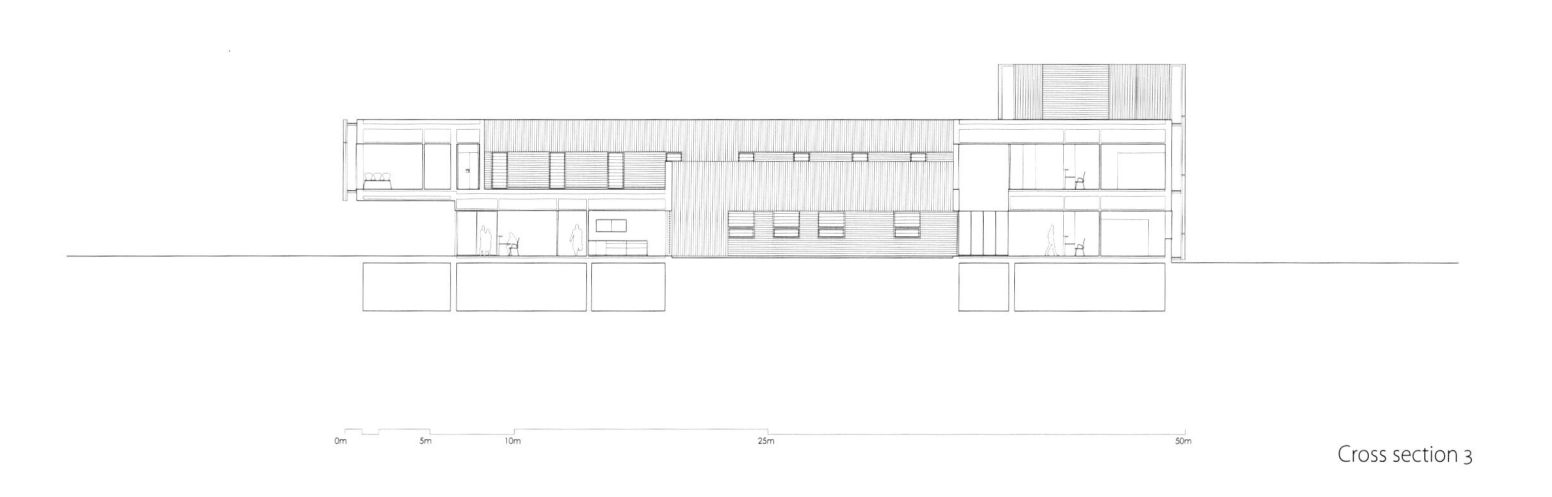

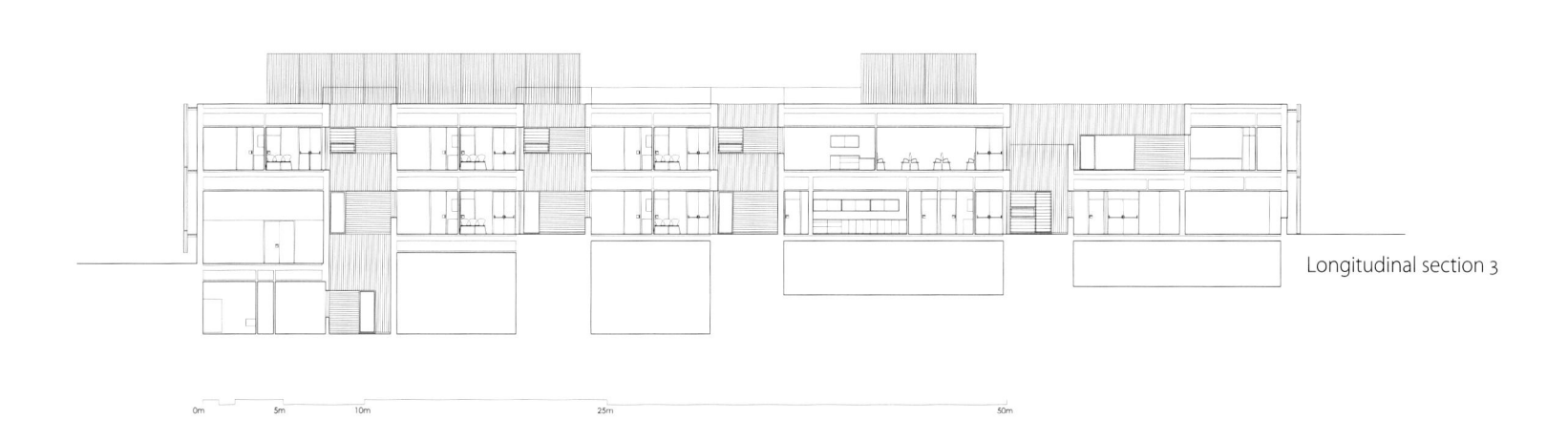

Cross section 3

Longitudinal section 3

Cross section 4

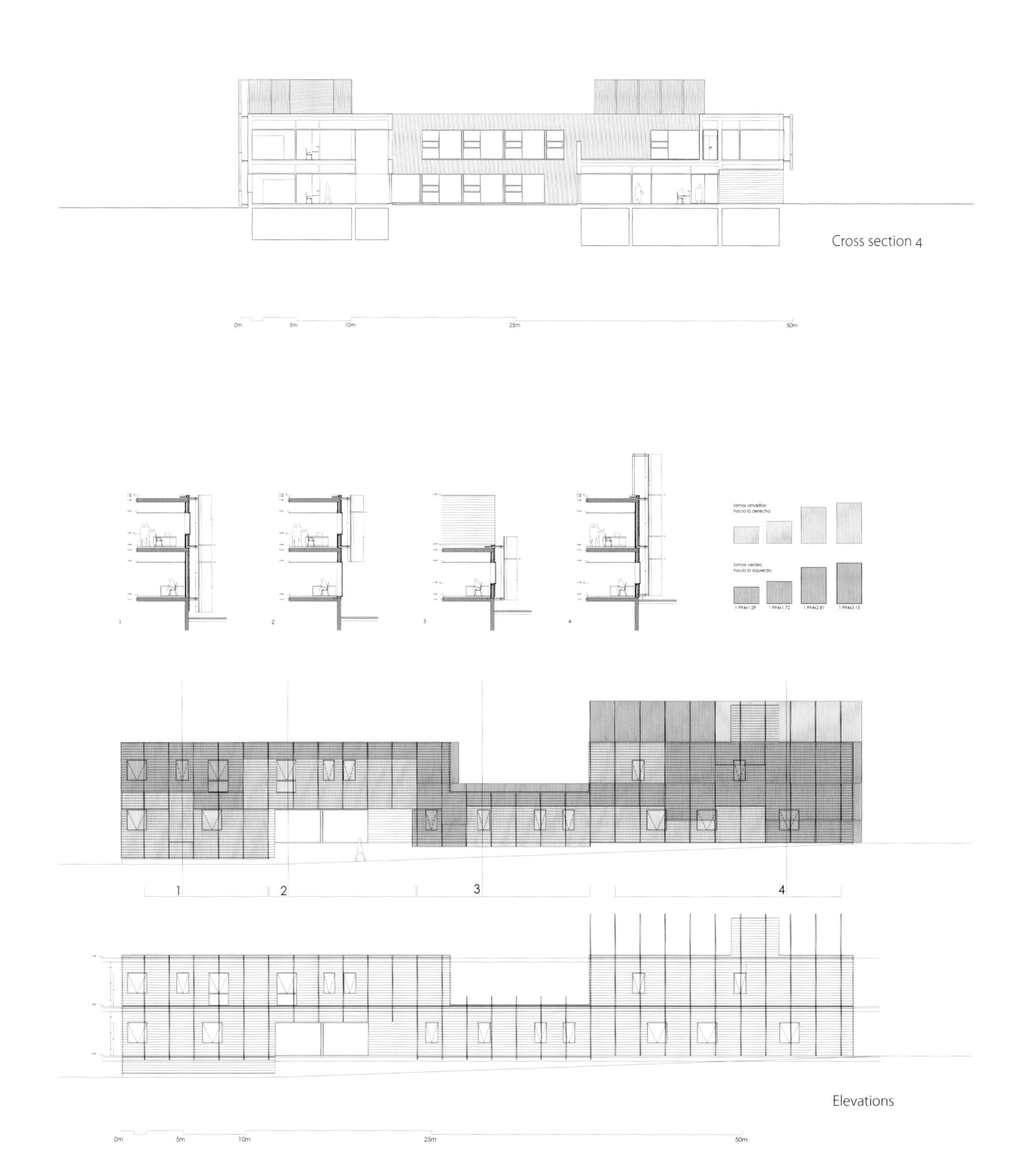

Elevations

230

Longitudinal section 4

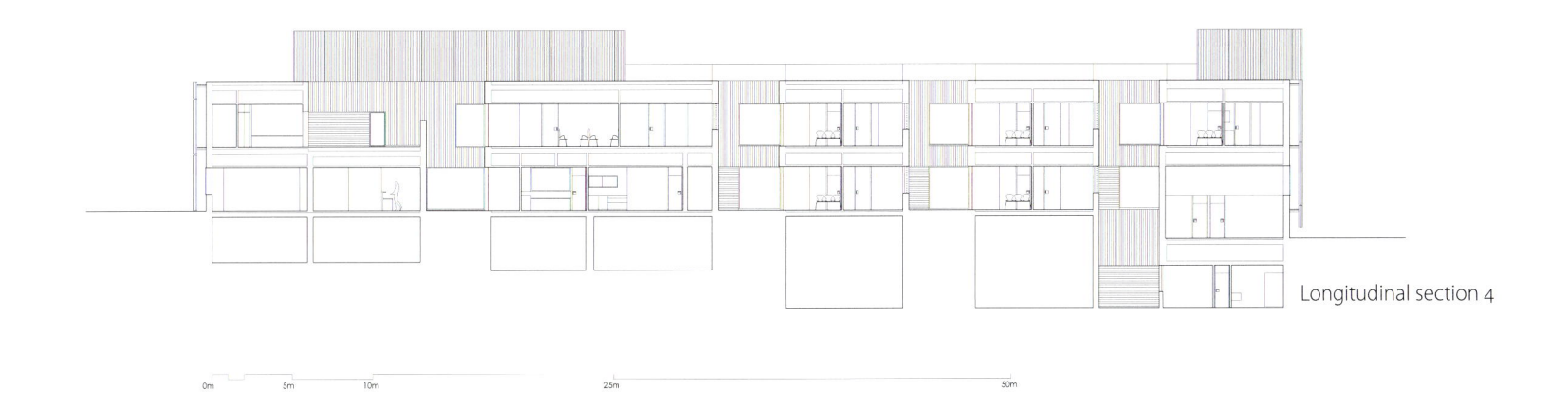

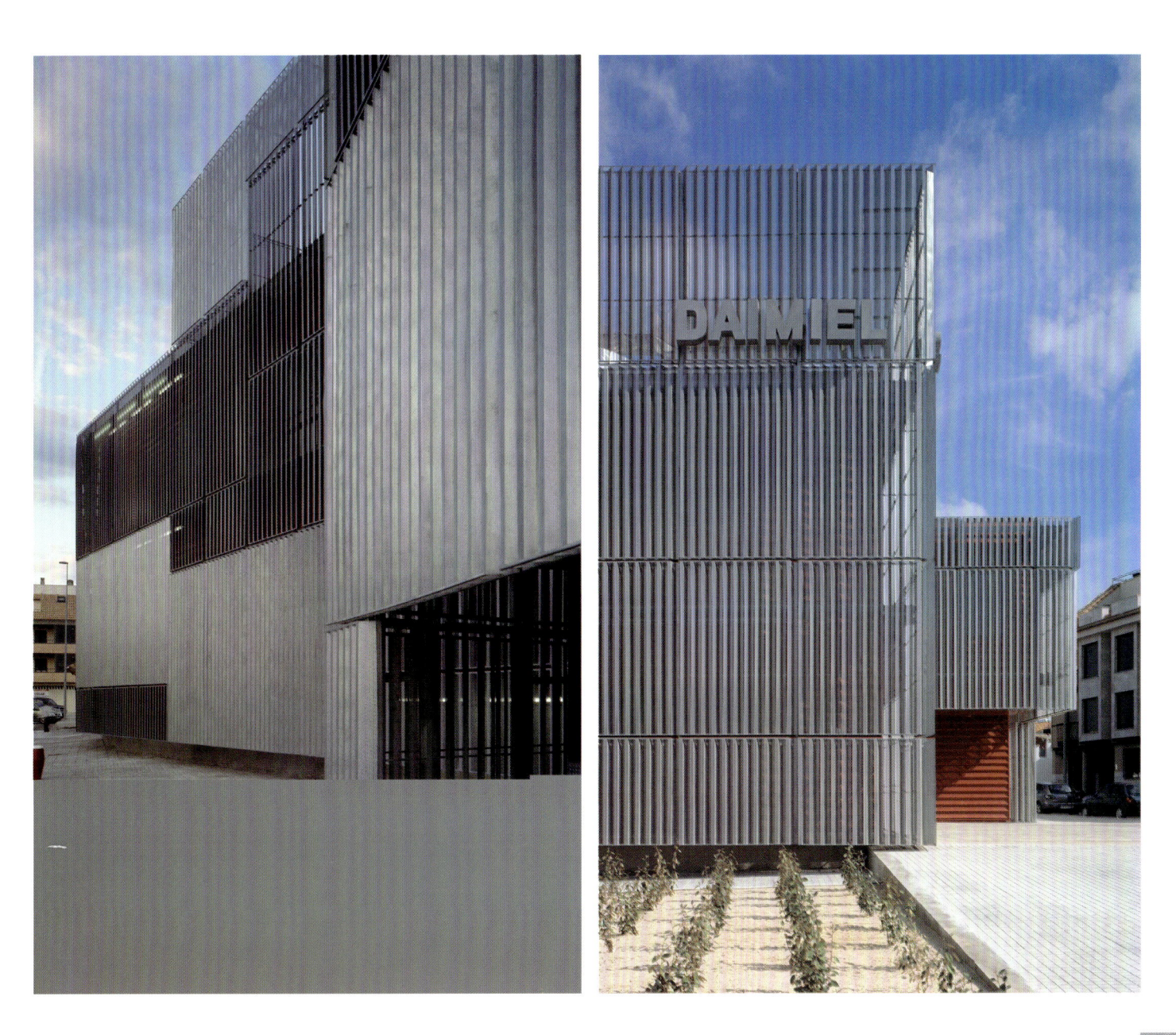

+7,83
+7,58
+7,28

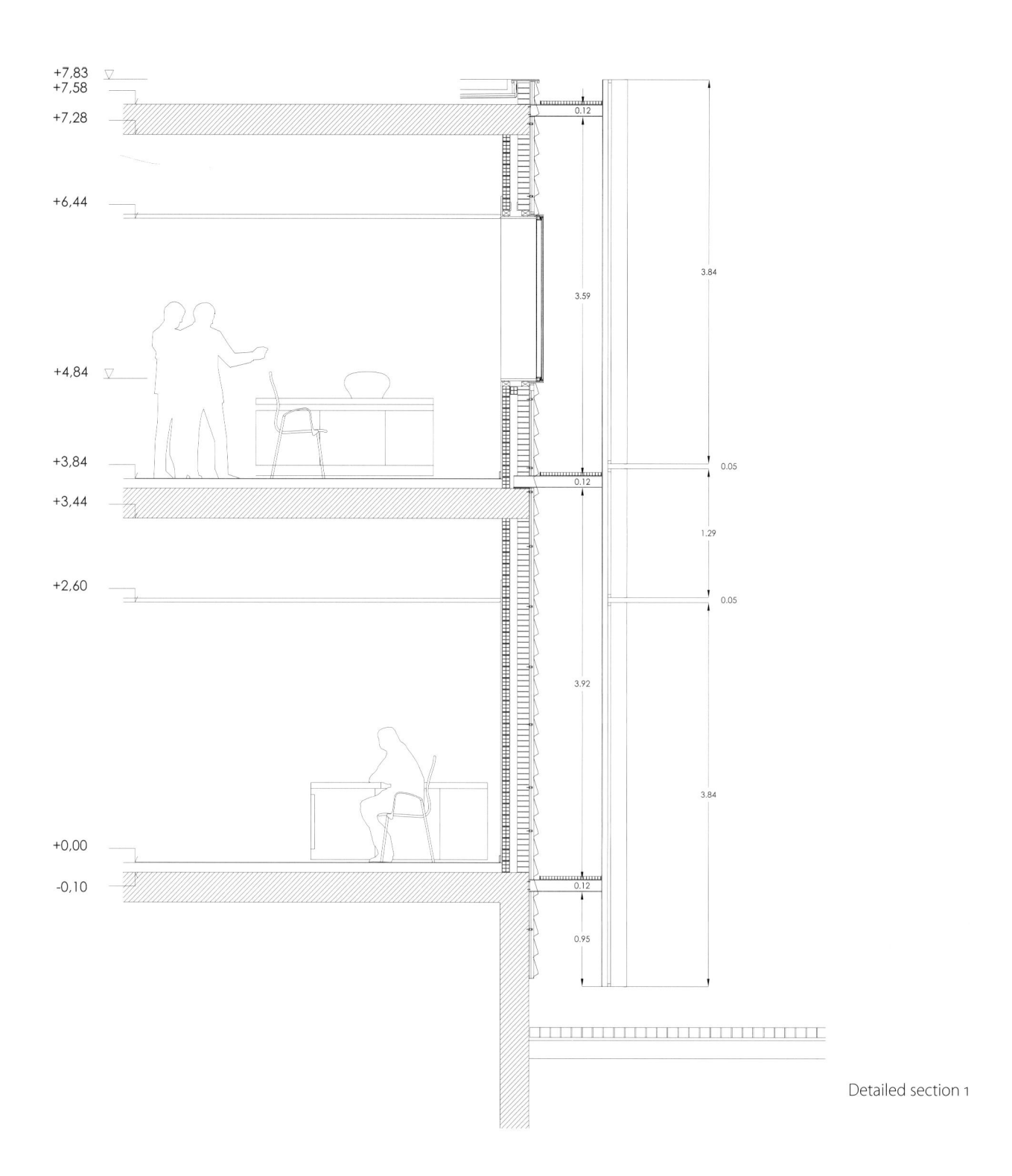

0.12

3.84

+6,44

3.59

+4,84

+3,84
+3,44

0.05

0.12

1.29

+2,60

0.05

3.92

3.84

+0,00
−0,10

0.12

0.95

Detailed section 1

0m 0.5m 1.0m 2.0m 5.0m

Detailed section 2

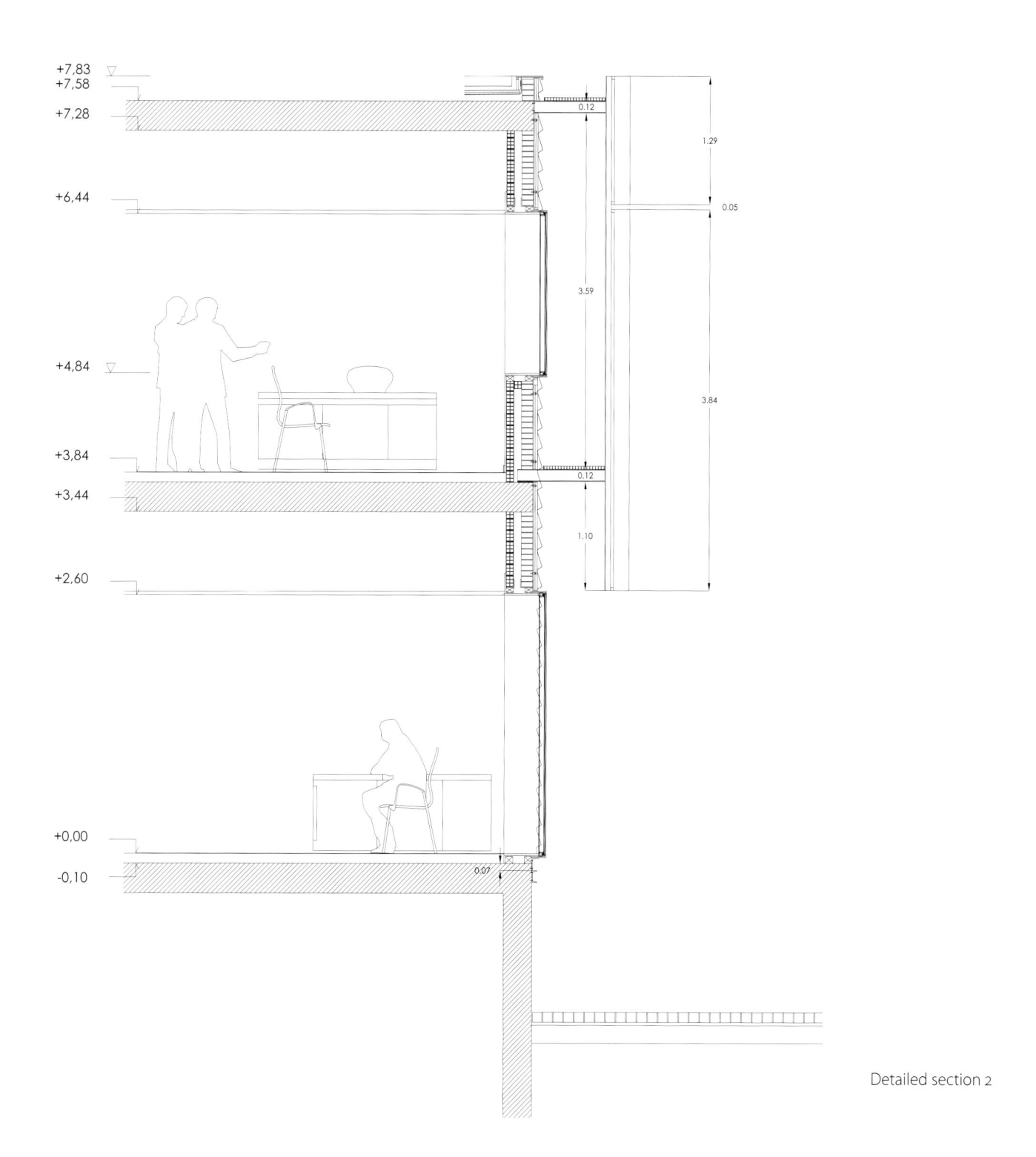

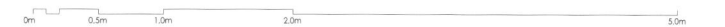

Detailed Lamas

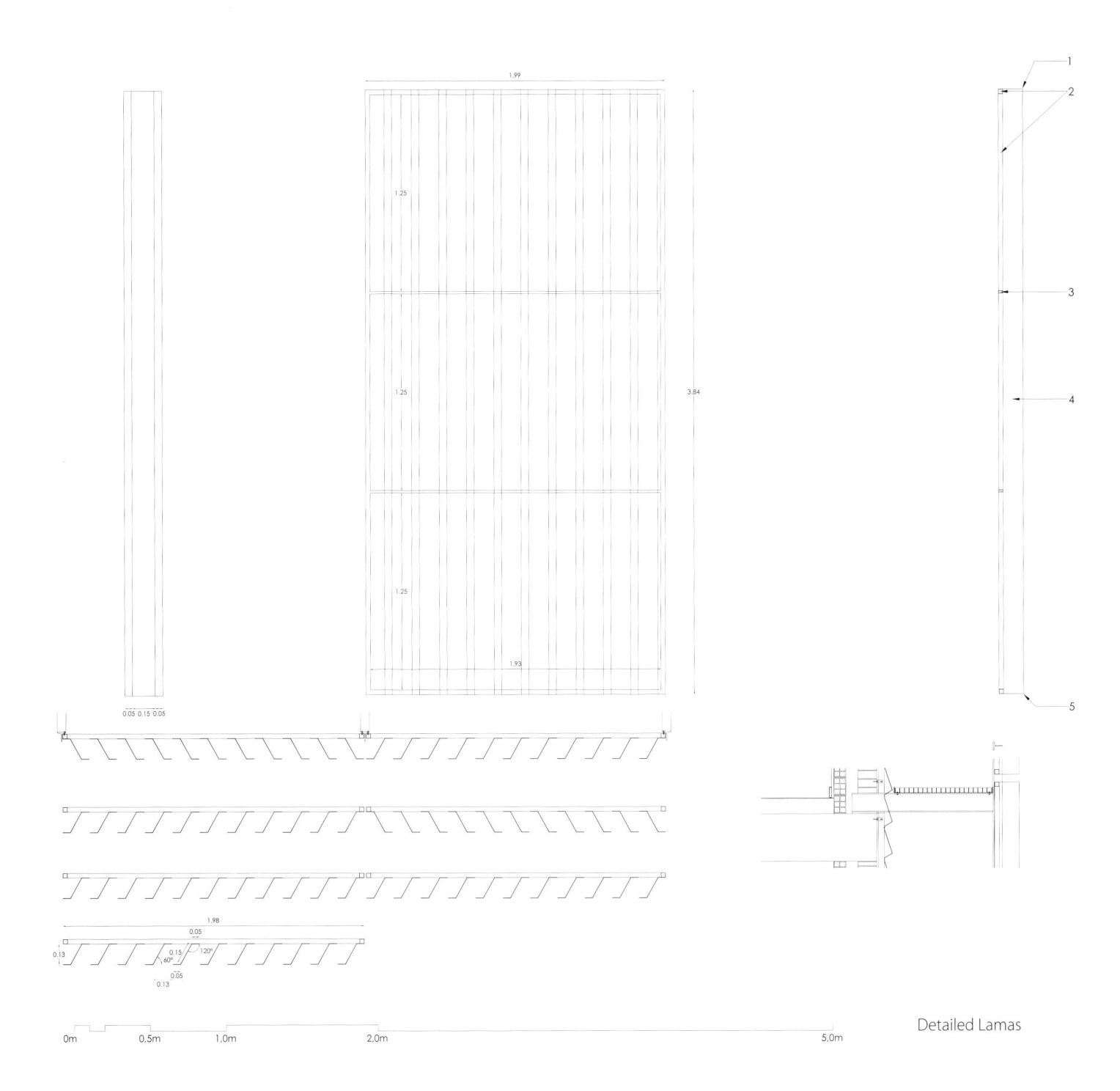

+7,85

+3,99

+3,44

+2,60

+1,00

+0,00

-0,10

0.12

1.72

0.05

3.92

3.15

0.07   0.12

Detailed section 3

0m   0.5m   1.0m   2.0m   5.0m

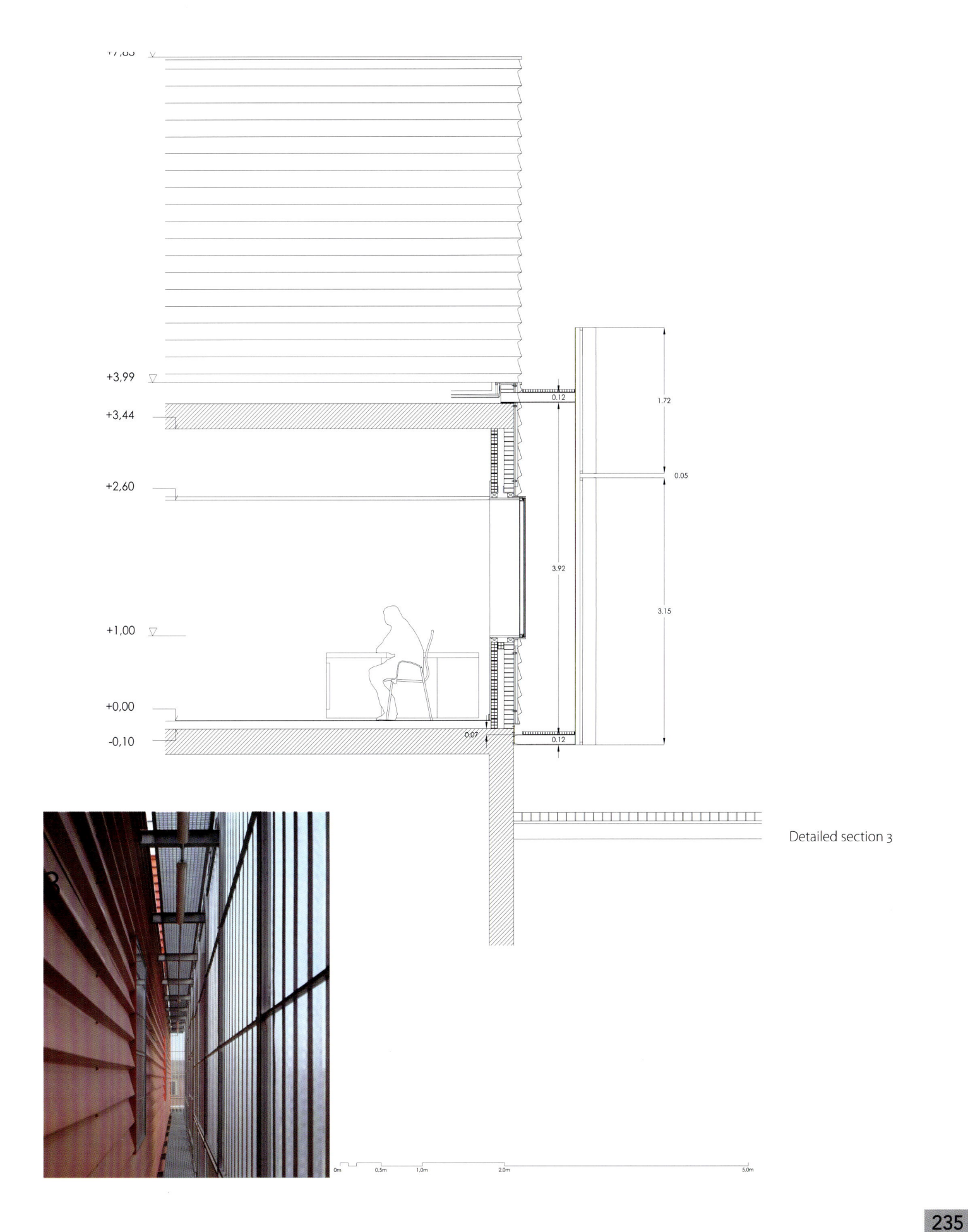

235

Detailed section 4

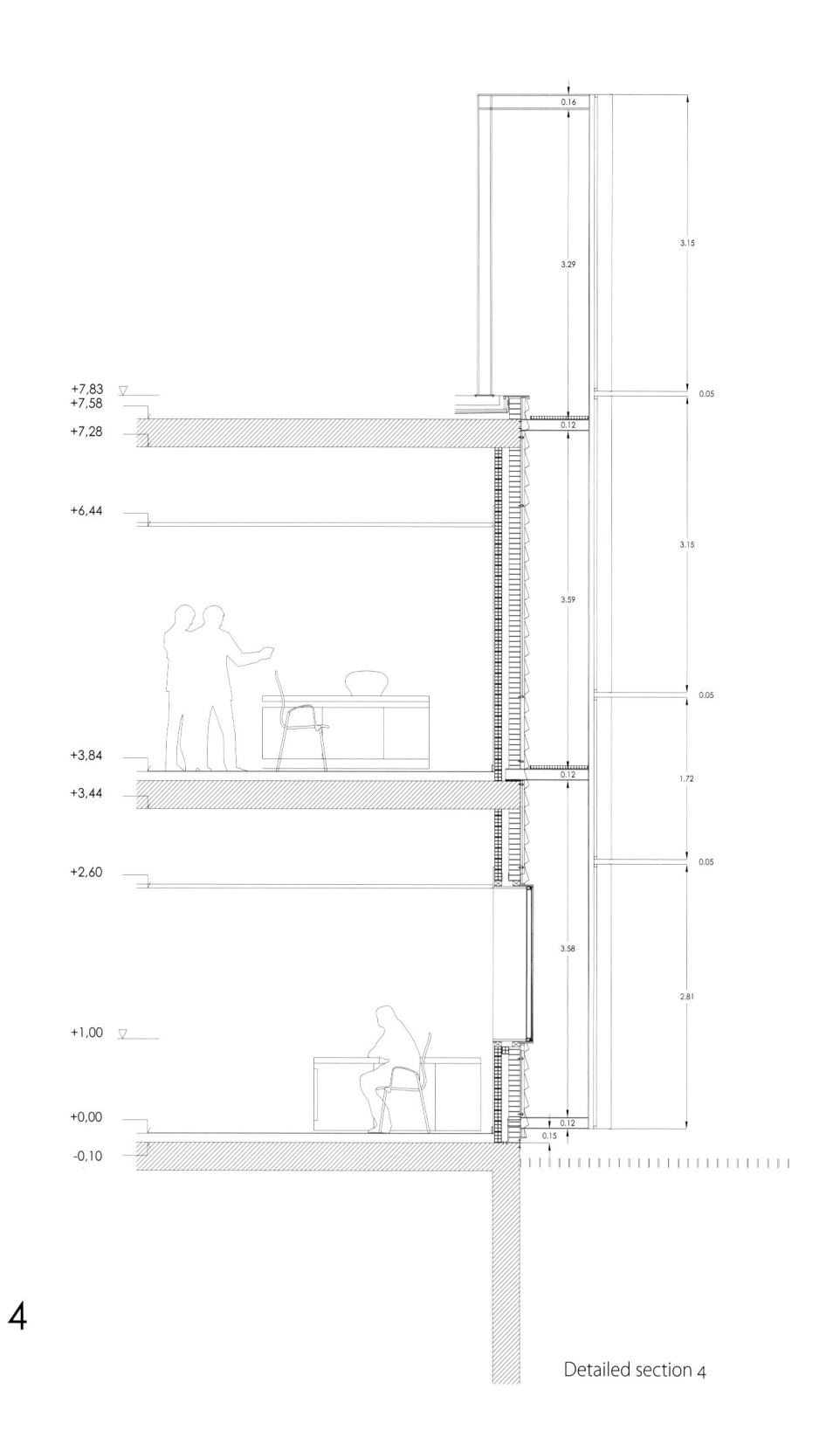

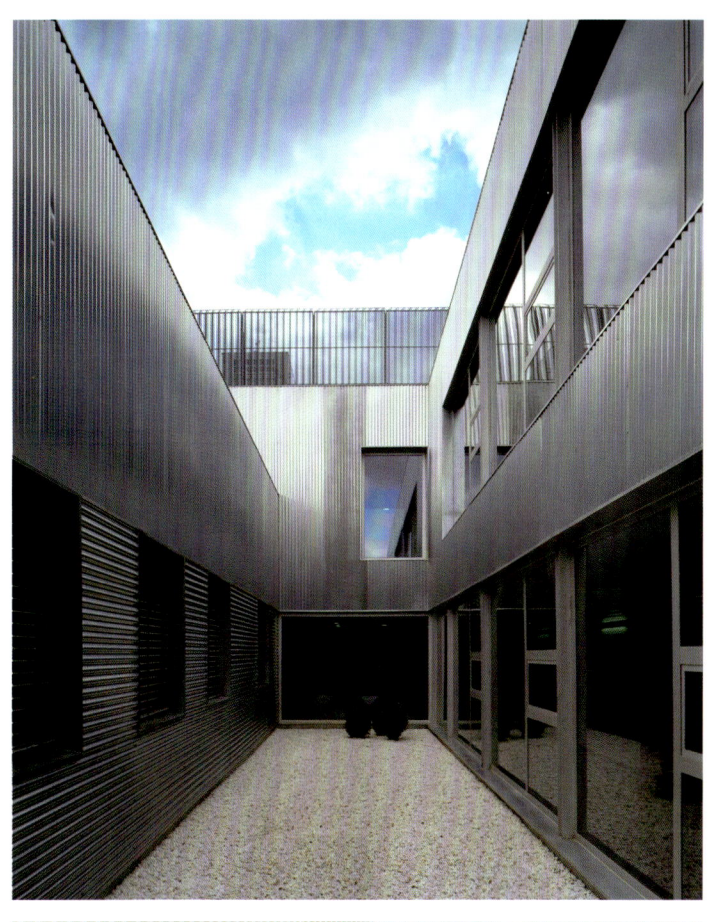

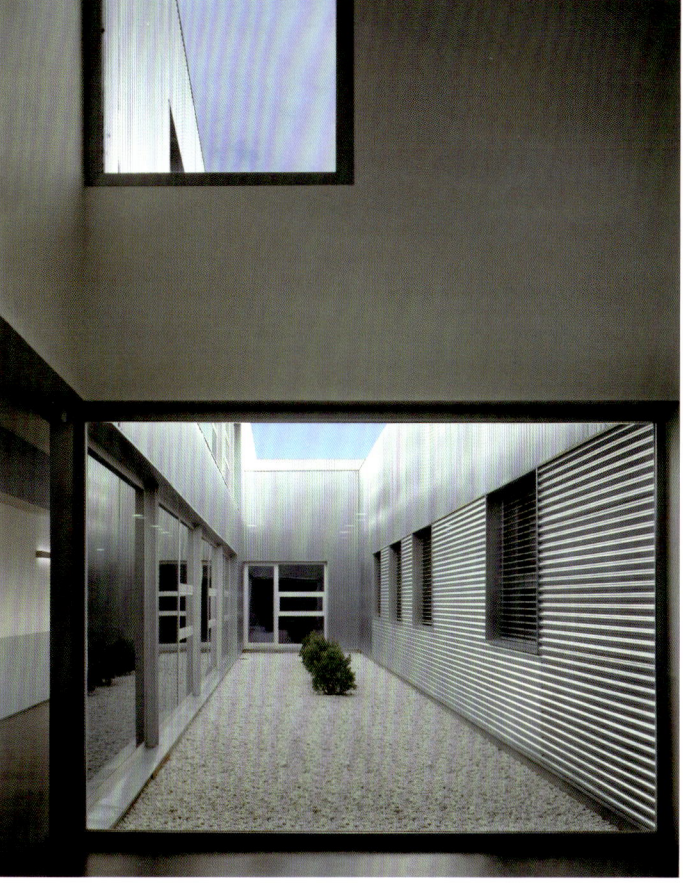

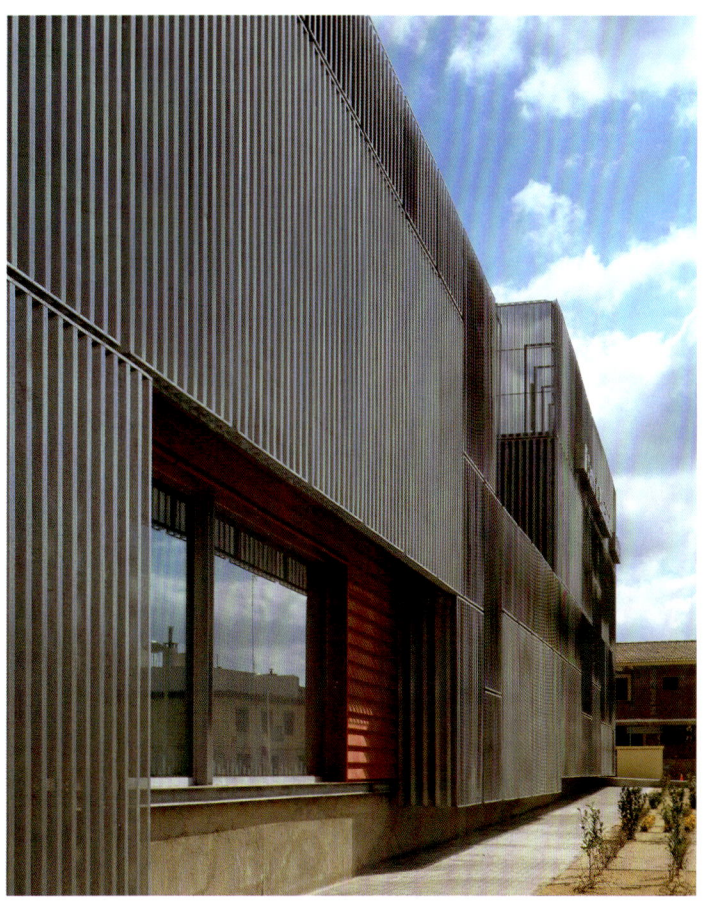

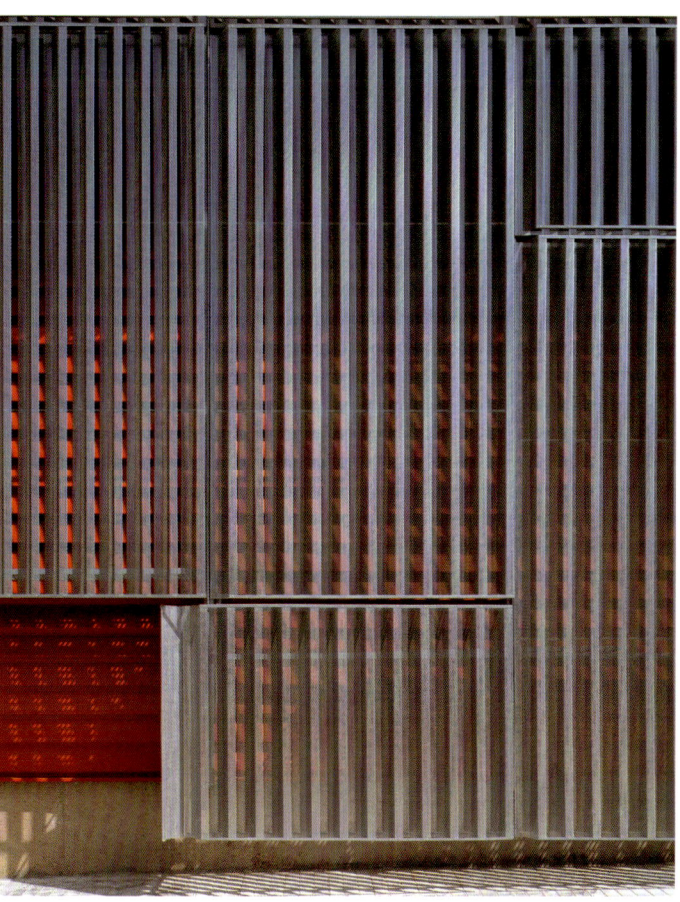

Groupe-6

Arras Hospital

Arras, France

Photographs: Groupe-6

Groupe-6, France's third largest architectural practice completed the restructuring and extension of the Arras Hospital, which now covers a surface area of 84,000 sqm (904,000 sqft) and contains 560 beds, in December 2008.

The Arras Hospital is a precursor of a new generation of hospitals which promise high architectural, spatial and social values, combining modernity and humanity.

The building is inserted into a dense urban environment. Stretching out into a landscaped park, it borders and faces the old fortifications allowing the patients spectacular views of the historic town.

The primary preoccupation was to optimize the relationship between the staff and the patient, serving and enhancing notions of caring, efficiency, welcome and dialogue.

A new bedroom organization with bathrooms on the external façade creates more space, more efficiency and time spent with the patients.

Logistics are maximized through NTIC, introducing the concept and reality of a networked hospital.

Transparent bridges connect the three main buildings ventilated with punctual green patios and water pools. Lightness, openness and transparency are accentuated by a flat roof floating over the architectural mass.

Public and mixed-use spaces are generously distributed, filled with natural light, allowing interaction and dialogue, and reinforcing the definition of the hospital as a living space.

The Arras Hospital pays particular attention to environmental quality through a system of natural renewable energy systems – the double skin façade creates a ventilating buffer space between the interior and the exterior. Closed in winter, opened in summer, the louvers allow natural heating and aeration according to the seasons.

Client:
Centre Hospitalier d'Arras
Surface area:
84,000 sqm (904,000 sqft)
Start Date:
2003
Finish Date:
2008
Cost:
€ 98 million

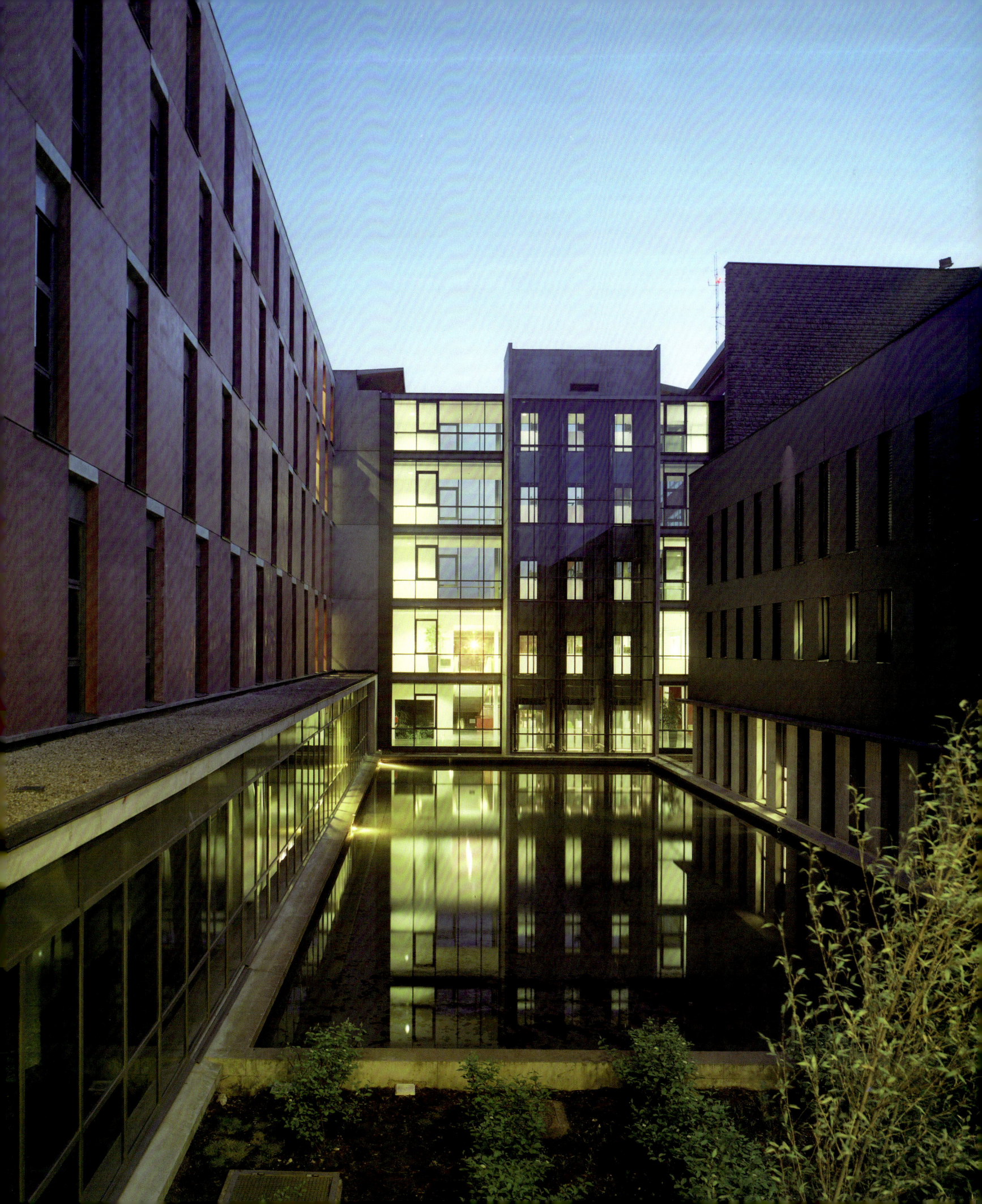

240

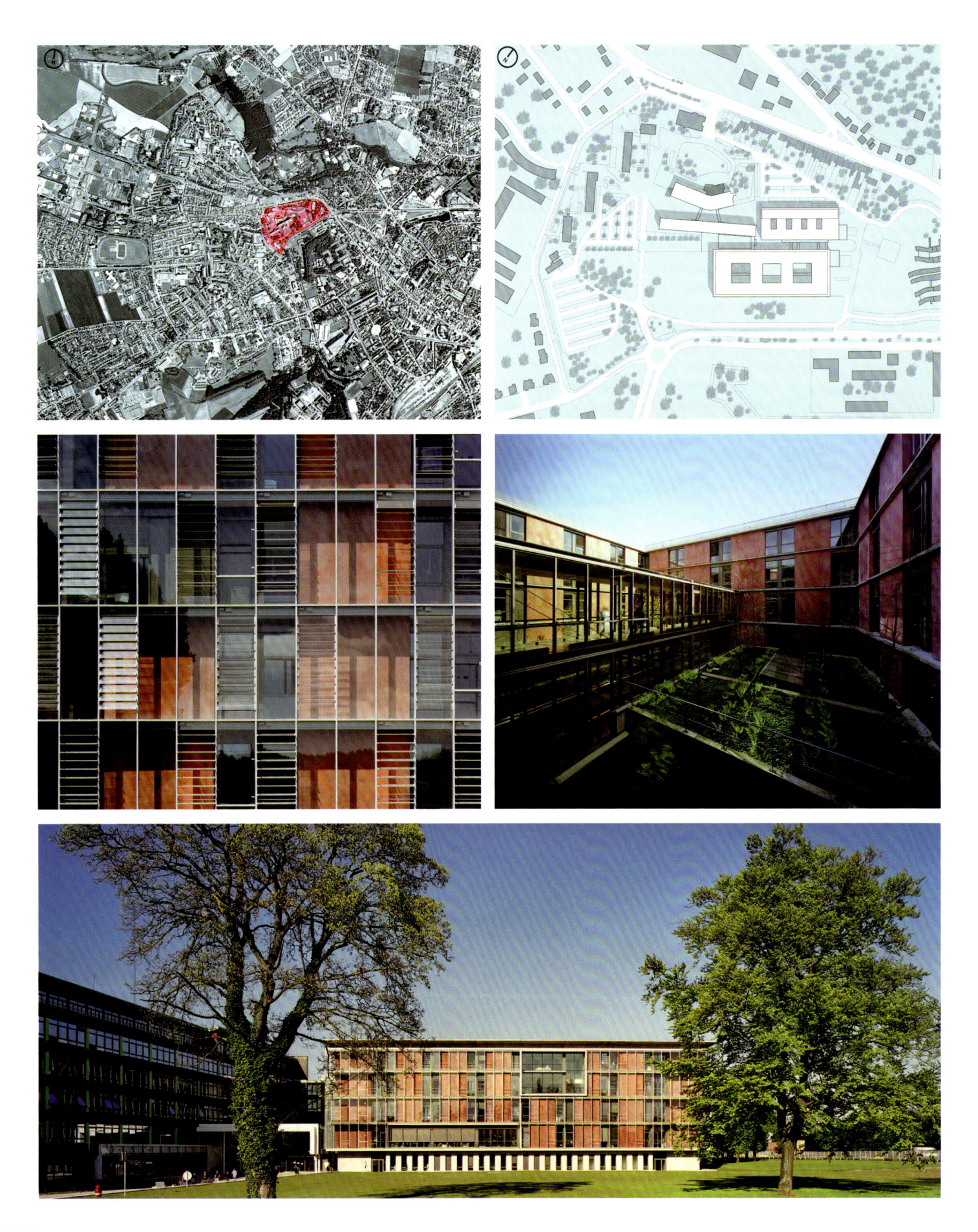

Ground floor plan

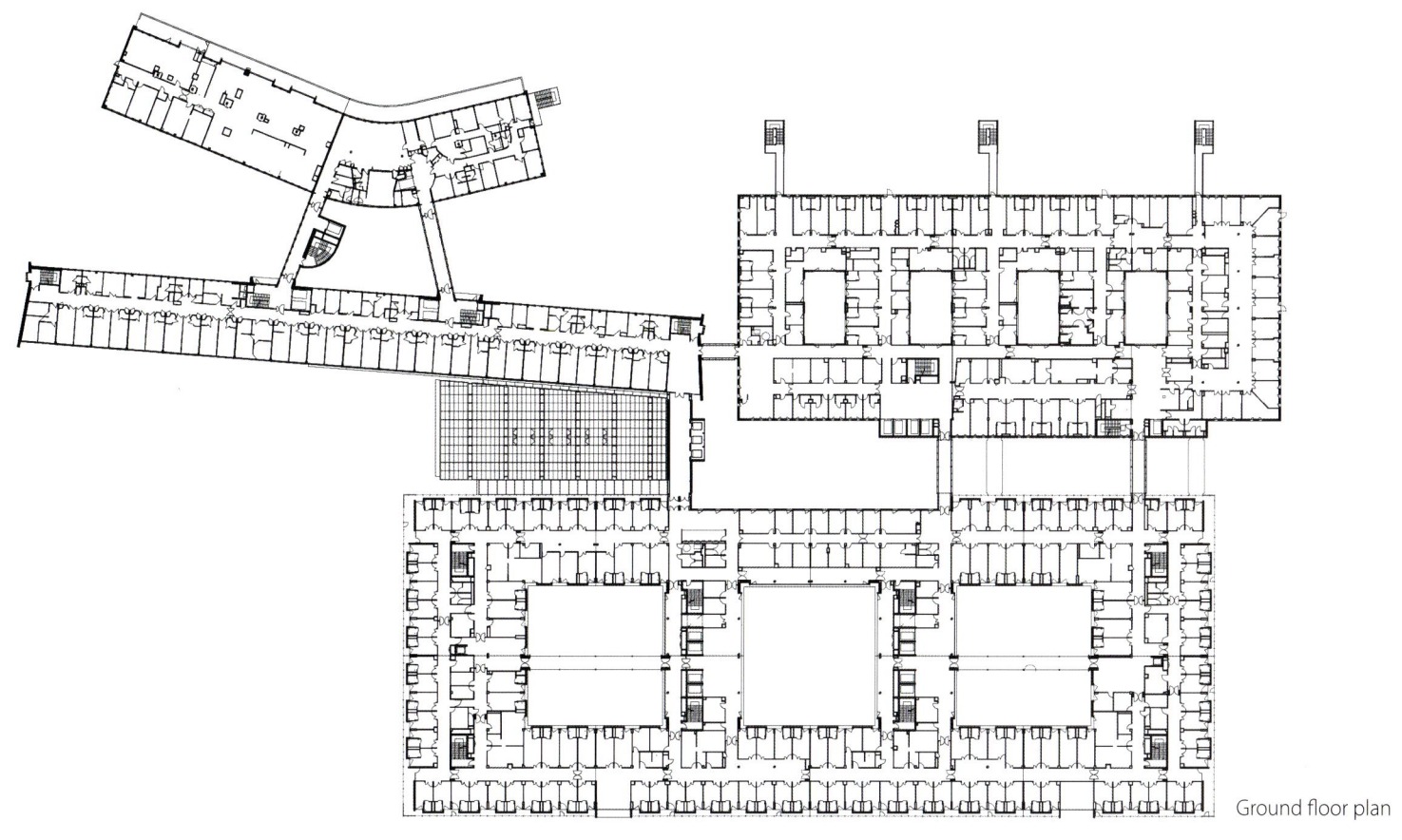

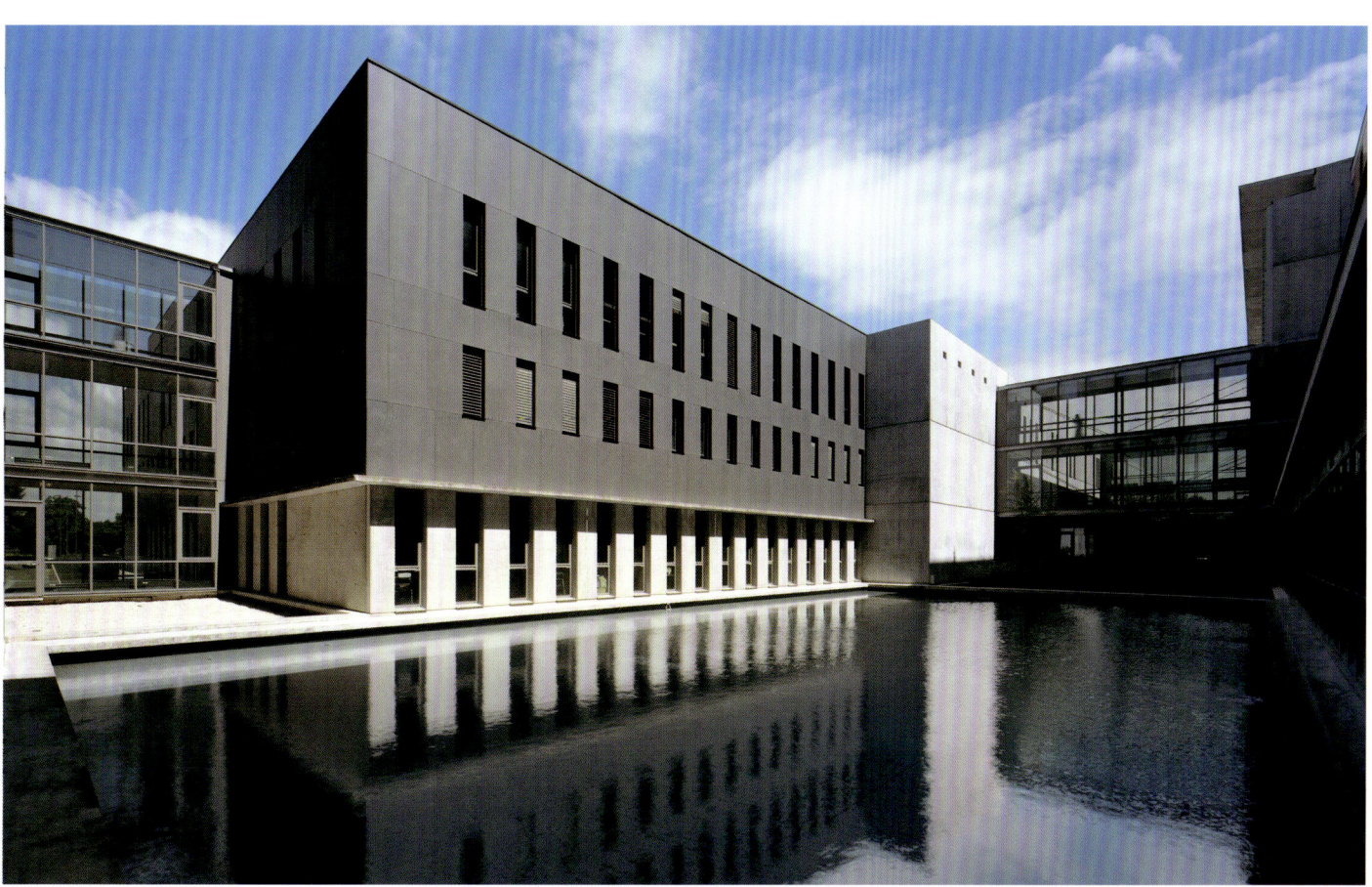

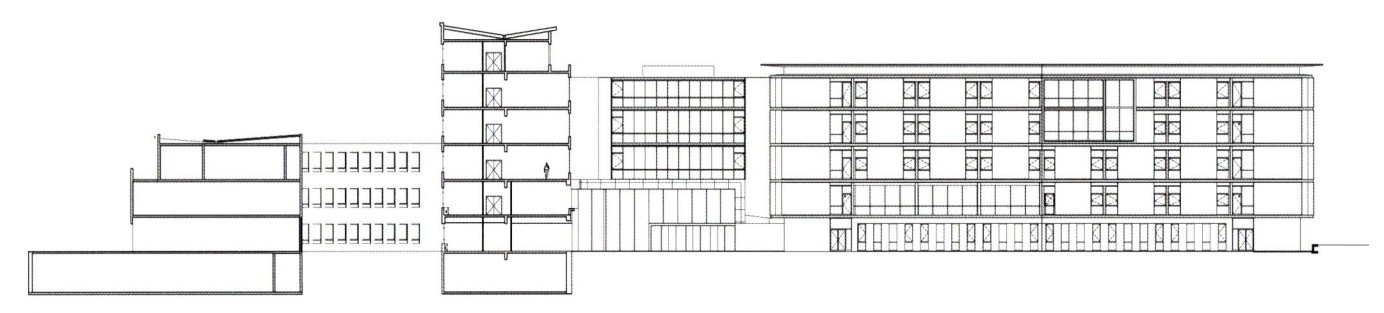

Section

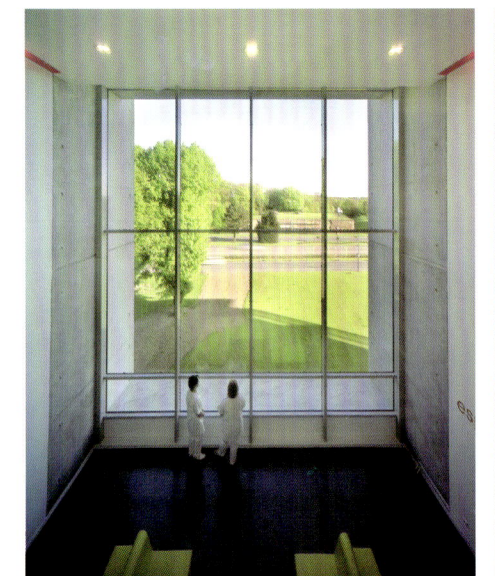

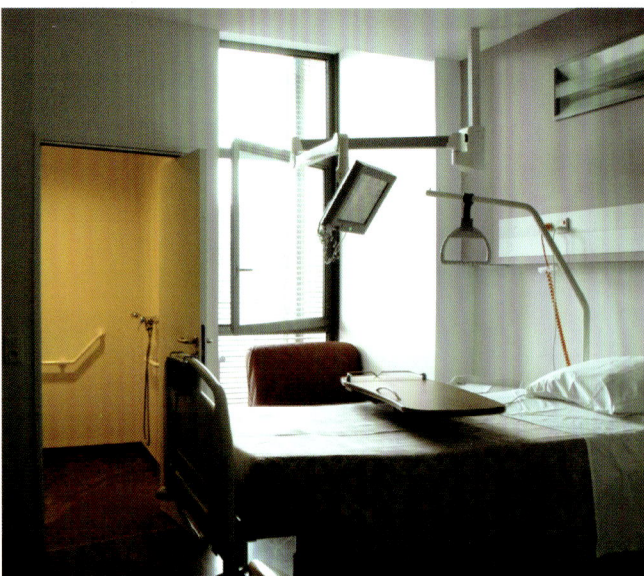

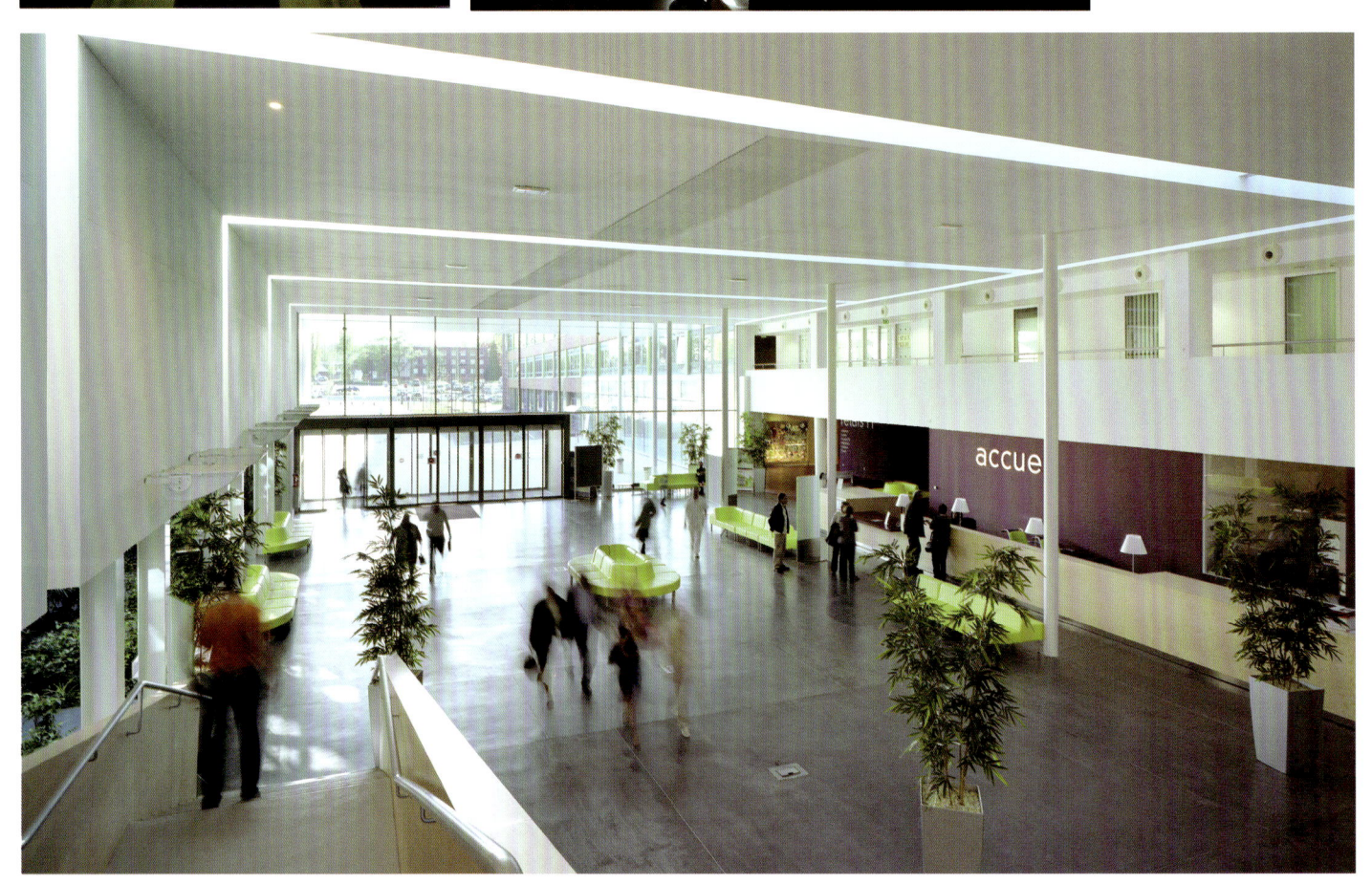

242

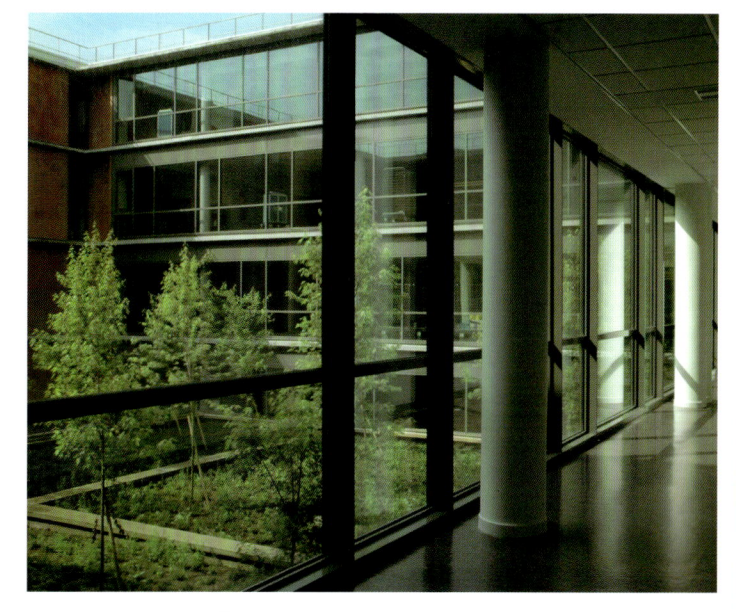

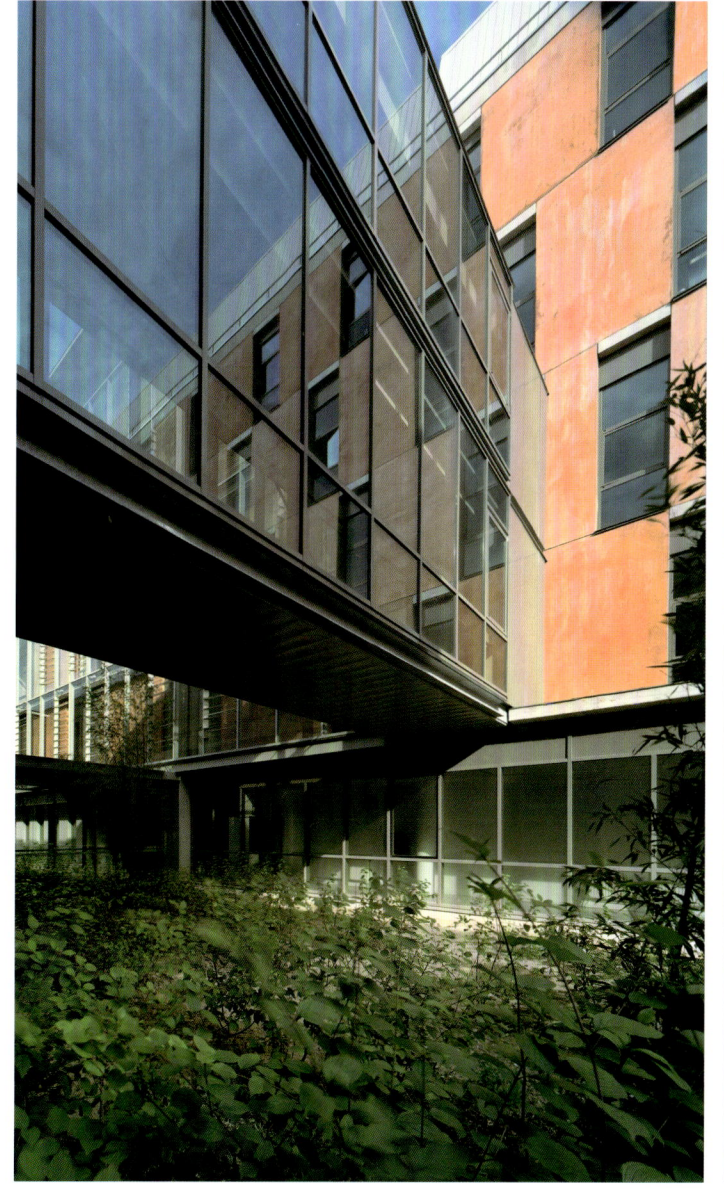

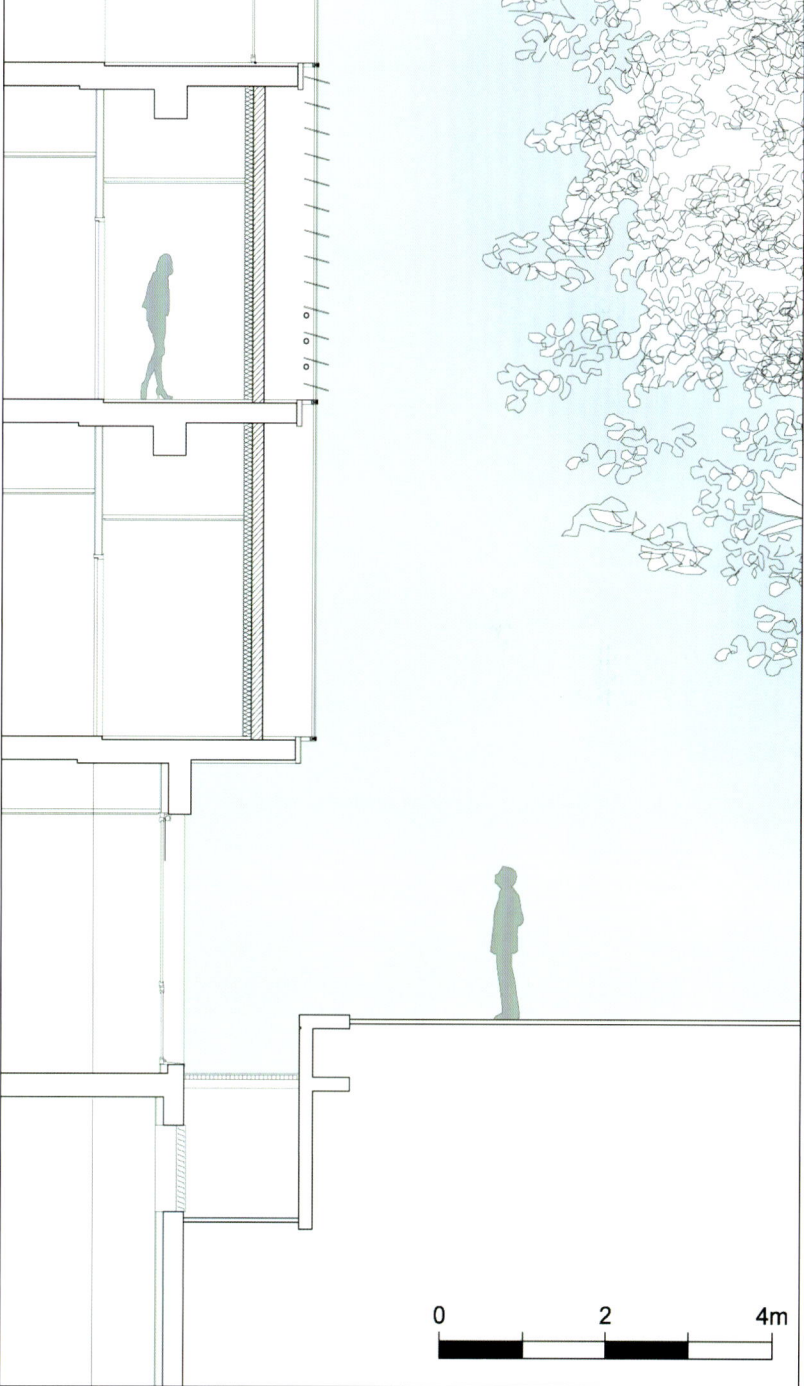

Façade detail 1

243

Stantec Architecture Ltd.

Peterborough Regional Health Centre

Peterborough, Canada

Photographs: Richard Johnson

The new Peterborough Regional Health Centre in the City of Peterborough is located one and a half hours north east of Toronto, Canada in a region known as Kawartha Lakes. Characterized by rolling hills, lakes and marshland, communities within the Kawarthas grew around crossroads or corners. Peterborough's industrial roots have influenced the city's rich architectural traditions rendered in masonry and local stone. The City is strongly influenced by its rolling geography, colliding street grids, its varied elevations, and the Ontonabee River with its associated bridges.

The design concept is focused on central issues of healing, community, people and connections. These fundamental issues raised questions about the kind of place that could address the unique attachment the community had to their local hospital. The key design objectives were to create: a family and patient-centered healing environment, a positive work environment and positive community connections.

The geographical elevation of the site provides the facility with a commanding panoramic view of the city and regional geography beyond. The concept utilizes this natural topography to break down the mass of the building, establish an appropriate community scale and provide multi-level entrances to foster public connection. It demonstrates that large-scale buildings can be designed to provide intimate moments and with an accessible scale that is understood at pedestrian level.

The architectural concept is rooted in the idea of 'crossroads' – the intersection of two paths. The east-west path establishes the main entrance and lobby space, defined by a stone wall. Upon entrance from the west, visitors are immediately visually reconnected to the panoramic view of the city and surrounding countryside through the fully glazed eastern lobby wall. The north-south path provides the prime circulation spine on all six levels. The six levels of the program develop around these two 'crossroad' elements leaving them legible as the principle organizing device. Interior courtyards punctuate the building mass along the north-south circulation spine drawing natural light deep into the building and providing further visual connection to the landscape. Throughout the facility, glazing is used to connect patients, family, visitors and staff to the community. Floor-to-ceiling windows in patient rooms provide a full spectrum of views from ground to sky. Clinical program areas where patient visits are frequent or lengthy enjoy spectacular views of the seasonally changing landscape of the Kawartha Lakes. The north-south spine passes through the courtyards, echoing the 'Bridges of Peterborough' while providing light, view and orientation. The materiality of the project, locally quarried stone, red clay brick with steel channel inserts and corrugated metal siding reflect the rich industrial architectural heritage of Peterborough. This together with the fundamental indoor/outdoor visual connections firmly roots the project in the community it serves.

Client:
Peterborough Regional Health Centre
Surface area:
66,425 sqm (715,000 sqft)
Completion:
August 2008
Project Design Principal:
Michael Moxam
Design team members:
Michael Moxam, Norm Crone, Stephen Phillips, Anthony Cho, Eugene Chumakov, Brian Moeller, George Bitsakakis, Lisa Gregg, Grant MacEachern, Ko Van Klaveren, Kevin Plant, Tommy Ong, Norma Angel, Terence Tam, Gordon Martyshuk, Christine Andrews, Sandy Park, Stacy Fleming, Shannon Crossman, Vanessa Vilic-Evangelista, Dana Tapak, Betty James, Chi-Ae Goodman
Contractor:
EllisDon Corporation
Cost:
$ 220 million

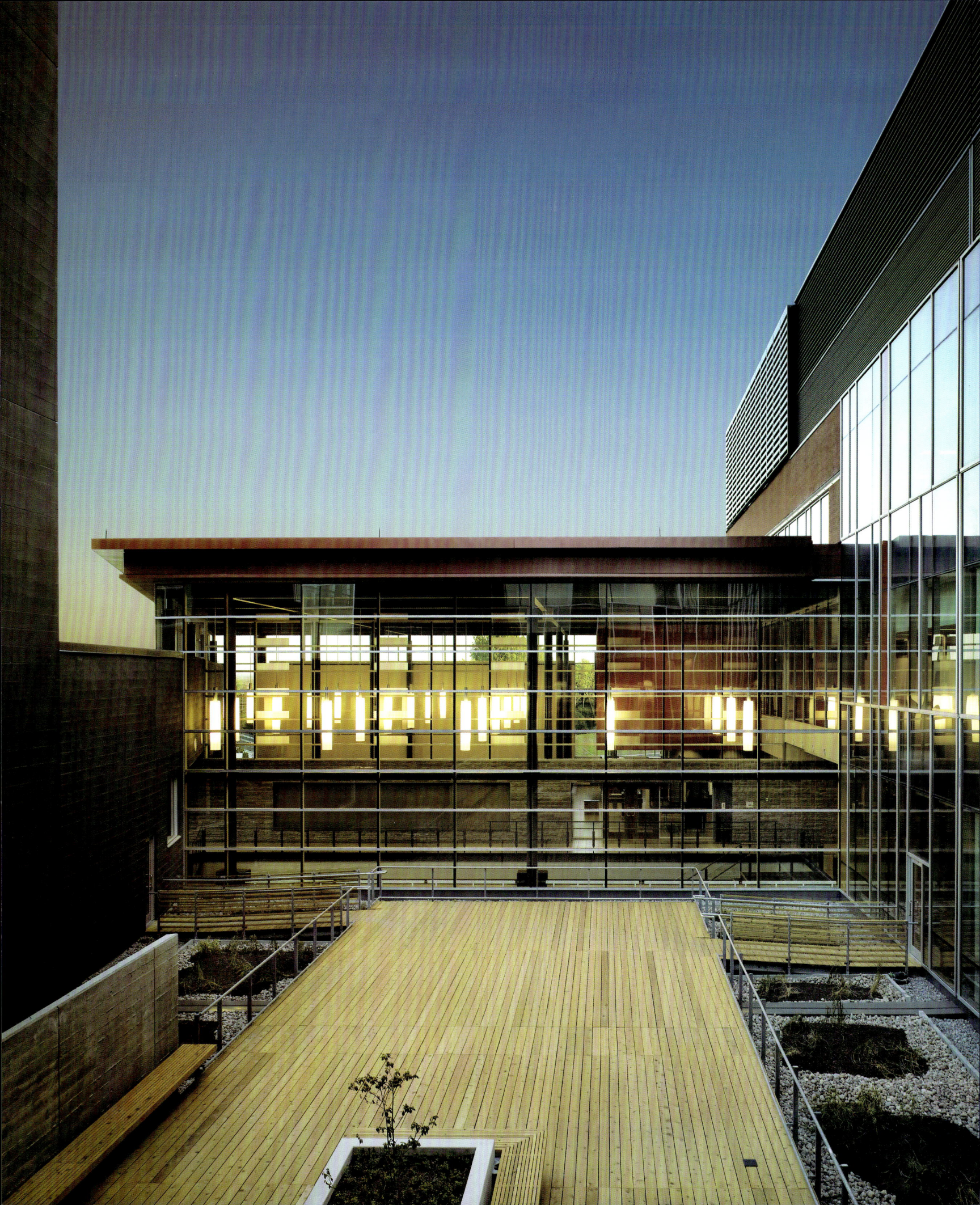

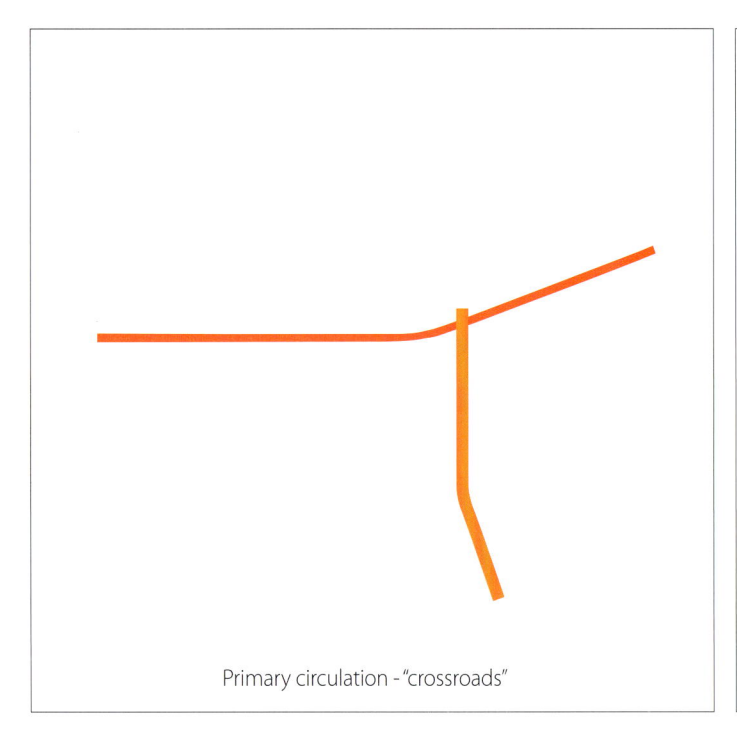

Primary circulation - "crossroads"

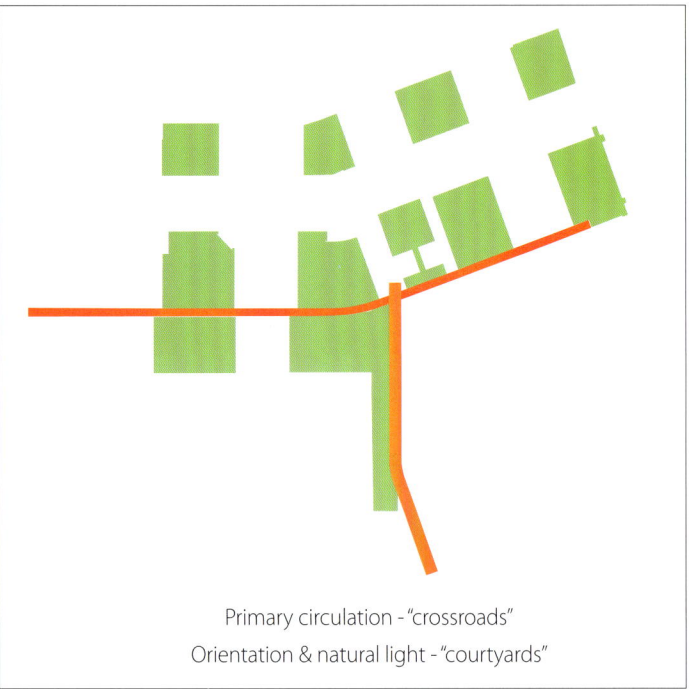

Primary circulation - "crossroads"
Orientation & natural light - "courtyards"

1. Main entrance 2. Public lobby 3. Courtyard 4. Library 5. Cafeteria 6. Admitting 7. Multi faith centre 8. Mental health inpatient 9. Medical inpatient 10. Surgical inpatient 11. Rehabilitation inpatient 12. Palliative care inpatient 13. Complex continuing care 14. Maternal child 15. Critical care respiratory services 16. Surgery 17. day surgery & ambulatory procedures 18. Ambulatory services 19. Dialysis 20. emergency 21. Diagnostic imaging 22. Rehabilitation therapy 23. Orthopaedics 24. oncology 25. Breast assessment 26. Cardiac cathertization 27. Pharmacy 28. Laboratory 29. Sterile processing 30. Kitchen 31. Nutrition services 32. Health records 33. Facility services 34. Staff facilities/Services 35. Offices 36. Materials management 37. Information technology 38. Morgue

Floor Plans A

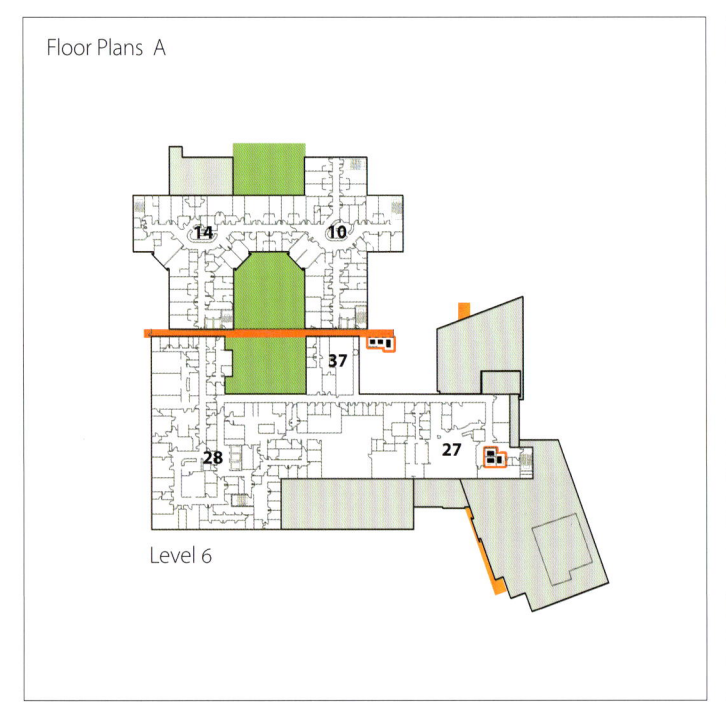

Level 6

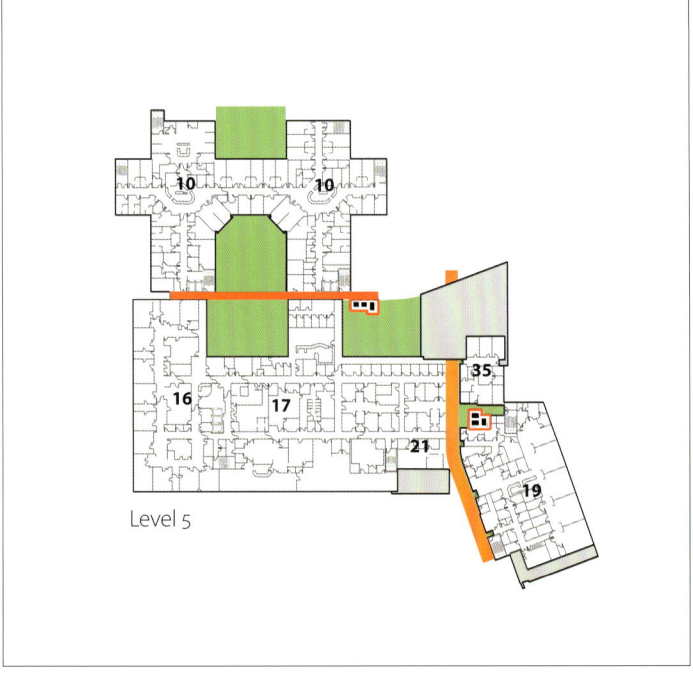

Level 5

level 1

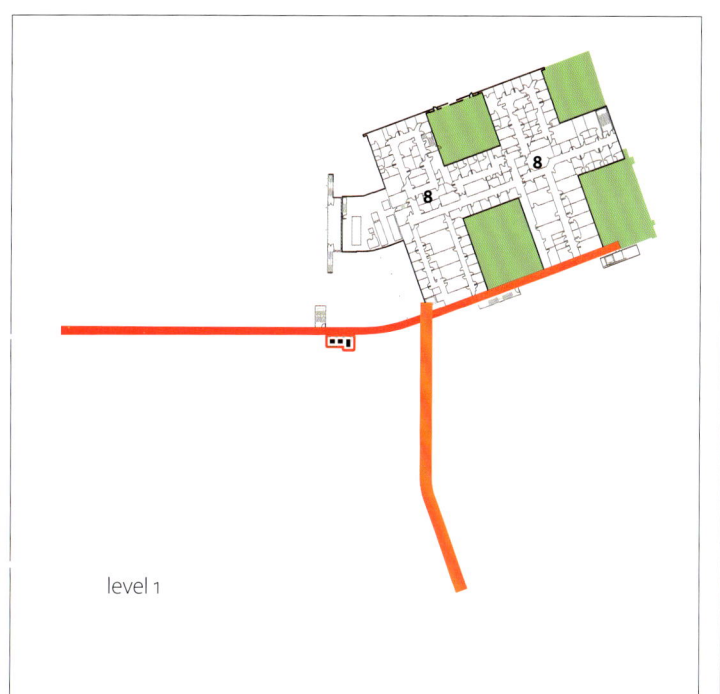

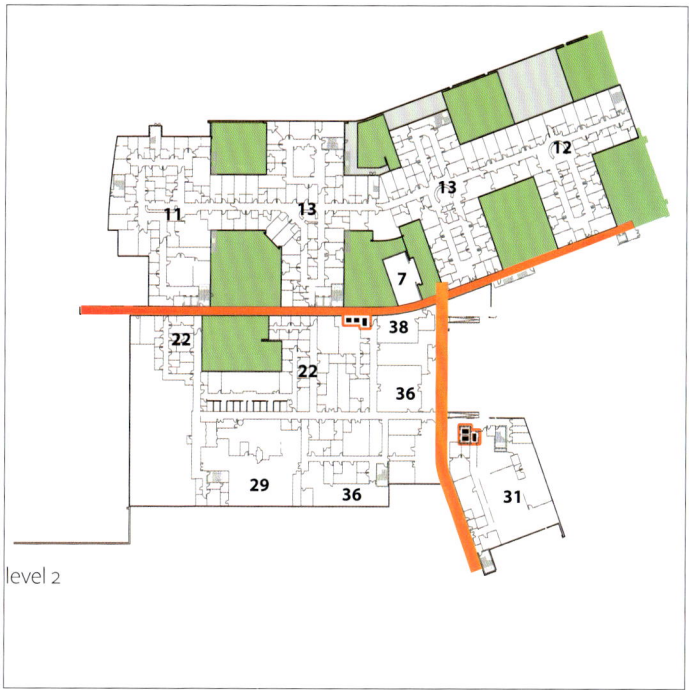

level 2

1. Main entrance 2. Public lobby 3. Courtyard 4. Library 5. Cafeteria 6. Admitting 7. Multi faith centre 8. Mental health inpatient 9. Medical inpatient 10. Surgical inpatient 11. Rehabilitation inpatient 12. Palliative care inpatient 13. Complex continuing care 14. Maternal child 15. Critical care respiratory services 16. Surgery 17. day surgery & ambulatory procedures 18. Ambulatory services 19. Dialysis 20. emergency 21. Diagnostic imaging 22. Rehabilitation therapy 23. Orthopaedics 24. oncology 25. Breast assessment 26. Cardiac cathertization 27. Pharmacy 28. Laboratory 29. Sterile processing 30. Kitchen 31. Nutrition services 32. Health records 33. Facility services 34. Staff facilities/Services 35. Offices 36. Materials management 37. Information technology 38. Morgue

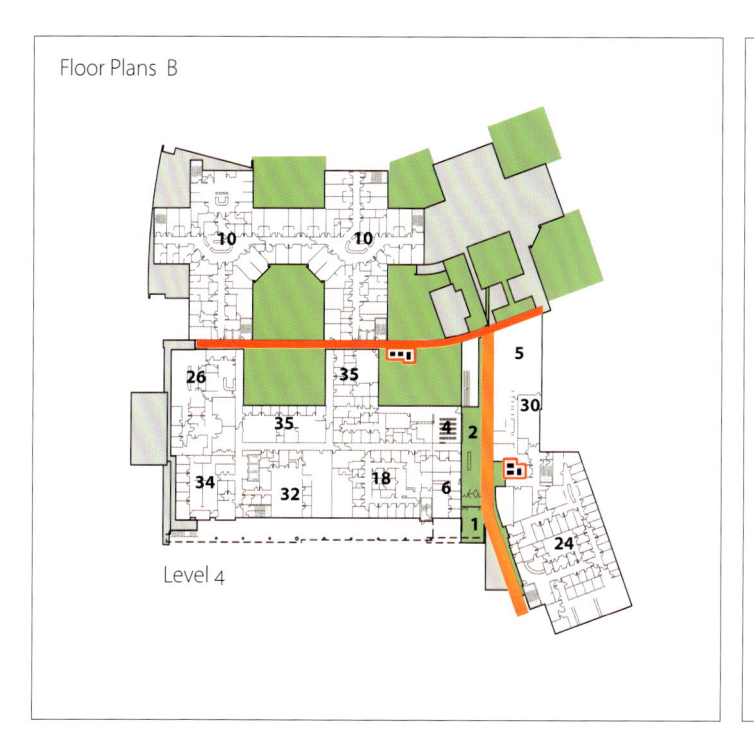

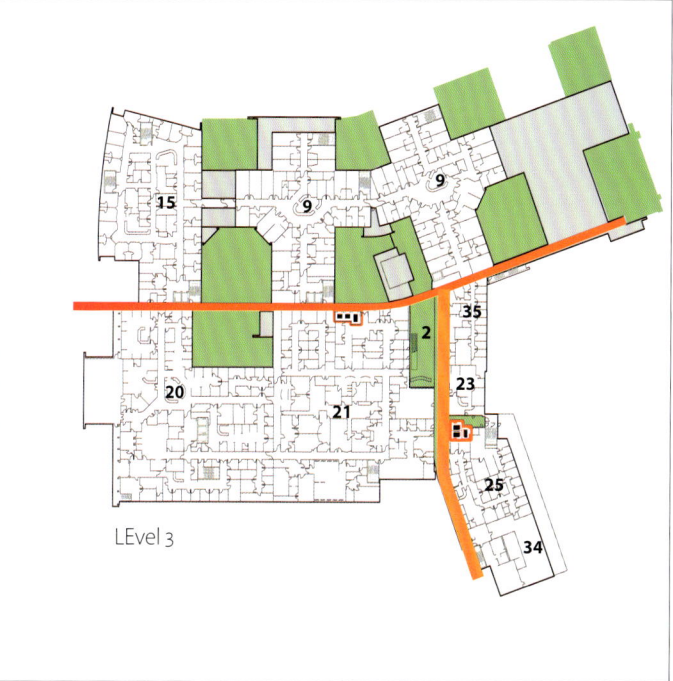

Floor Plans B

Level 4

LEvel 3

247

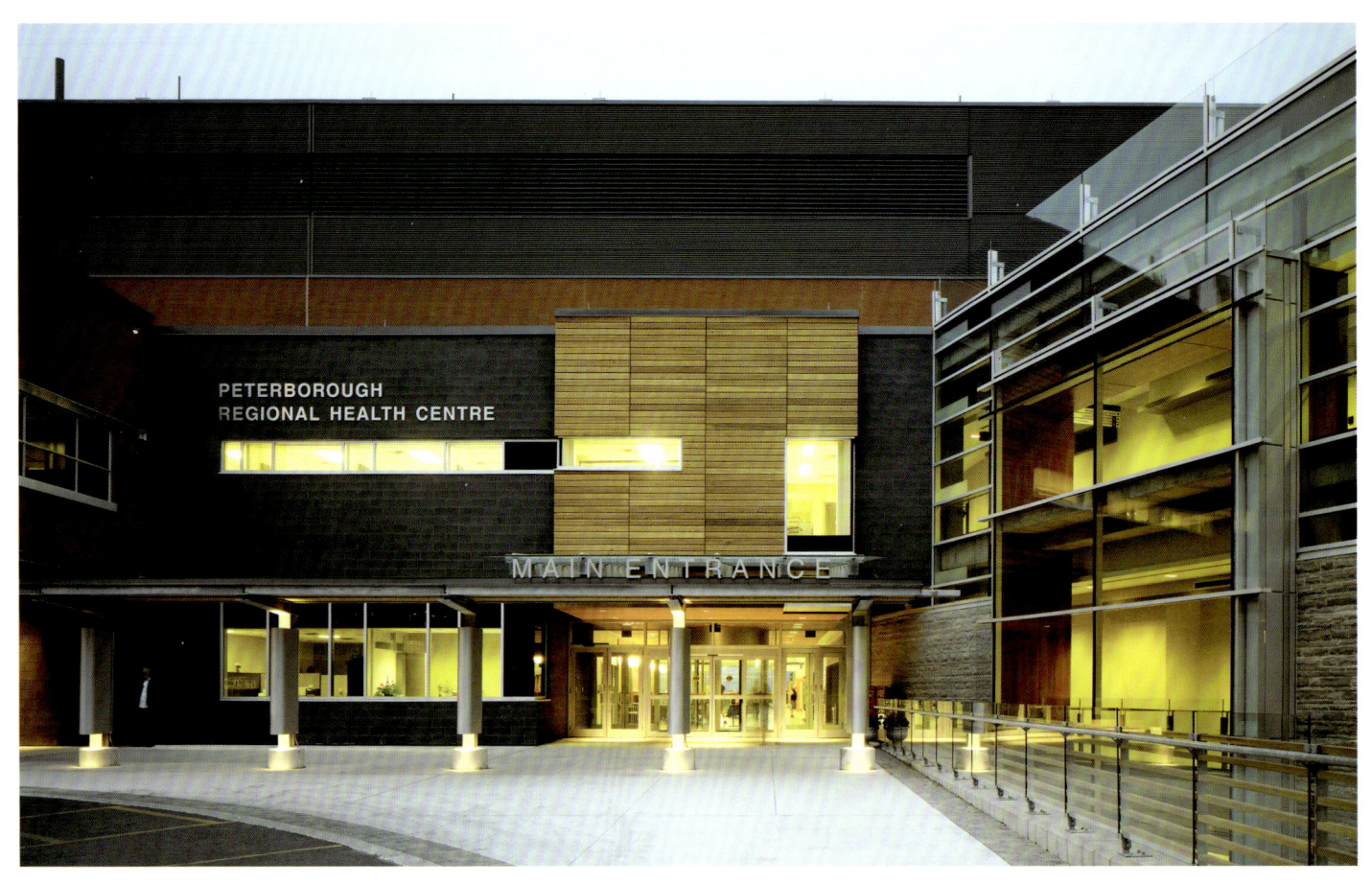

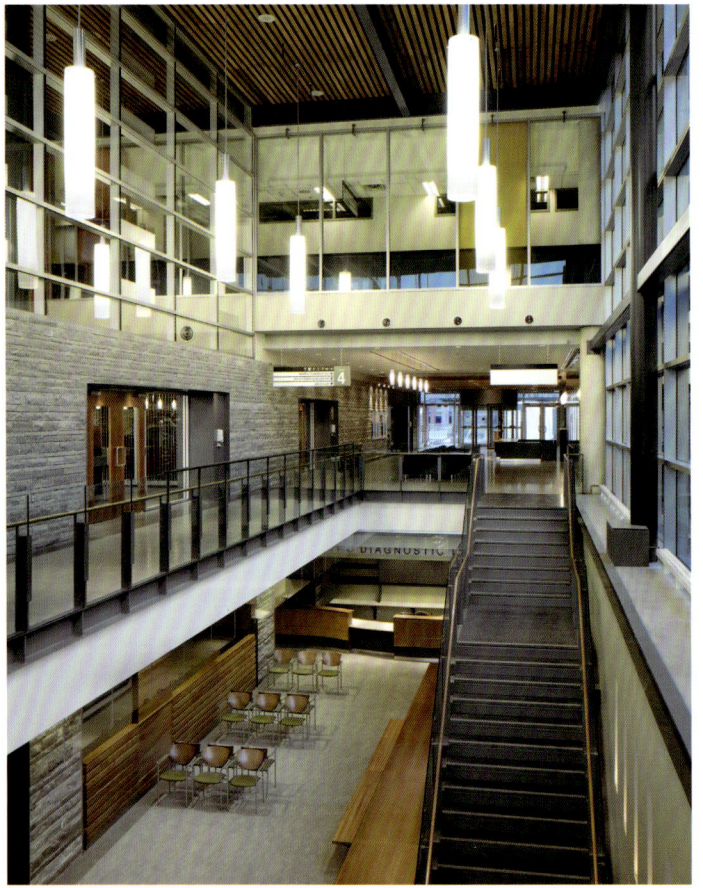

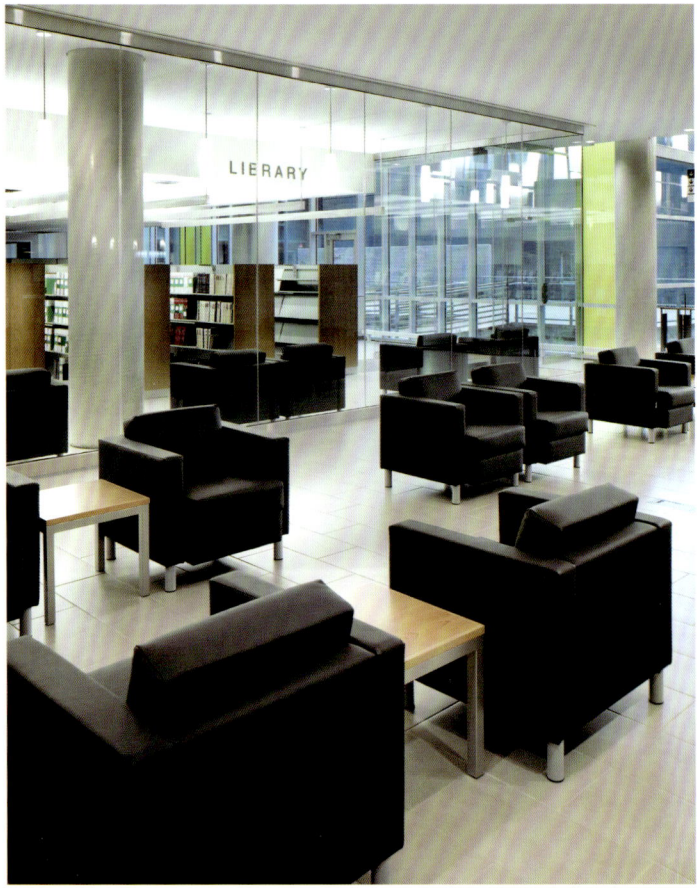

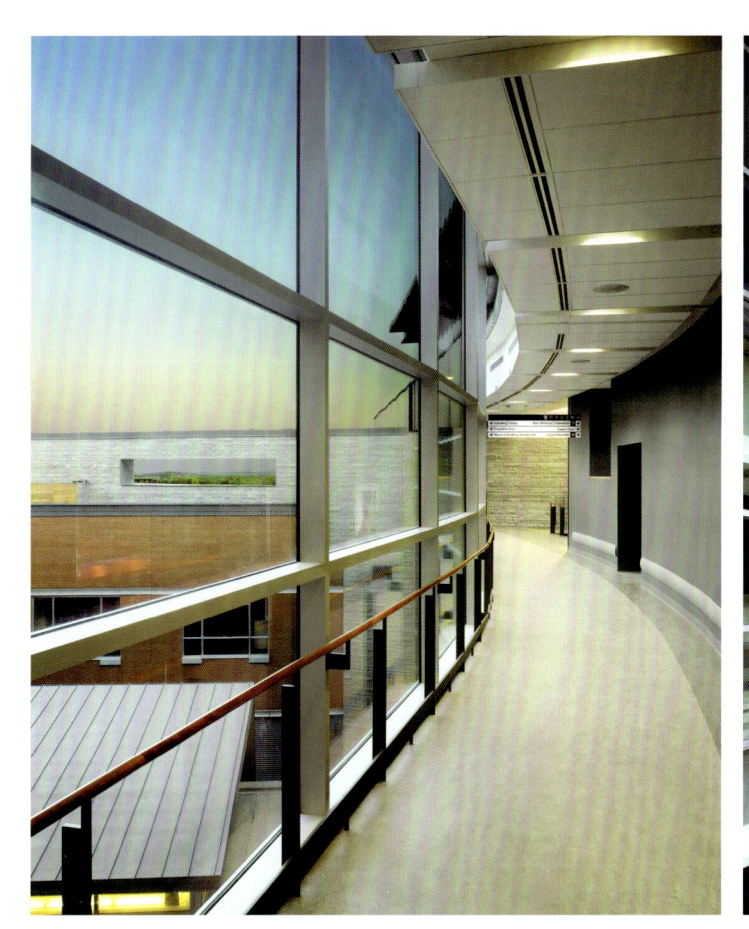

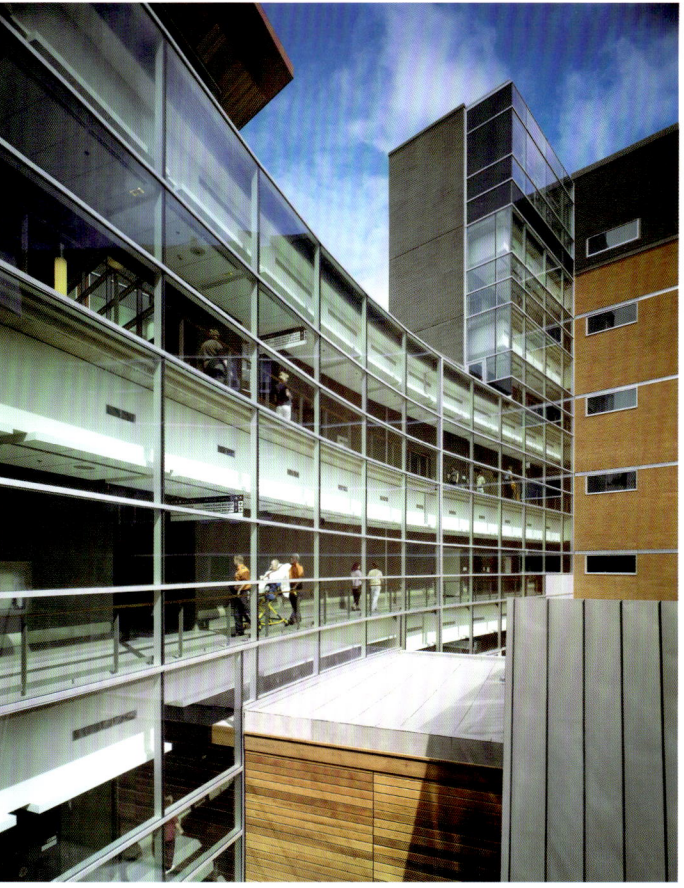

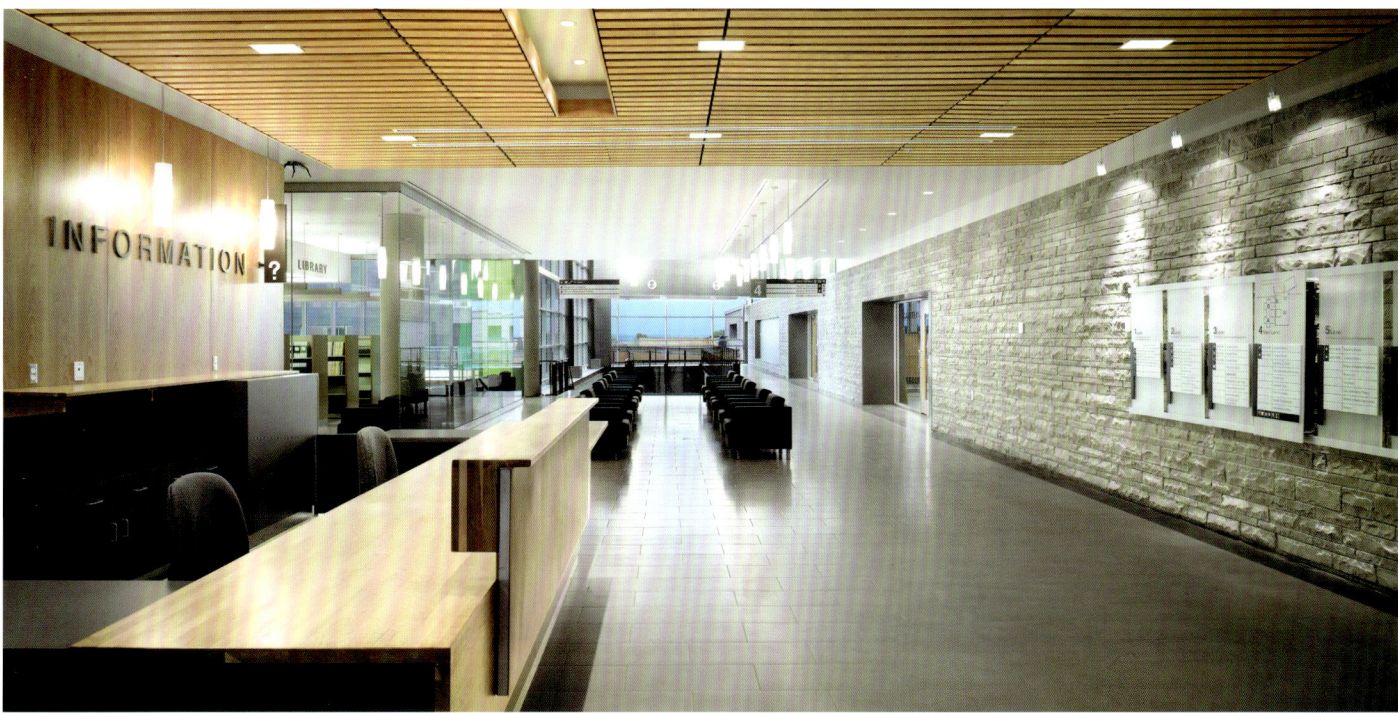

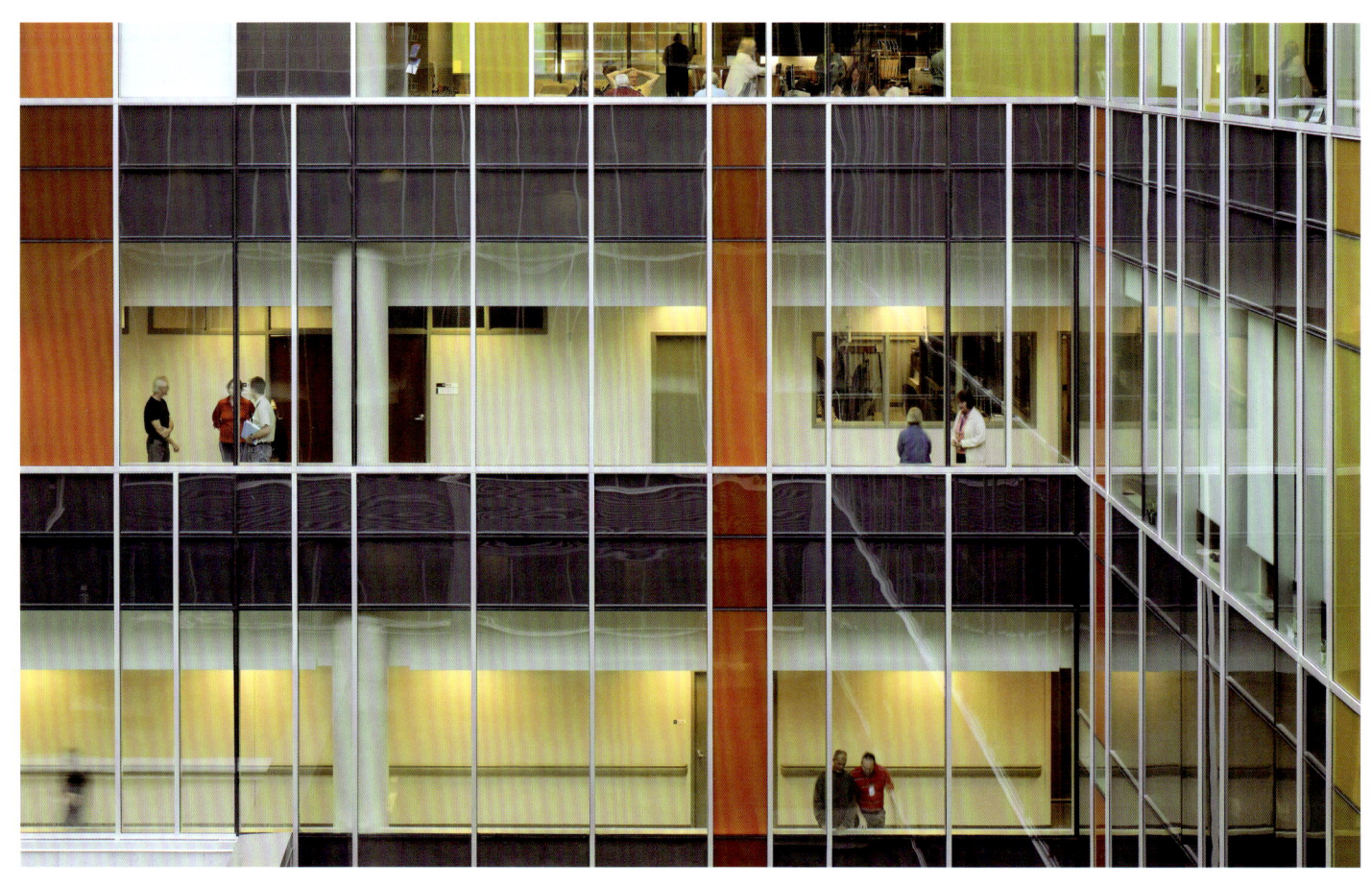

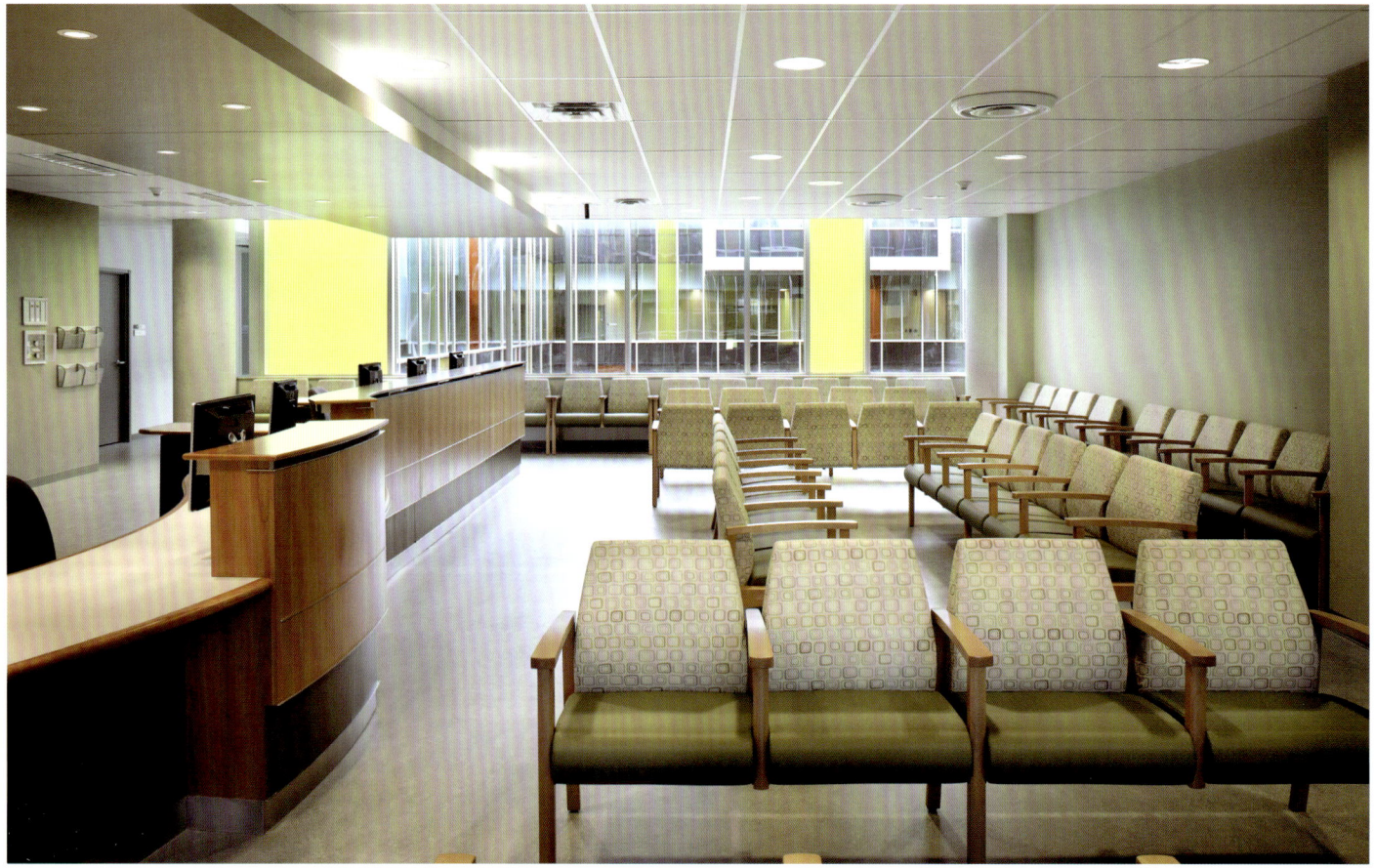

251

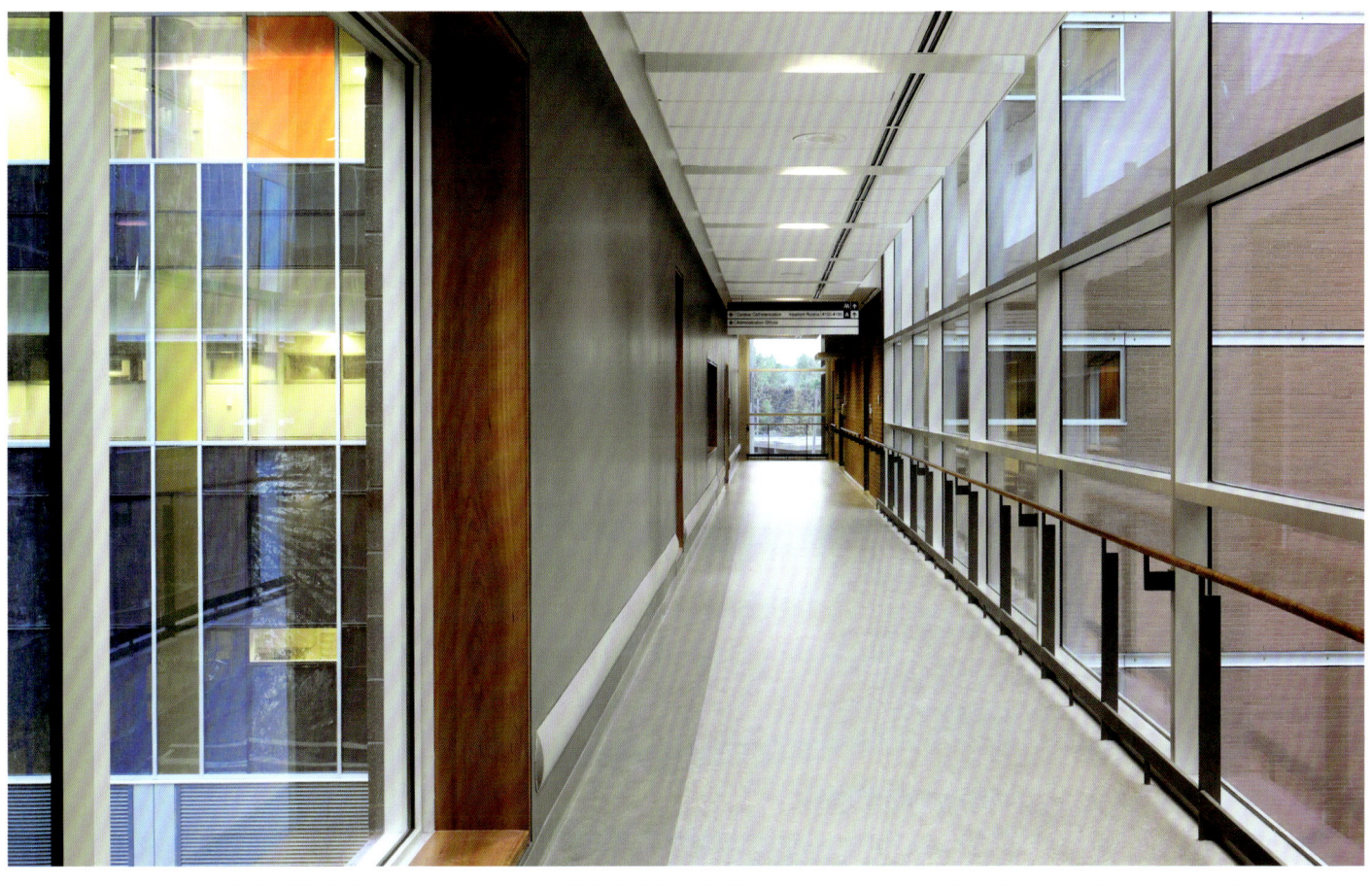

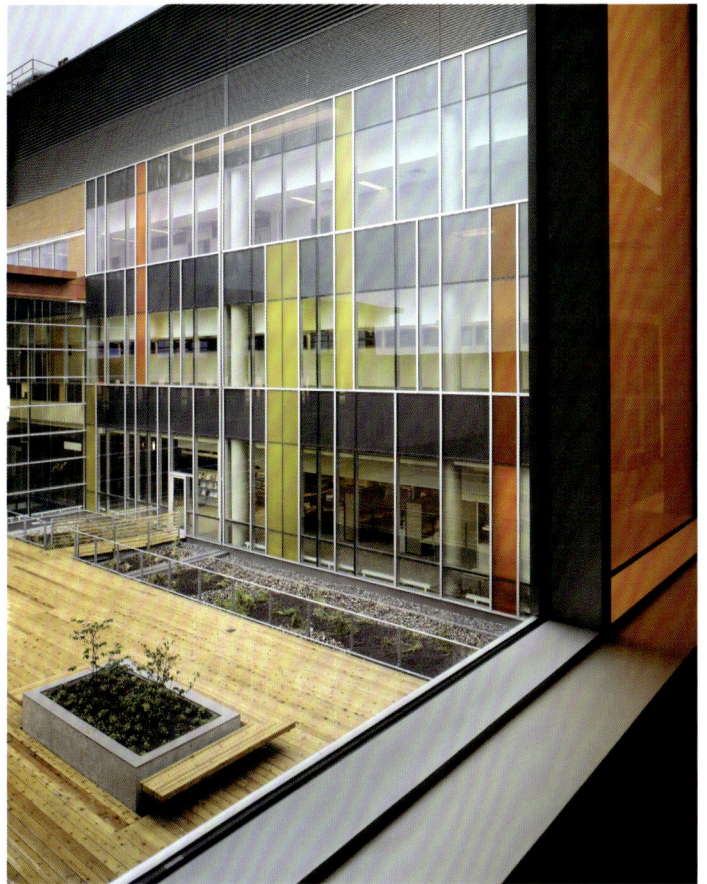

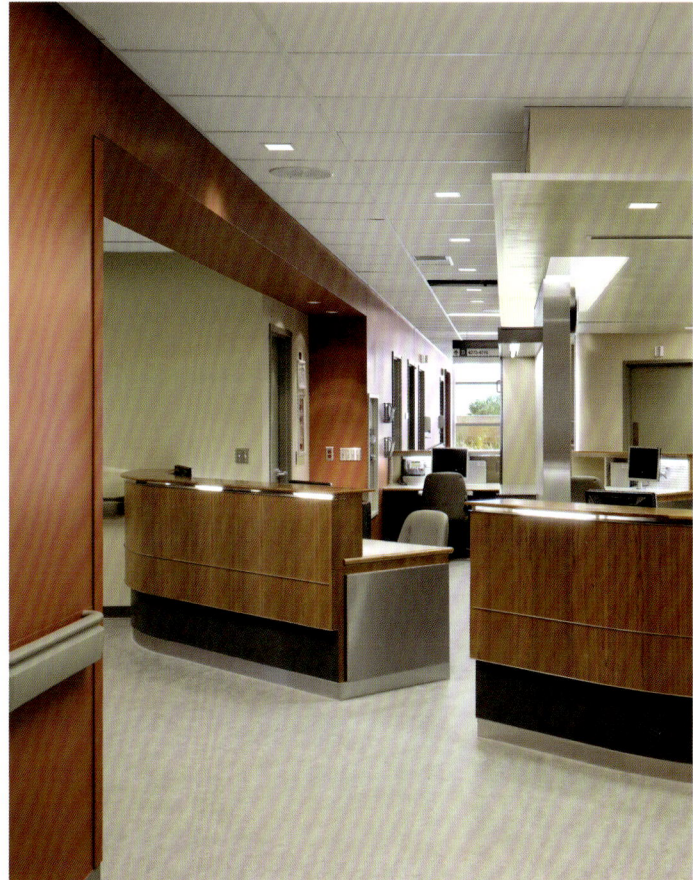

252

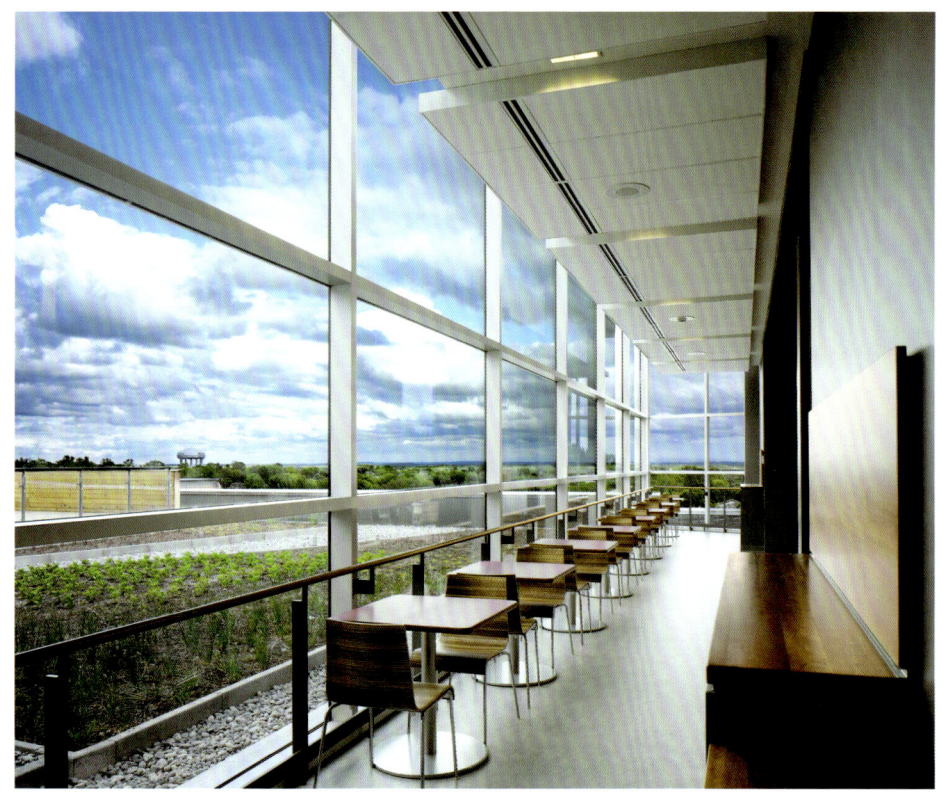

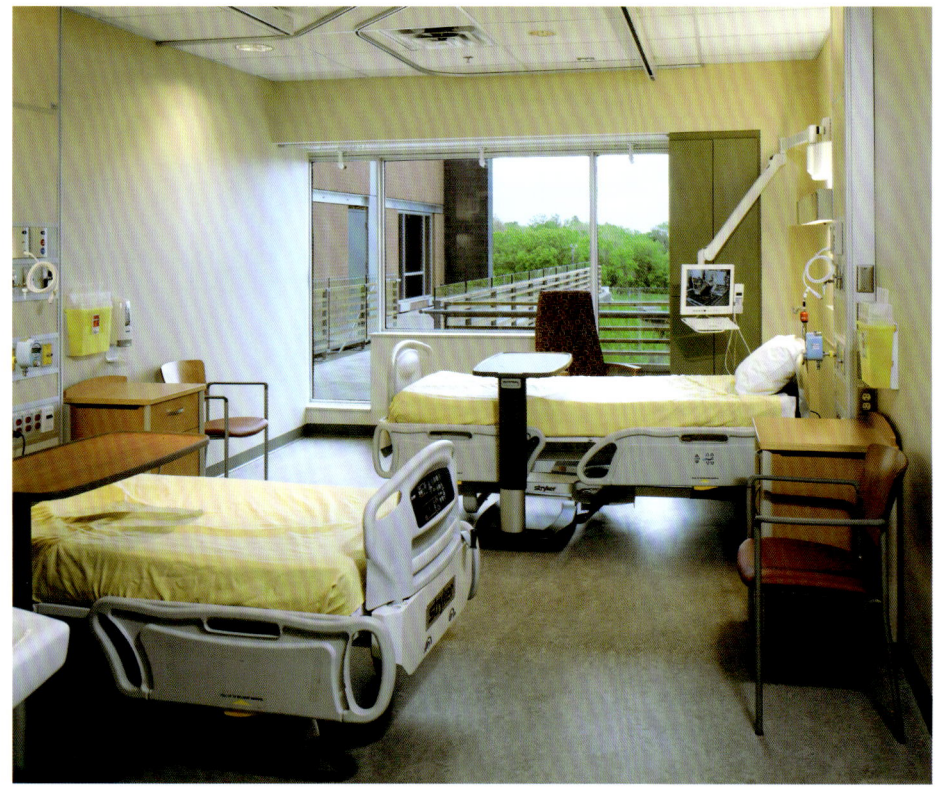

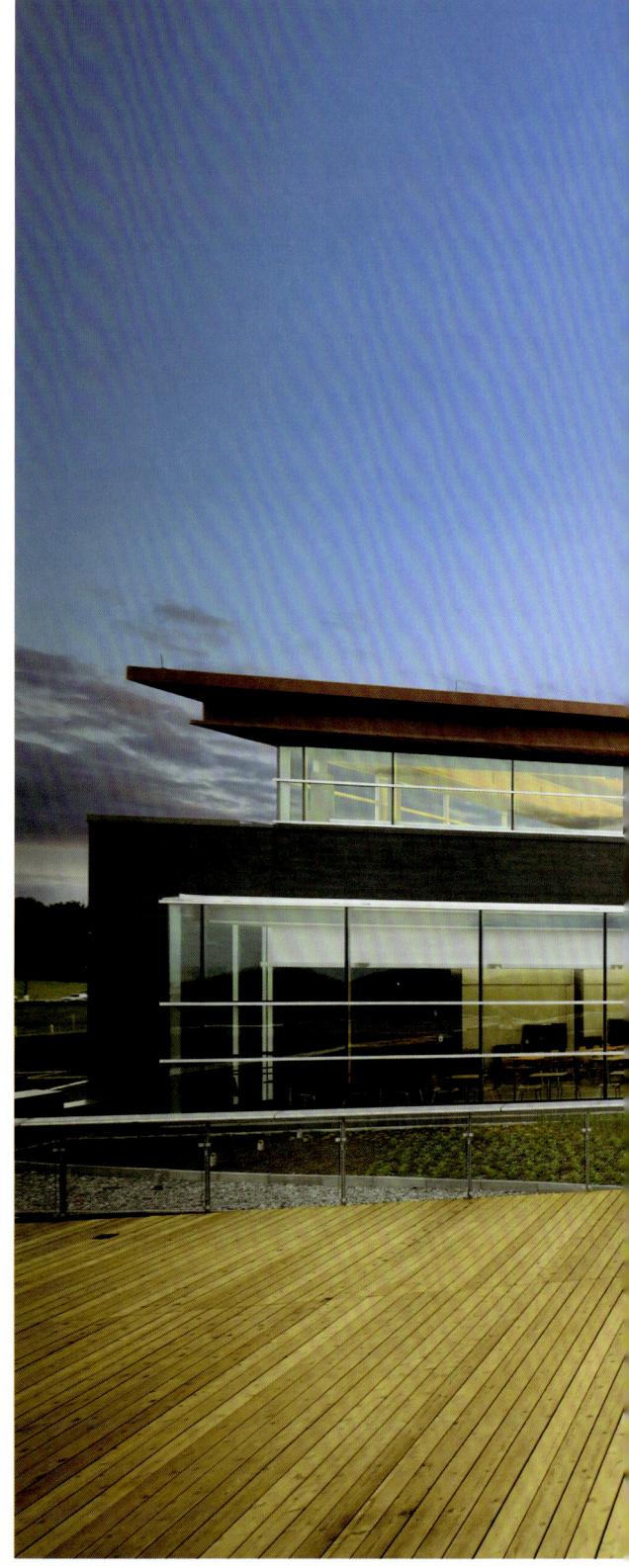

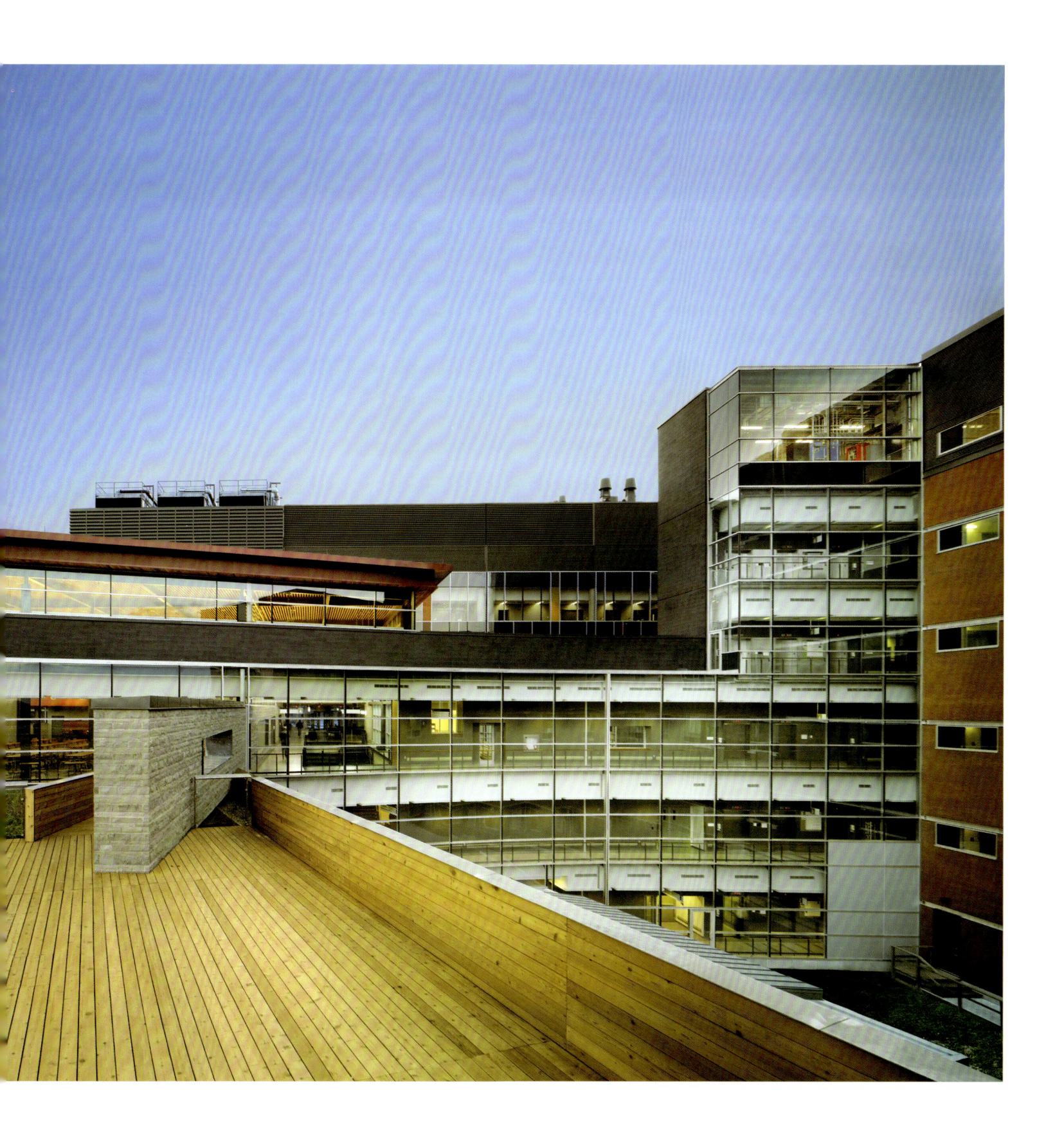

Carvajal + Casariego Baquerizo Cruz Petrement

Marqués de Valdecilla Hospital

Santander, Spain

Photographs: *Luis Asín and Carvajal Casariego*

The site was originally occupied at its northern end by a large building which, as a consequence of its unstructured development, joined all the hospital services in a disordered manner. In the central area is a series of pavilions developed for administration and outpatient treatment. With the exception of the restored pavilion used for management and as a funeral home, the southern section of the plot was used for installations like laundry services, energy centers and water tanks.

A series of ideas formed the basis for the general restructuring of the hospital. The general image of the hospital needed to be transformed, reducing the existing spatial confusion and improving the poor quality constructions. All work needed to be carried out allowing the hospital to continue to operate with as little interference as possible.

It was decided to preserve all the central pavilions for both historical and compositional reasons. A large plinth was created to house the general services crowned by a landscaped roof. The pavilions emerge from this area recovering their lost aesthetical value. The plinth contains the basements of the pavilions and allows for close proximity between the general services, while the large terrace injects tranquility into the heart of the hospital. The slope of the plot was used to order the different entrances and stagger the buildings, thereby softening the impact the hospital has on its urban surroundings.

The circulation system develops on different levels. A network for internal services, including delivery of food and supplies and for staff circulation, connects with areas such as the kitchens, pharmacy, storage rooms etc. A separate external network is intended for outpatients and visitors and begins with the large entrance hall to the north, where elevators lead to the wards, and develops into a passageway that penetrates the hospital in a north-south direction

The plot is organized into three parallel, staggered areas: the wards to the north, where galleries establish links between all the pavilions; general services in the center of the site inside the plinth that incorporates the basements of the pavilions and the outpatient departments to the south which overlook a landscaped square above the parking. The entrance hall is located within the rectangular floor plan to allow for the outpatient areas to be positioned on one side and the consulting rooms and surgeries on the other.

The location of the wards around the periphery permits easy access to the central services from the wards and from the outpatient departments in an ordered way, and with exclusive circulation routes that avoid crossovers between internal and external routes.

Client:
Cantabria Health Service
Surface area:
110,000 sqm (1,180,000 sqft)
Start date:
2000
Finish date:
2007
Project team:
Pedro Casariego, Genaro Alas, Jose Manuel Baquerizo, Fernando Cruz, Carlos Petrement, Gádor de Carvajal, Juan Casariego
Collaborators:
Victoriano Gorostegui, Patricia Reznak, Alicia Montero, Francisco López, Mario Pascual, Alfredo Navarro, Iñigo Prieto, Virginia Aguilar
Contractor:
FCC, UTE. OHL, S.A. - Arruti Santander S.A.

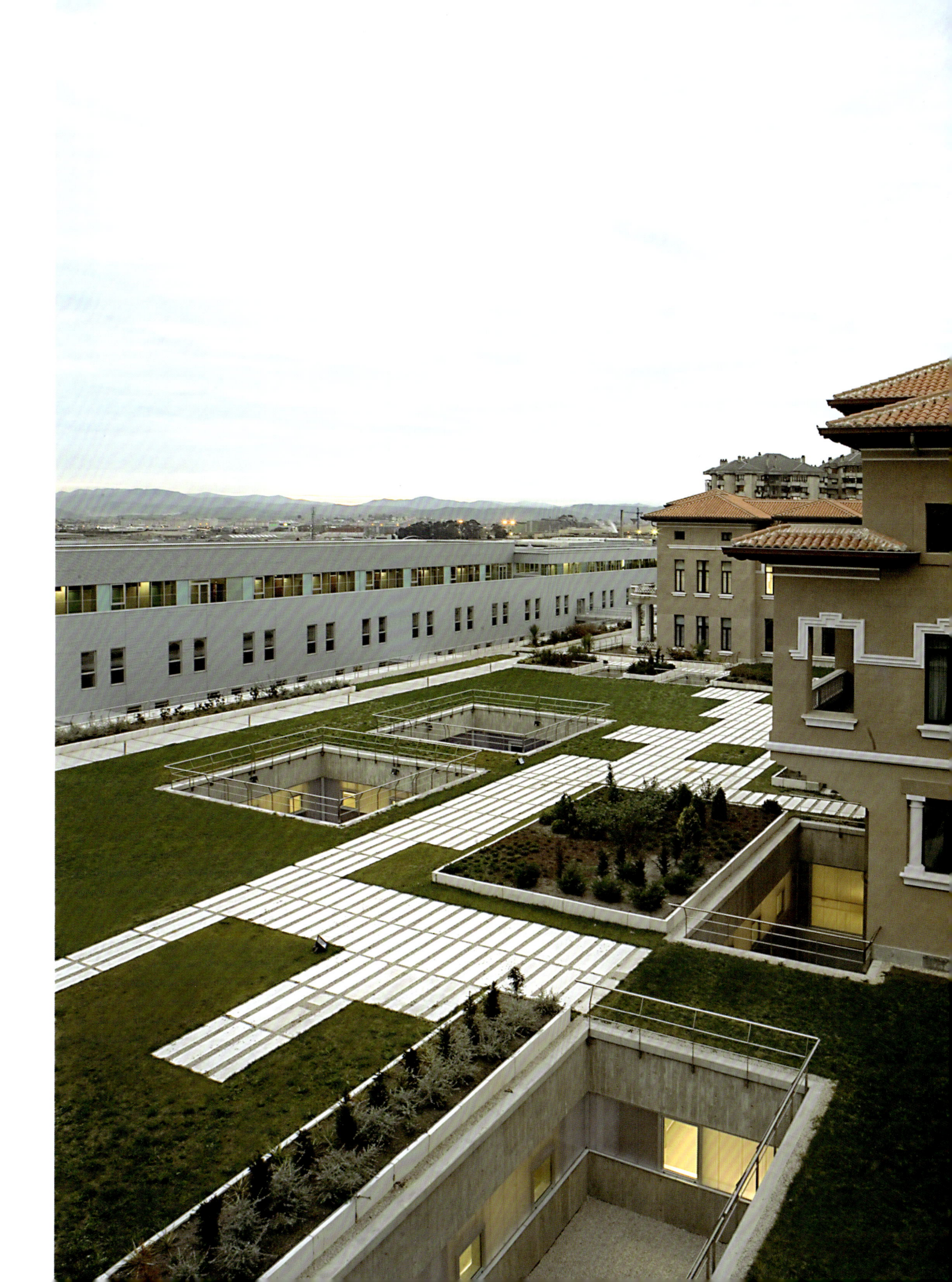

PHASE 1

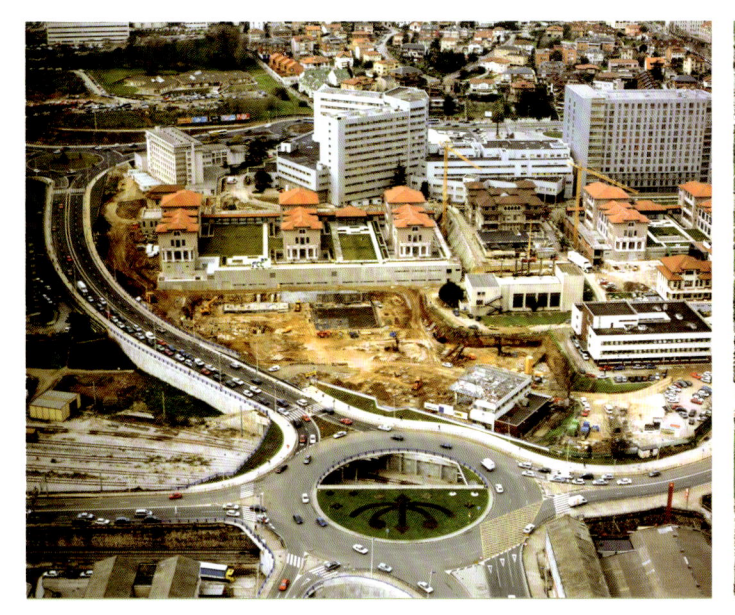

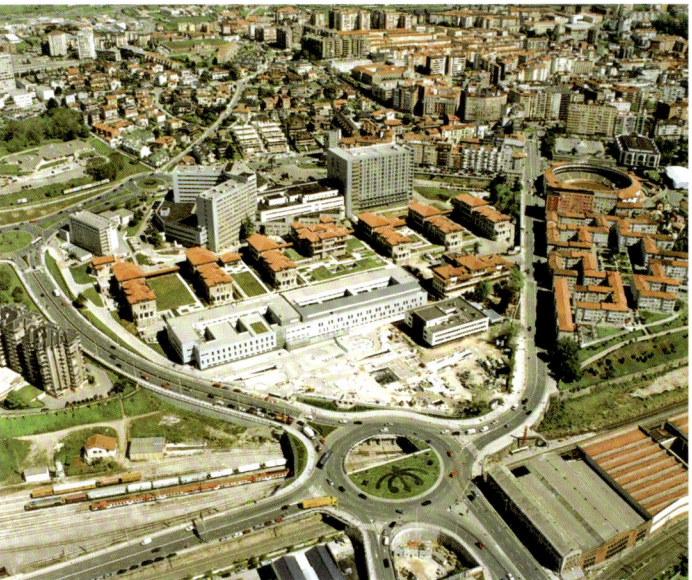

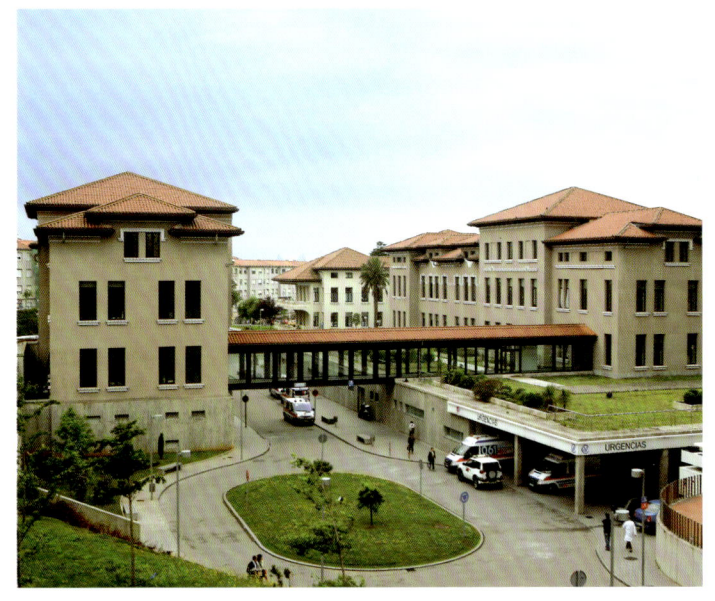

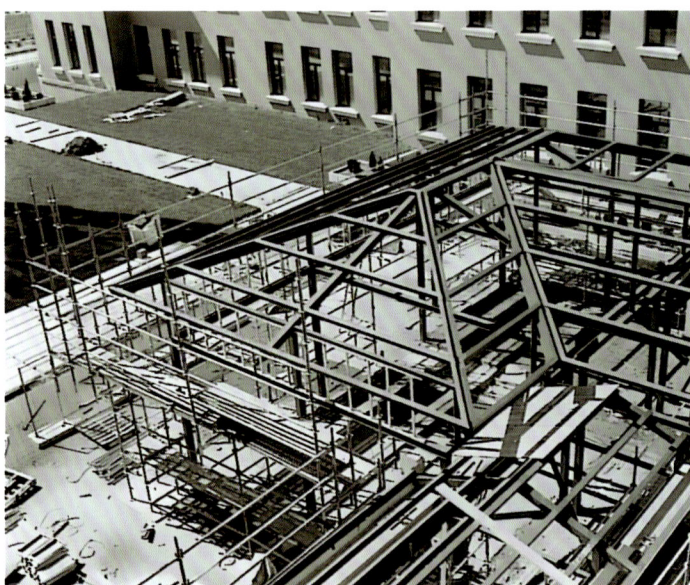

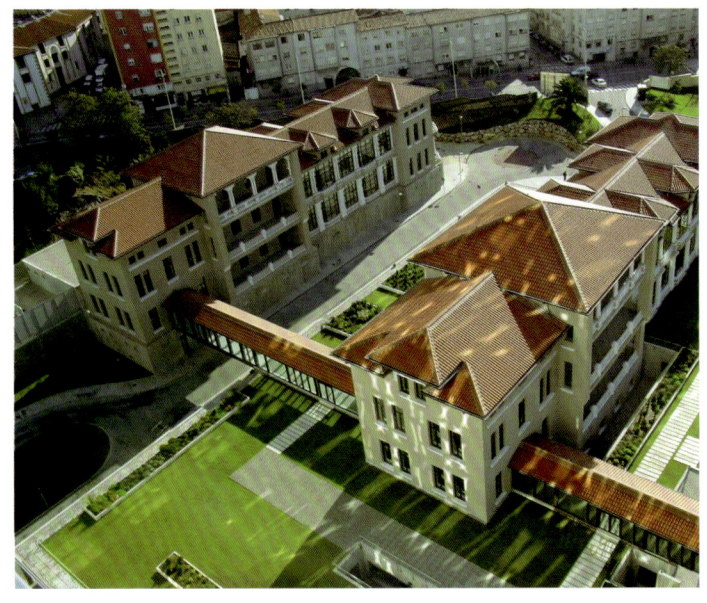

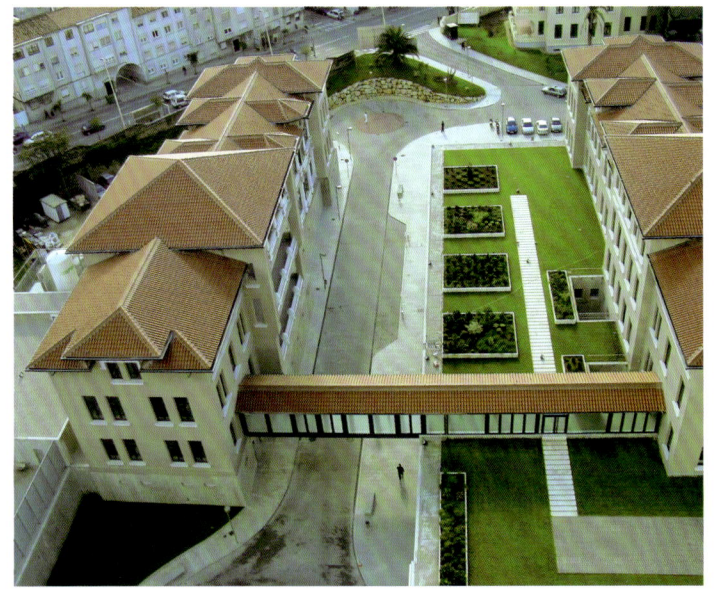

256

257

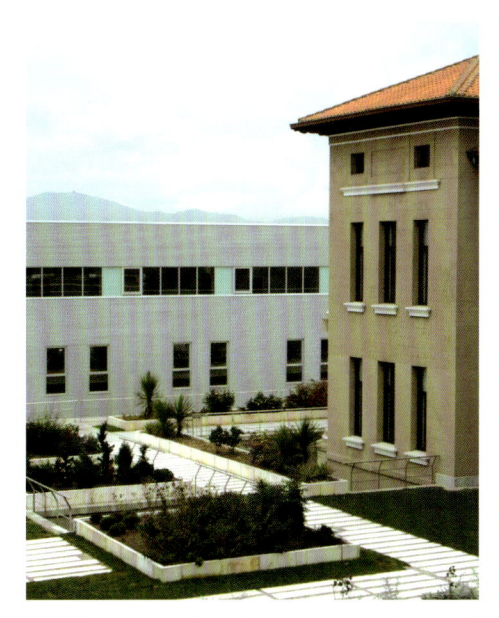

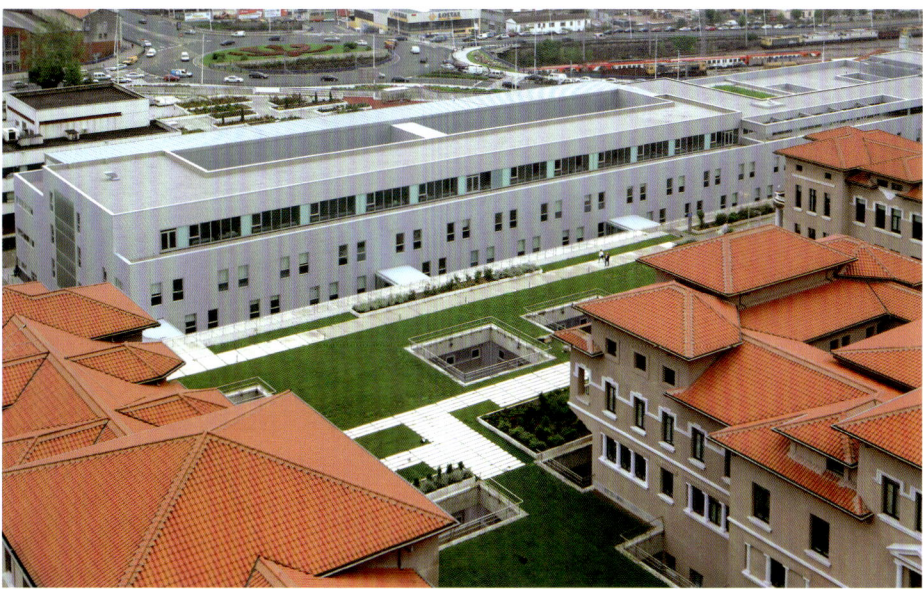

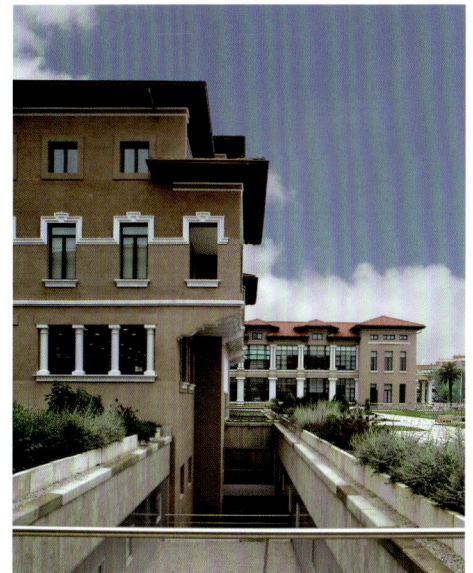

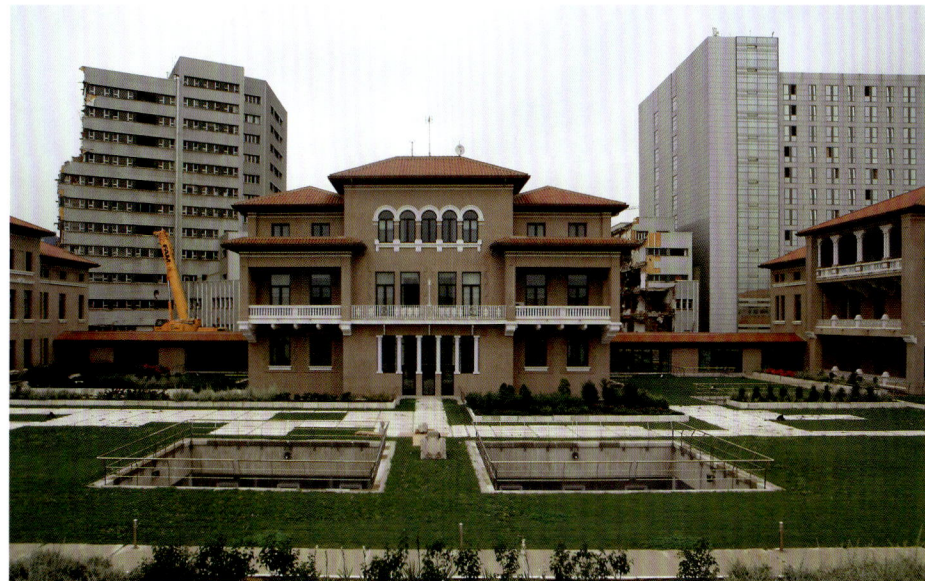

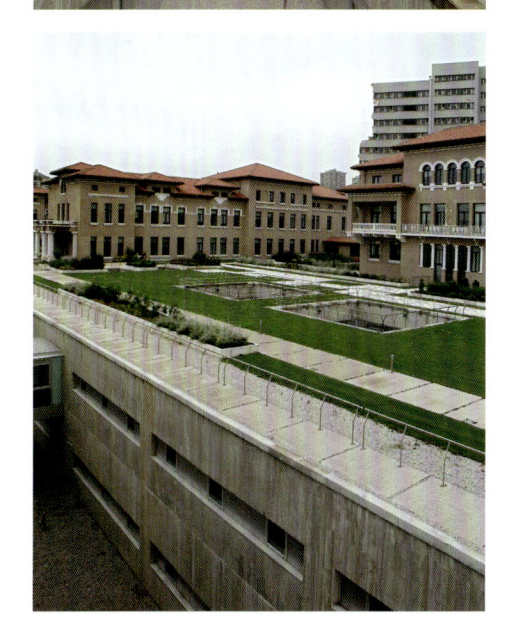

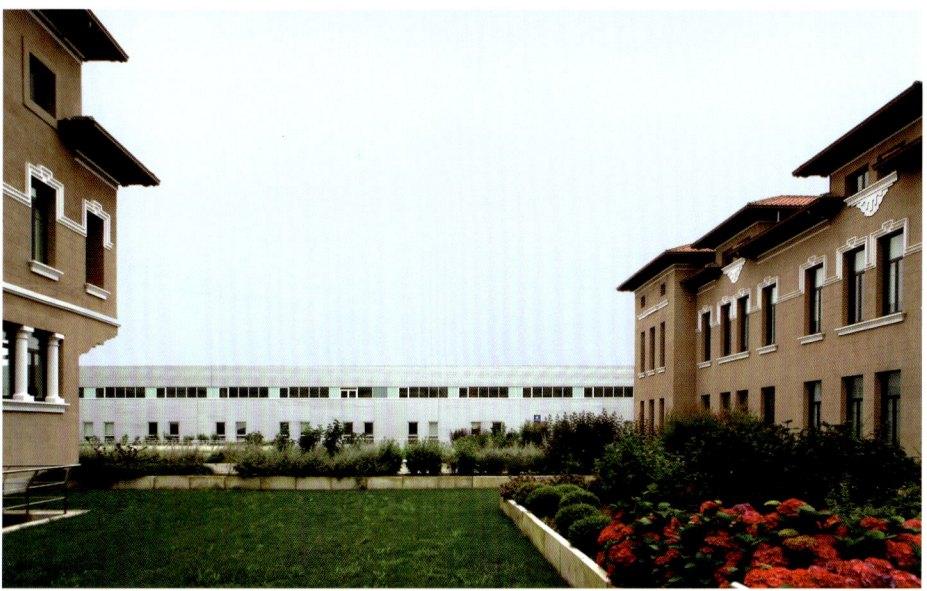

258

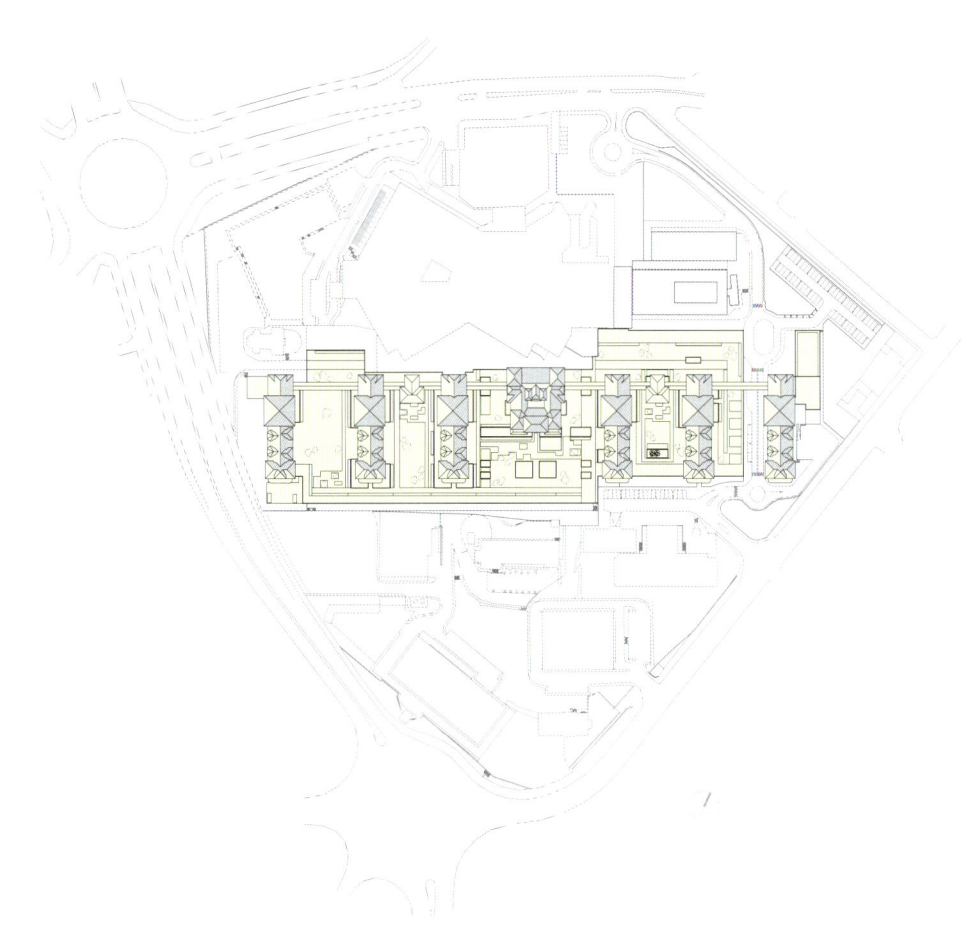

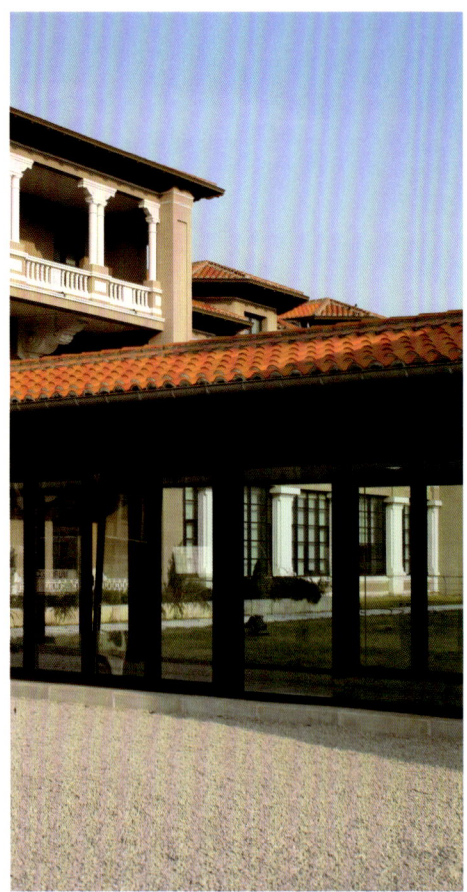

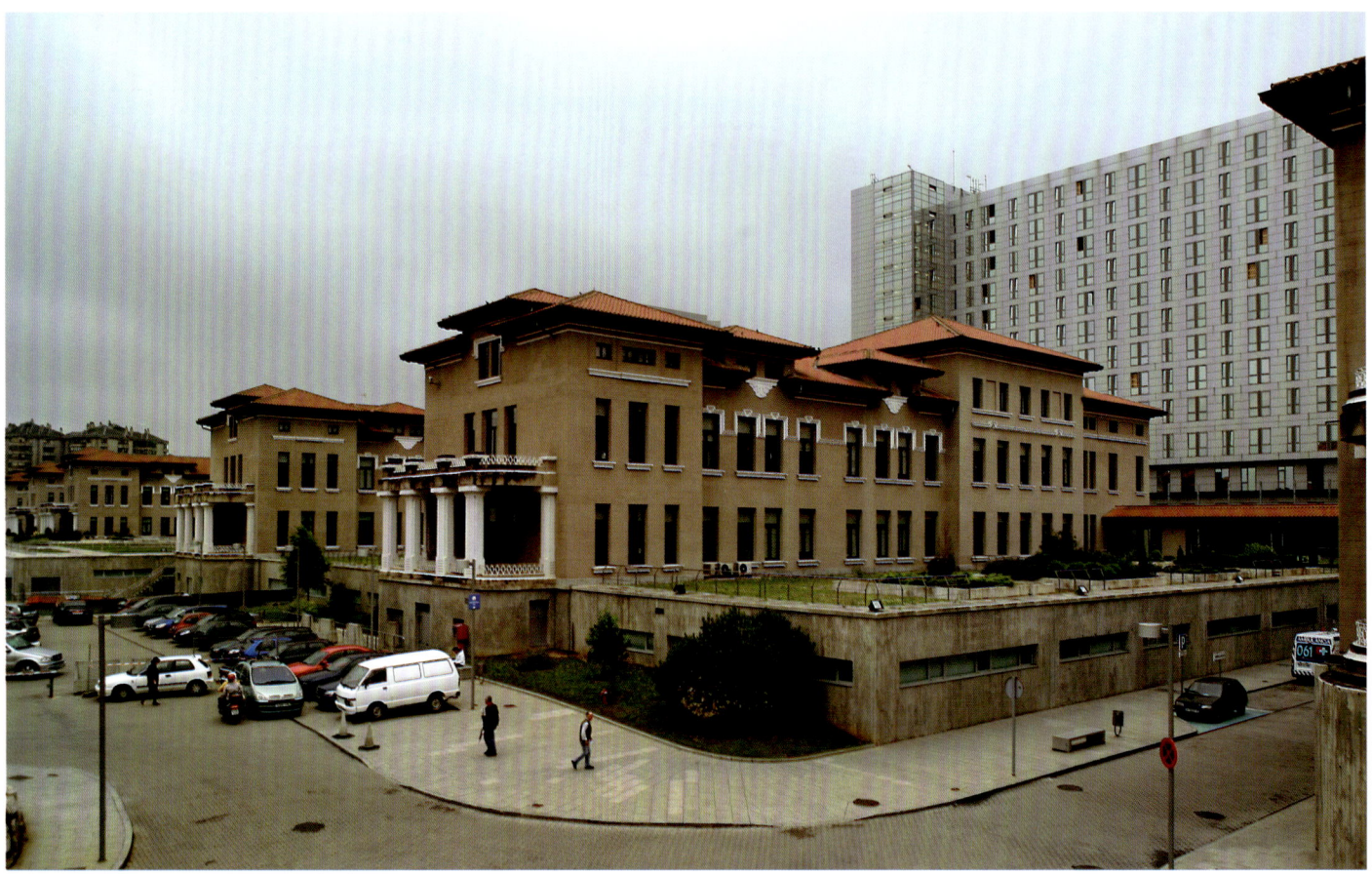

It was decided to preserve all the central pavilions for both historical and compositional reasons. A large plinth was created to house the general services crowned by a landscaped roof. The pavilions emerge from this area recovering their lost aesthetical value. The plinth contains the basements of the pavilions and allows for close proximity between the general services, while the large terrace injects tranquility into the heart of the hospital.

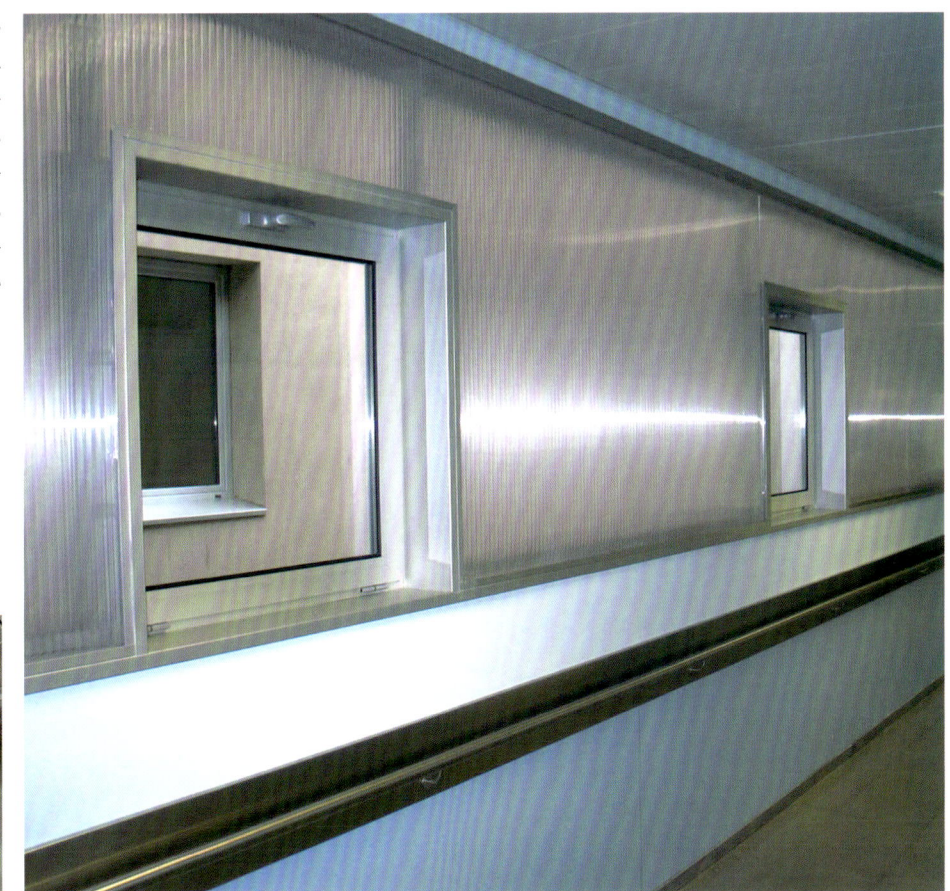

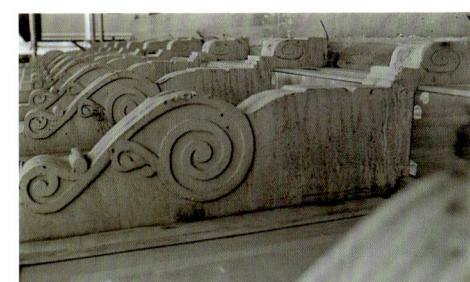

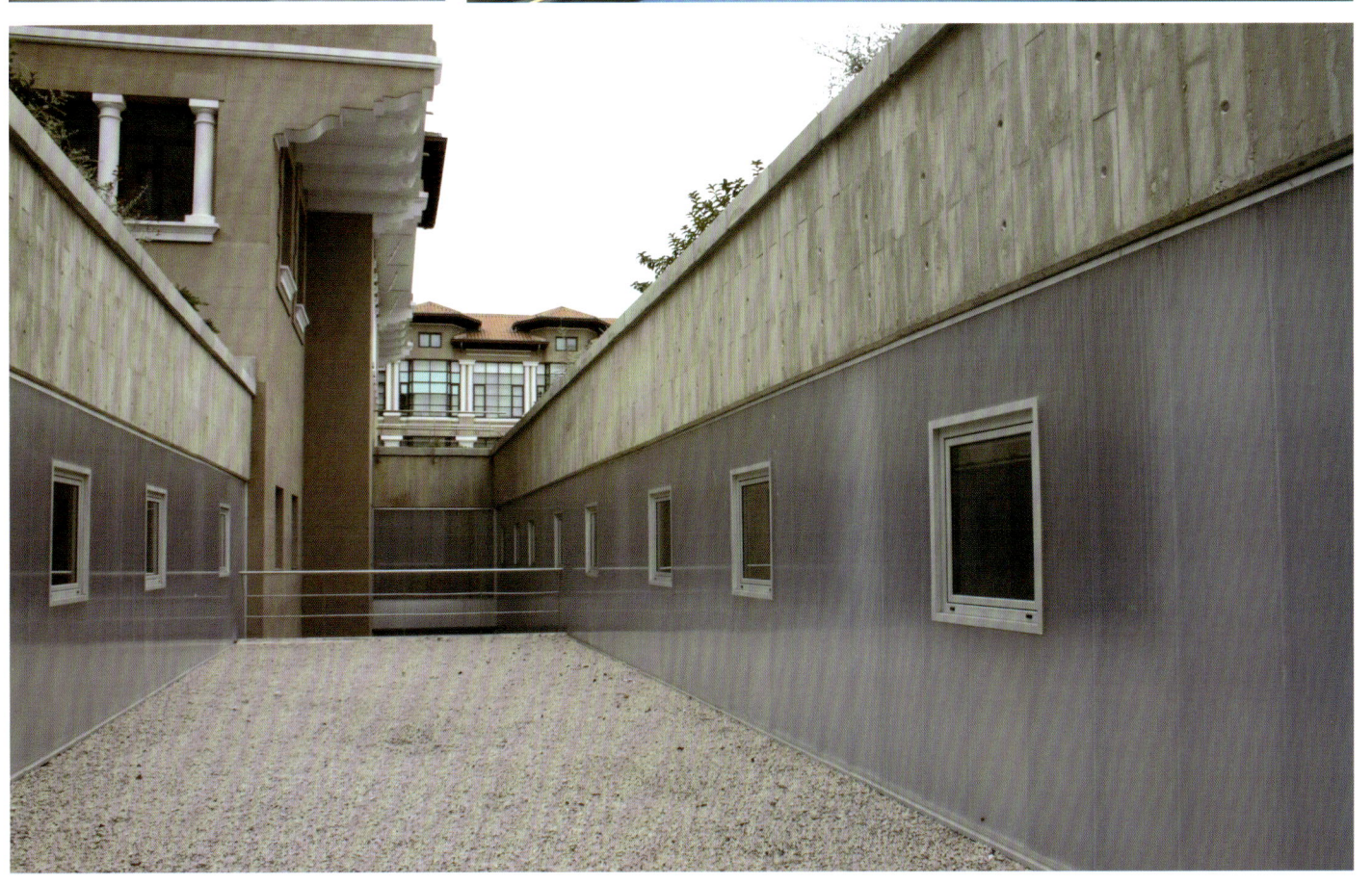

Roof plan

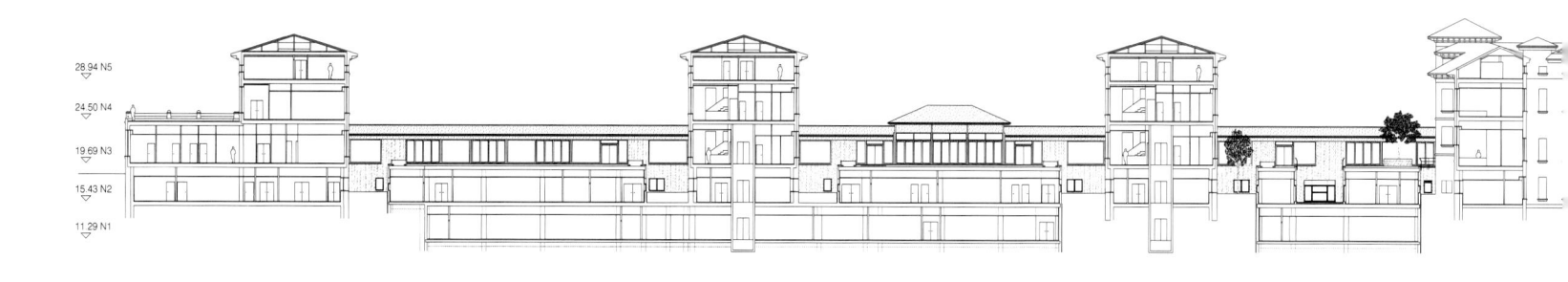

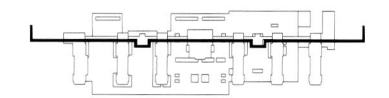

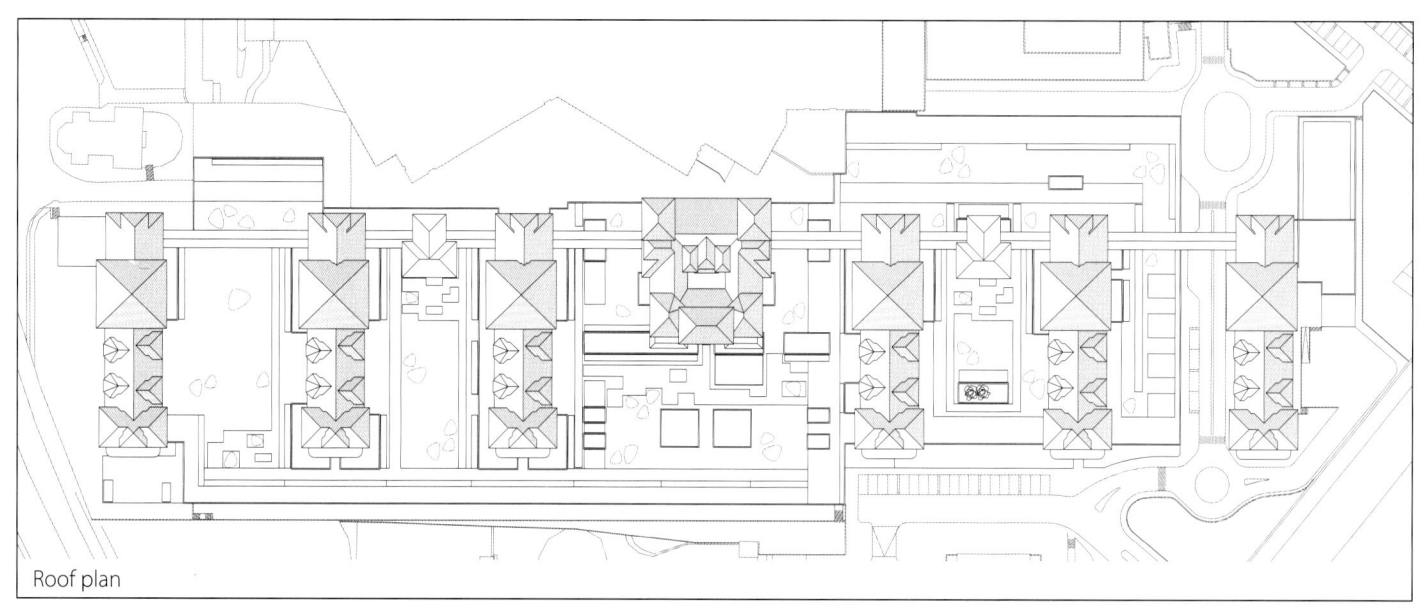

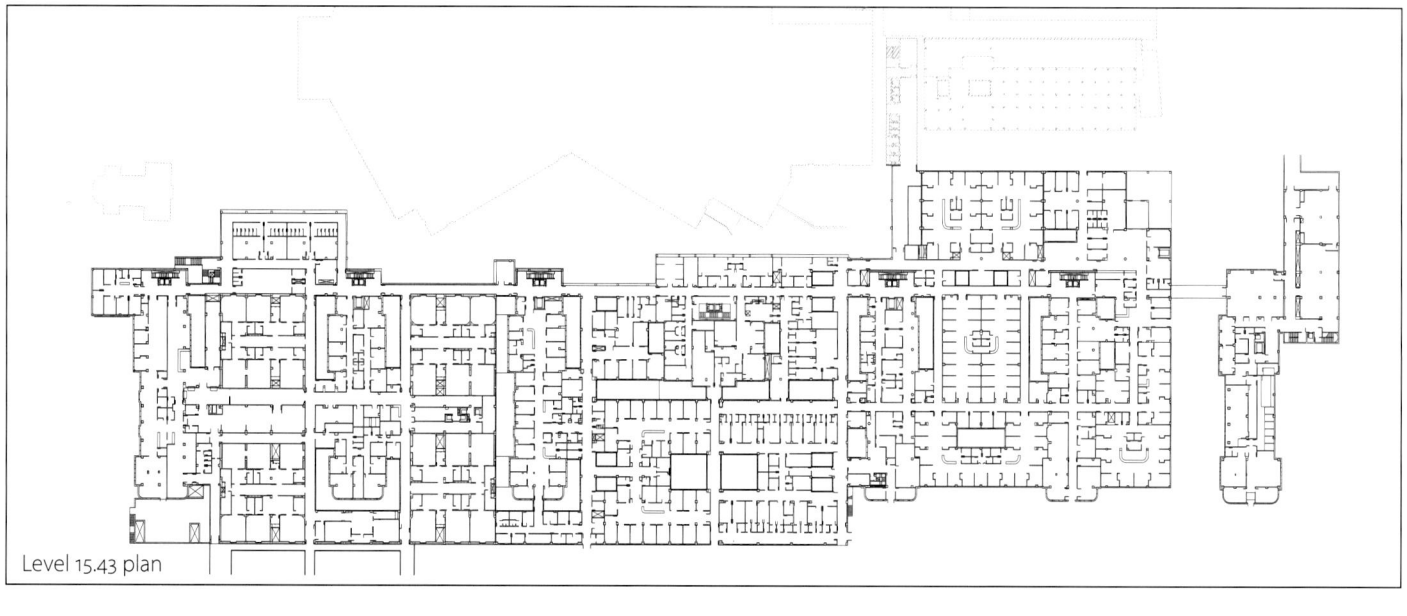

Level 15.43 plan

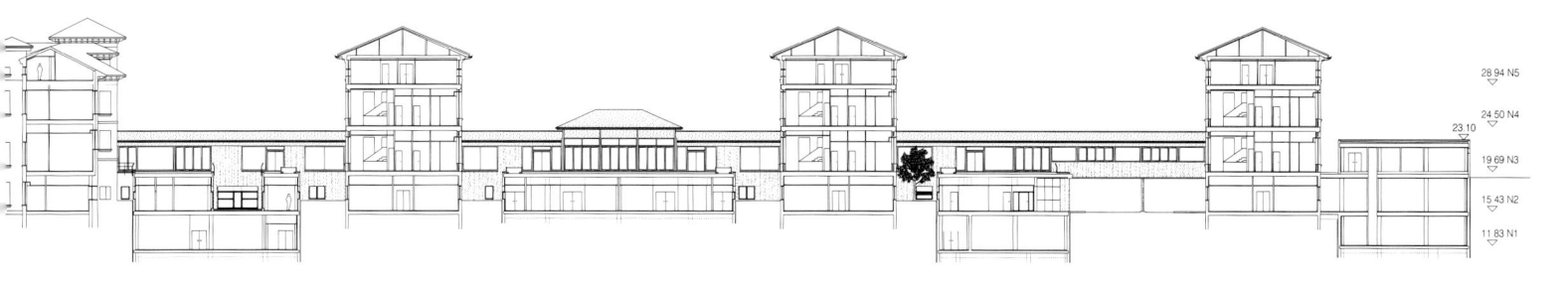

Cross section

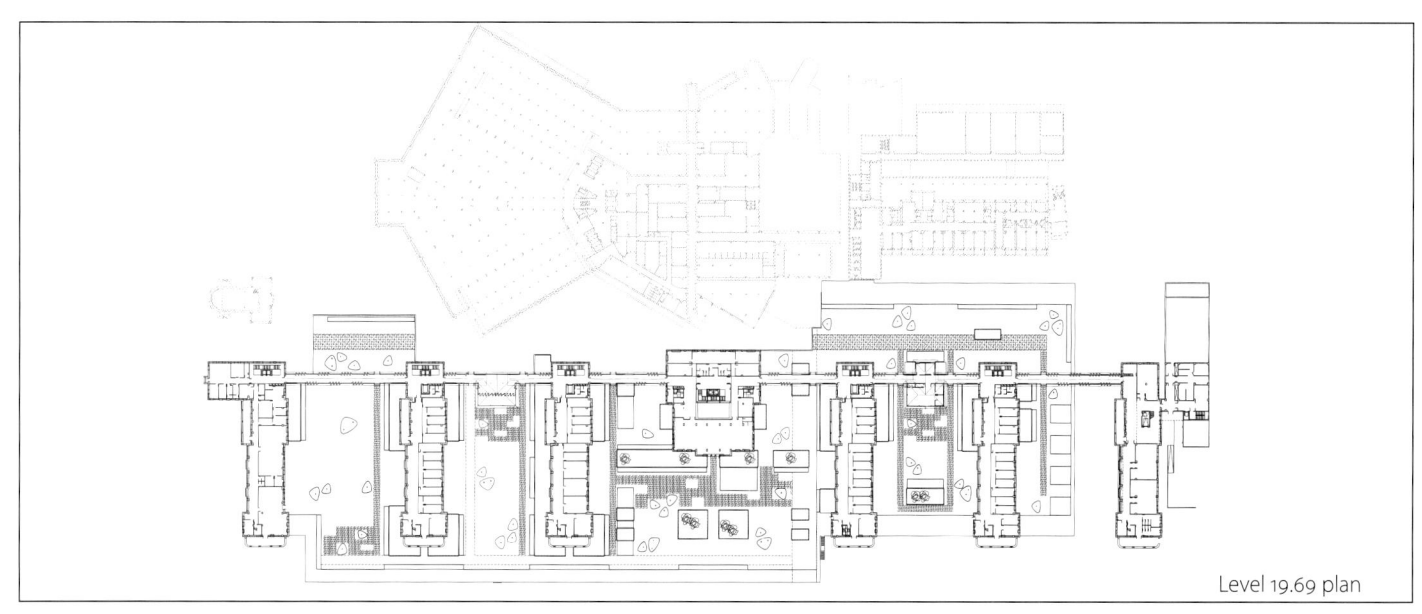

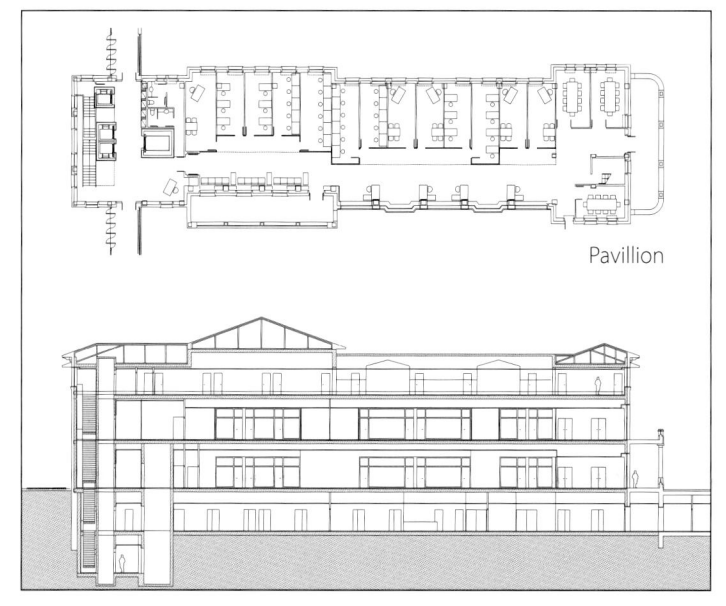

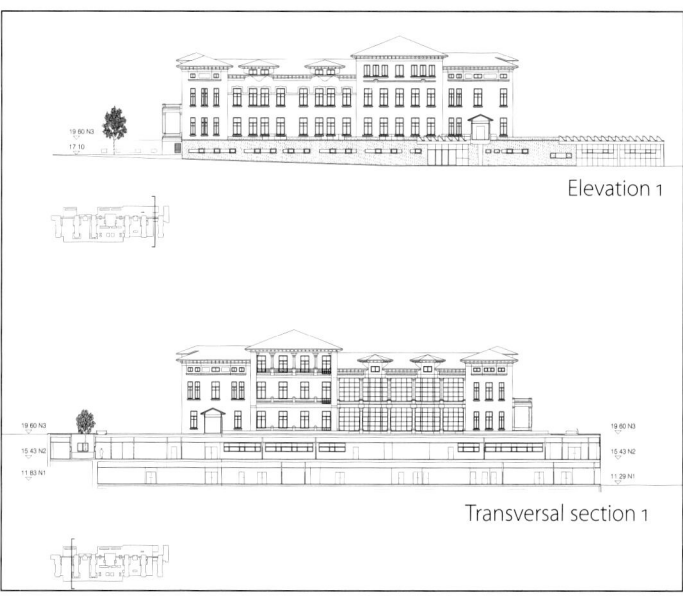

Level 19.69 plan

Pavillion

Elevation 1

Transversal section 1

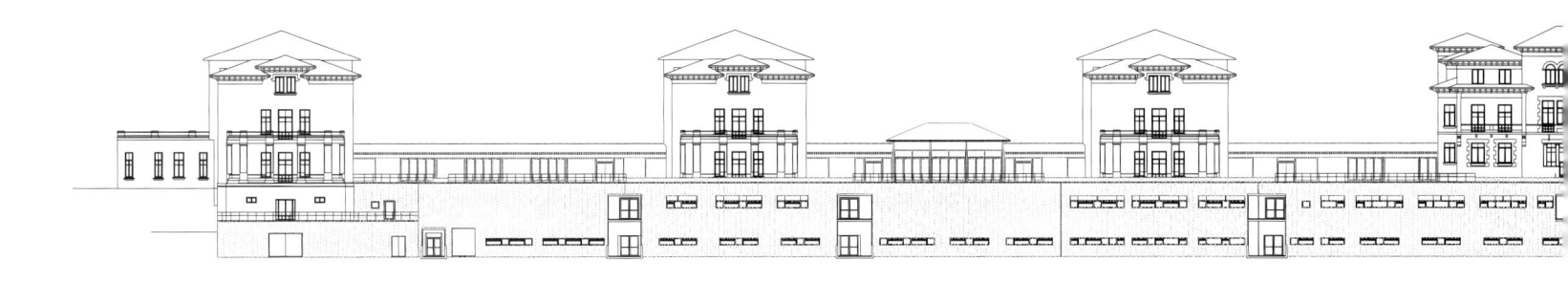

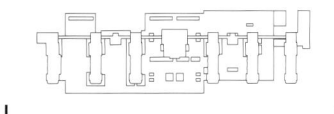

Elevation 2

Details of South elevation

1. Plantation of shrub-like species
2. Enriched organic soil: terracotem min. 50cm
3. Felt: geotextile 150 G/M2ç
4. Membrane: drentemper H:60mm
5. Waterproof layer: PVC P 1.2mm
6. Felt: geotextile 300 g/m2
7. Self-leveling mortar: no slope, min. 2cm
8. Concrete planter: pre-fabricated
9. Slab: reinforced concrete 40 cm
10. Sprayed insulation: 4cm
11. Conditioned space for duct installation
12. Dropped ceiling: pladur N15
13. Floor tiles: agglomerate cement: T.Vacutile EQ. 60x40
14. Fixing mortar
15. Hollow core slab
16. Sanitary airspace
17. Non-structural wall: reinforced concrete, thickness 30cm, metal formwork.
18. Gravel: marble
19. Imprinted pavement: reinforced concrete, 8cm thick, with 1.5% slope.
20. Flashing: concrete. Pre-fabricated
21. Wall: reinforced concrete. 22cm textured wooden formwork
22. Insulated double wall panel: type Pladur-metal or alike (15+15+50)
23. Exterior door jam, reinforced concrete, formwork unconcealed
24. Aluminum carpentry, transparent and translucent glass+opaque areas of Trespa panel
25. Velthec glass (6/25/4+4) with venetian blind inside the airspace between the panes
26. Substructure of carpentry of #150.50.4mm every 1.80m fixed to outside wall of reinforced concrete
27. Baseboard: polyester resin agglomerate 100x8mm.
28. Trespa panel suspended from substructure of the carpentry
29. Substructure of carpentry of #150.50.4mm every 1.80m fixed to outside wall of reinforced concrete and edge of slab
30. Gutter of lacquered sheet-metal +soundproofing
31. Mouth of opening finished with lacquered DM board, thickness:15mm.
32. Drip flashing of folded sheet metal, with waterproof beading
33. Wall of reinforced concrete, 30cm., cast, fairfaced.
34. Waterproof layer, double
35. Drainage membrane
36. Flooring: clinker blocks, thickness: 5cm.
37. Trespa panel, thickness: 1cm.

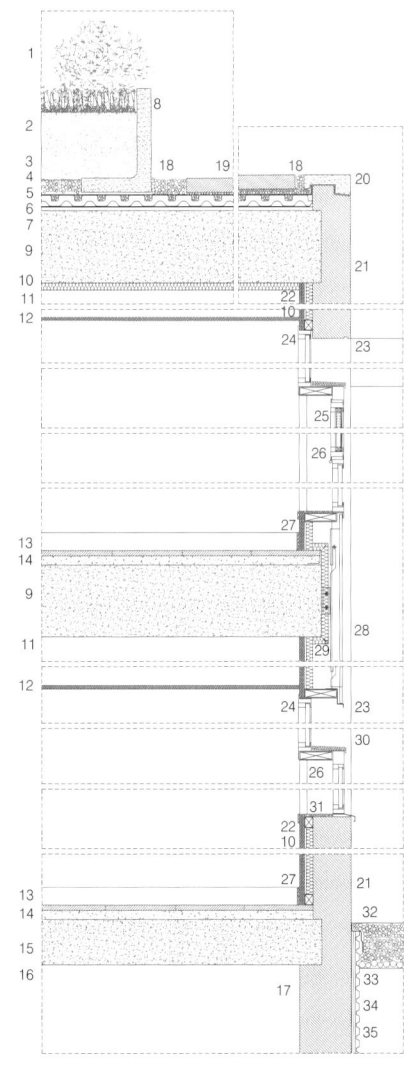

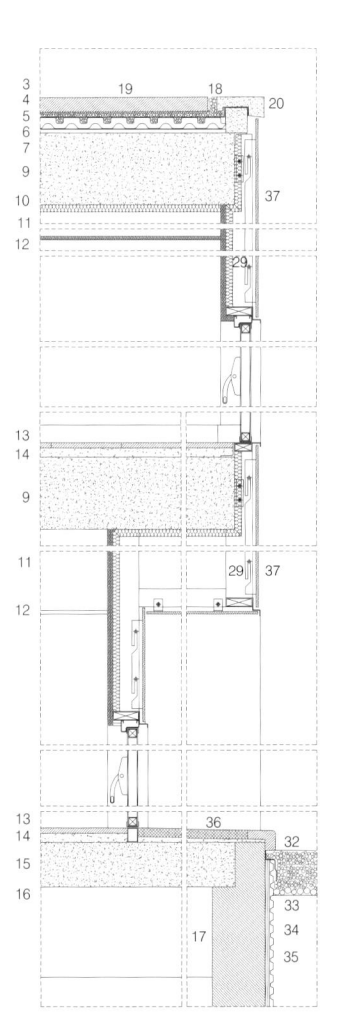

D4 Tipo

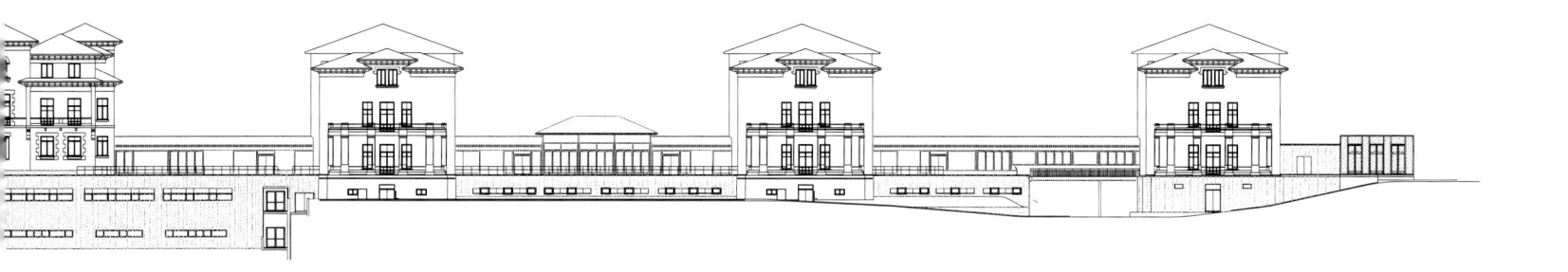

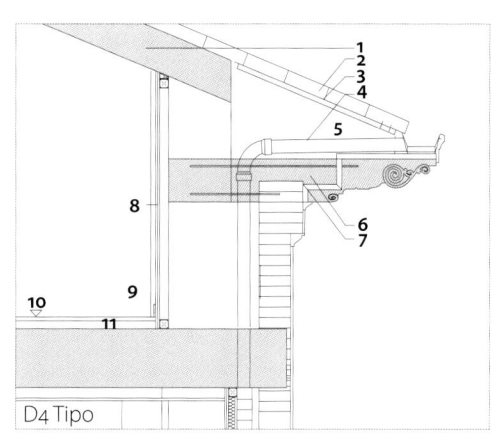

1. Slab, inclined, reinforced concrete cast in situ
2. Tiles, pre-existing
3. Prefabricated concrete flashing
4. Storm-water drainage pipe
5. Slope 1.5%
6. Prefabricated concrete flashing
7. Wooden board, as pre-existing
8. Pladur (1.5+1.5) on angles 70mm
9. Floor-tiles
10. Level +28.94 P.A
11. Fixing mortar (6cm)

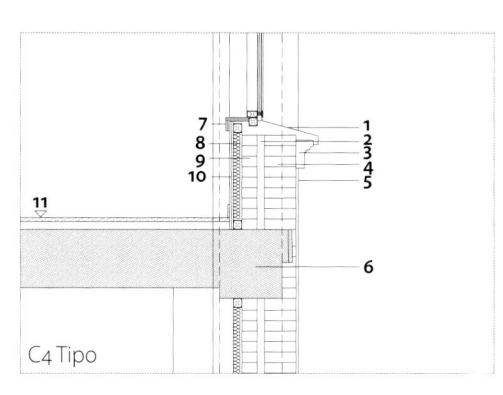

C4 Tipo

1. Prefabricated molded concrete piece
2. Ventilation chamber. Width: 11cm
3. Prefabricated molded concrete piece
4. Solid masonry foot
5. Rendering 2cm
6. Prefabricated slab
7. DM board 2cm
8. Sprayed insulation. Thickness: 4cm
9. Backing, 1/2 reinforced concrete foot. Thickness: 4 cm
10. Pladur (1.5+1.5) on angles 70mm
11. Level 4 +24.50 p.a

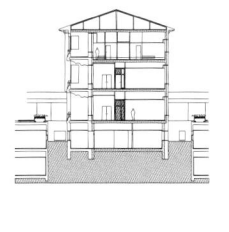

B4 Tipo

1. Slope formation
2. Molded concrete piece
3. Concrete wall
4. Level 3 +19.69 p.a.
5. Backing: Pladur metal (5.0+1.5+1.5)
6. Suspended ceiling

263

PHASE 2

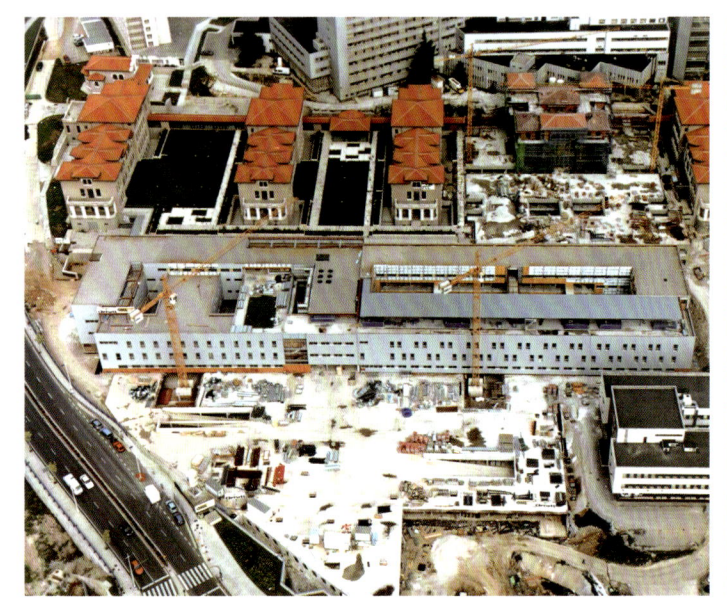

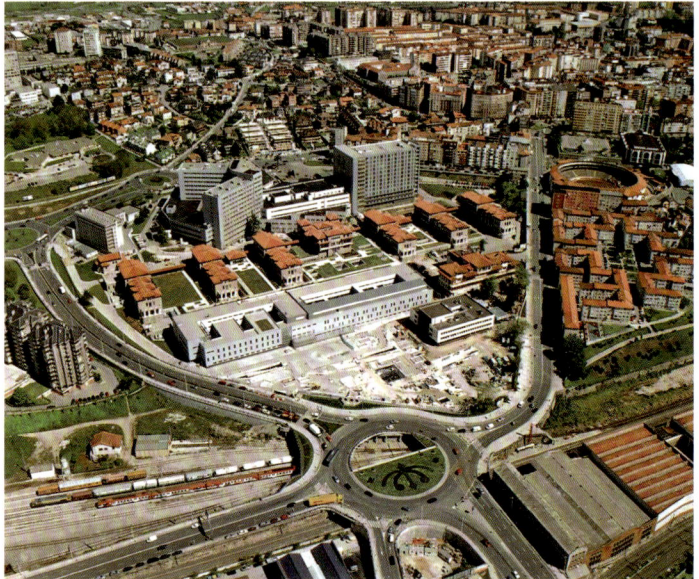

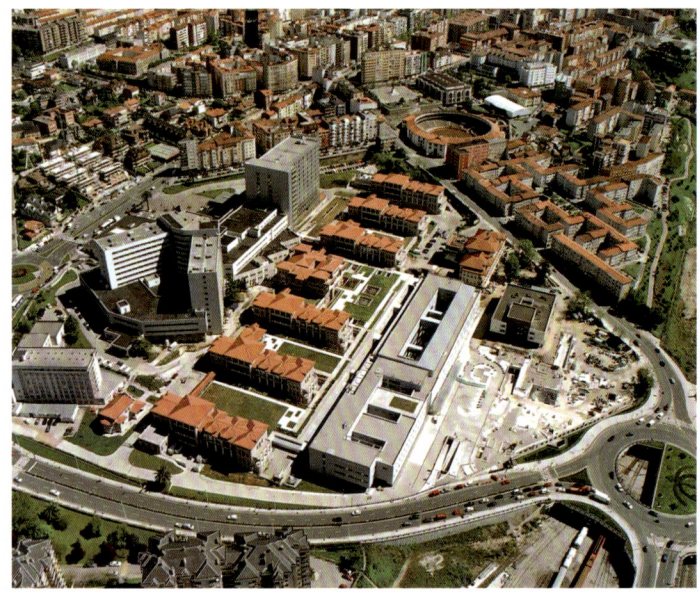

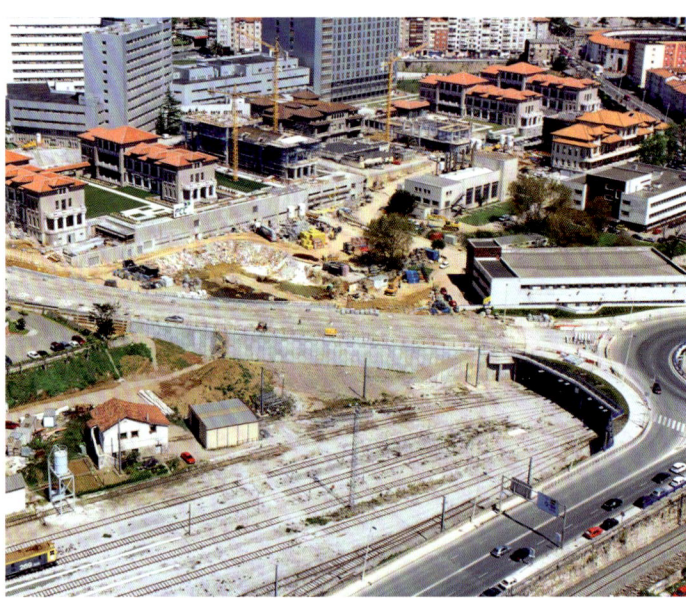

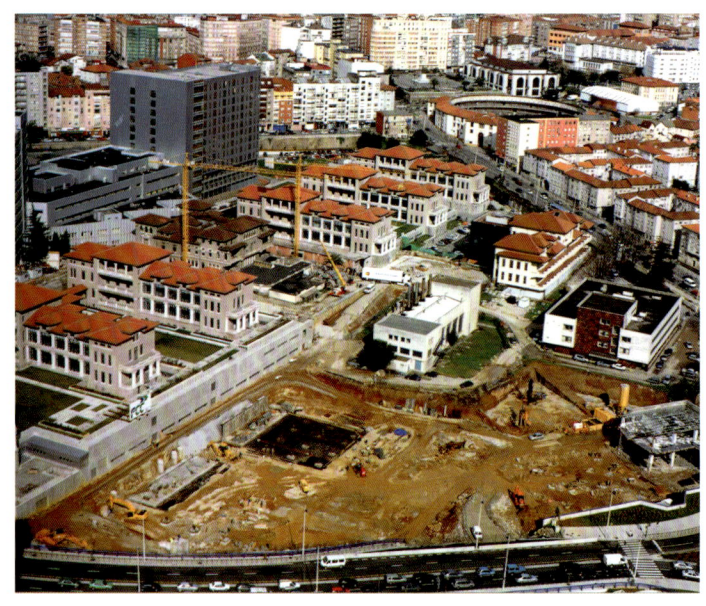

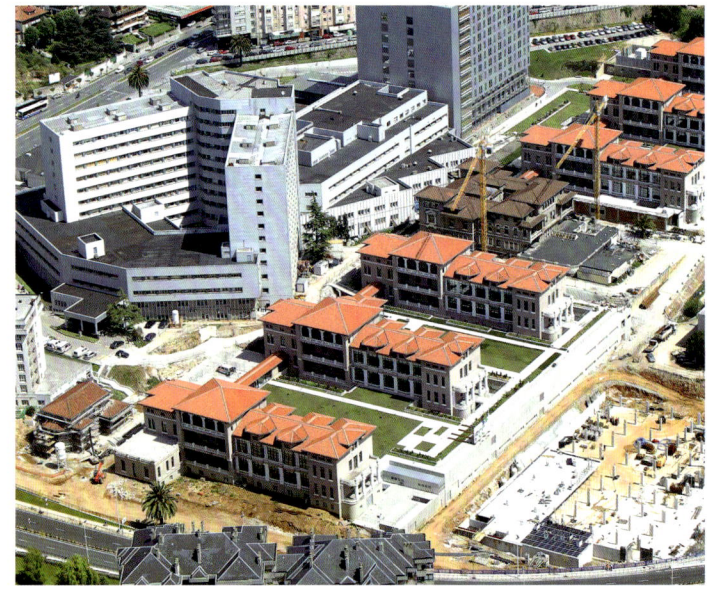

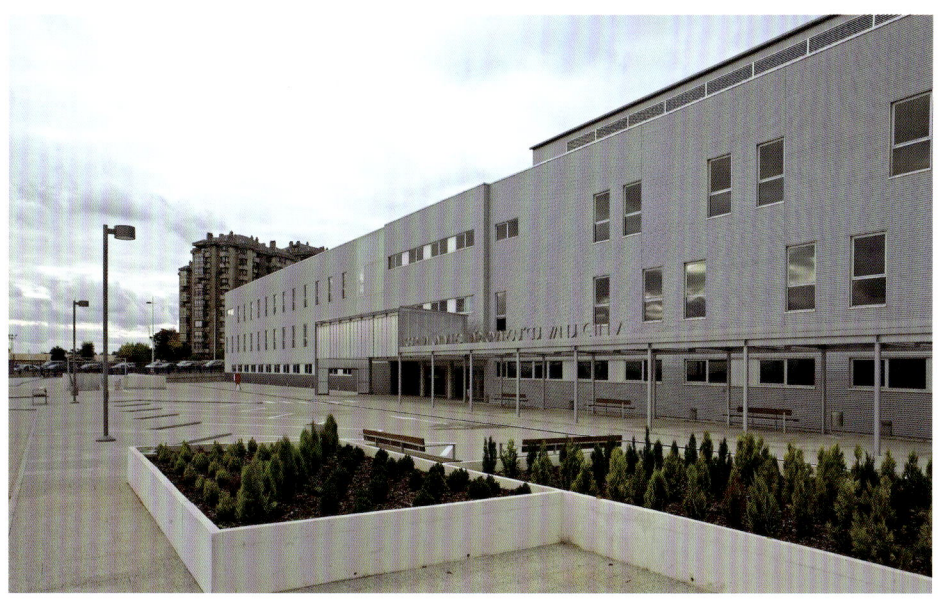

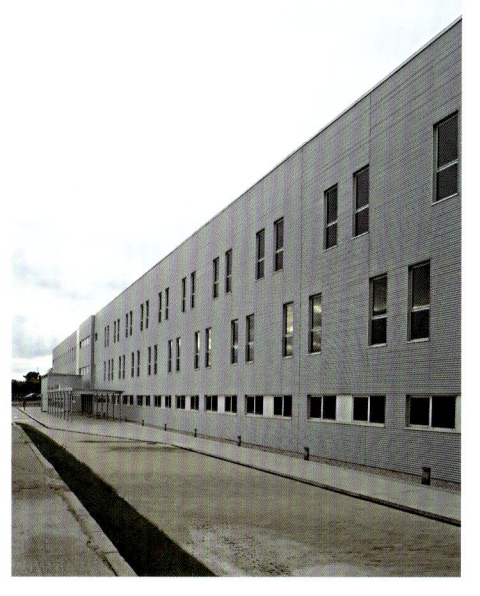

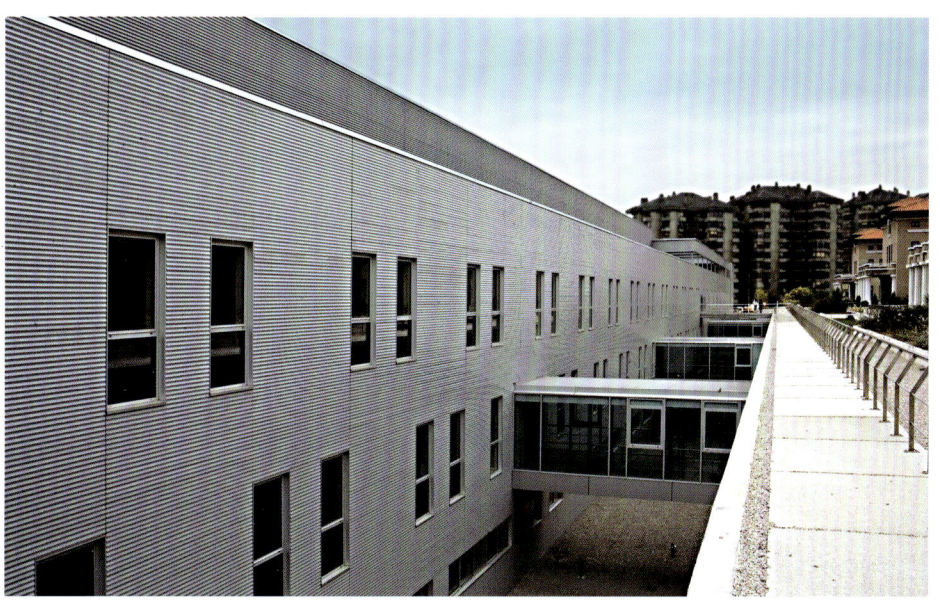

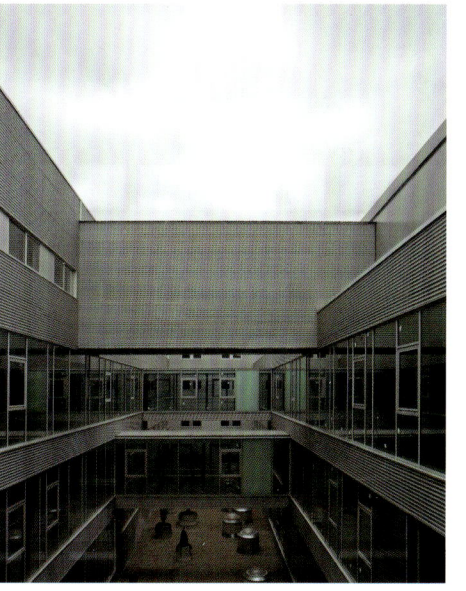

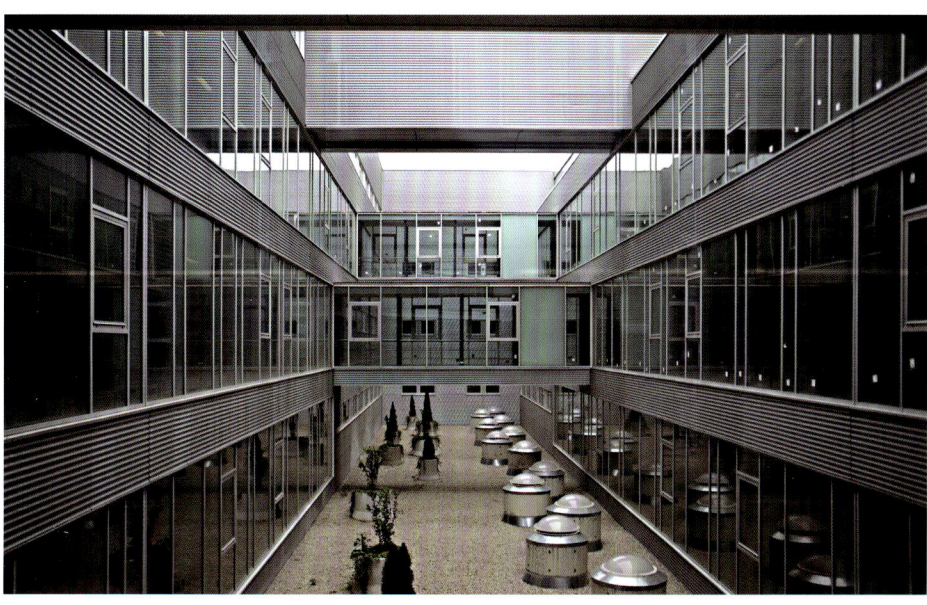

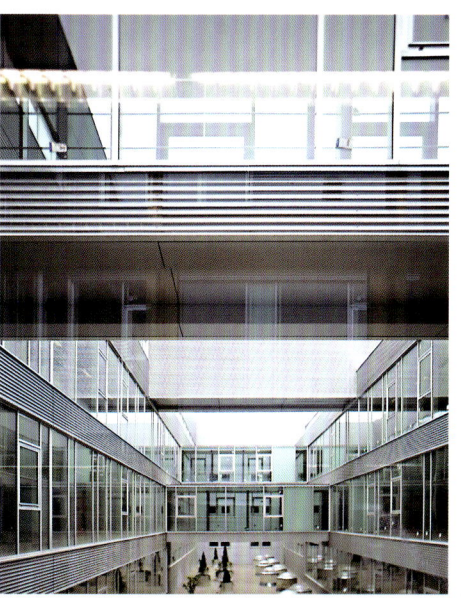

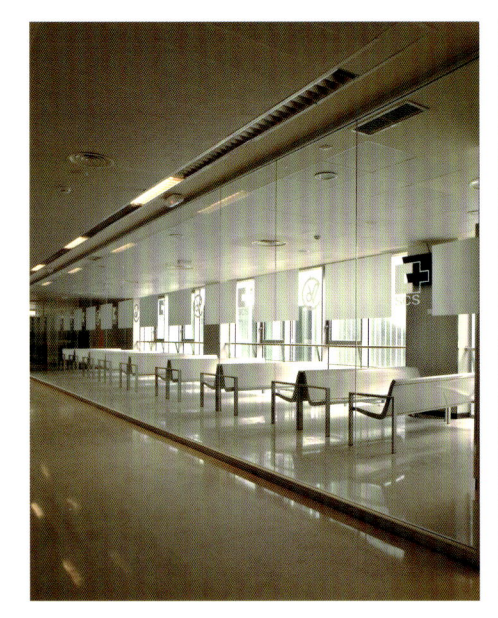

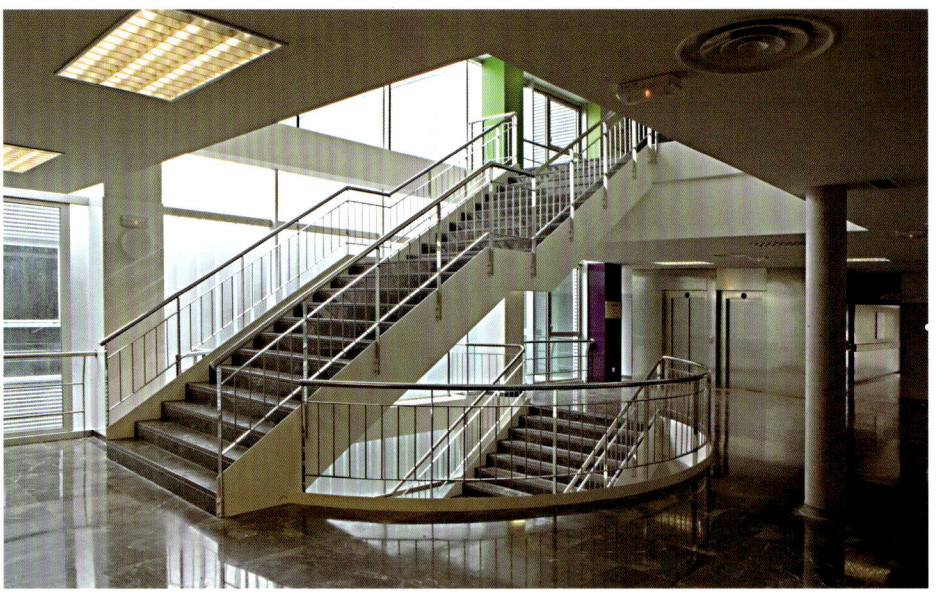

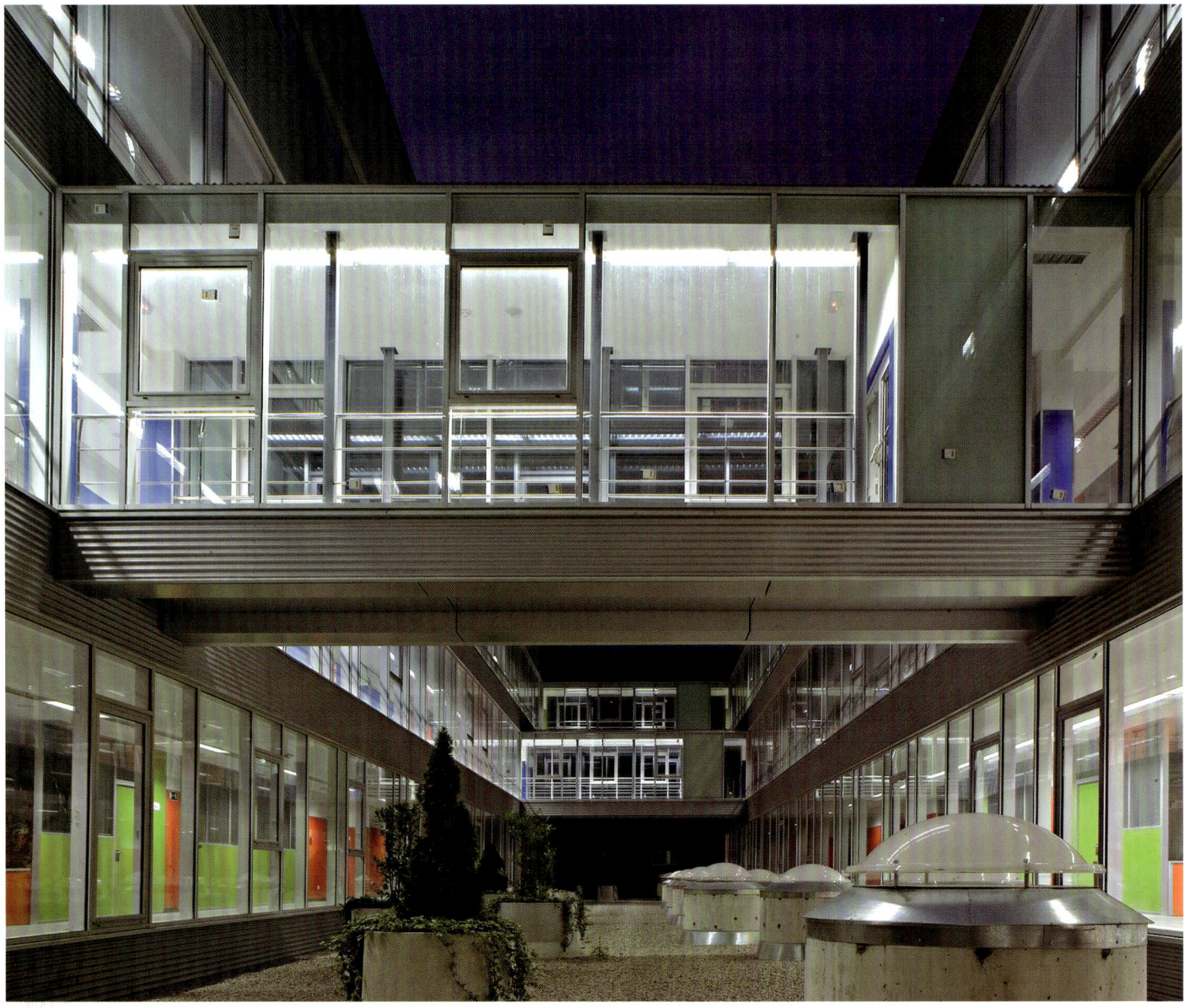

267

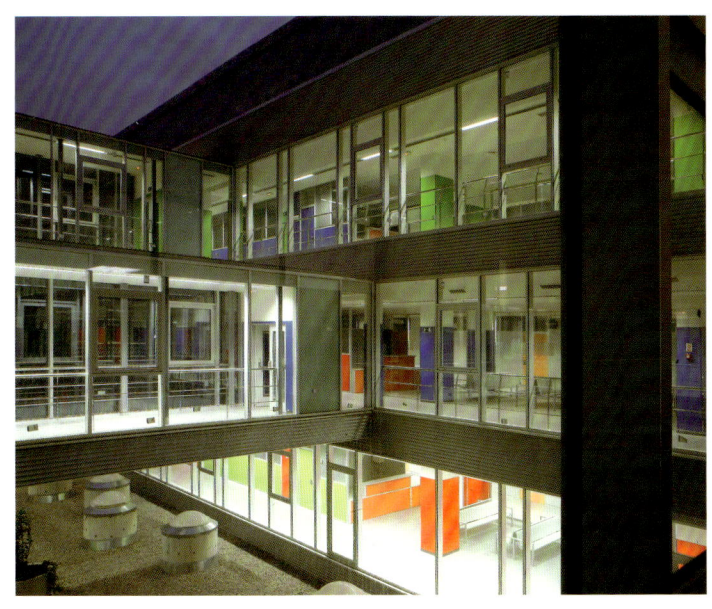

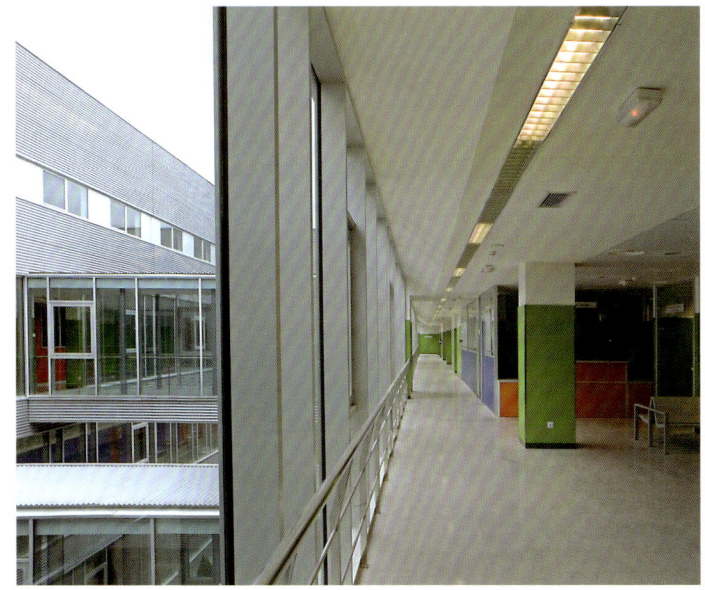

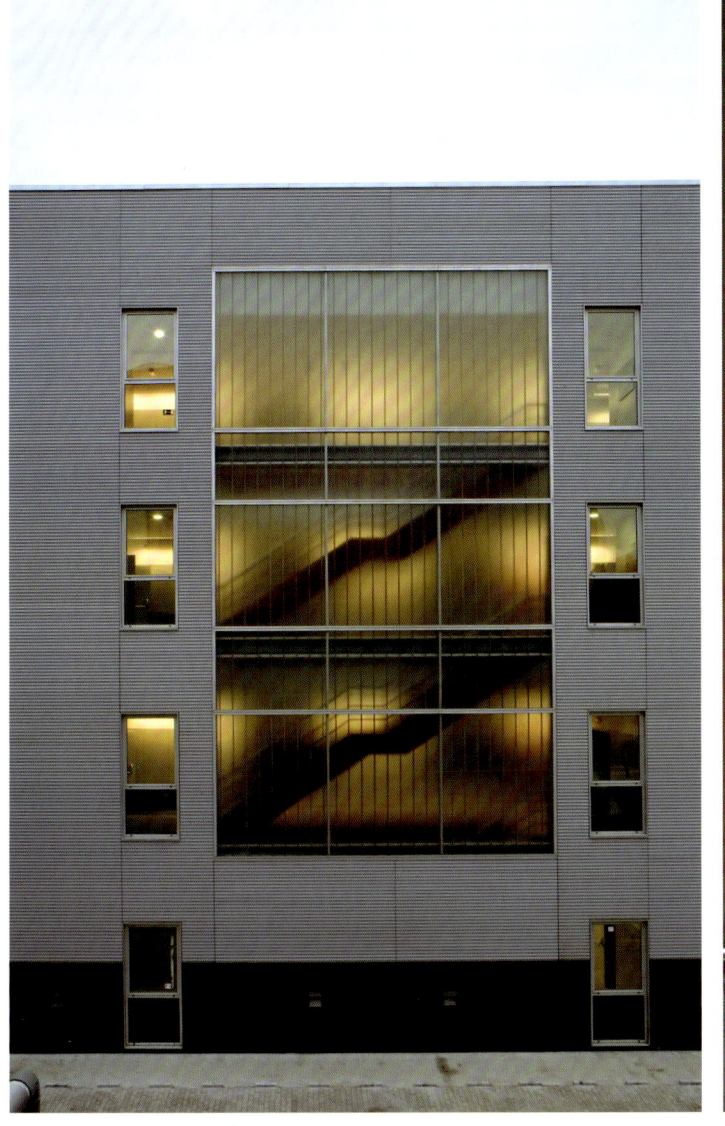

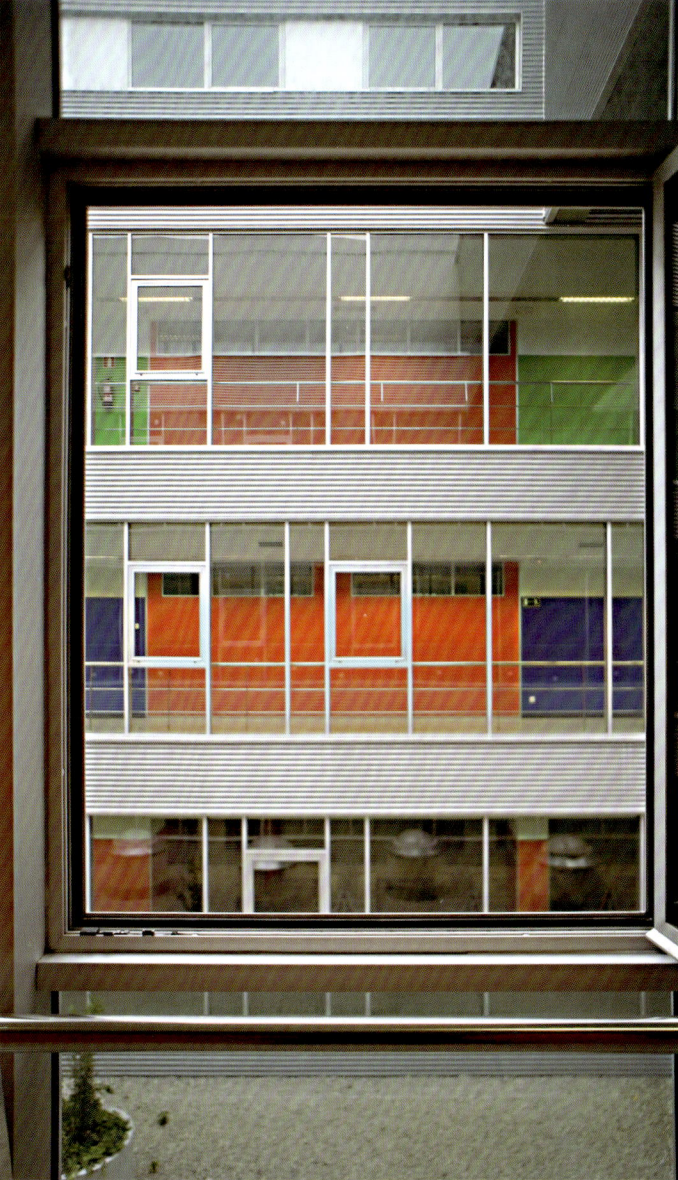

268

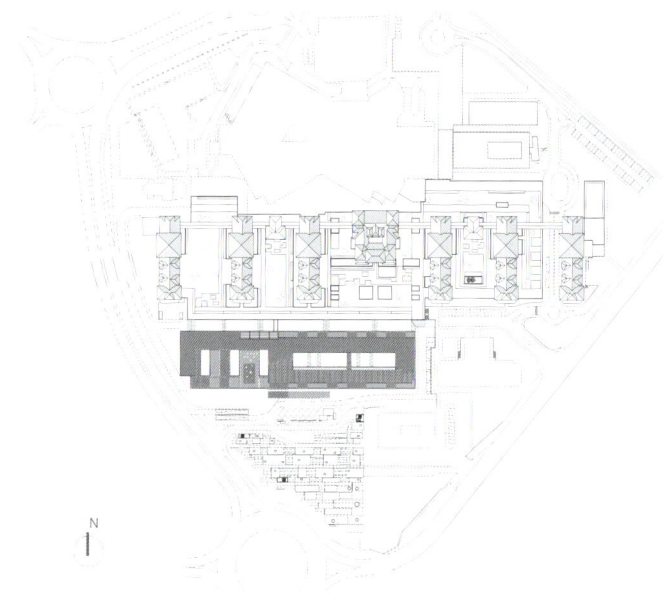

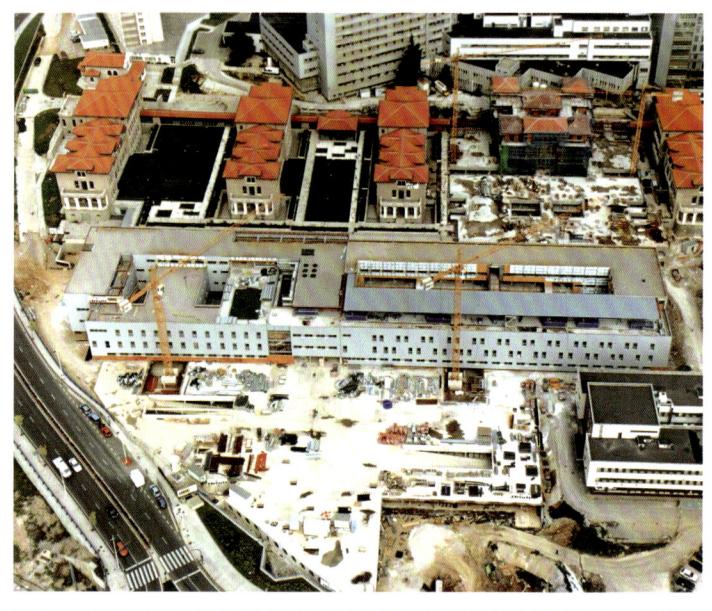

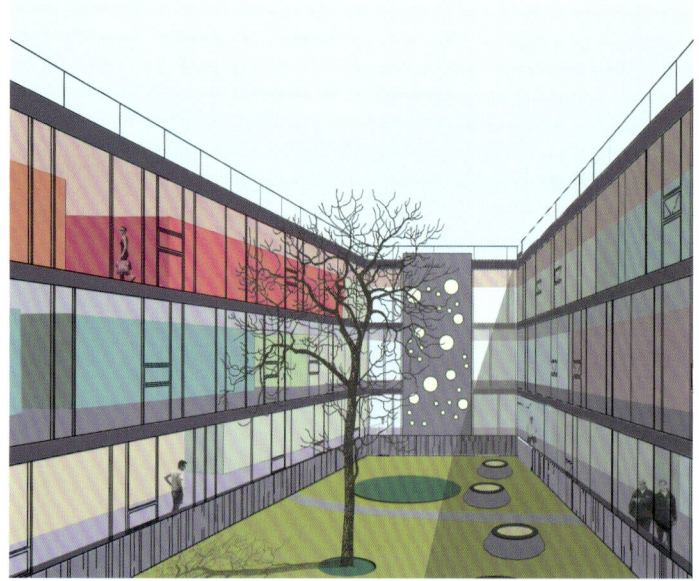

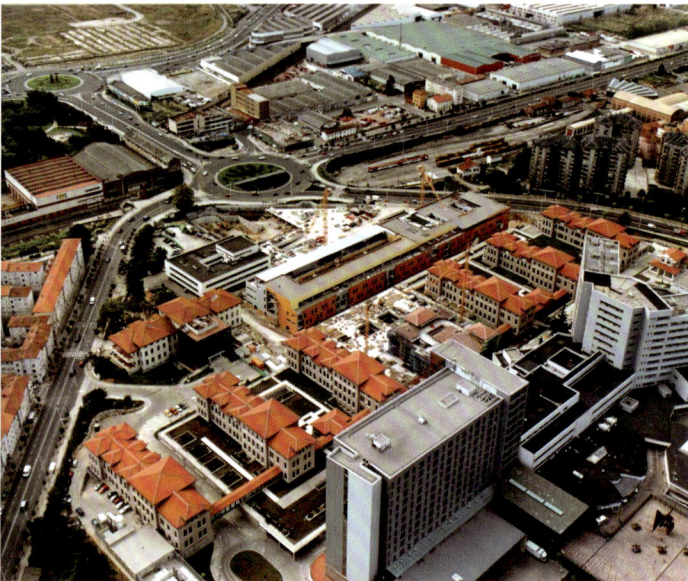

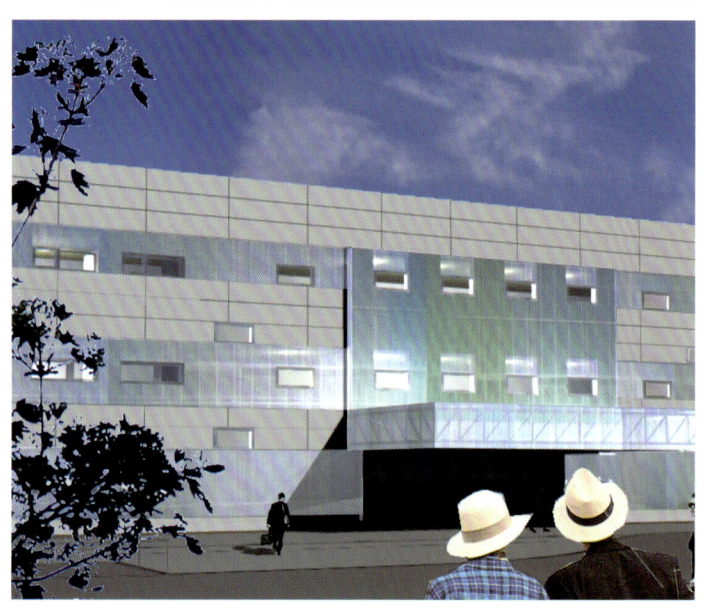

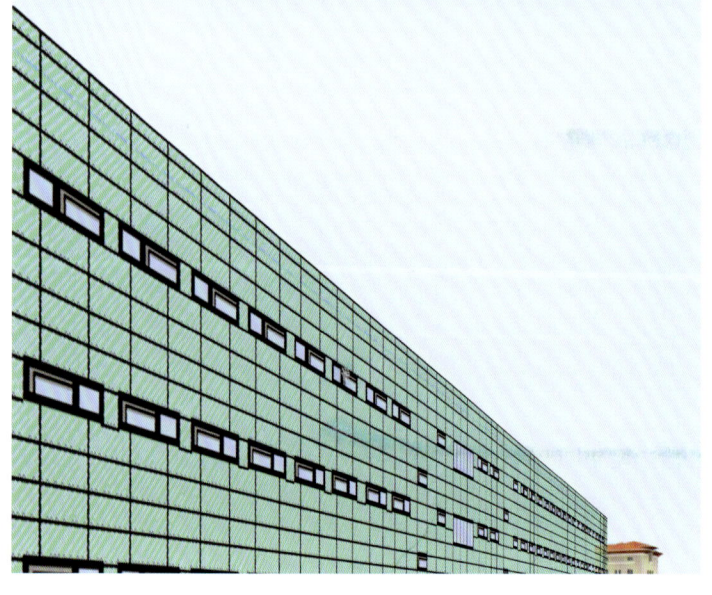

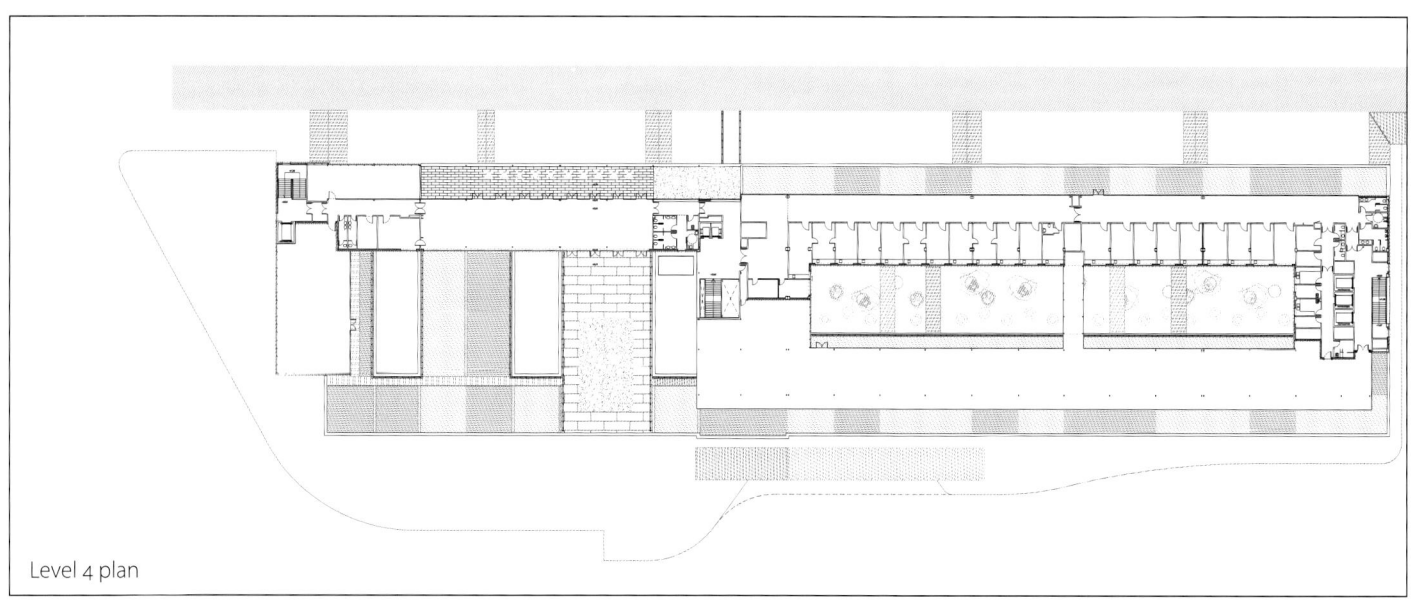

Level 4 plan

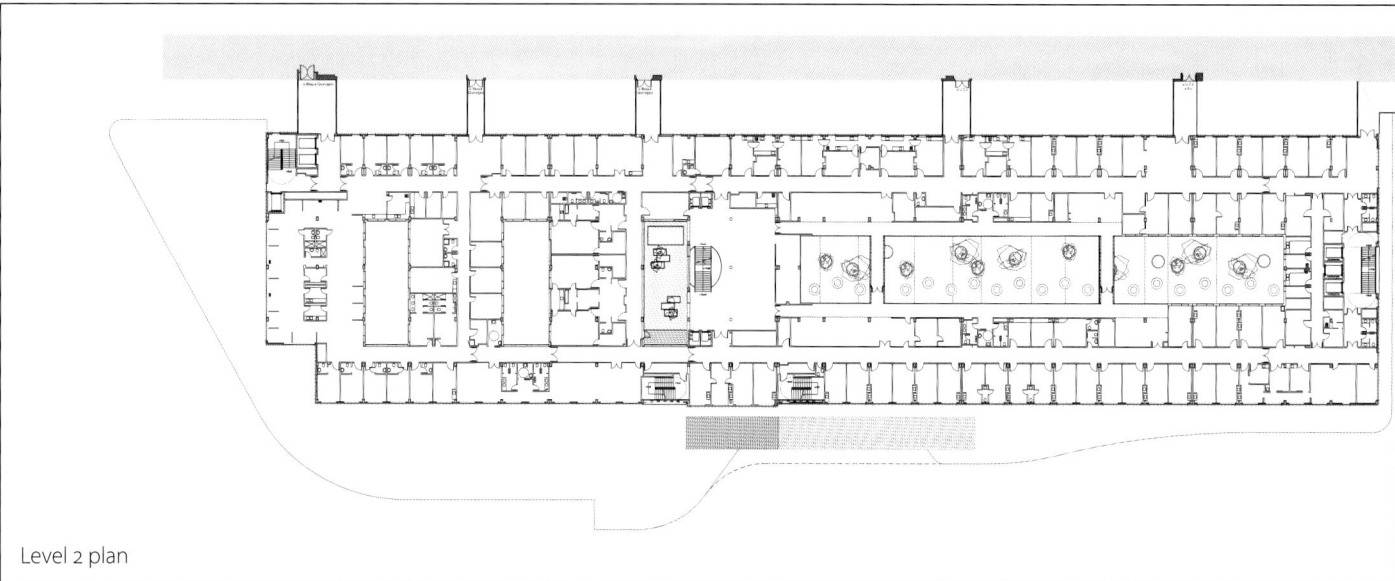

Level 2 plan

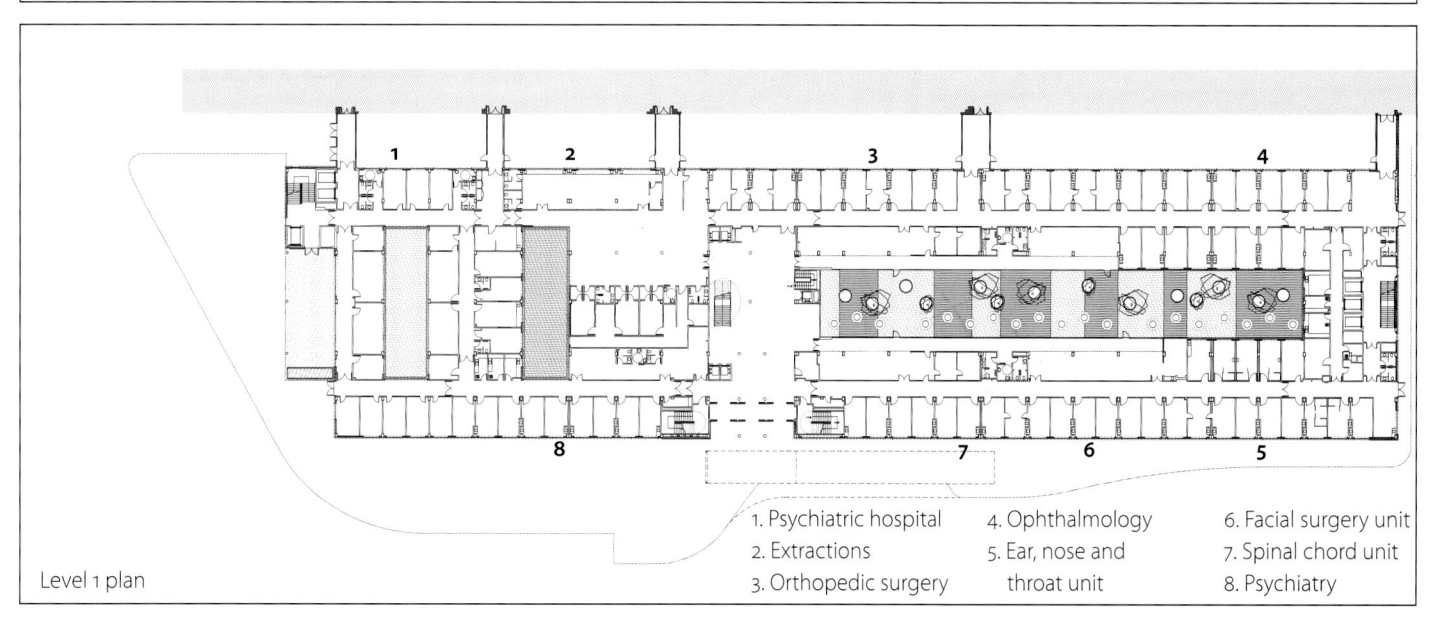

Level 1 plan

1. Psychiatric hospital
2. Extractions
3. Orthopedic surgery
4. Ophthalmology
5. Ear, nose and throat unit
6. Facial surgery unit
7. Spinal chord unit
8. Psychiatry

South elevation

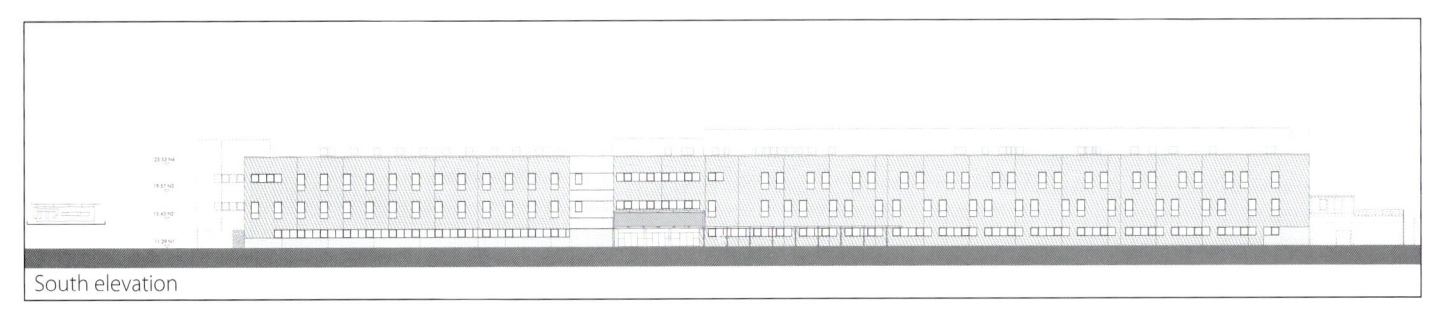

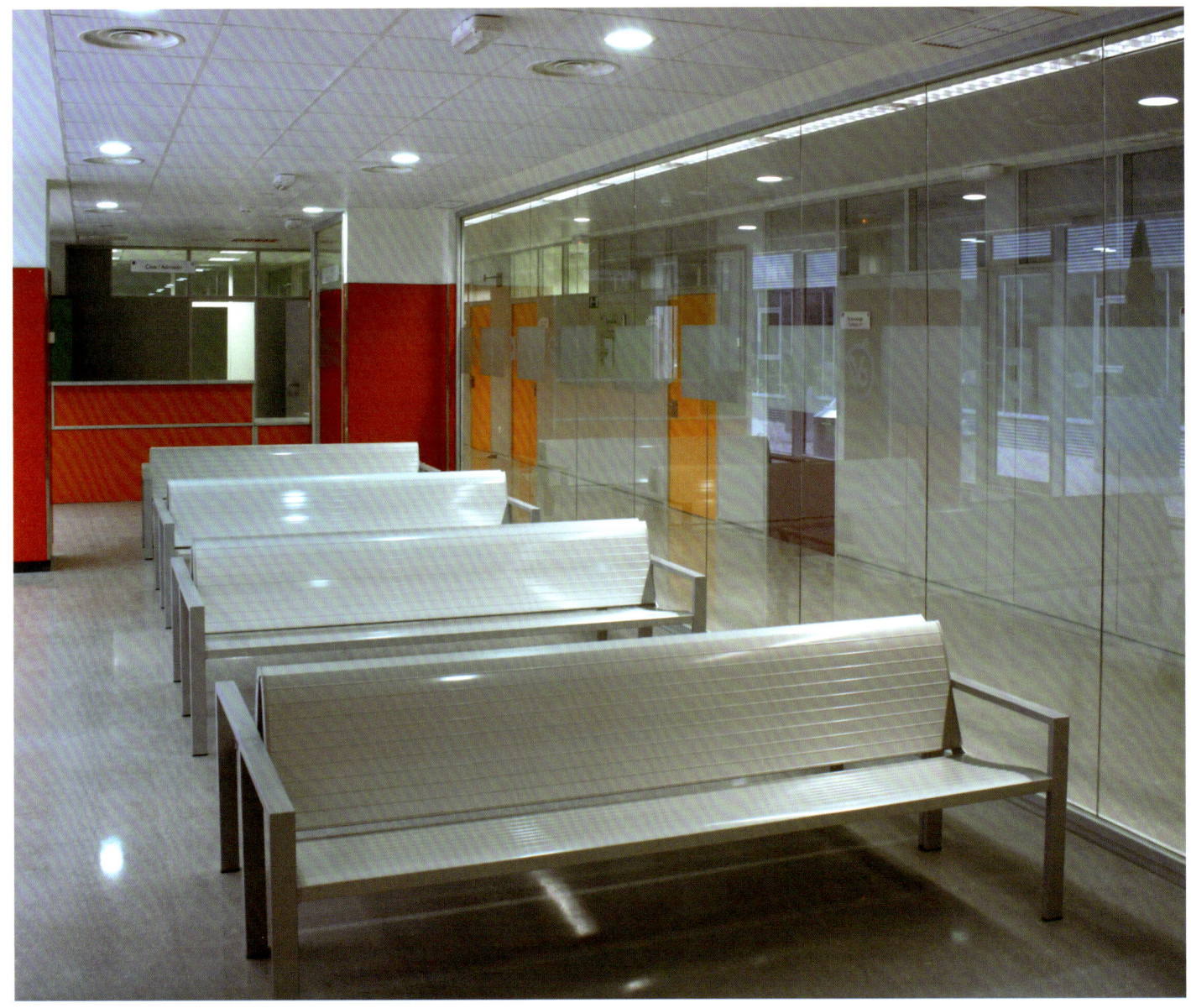

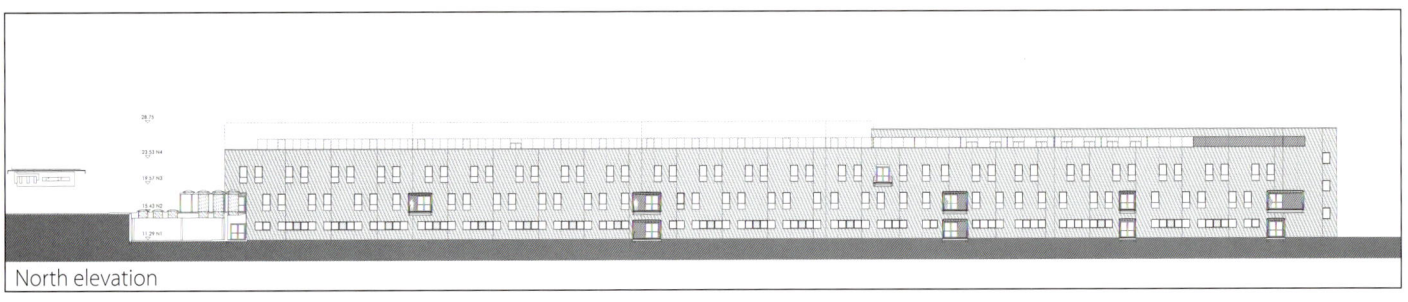

North elevation

| West elevation | East elevation |

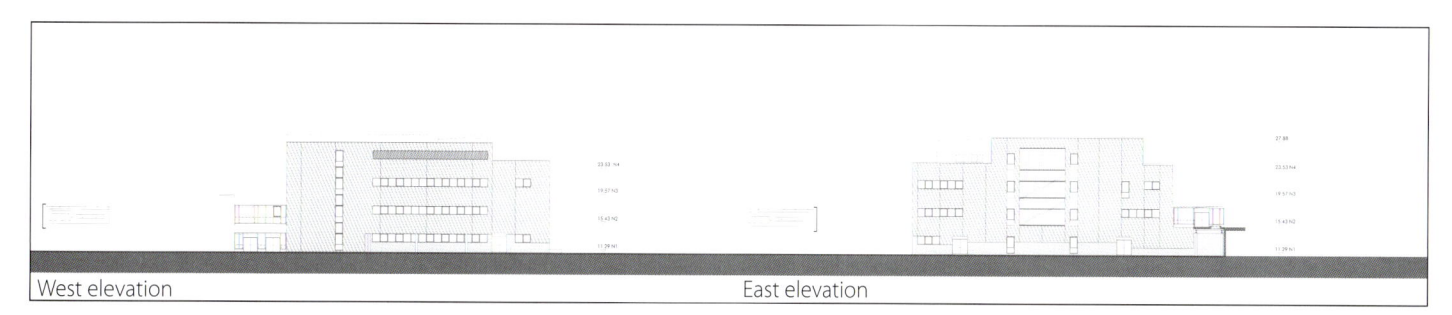

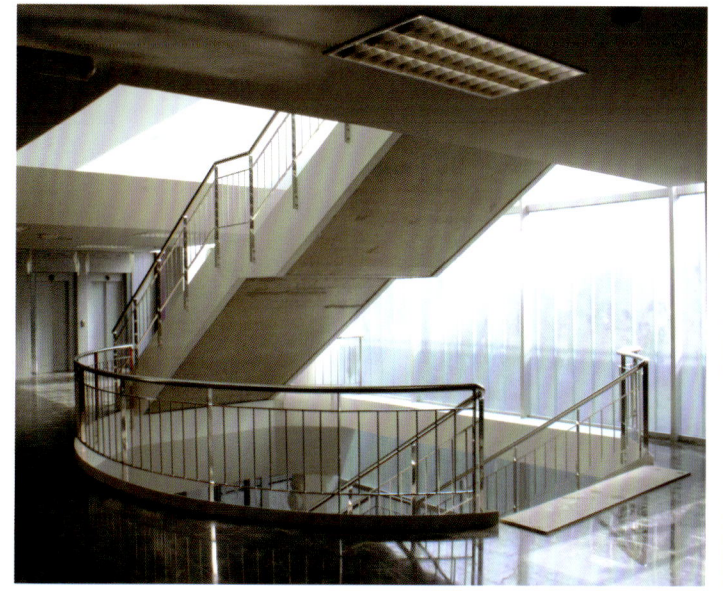

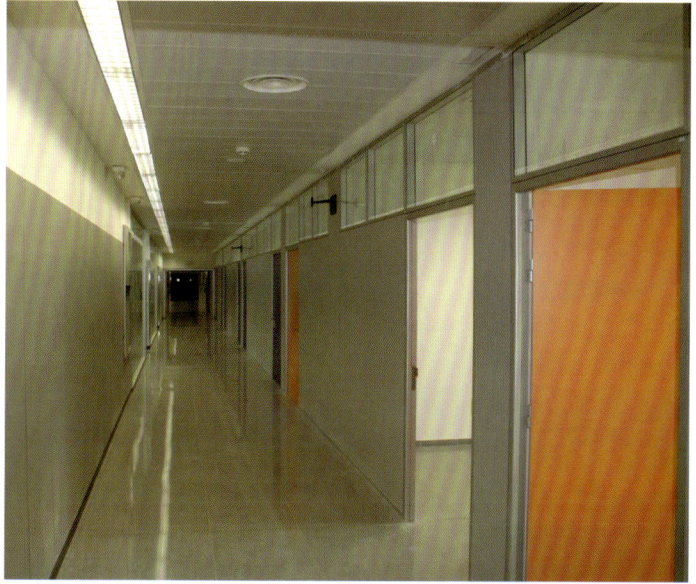

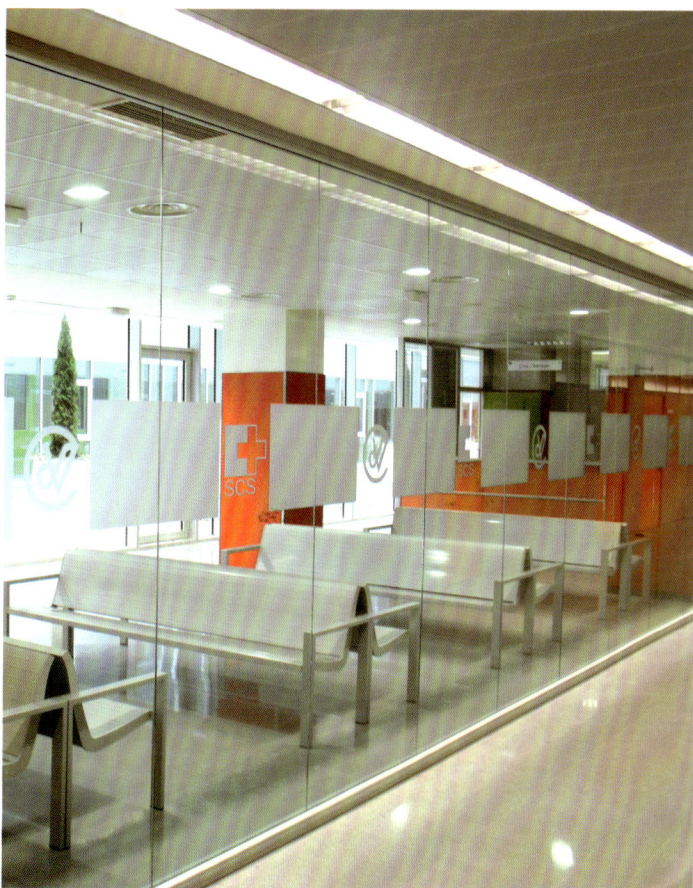

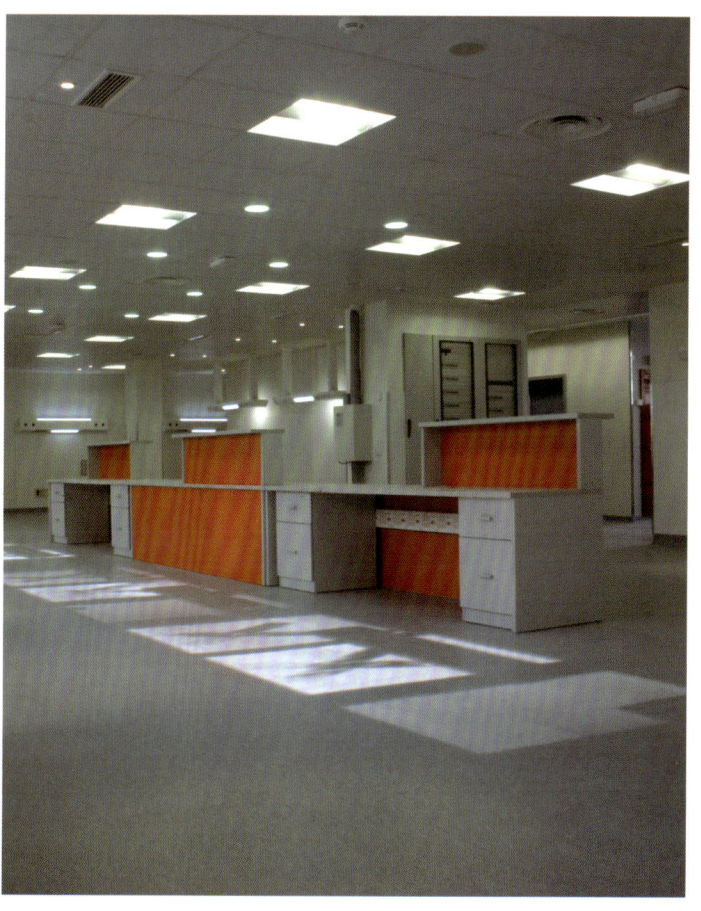

271

Section 1

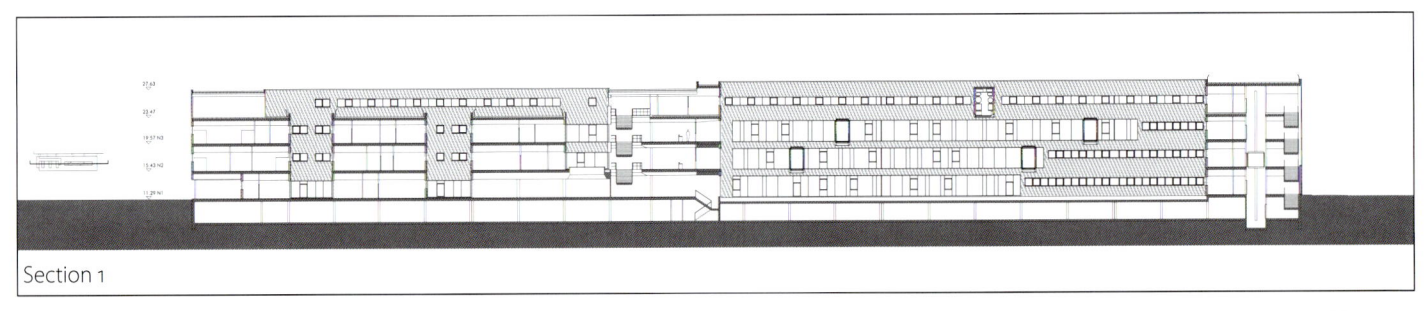

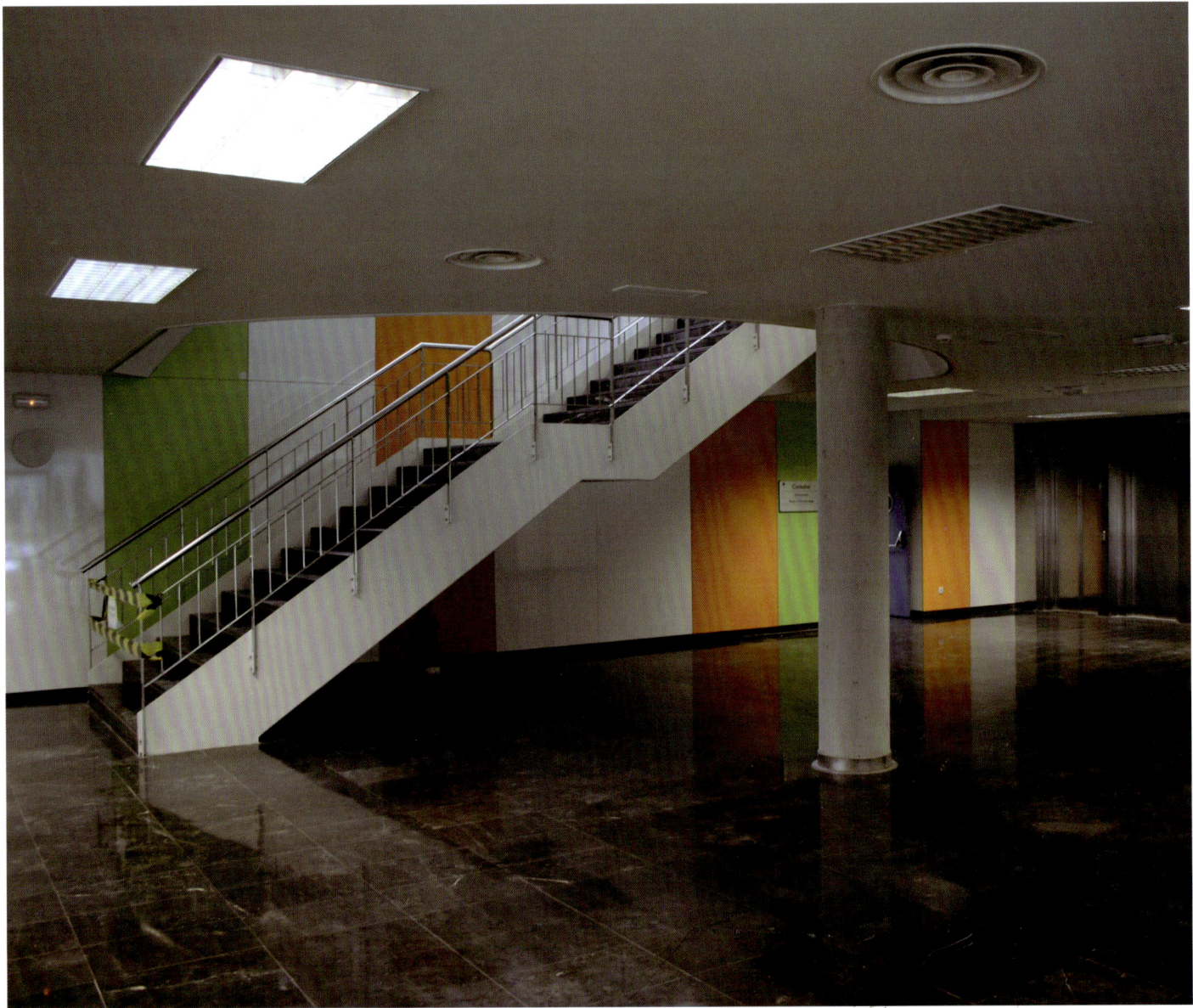

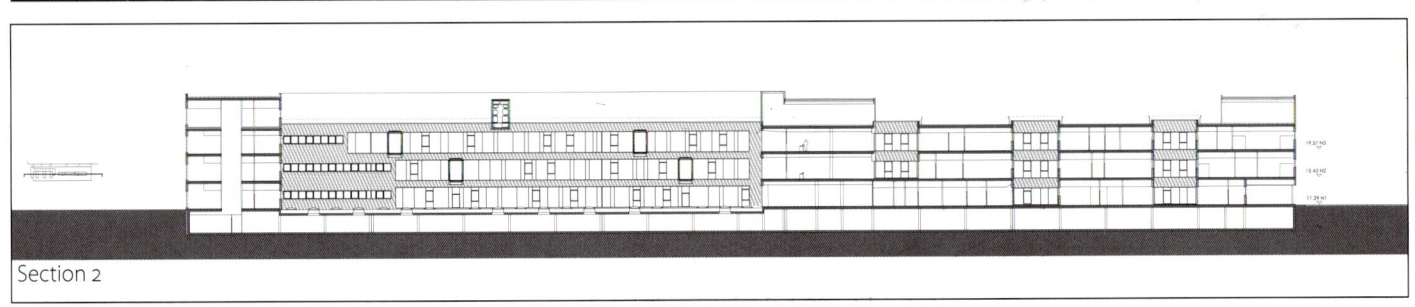

Section 2

Section t1 Section t2

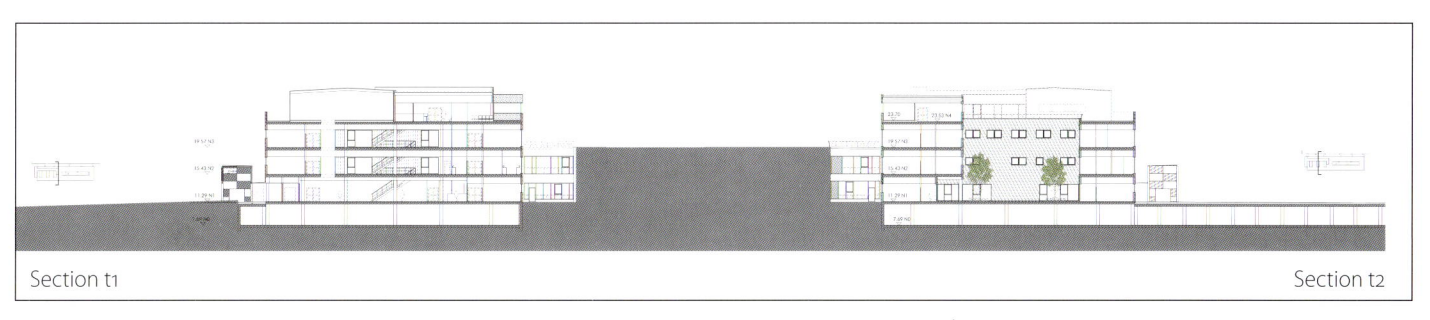

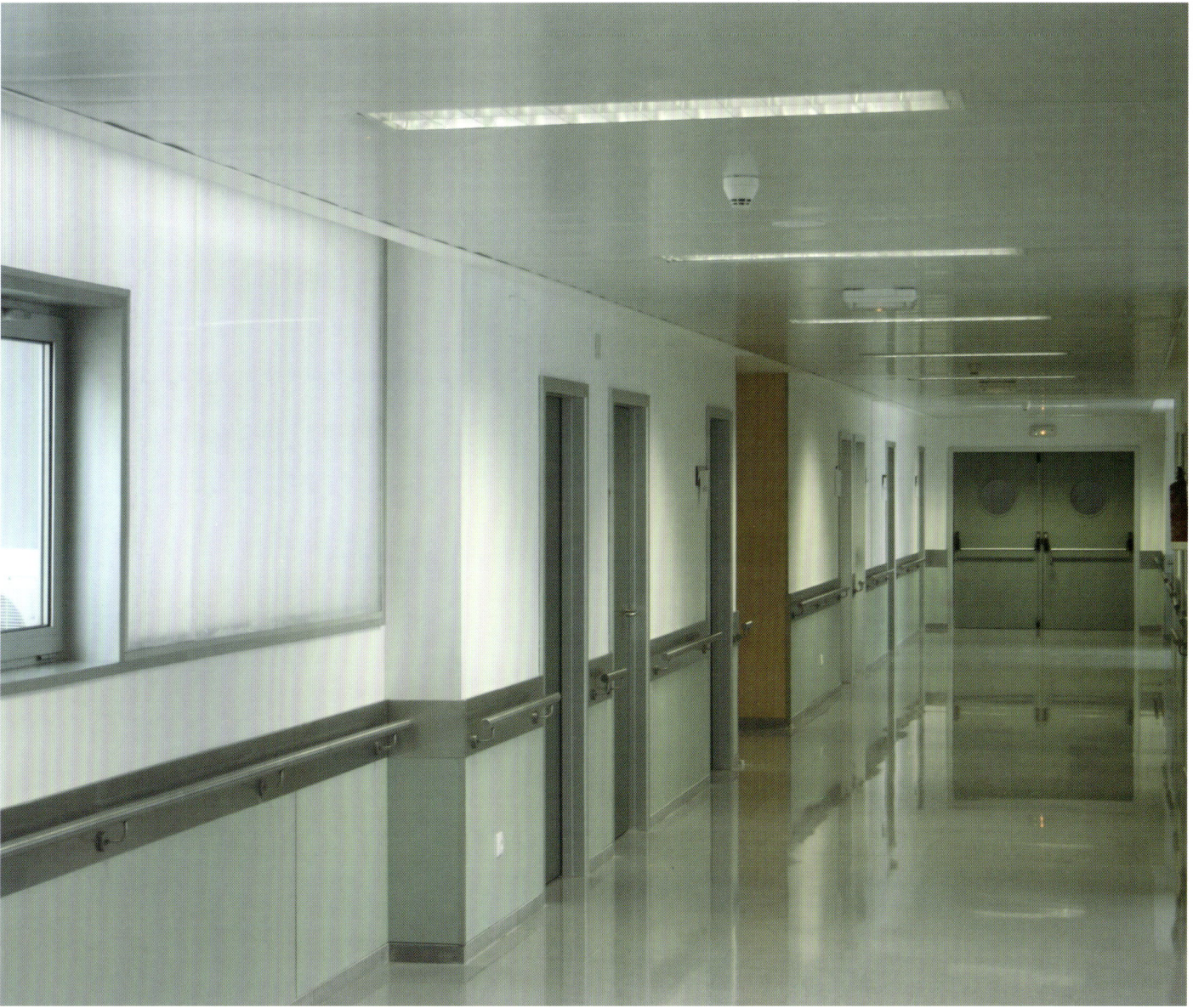

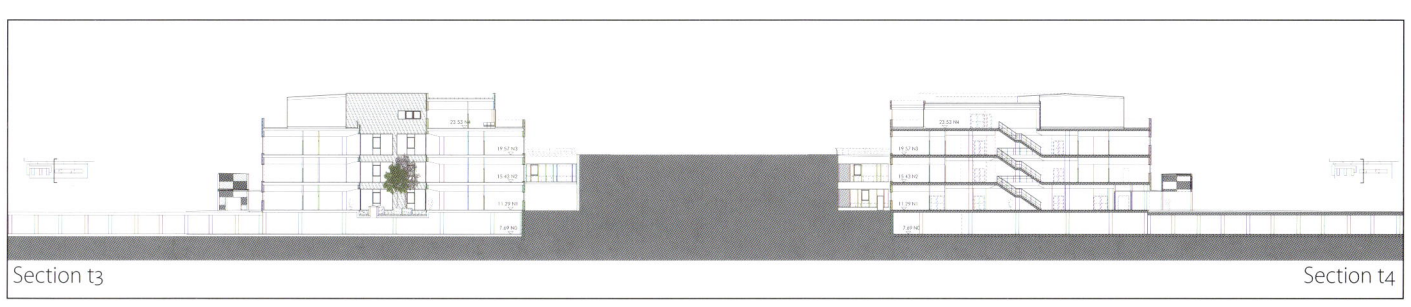

Section t3 Section t4

273

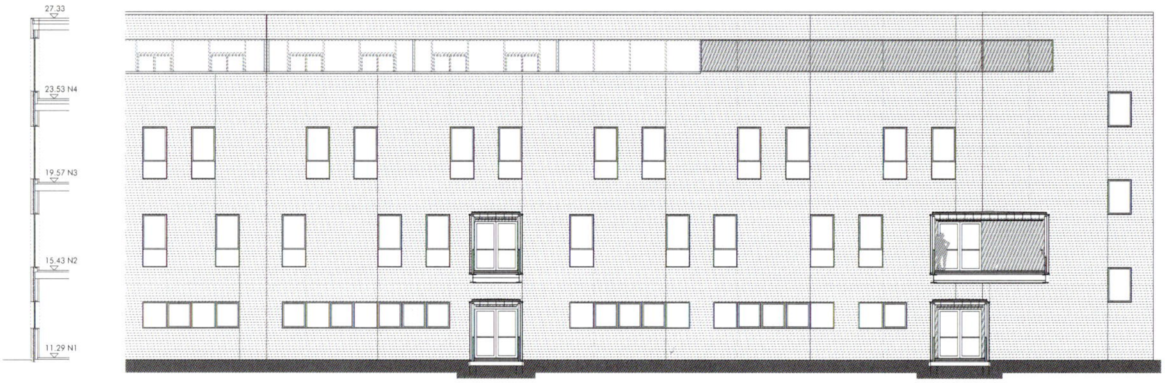
27.33
23.53 N4
19.57 N3
15.43 N2
11.29 N1

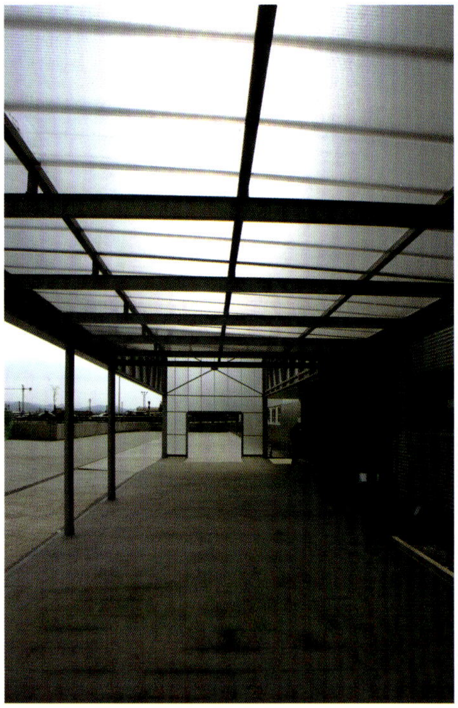

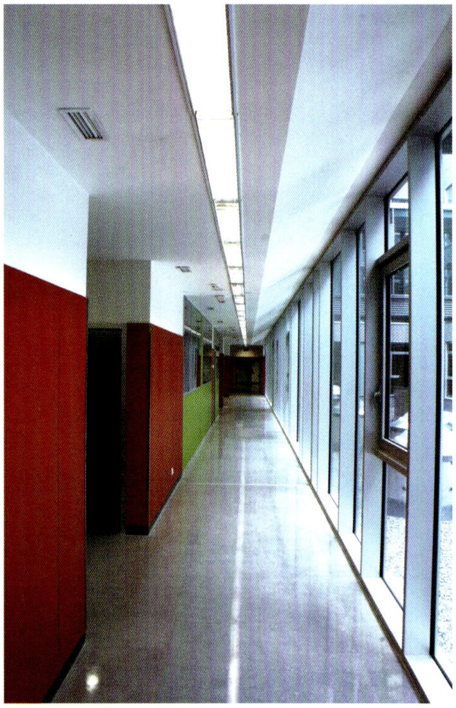

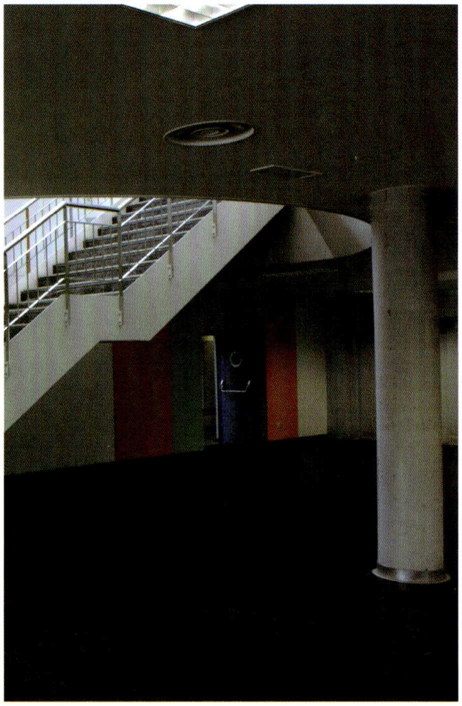

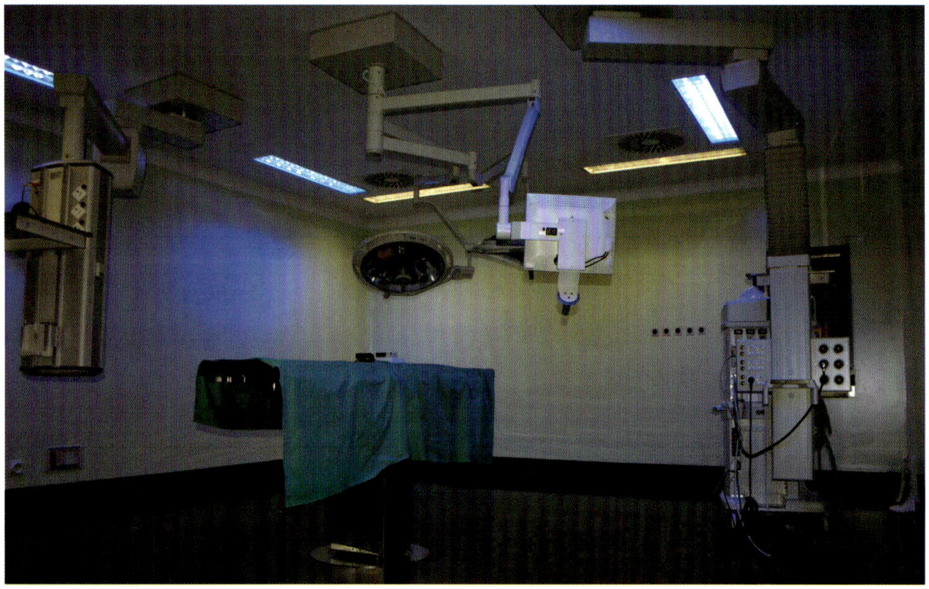

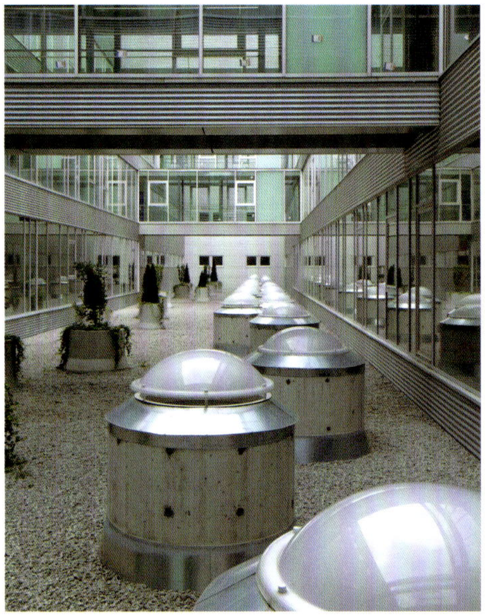

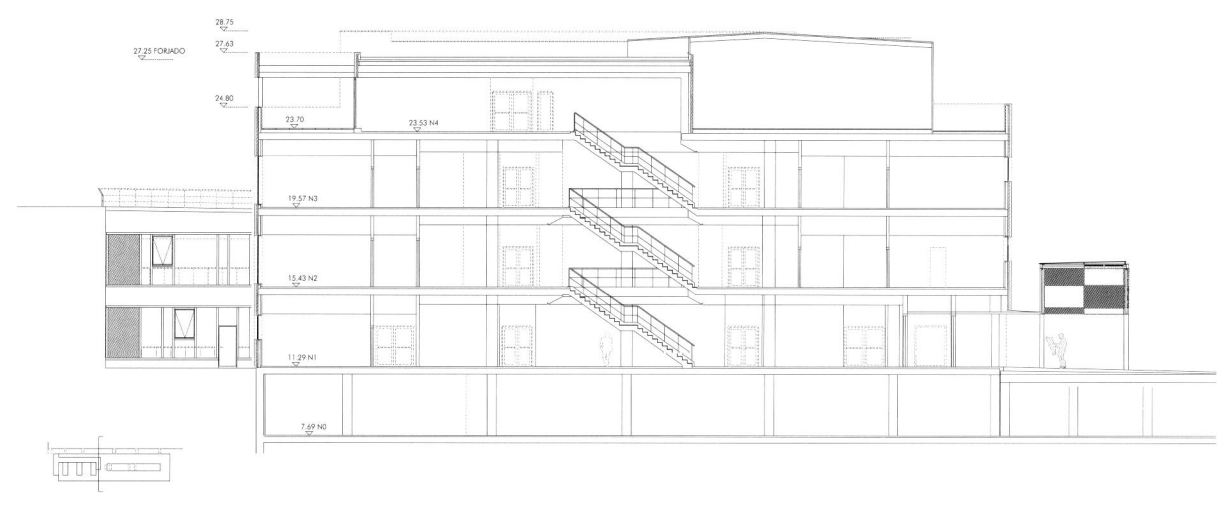

Transversal section T3

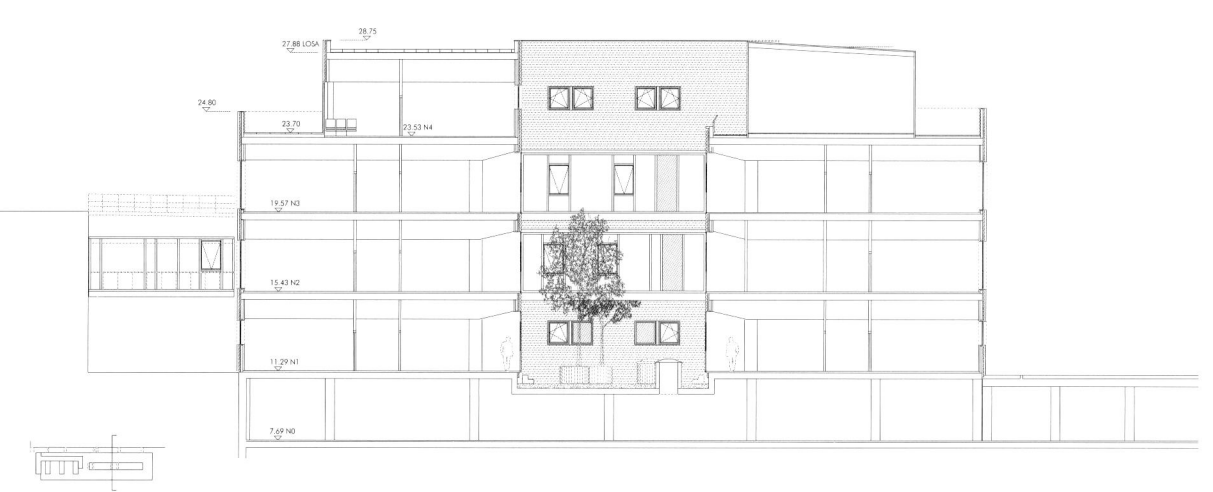

Transversal section T4

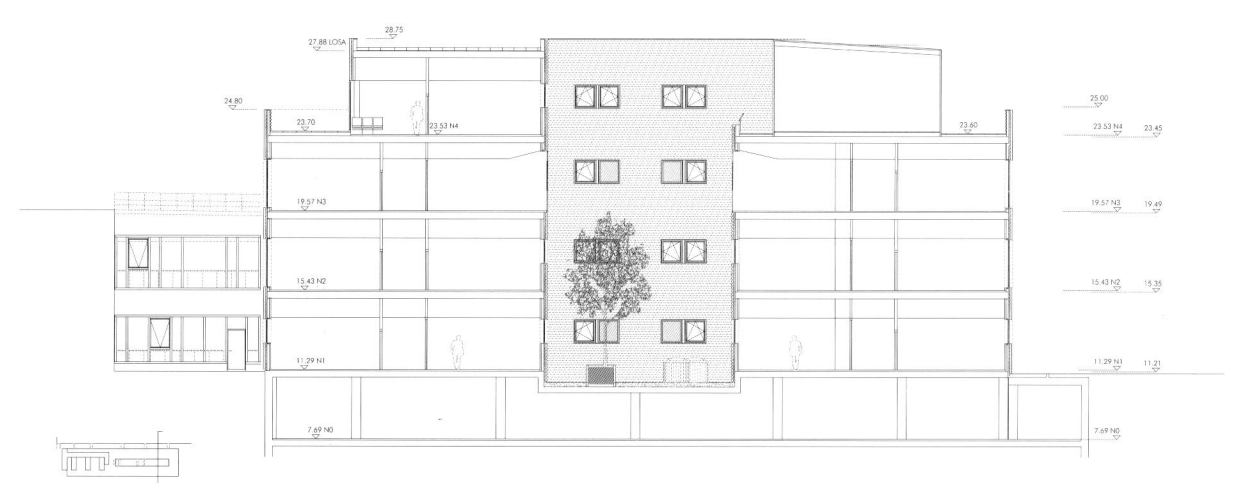

Transversal section T5

CSPE & Anshen + Allen

Meyer Children's Hospital

Florence, Italy

Photographs: *CSPE - Alessandro Ciampi and Pietro Savorelli.*

The new Meyer Children's Hospital in Florence is an international benchmark for children's hospitals – it represents an ideal and humanized healthcare environment for children. Its design returns the hospital as a building type to the mainstream of architecture, whilst recognizing that the architecture of healthcare, especially pediatric, has an absolute need to create a therapeutic environment.

The new facility has been designed within the framework of existing classical buildings and lush parkland. The masterplan respects this context by using the Villa Ognissanti as the main entrance, connecting it to the new hospital beyond by two galleria which enclose and define the landscape. The new building is embedded into the hillside at the rear and so is invisible from the street and, although is demonstrably modern with a settled plan form, it is axially centered on this entrance point. The design echoes the past whilst reducing the impact of a big structure.

To retain the well-loved historic buildings and keep cars out of the park, families now walk past the palazzo, down a long, glazed passageway that winds through a healing garden and into the sun-drenched atrium. The atrium, called the Serra, is a curved, triple-height space attached to the Villa Ognissanti pavilions. This is the hospital's public face and circulatory heart, connecting the old with the new. The Serra is a vast glass room dominated by a white laminated ceiling, evoking the ribs of a whale – it is the first of many architectural references to the Pinocchio story: colorful ceramic wayfinding devices mimic the shape of his conical cap, which also turns up as 'Pinocchio hat' skylights, which pierce the hospital's green roof.

Meyer's technological and environmental sensitivity can be seen in many of the building's features: the green roof is an innovative solution, which uses the German DAKU system; the SOS 'double-glass' system (the use of intelligent windows) is a further strategy which, in addition to reducing heat and allowing environmental control, ensures night-time ventilation through the use of electronic devices guaranteeing the advantage of passive cooling; the 47 'Pinocchio's hat' light wells enhance the building's integration into its surroundings and capture the maximum possible solar light available to 'enter' the hospital space.

Humanizing the patient environment is achieved in a number of ways. Waiting and play areas employ variations in shapes and colors to relieve visual monotony. Colors have been selected to create bright and stimulating play areas, and restful nursing and treatment areas. MeyerArt has developed an extensive public arts program, comprising paintings and sculpture, some by children and others referencing the Pinocchio theme.

Architects:
Anshen + Allen and CSPE (Centro Studi Progettazione Edilizia)

Client:
Meyer Children's Hospital

Area:
37,000 sqm (398264 sqf)

Cost:
£33,866,000

Contractor:
Itinera SPA,

Structural Engineer:
A&I Ingegneri Associati; Studio Tecnico Chiarugi

Mechanical Engineer:
CMZ (Cinelli – Marazzini – Zambaldi)

Electrical Engineer:
Studio Lombardini Engineering SRL.

Energetic experimentation:
Centro ABITA

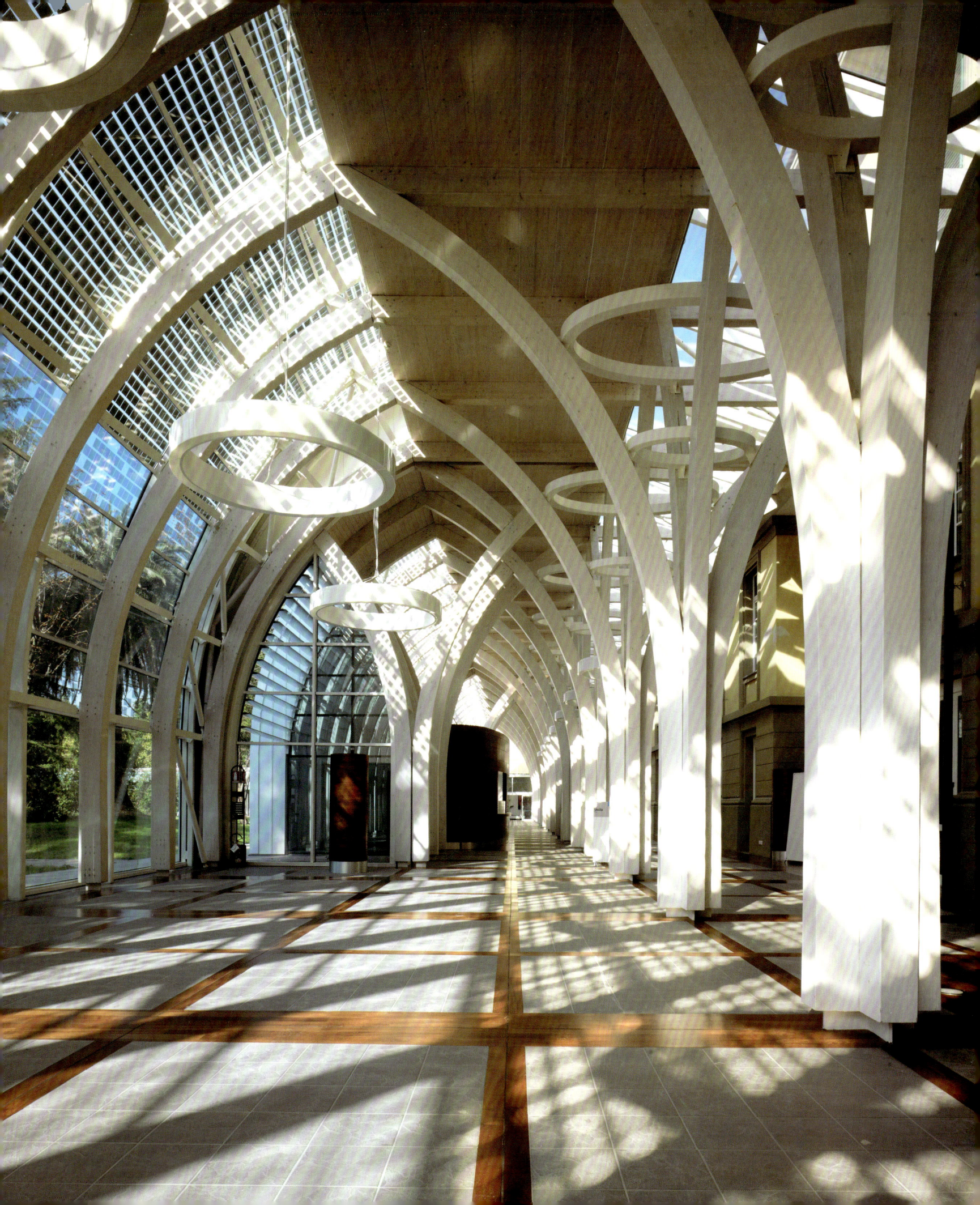

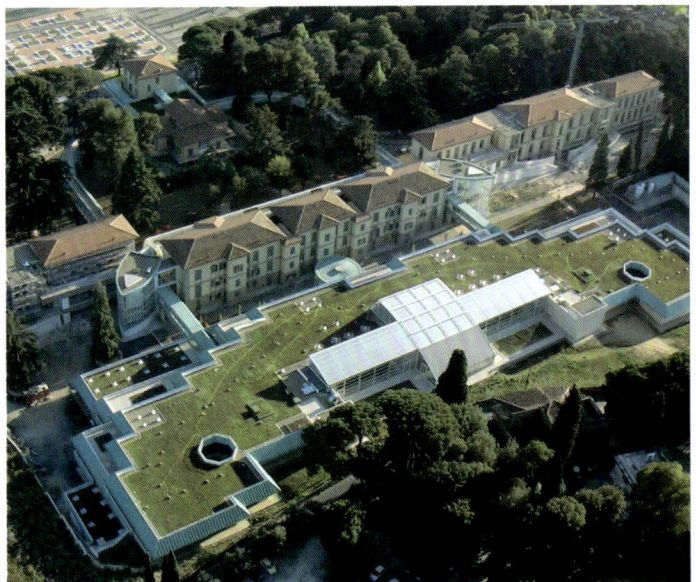

The design seeks to integrate state of the art medical services and design with an overall campus identity that will act as the catalyst to unify the existing disparate elements of the Hospital's already extensive campus.

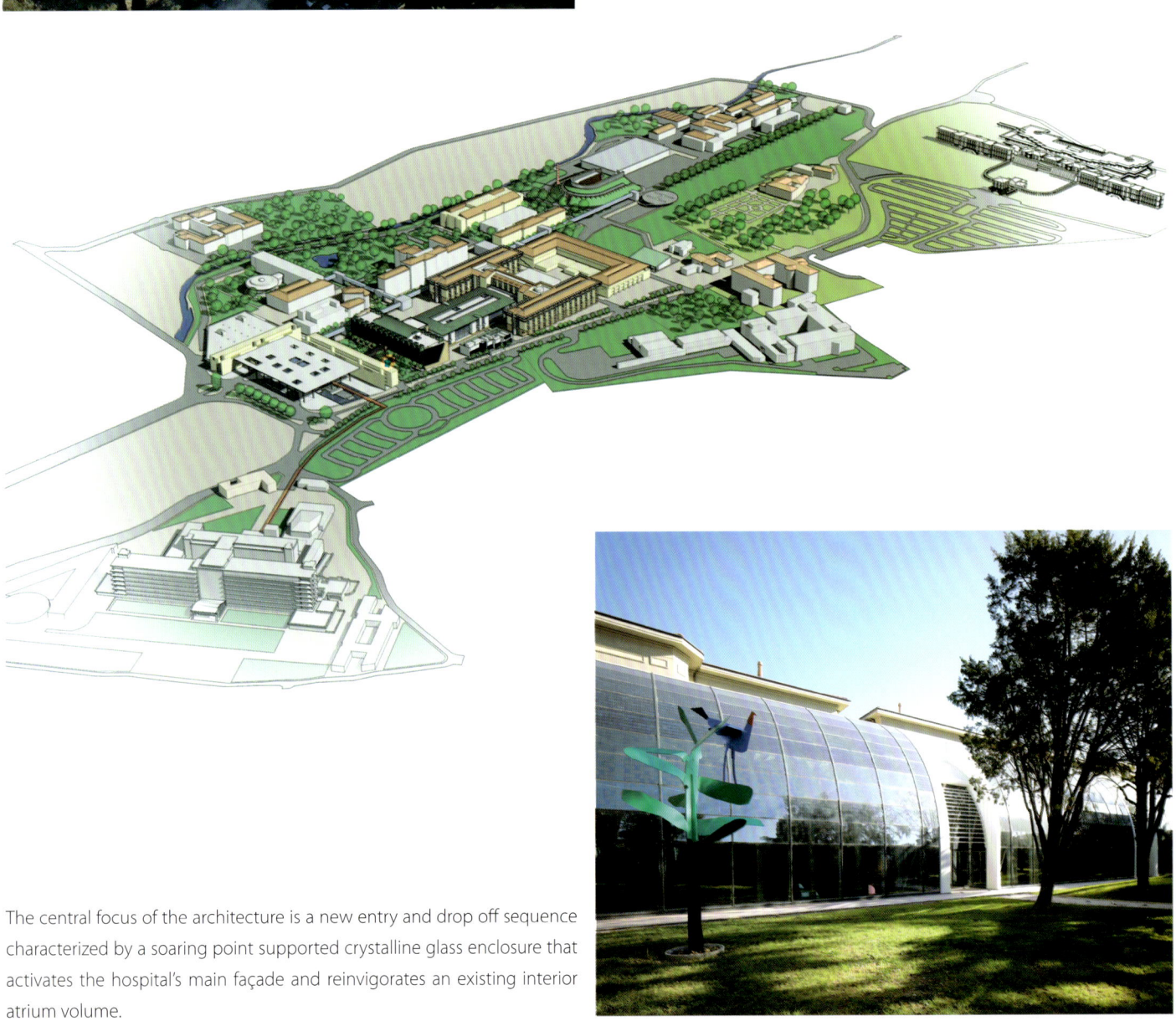

The central focus of the architecture is a new entry and drop off sequence characterized by a soaring point supported crystalline glass enclosure that activates the hospital's main façade and reinvigorates an existing interior atrium volume.

279

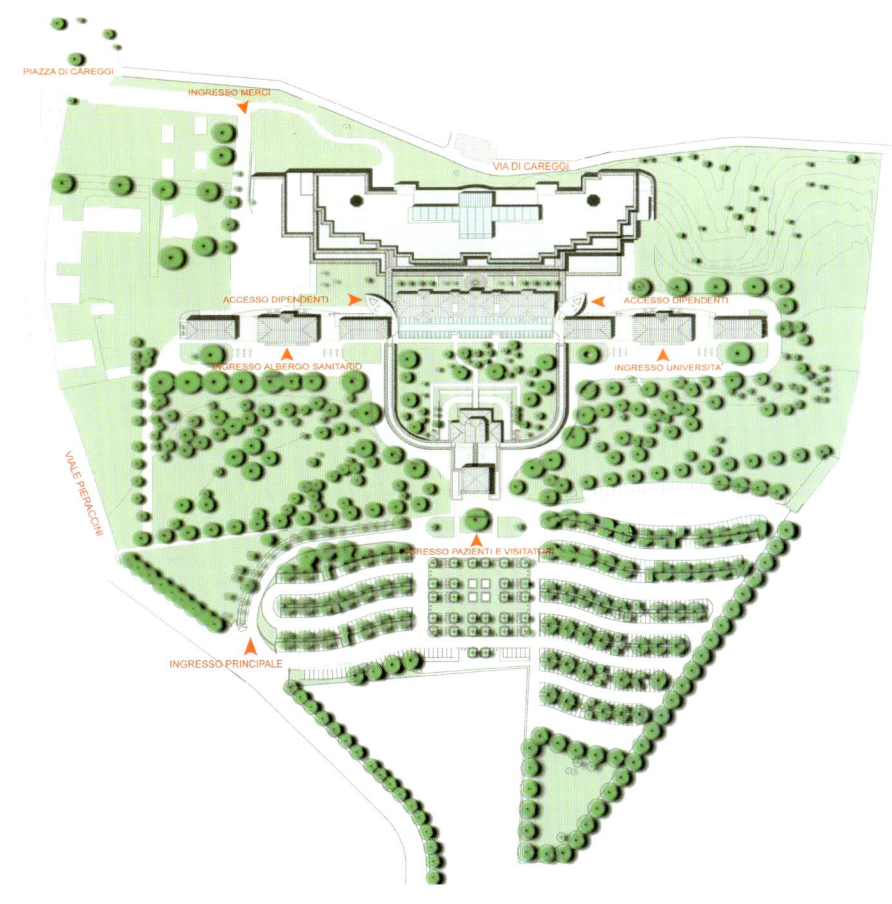

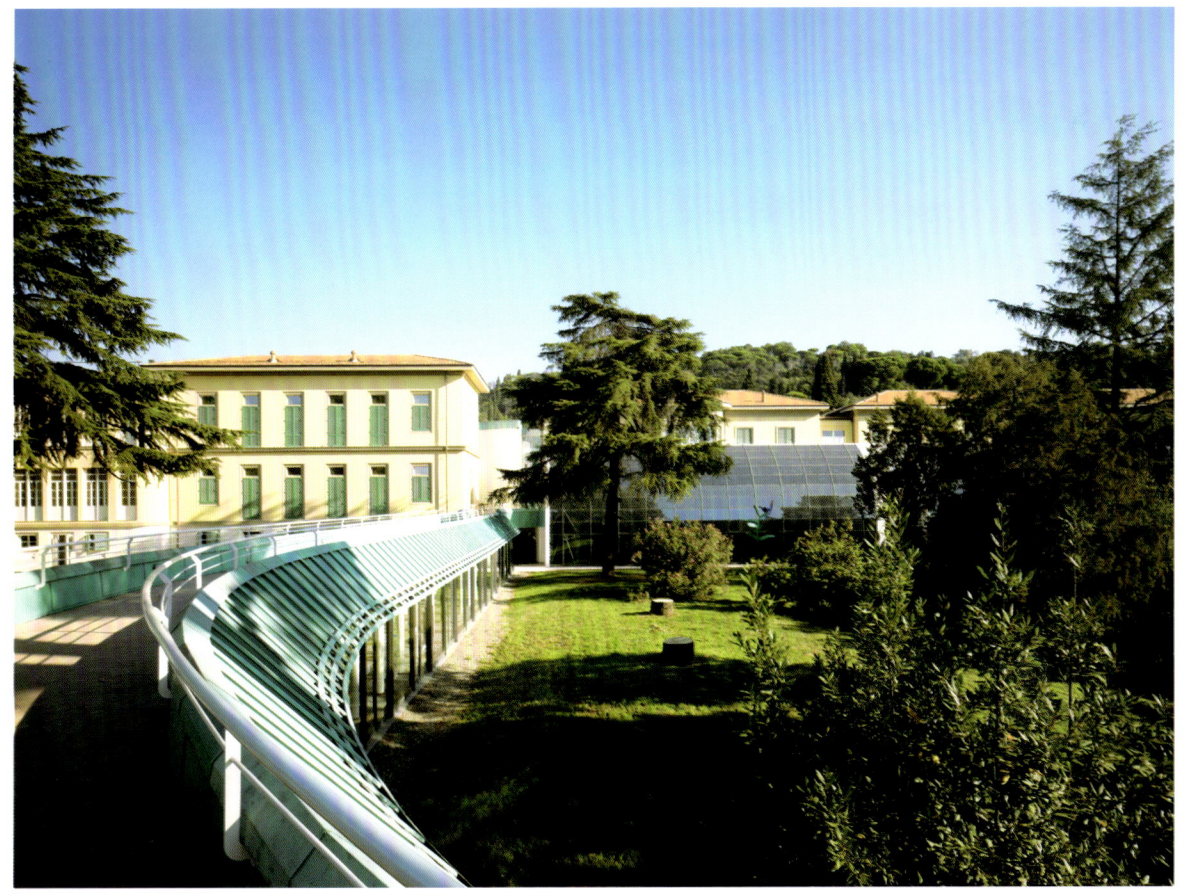

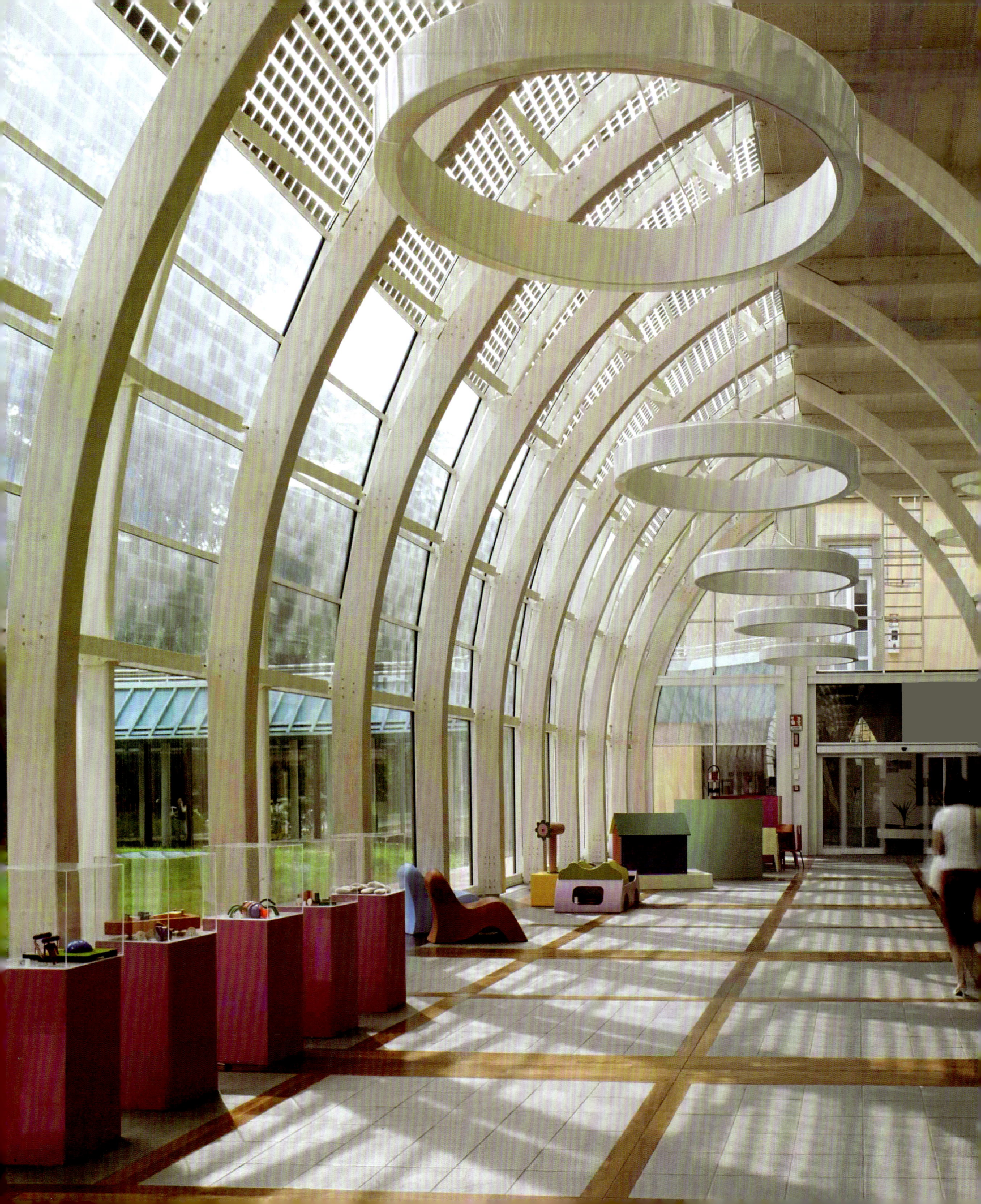

281

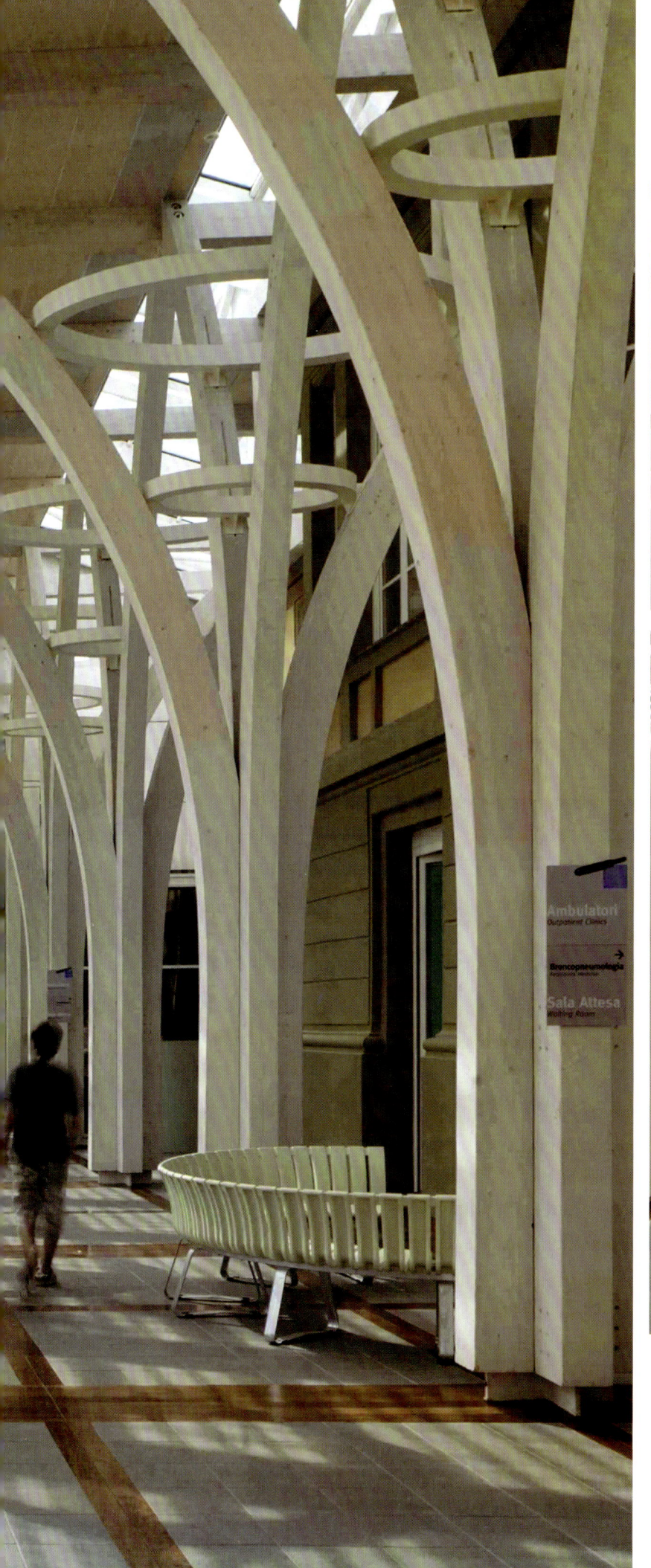

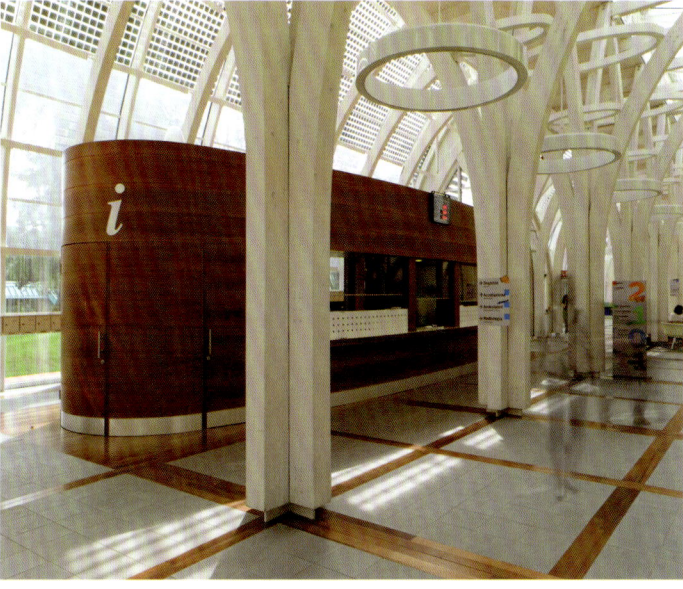

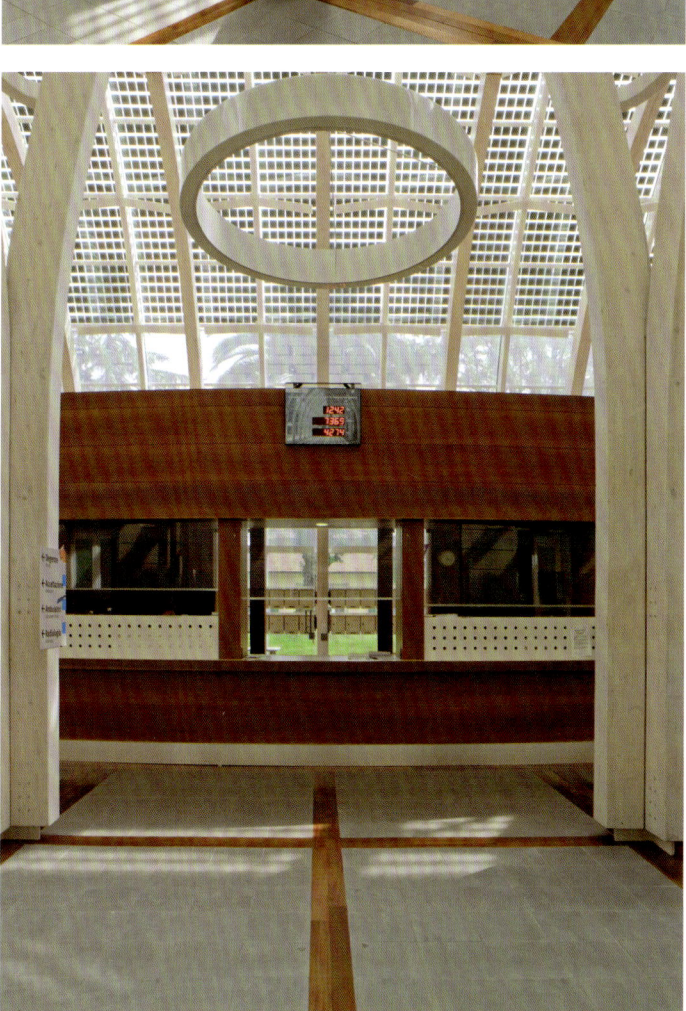

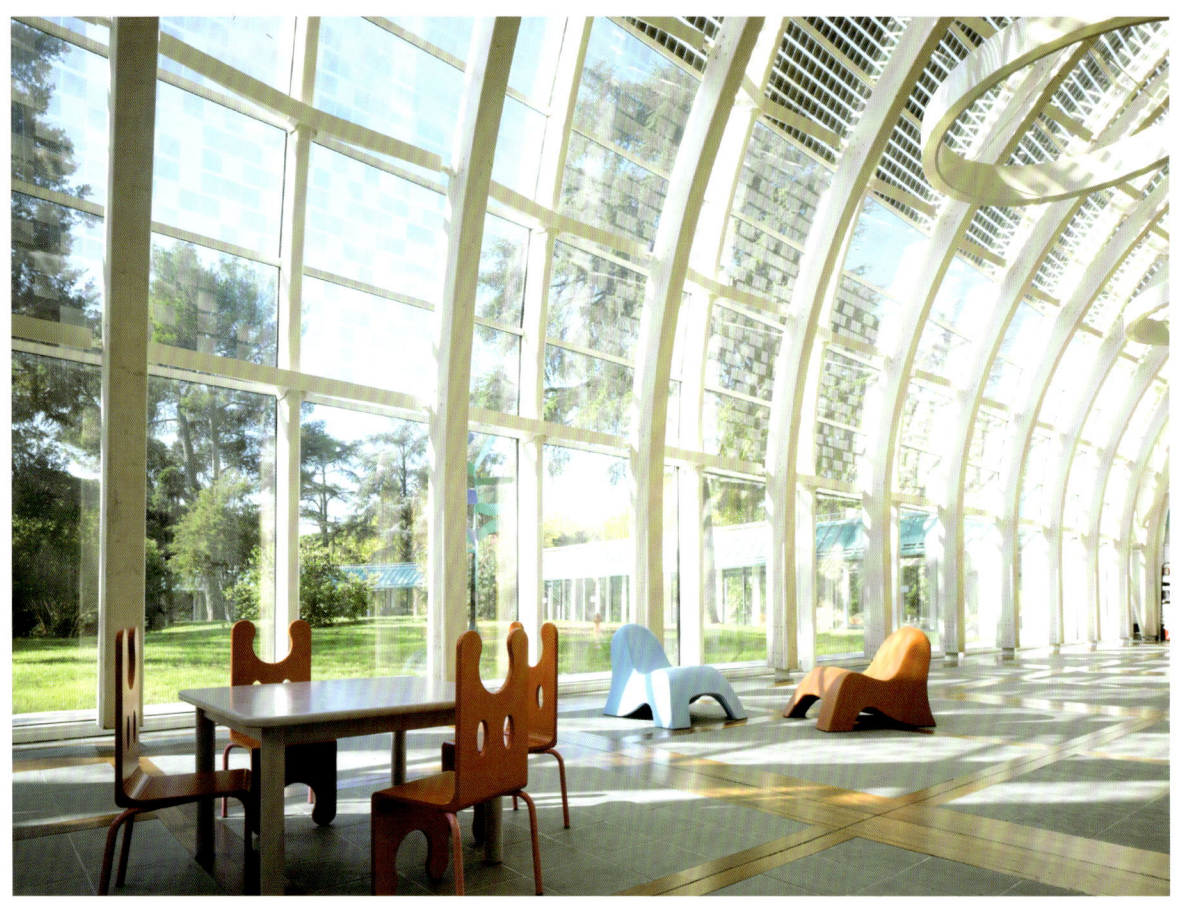

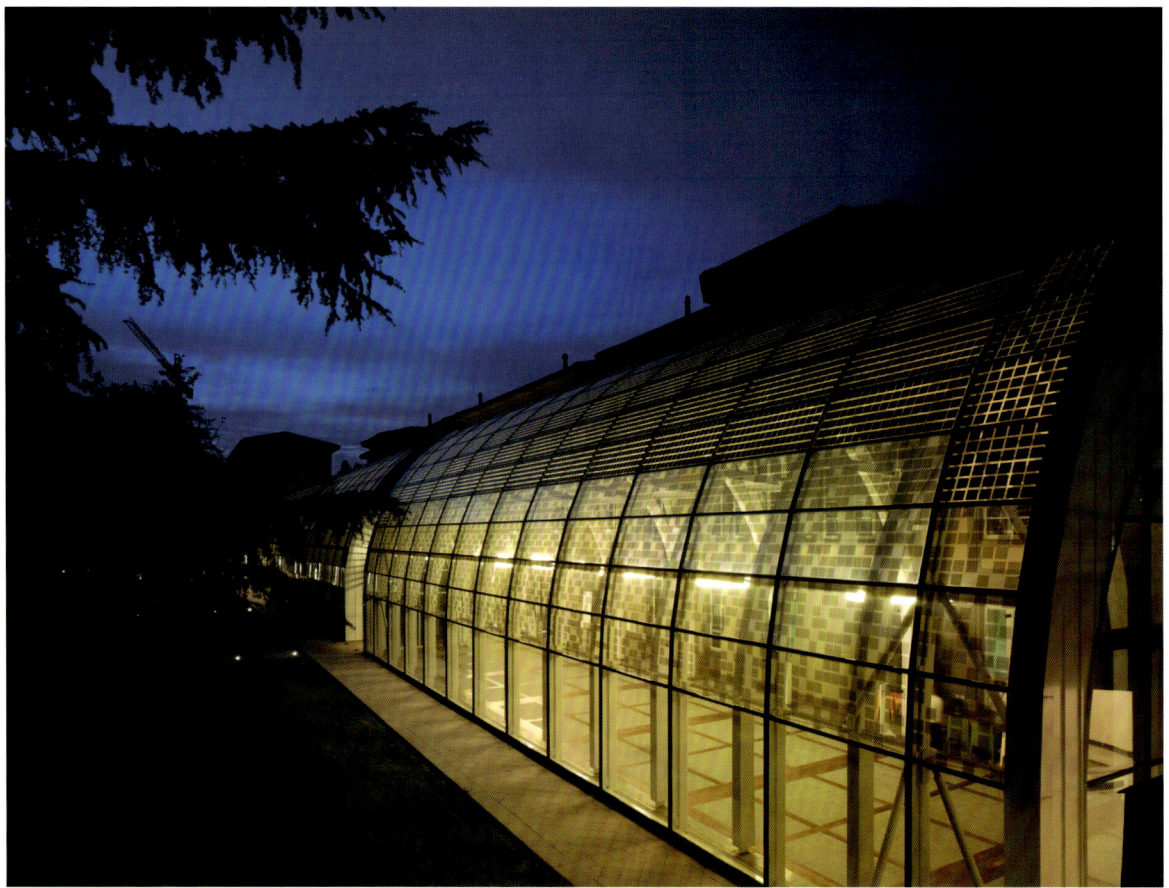

283

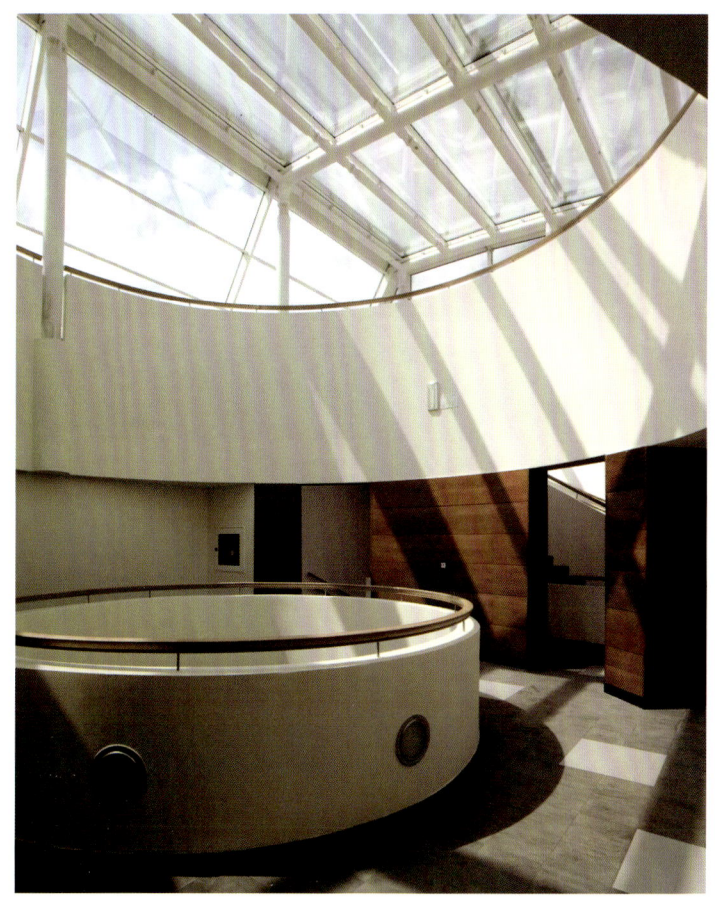

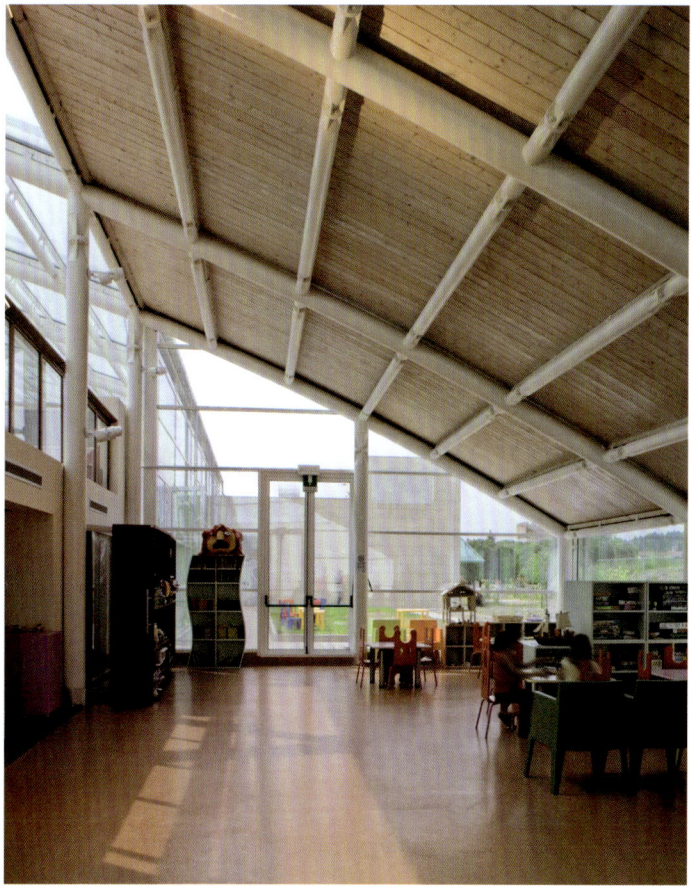

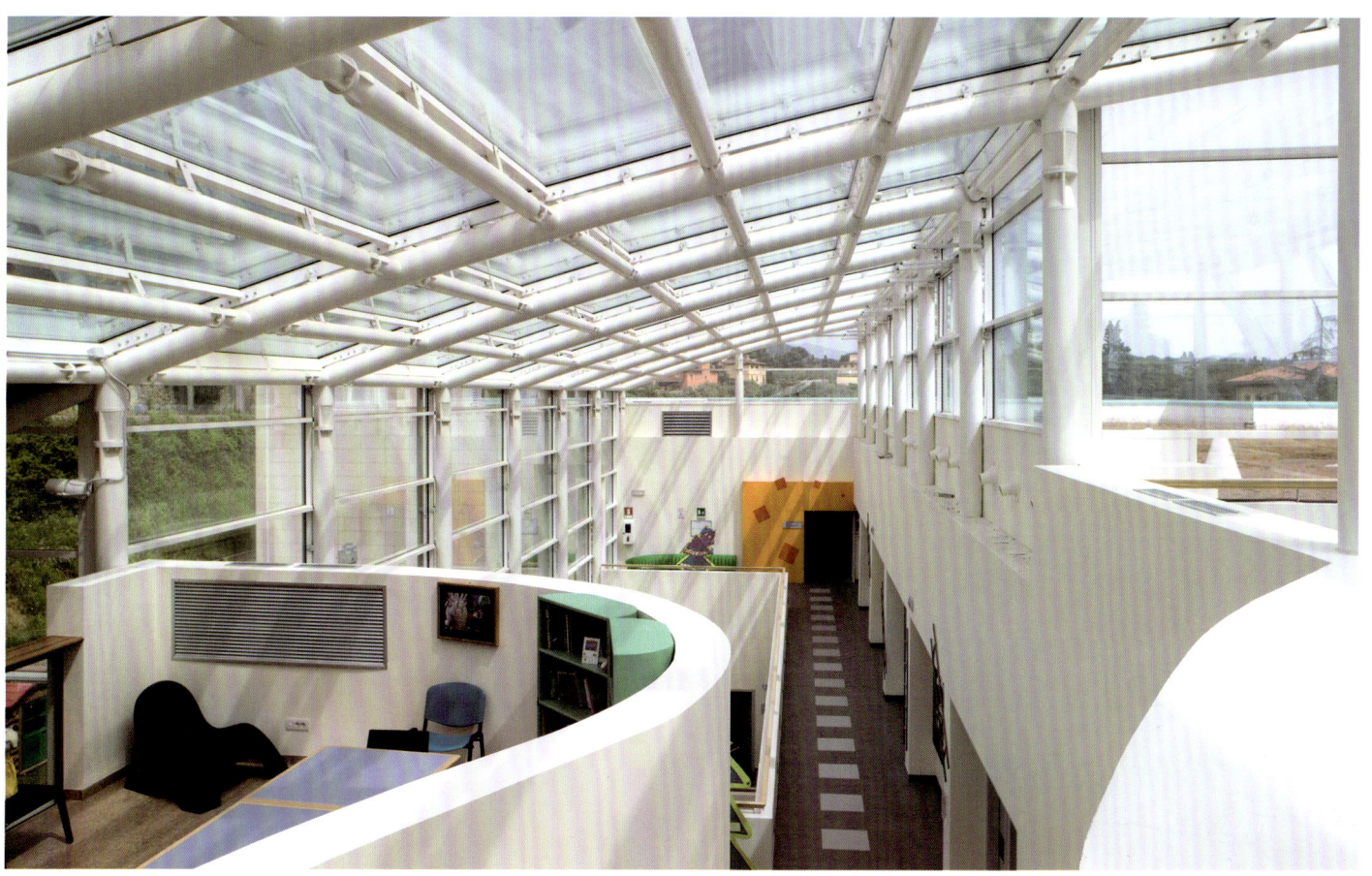

Ground floor

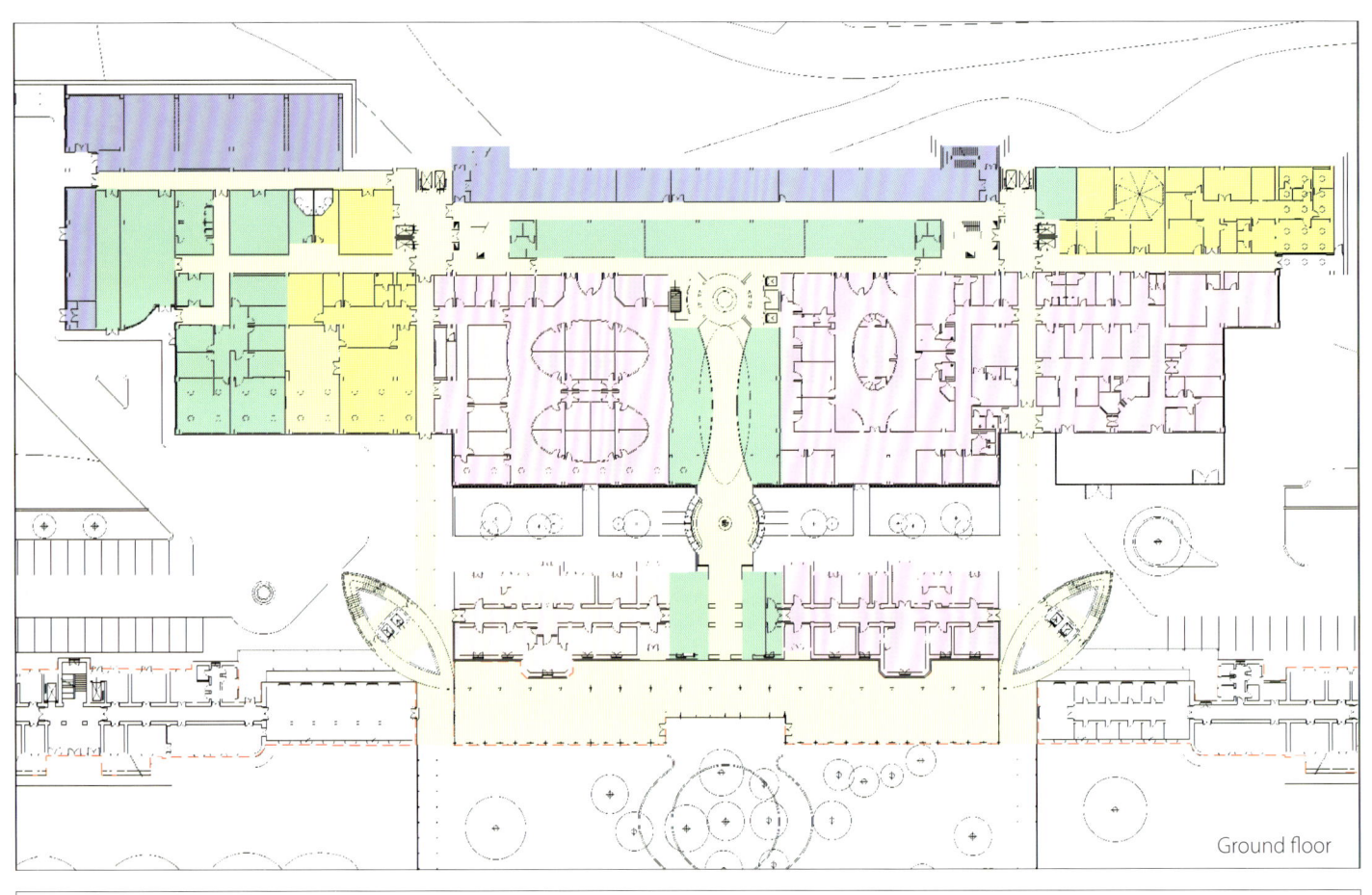

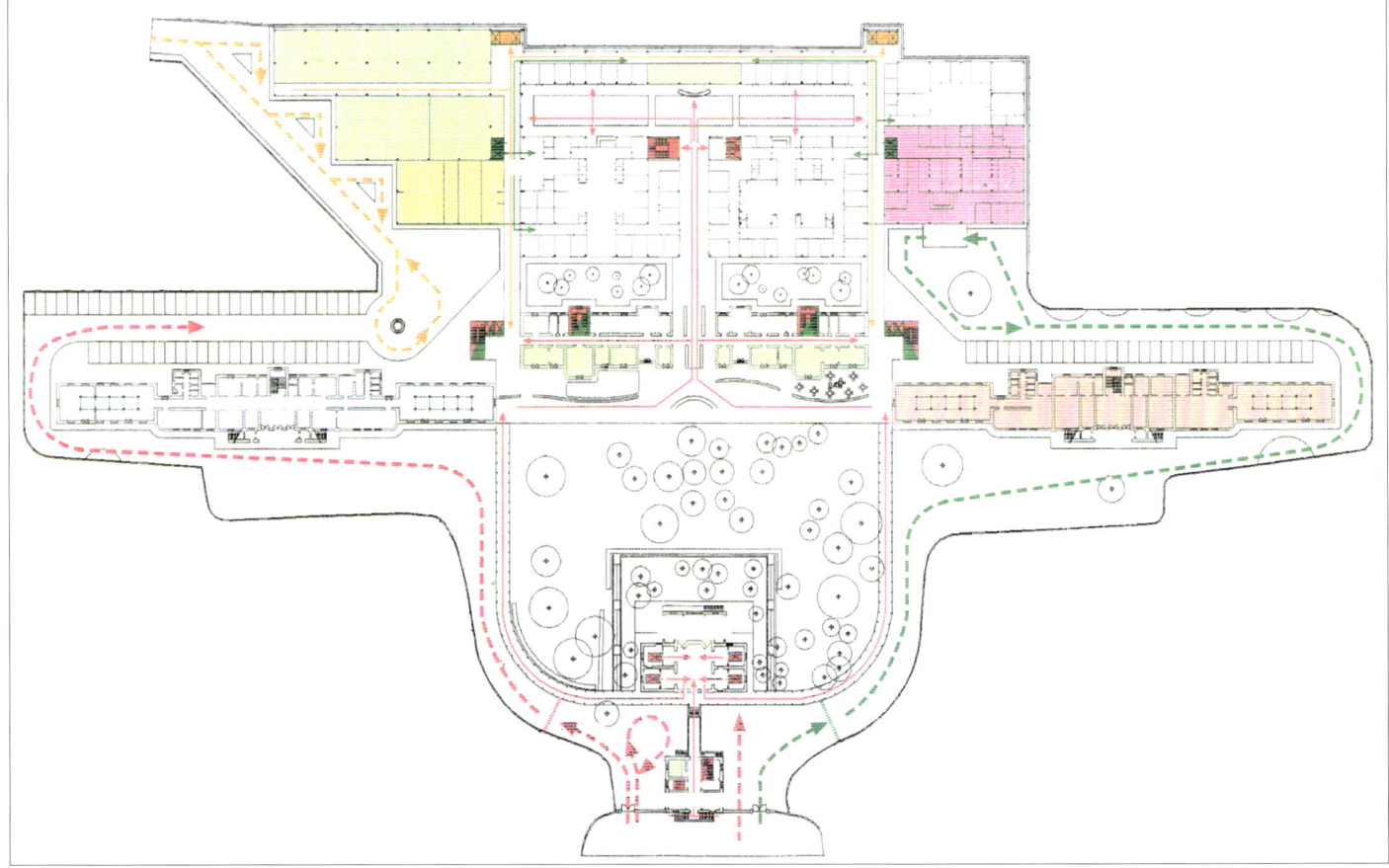

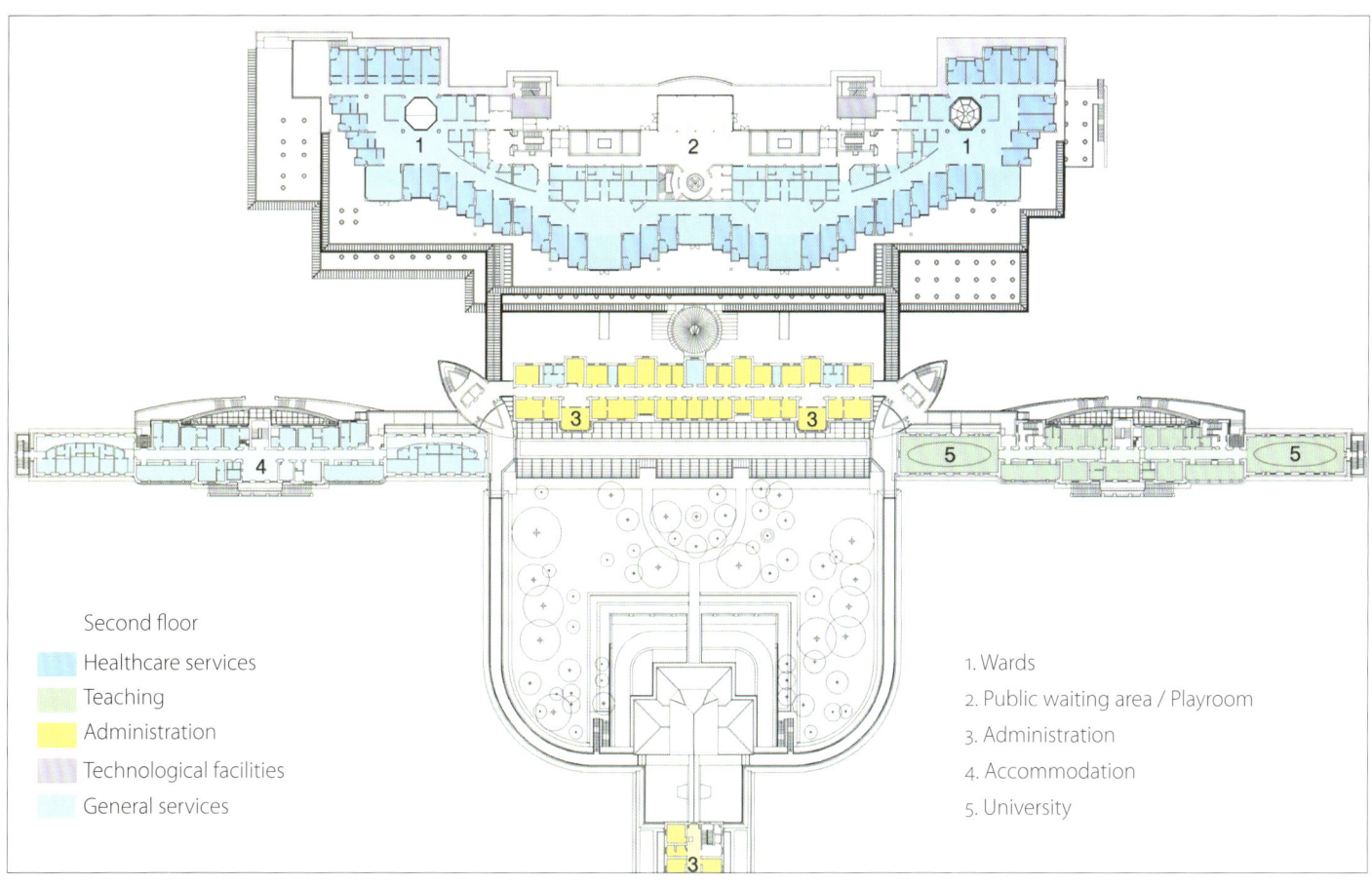

Second floor
- Healthcare services
- Teaching
- Administration
- Technological facilities
- General services

1. Wards
2. Public waiting area / Playroom
3. Administration
4. Accommodation
5. University

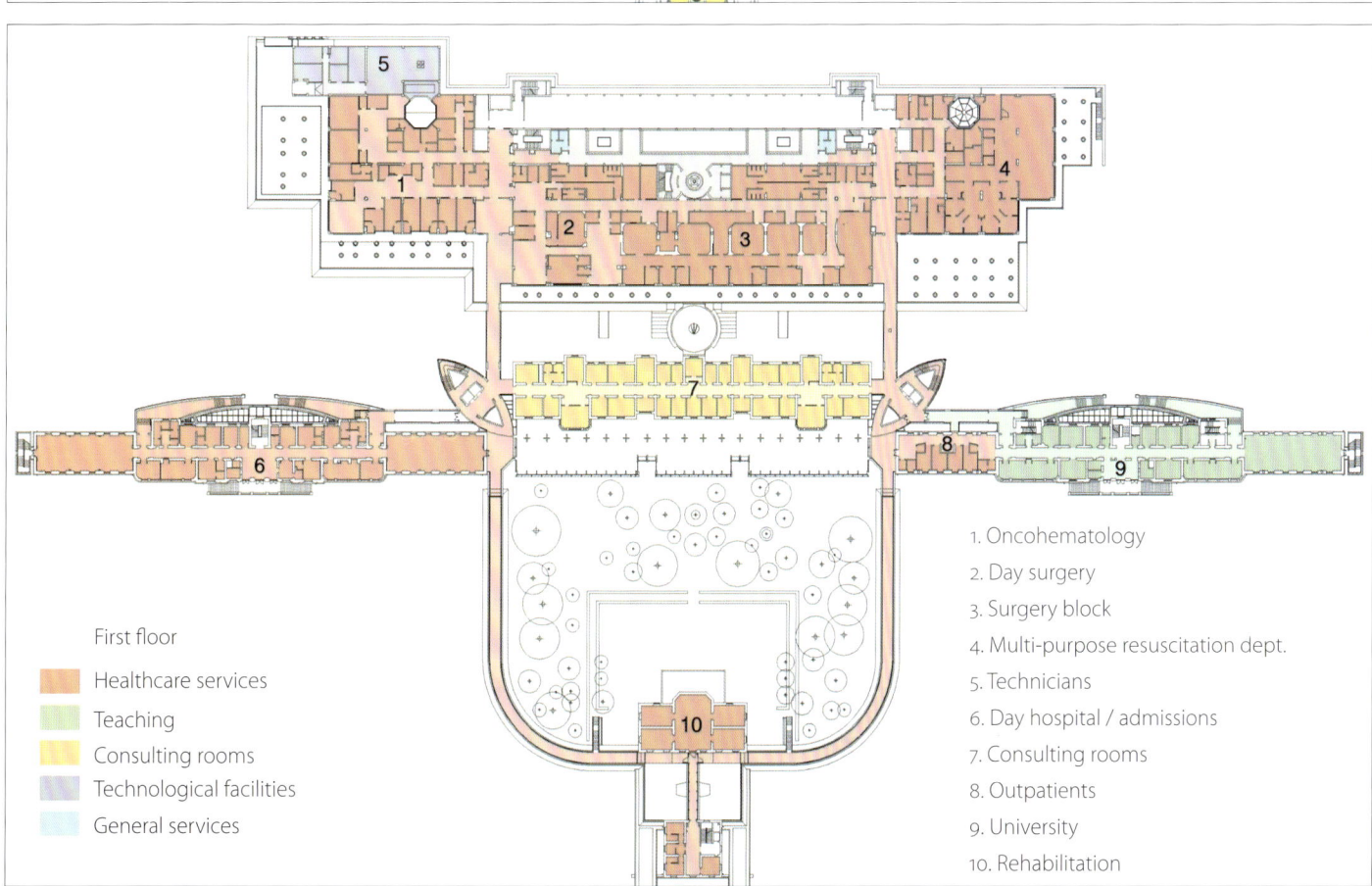

First floor
- Healthcare services
- Teaching
- Consulting rooms
- Technological facilities
- General services

1. Oncohematology
2. Day surgery
3. Surgery block
4. Multi-purpose resuscitation dept.
5. Technicians
6. Day hospital / admissions
7. Consulting rooms
8. Outpatients
9. University
10. Rehabilitation

285

NEW INTERVENTION

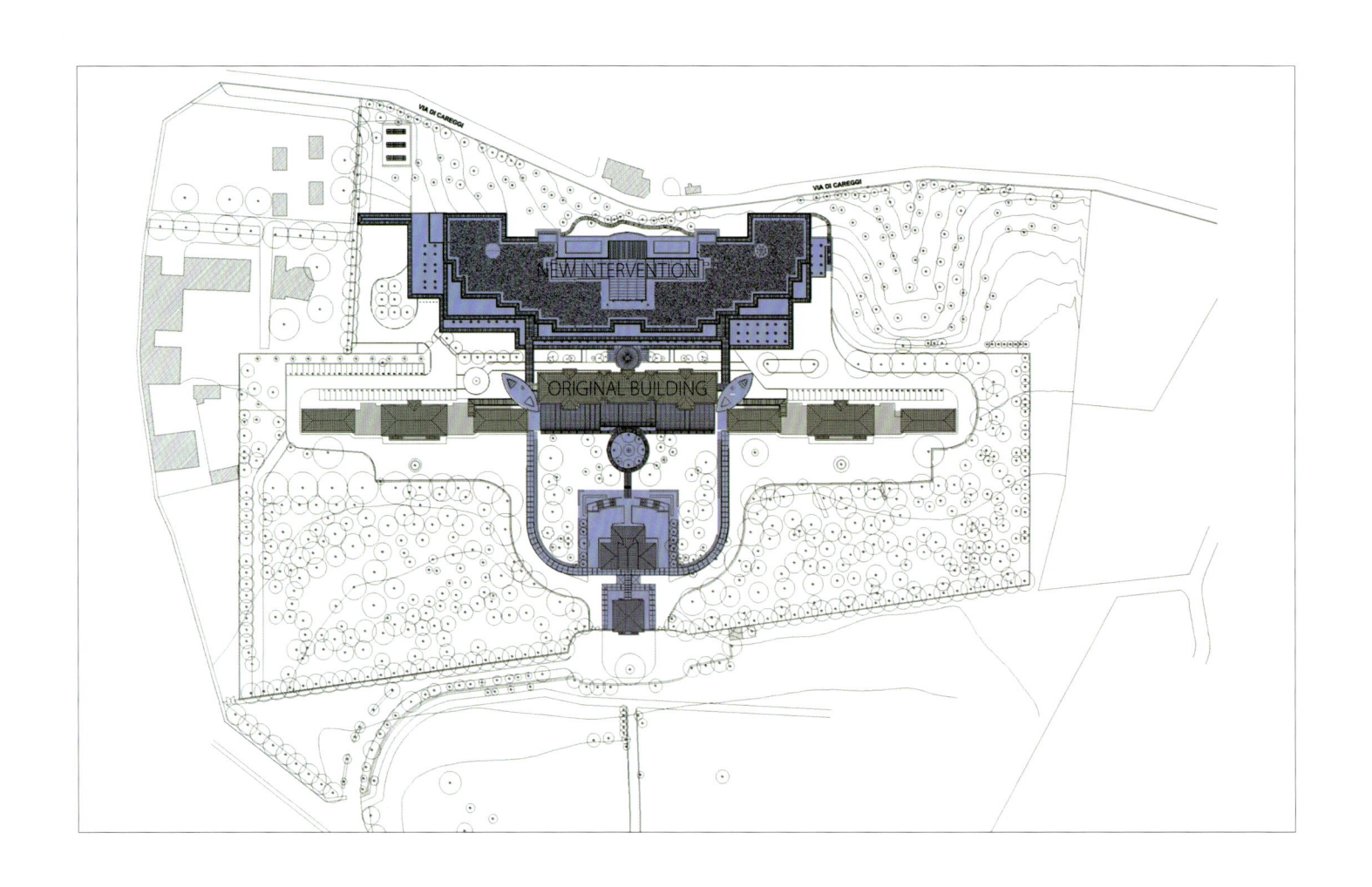

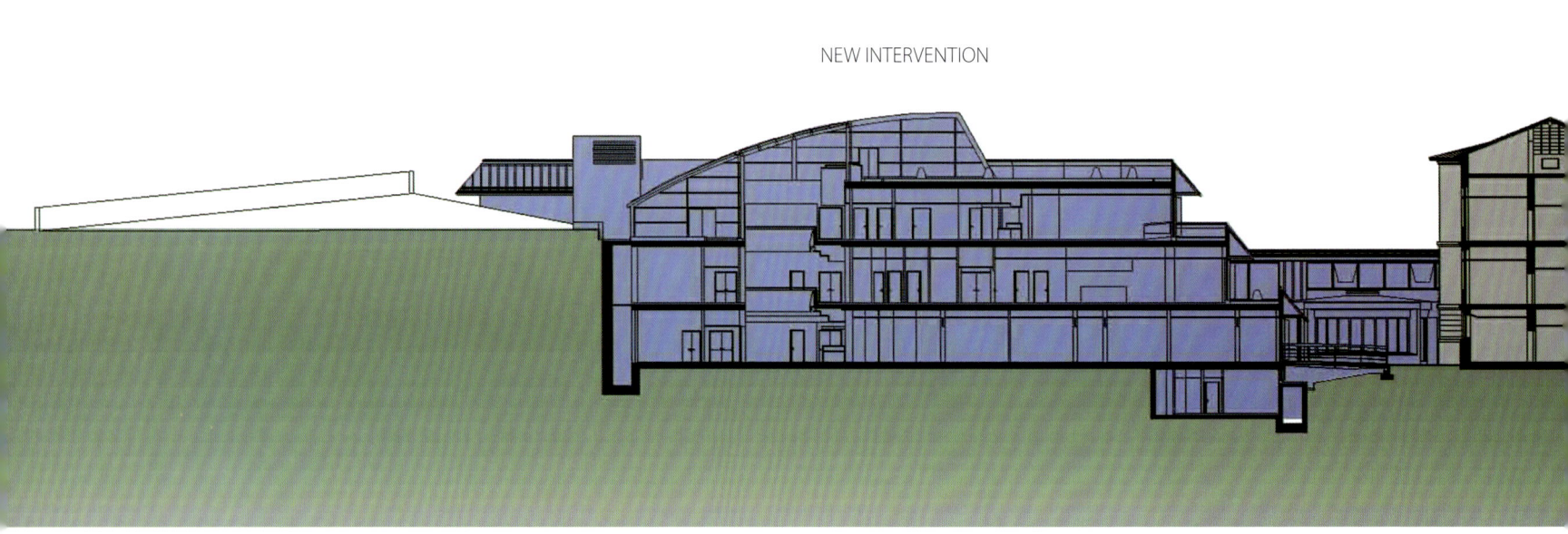

1. Wards
2. Administration
3. Medical hotel
4. Outpatients
5. Emergency room
6. University

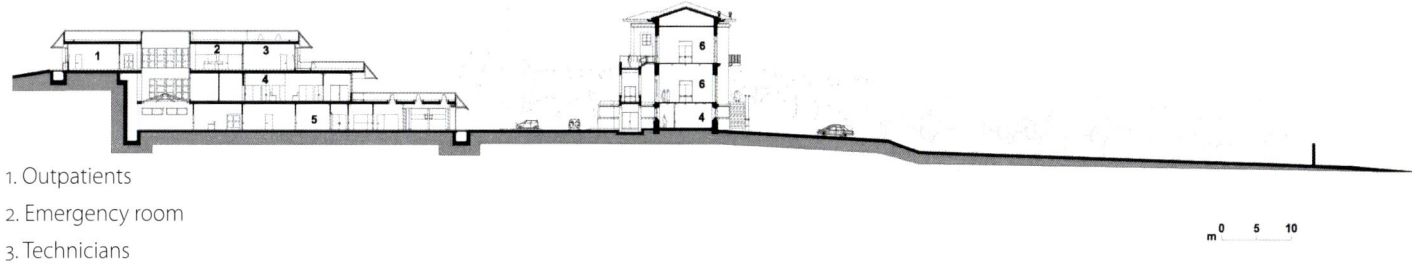

1. Outpatients
2. Emergency room
3. Technicians
4. Consulting rooms
5. Administration
6. Medical hotel
7. University
8. Conservatory

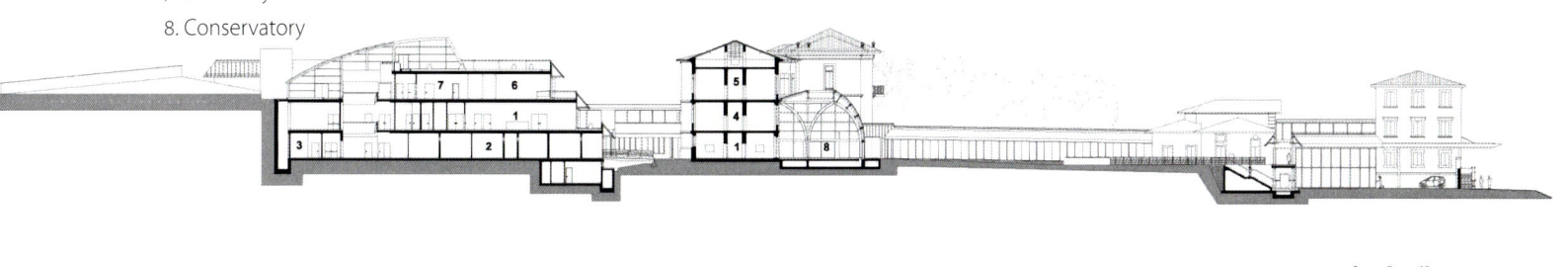

ORIGINAL BUILDING

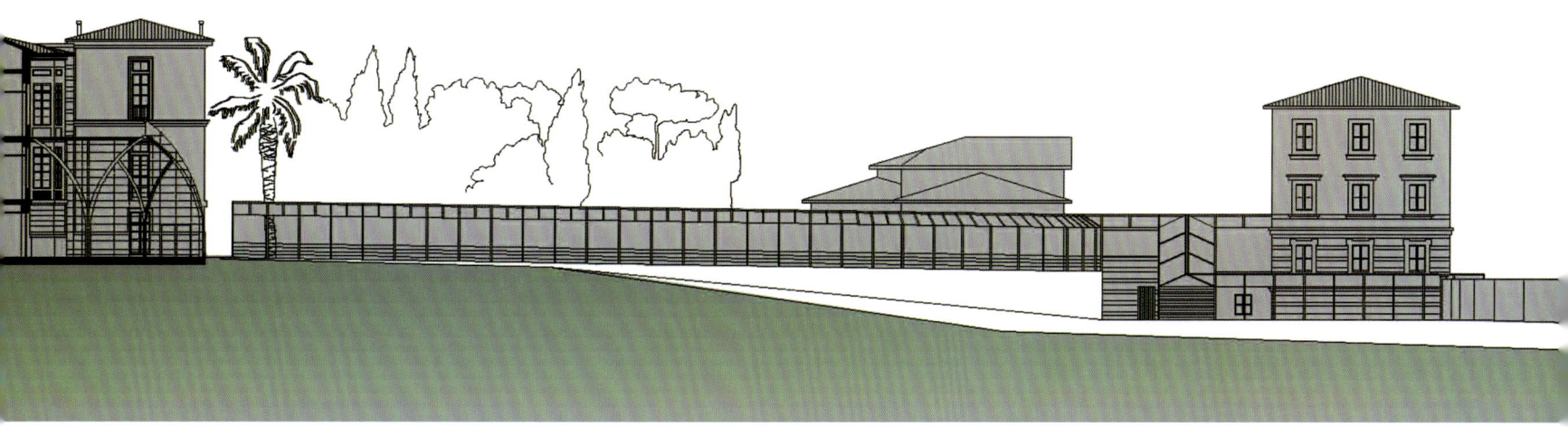

1. Wards
2. Personal work area
3. Medication room
4. Therapy preparation
5. Duty doctor's office
6. Kitchen
7. Ward manager's office
8. Parents' waiting room
9. Assisted bathroom
10. Pharmacy
11. Play area

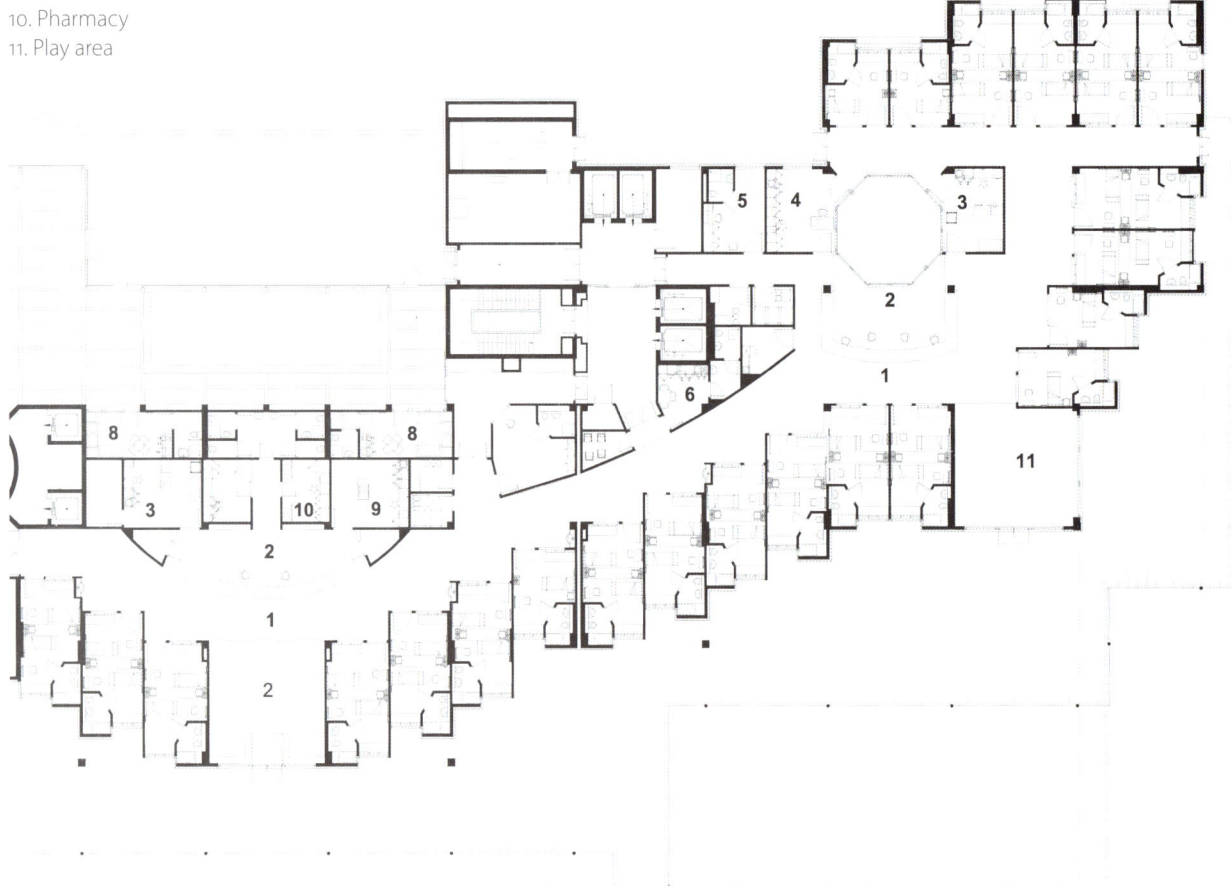

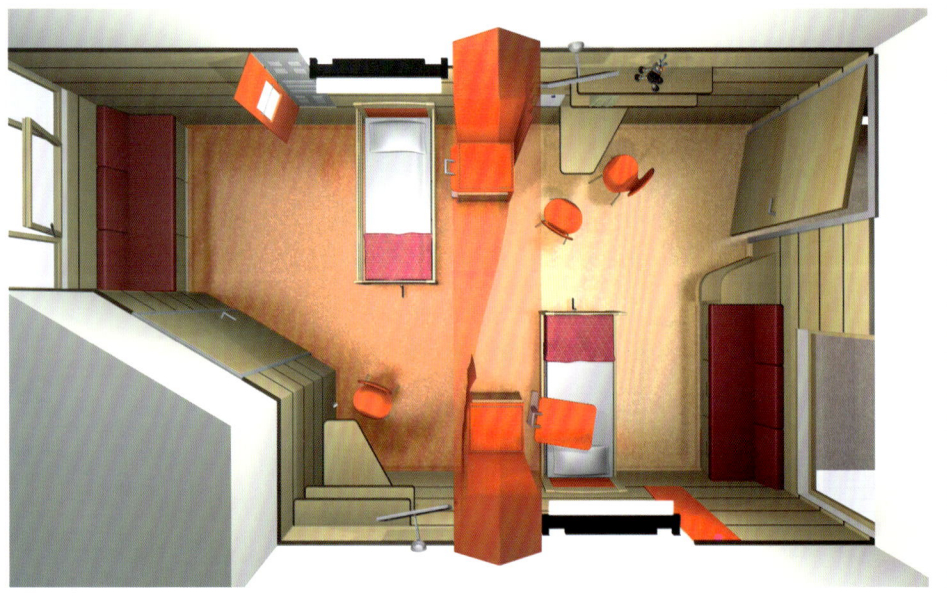

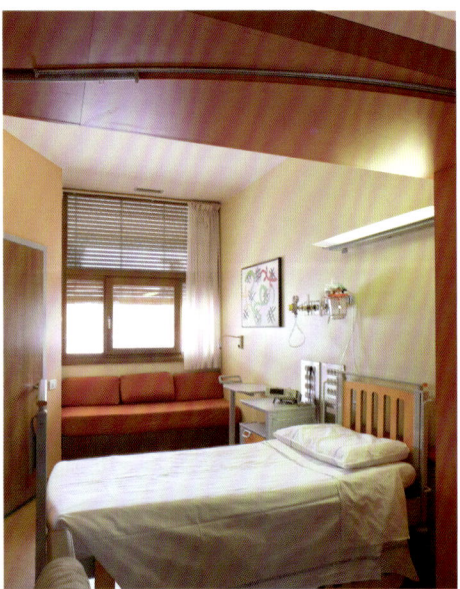

289

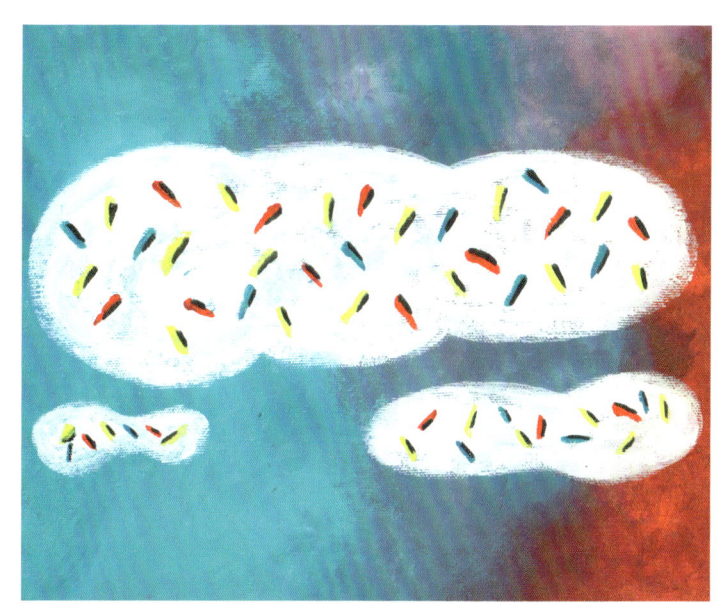

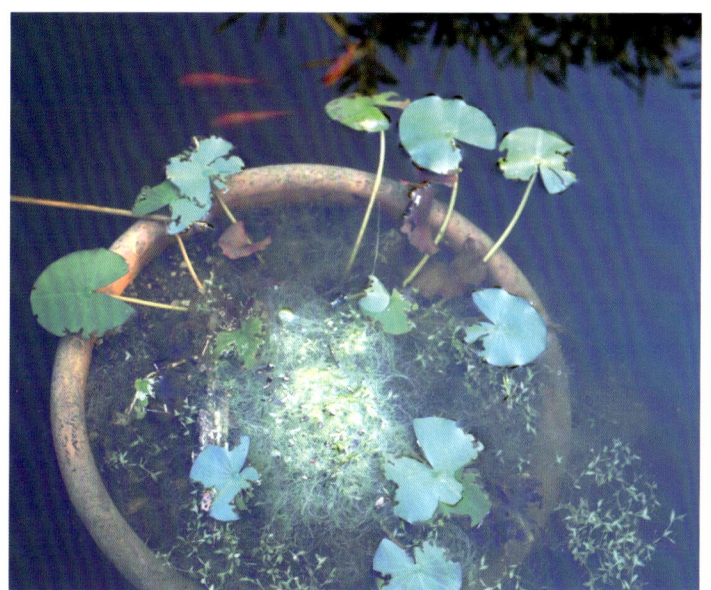

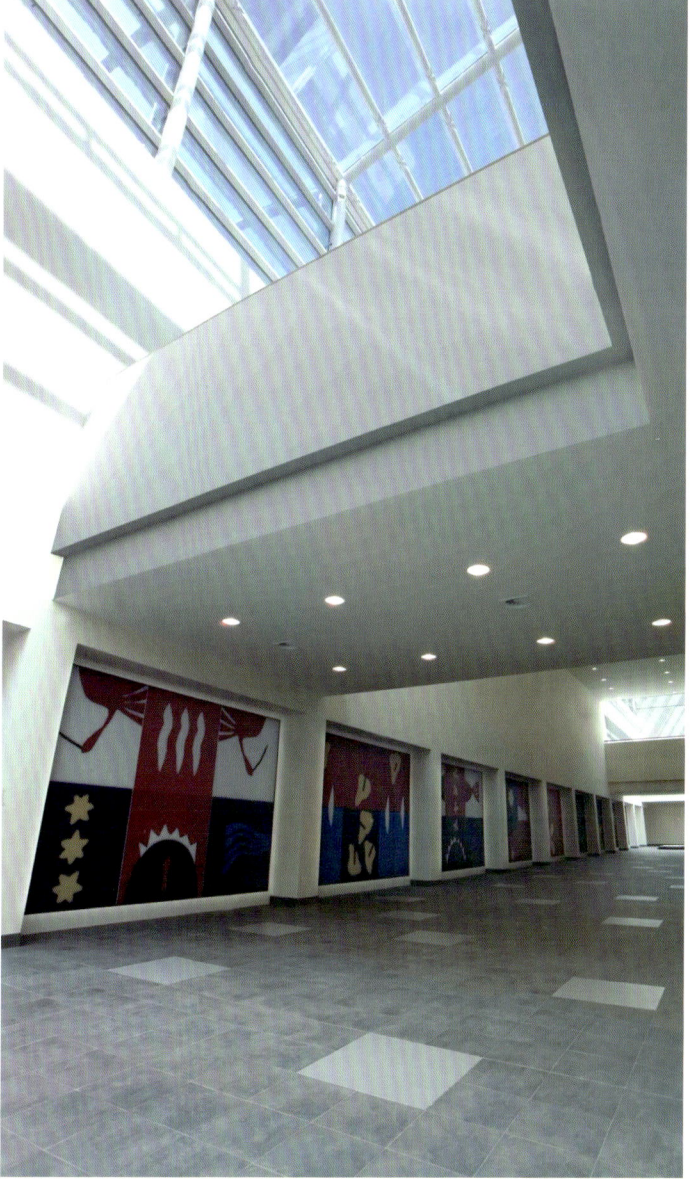

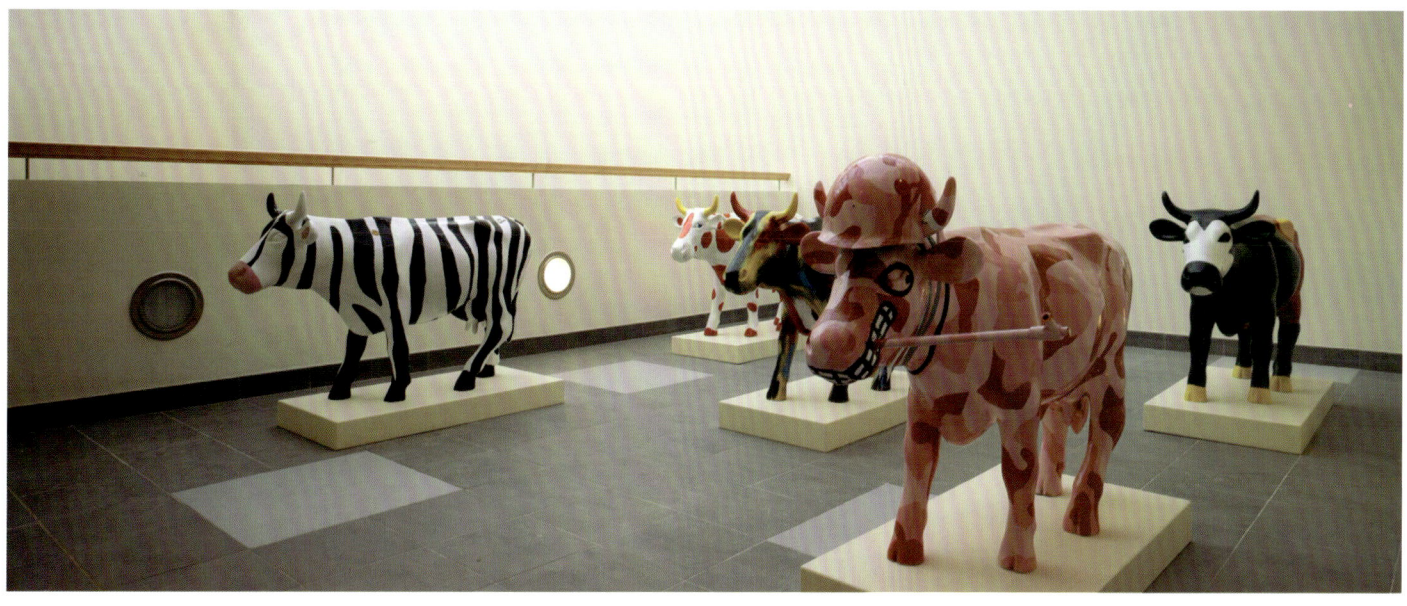

Anshen + Allen

The Bexley Wing, St James's Institute of Oncology

St James's University Hospital, Leeds, UK

Photographs: Fisher Hart

Located near Leeds city center on St James's University Hospital campus, the new Bexley Wing is the largest cancer research hospital in Europe. It has successfully centralized previously fragmented oncology services from dispersed locations to provide an impressive concentration of highly specialist and innovative clinical activities.

The principal architectural challenge presented by the site was organizing 67,000 sqm (700,000 sqft) of clinical and support space on a steeply sloping site of just 15,300 sqm (1650,000 sqft). To successfully integrate the building on this congested site, the issues of scale, massing and materials needed to be addressed. The design strategy broke down the massing of the building into vertical and horizontal elements, enabling natural light to penetrate deep into the hospital plan. The creation of an E-shaped block of three peninsula wings – comprising patient zone, outpatient, daycase and inpatient activity – is linked by a hi-tech spine of diagnostic and treatment facilities. The peninsular ward form breaks down the massing into a set of strongly modeled components that mitigate the density of the building on site. It also affords all patient bedrooms with views onto open-ended courtyards, many of which have distant views of the city skyline.

The wings and high-tech spine are linked by a glazed galleria that runs from the main entrance at the north to a secondary entrance at the south and which accommodates all public activity. Lifts take patients and visitors from the galleria to their designated floor and are strategically situated so that they are no more that 10 m (30 ft) away from the relevant treatment area. The integration of Cancer Research UK and the Yorkshire Cancer Network with the clinical areas encourages 'chance meetings' between researchers and clinicians, which in turn helps to promote translational research and effective bench-to-bedside treatment.

High quality materials were selected to create a sense of place within the community, and to act as a catalyst for the regeneration and reorganization of the campus. The size and scale of the building required a range of complementary materials. The design of the external envelope is based on a fully unitized system of copper, zinc and glazed panels, with brick and timber forming a podium at the lower levels and large expanses of curtain walling, all of which meets the strict energy targets for the new facility. The ward floors of the peninsular wings are clad in copper while the ambulatory floors below are glazed in curtain walling. The hi-tech spine is clad in zinc and aluminum rain screen paneling

Client:
Leeds Teaching Hospitals NHS Trust

Surface area:
37.000 sqm

Start date:
February 2002

Finish date:
December 2007

Contractor:
Bovis Lend Lease

SPV Lead:
Catalyst Lend Lease

Cost:
£232 million

Strategic Healthcare Planning:
RKW (now EC Harris)

Landscape Architect:
Plincke Landscape

Structural, Civil and Services Engineer:
Faber Maunsell

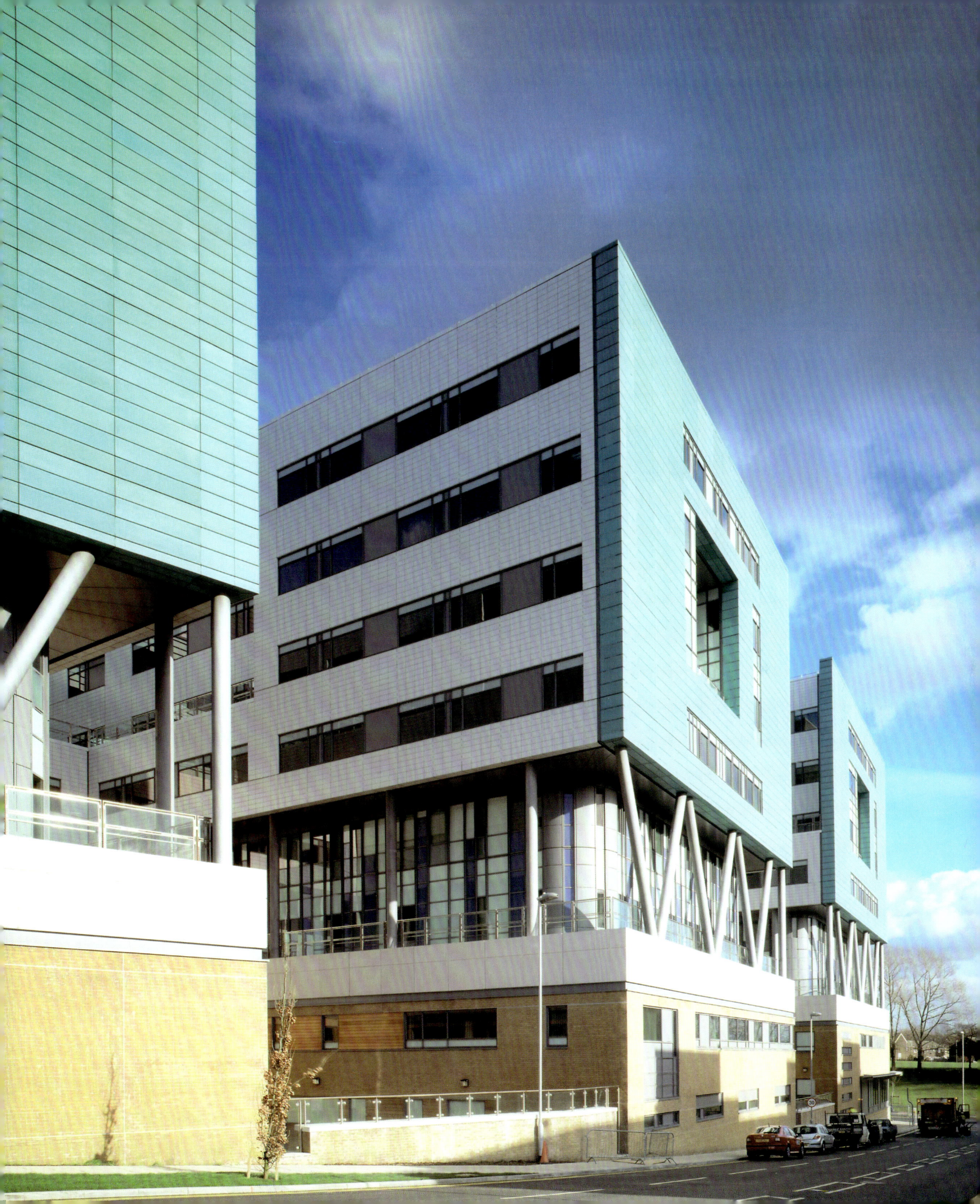

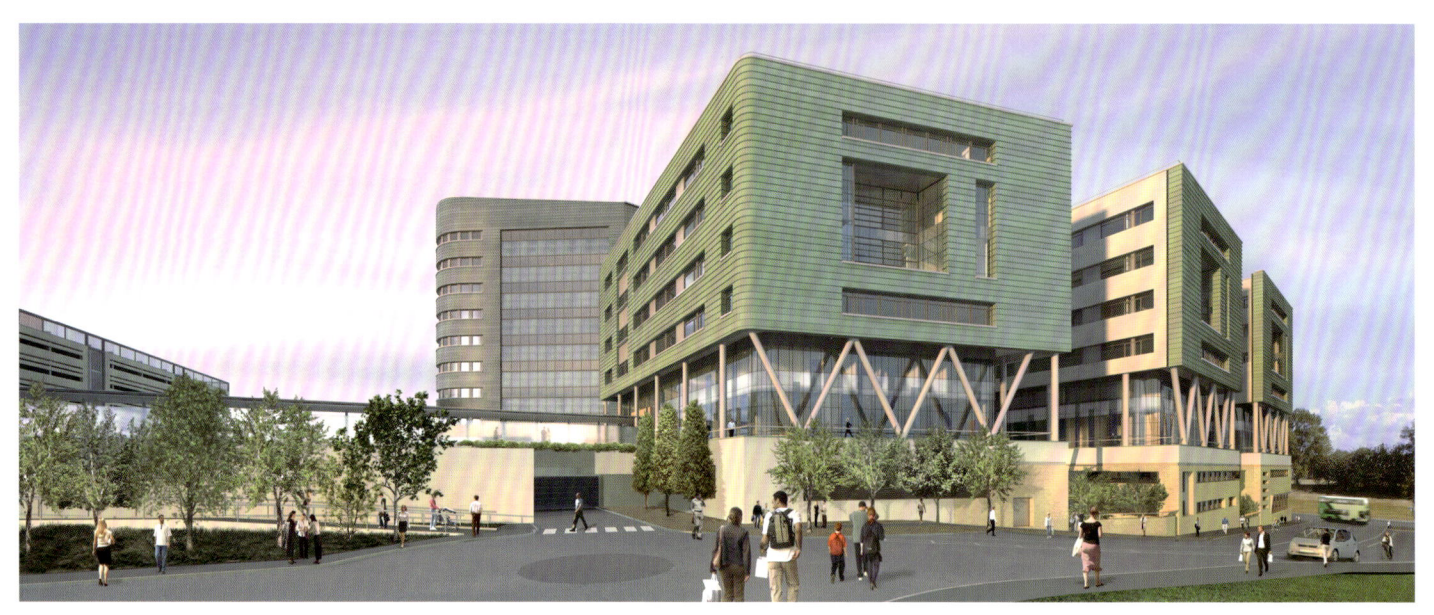

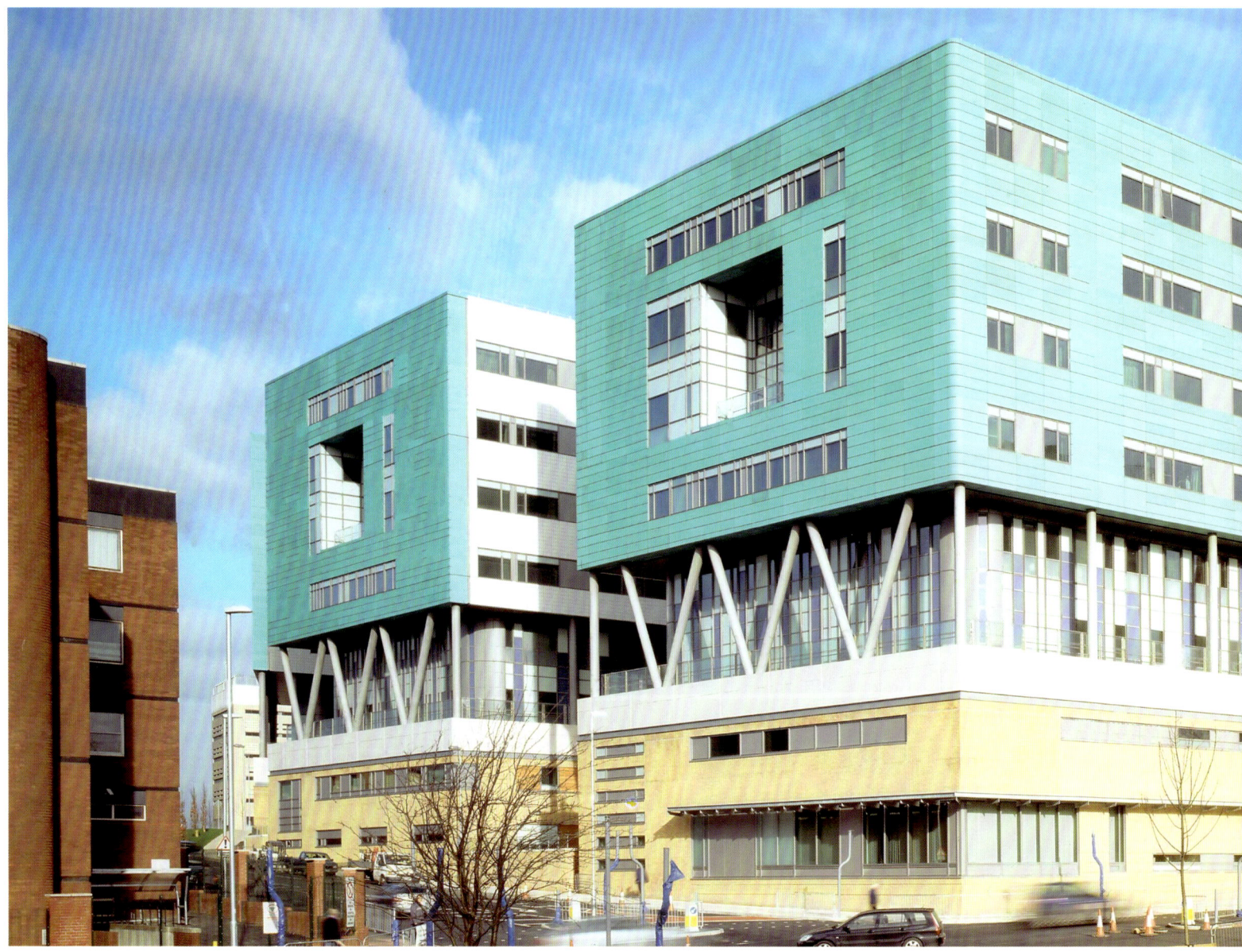

Site plan

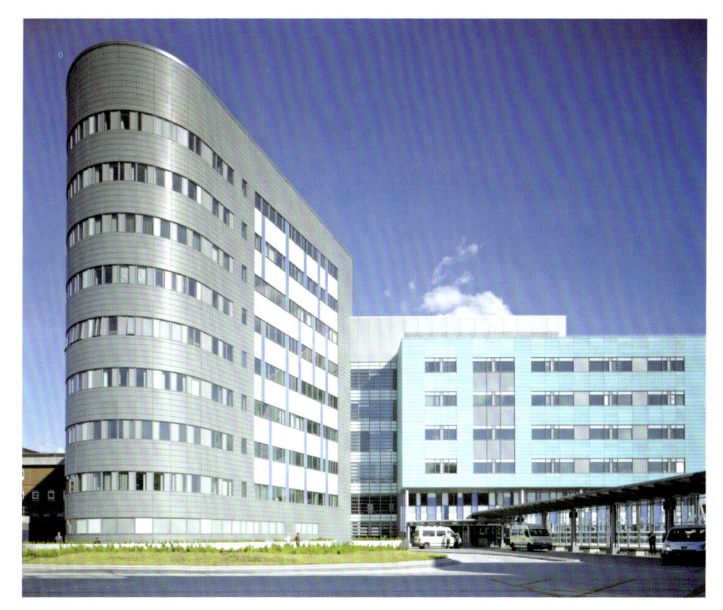

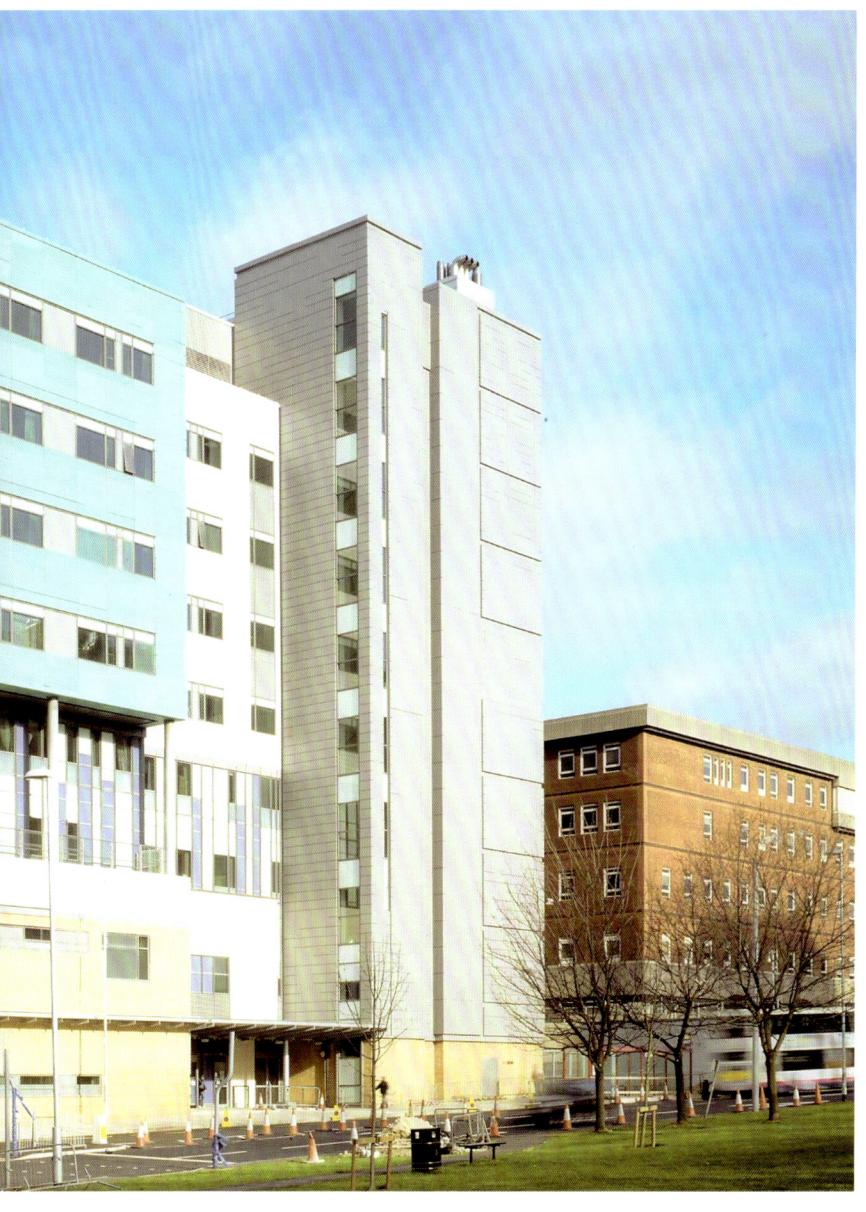

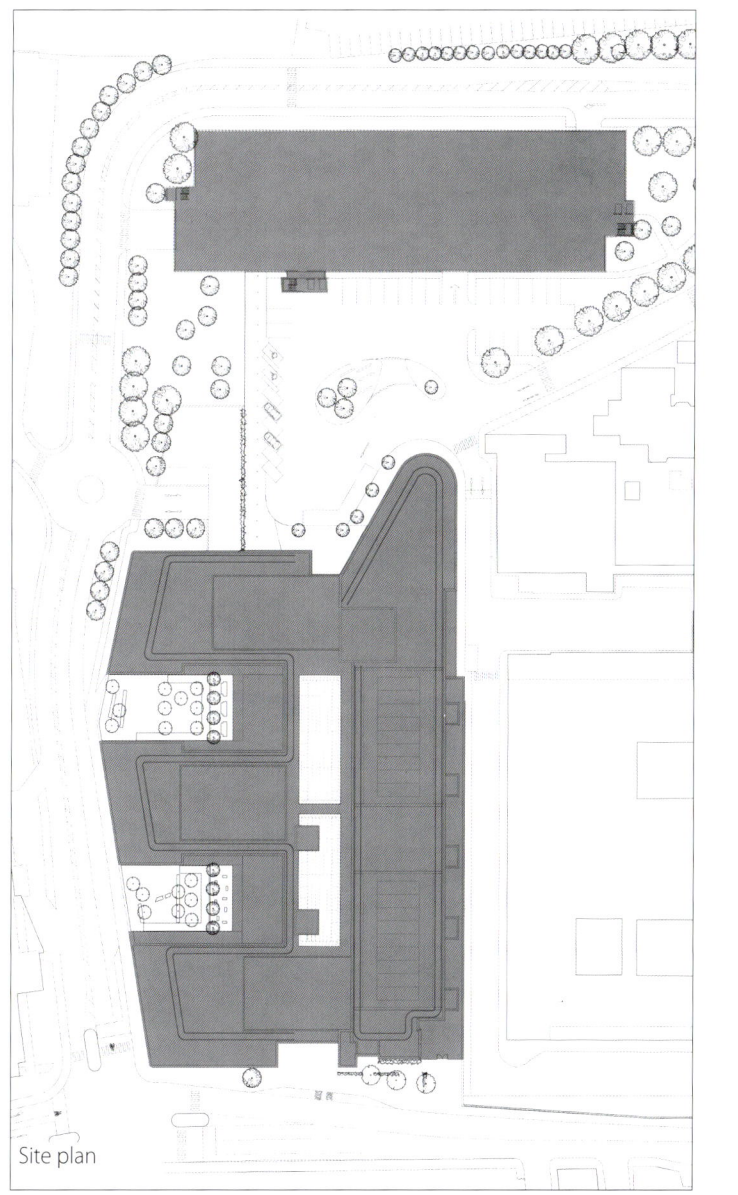

293

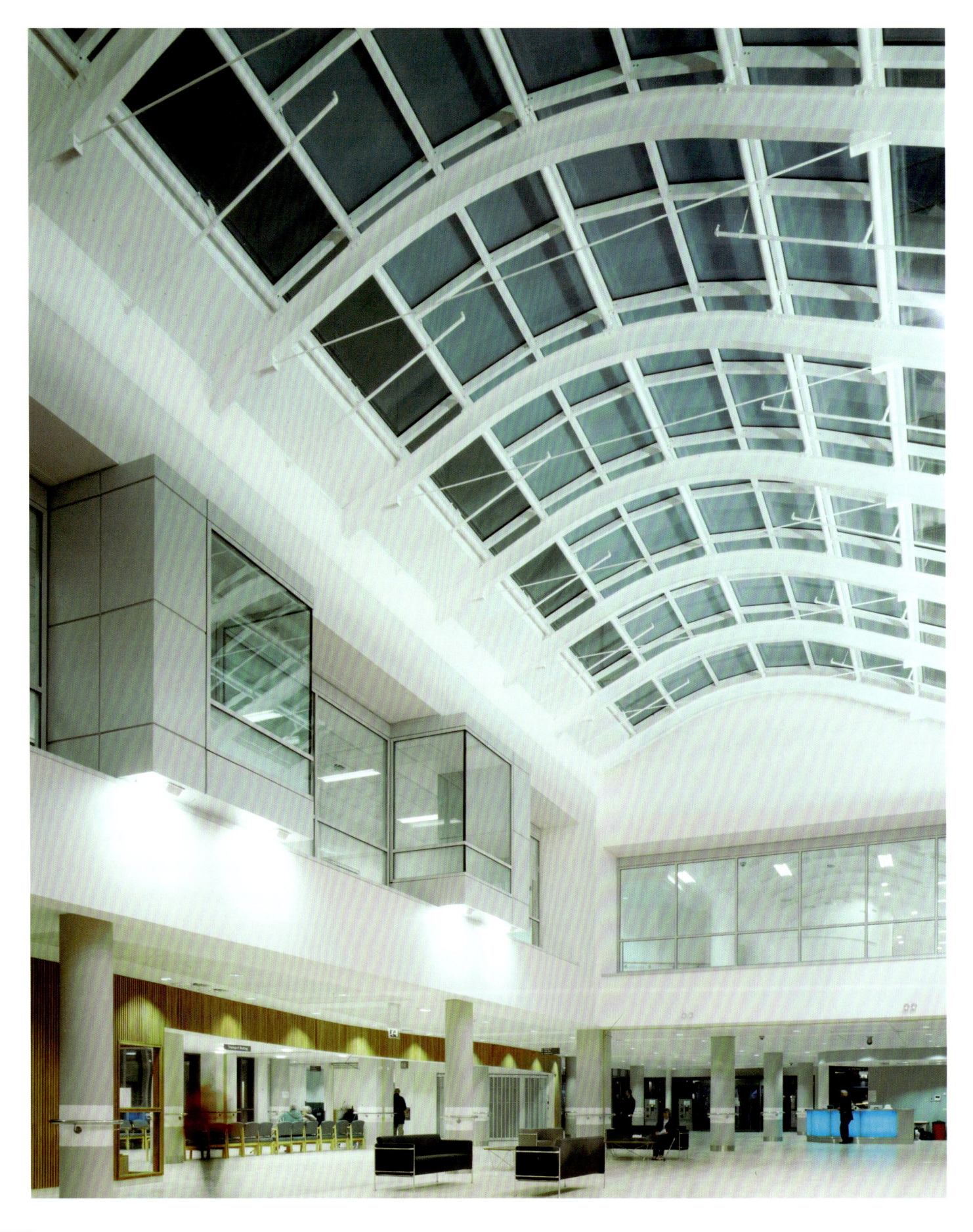

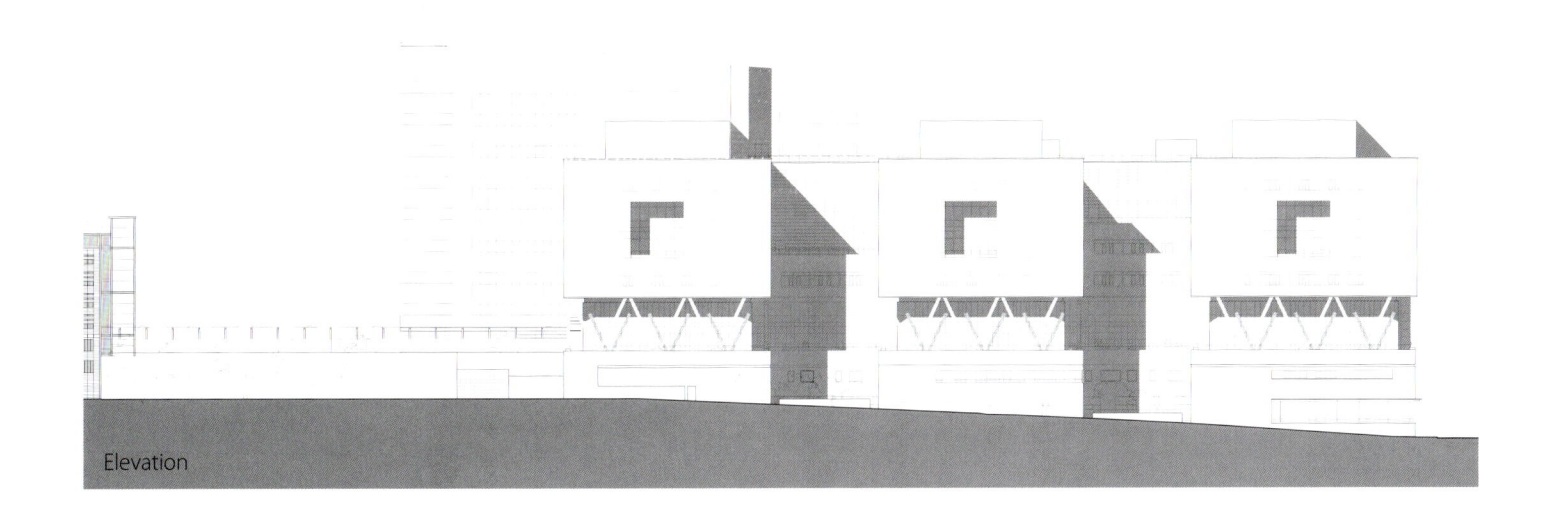

Elevation

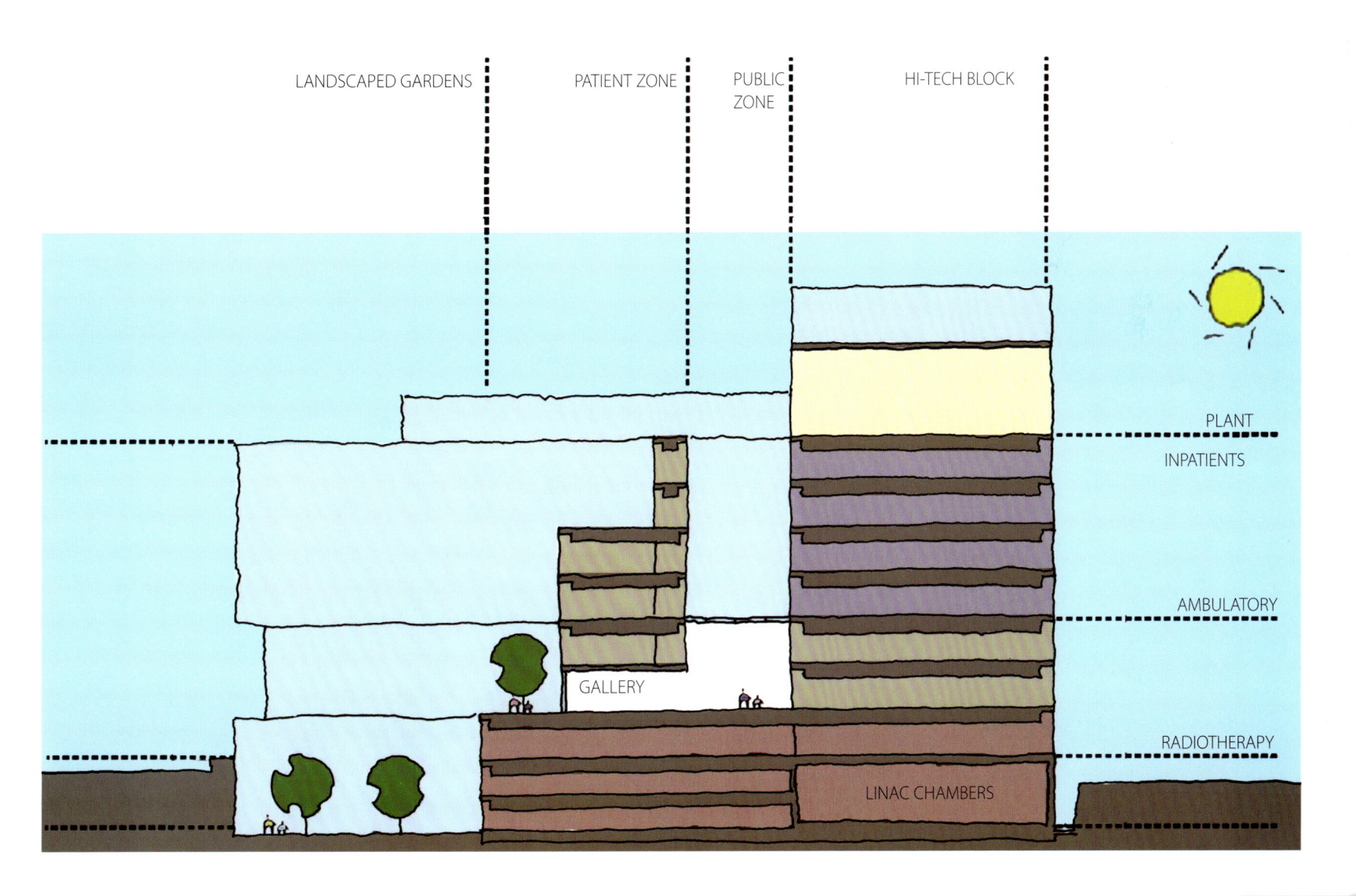

| LANDSCAPED GARDENS | PATIENT ZONE | PUBLIC ZONE | HI-TECH BLOCK |

PLANT
INPATIENTS
AMBULATORY
GALLERY
RADIOTHERAPY
LINAC CHAMBERS

295

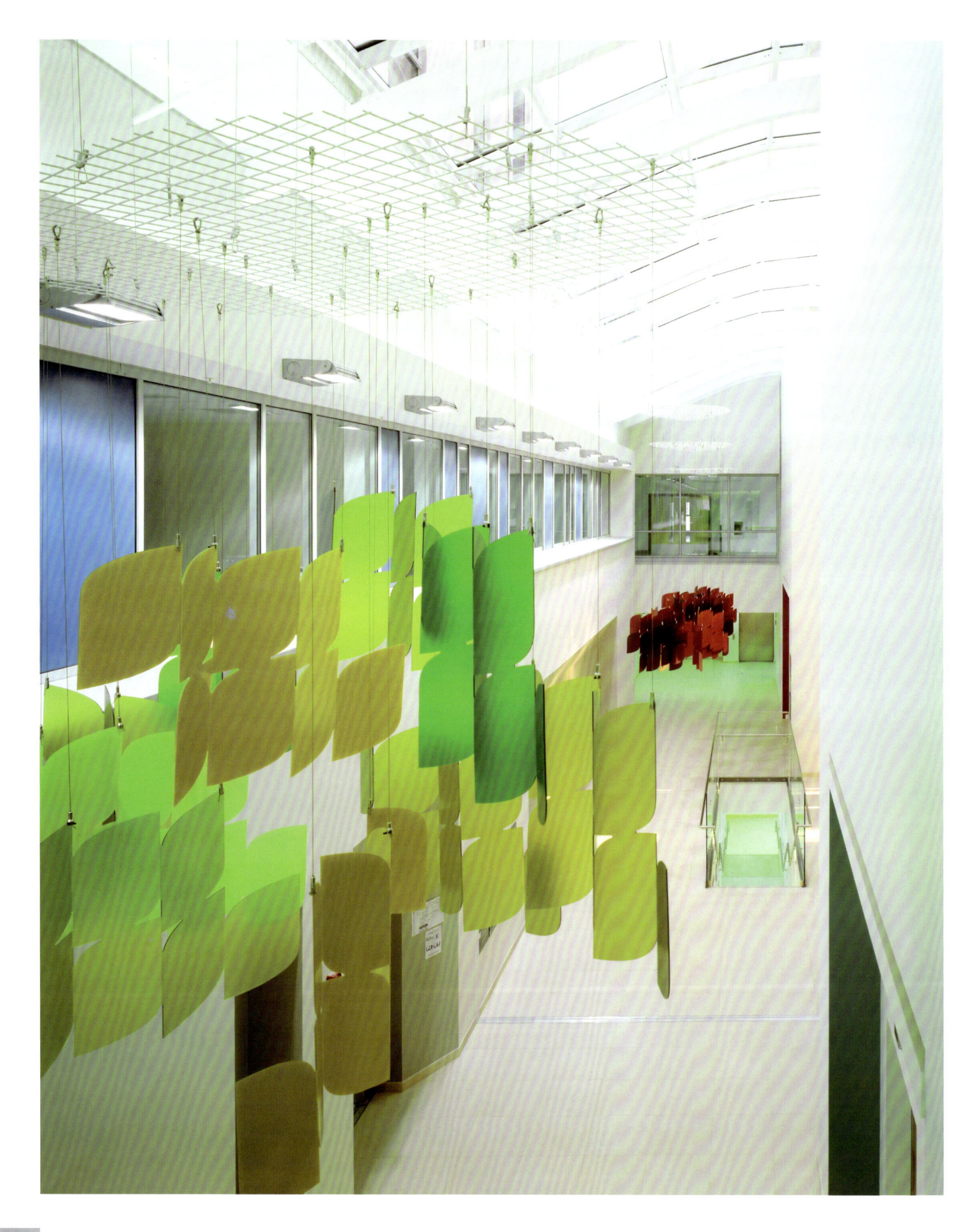

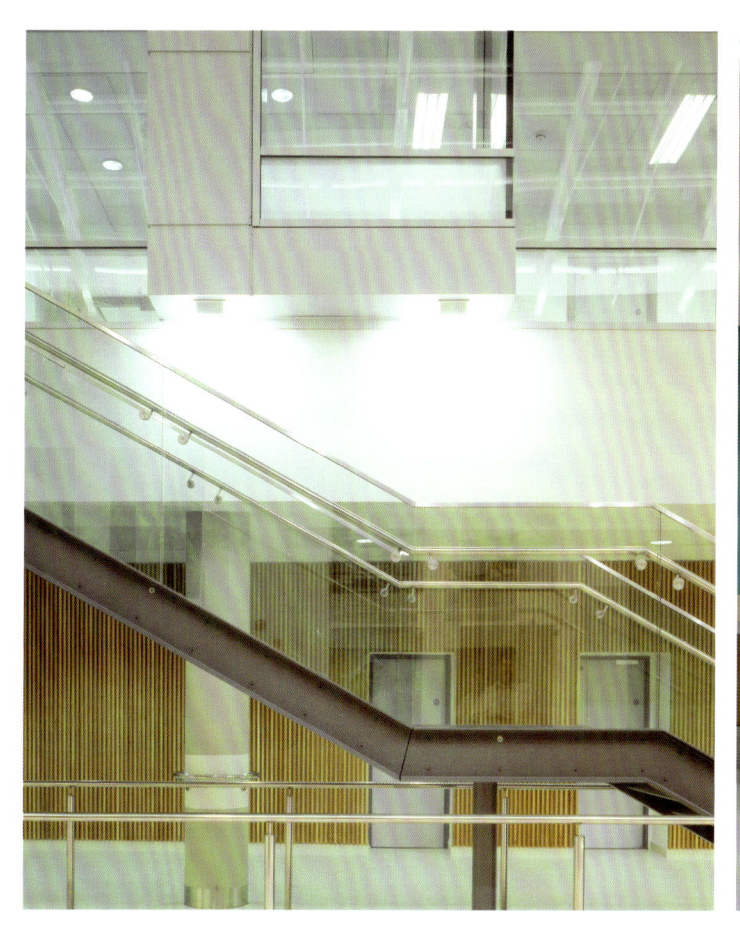

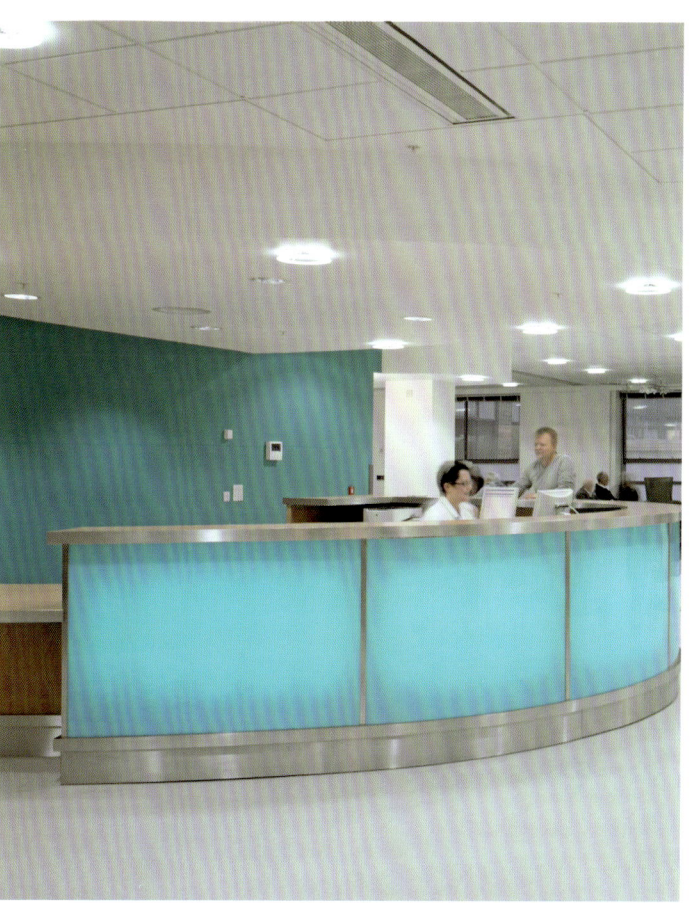

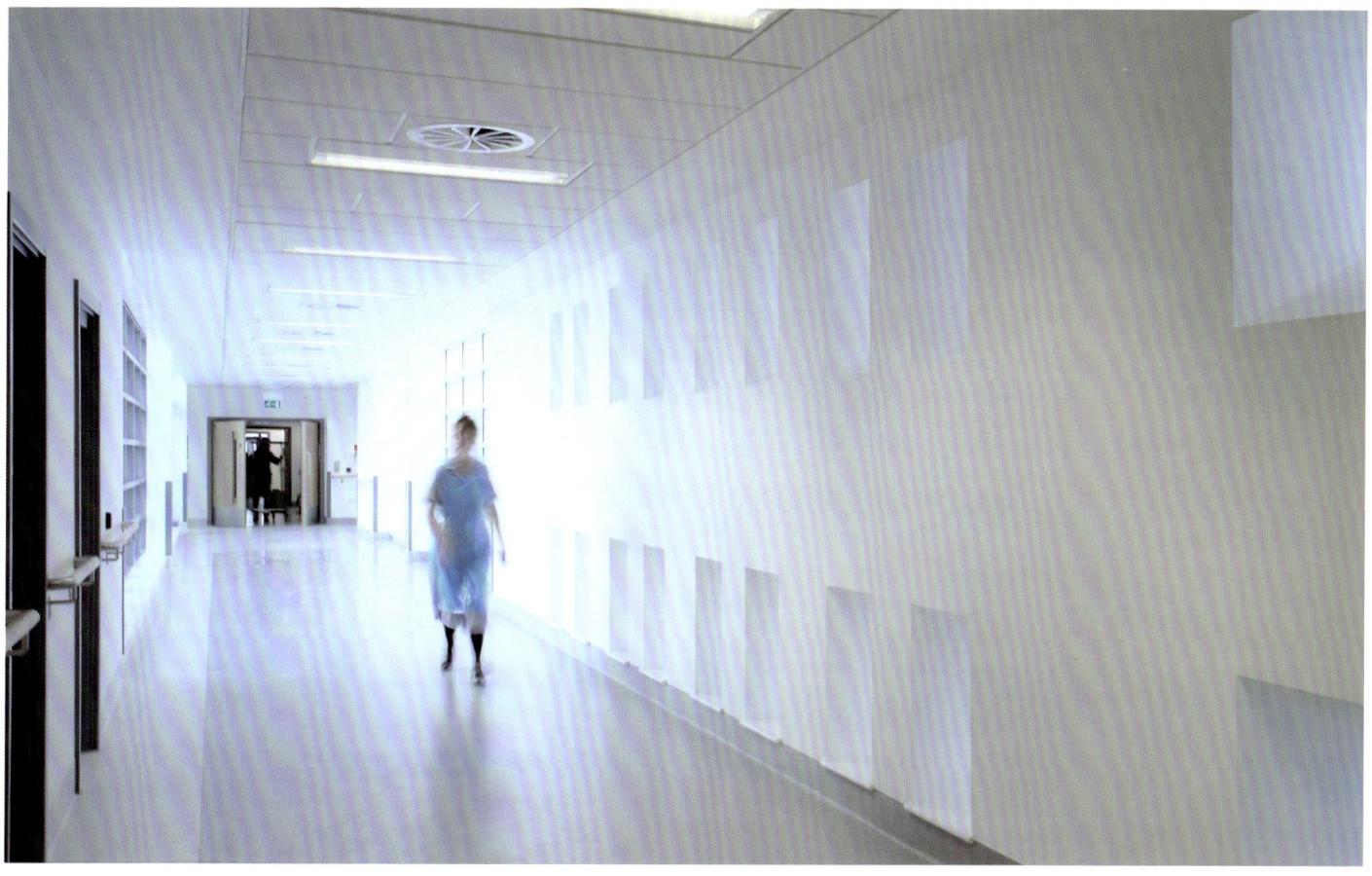

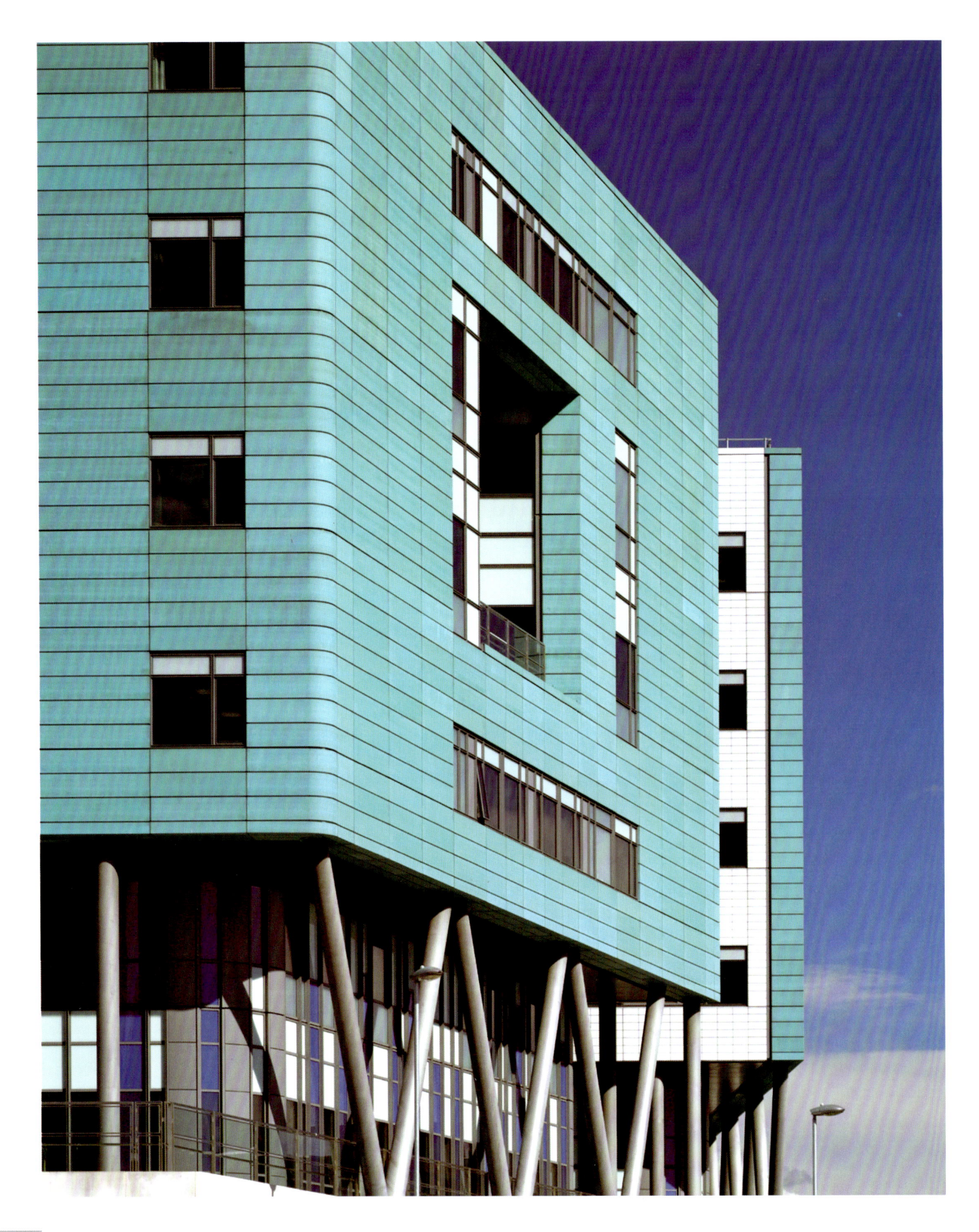

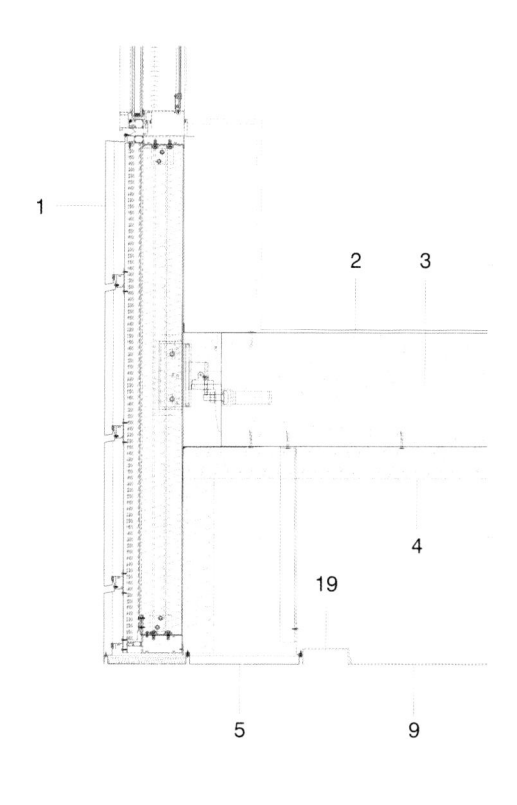

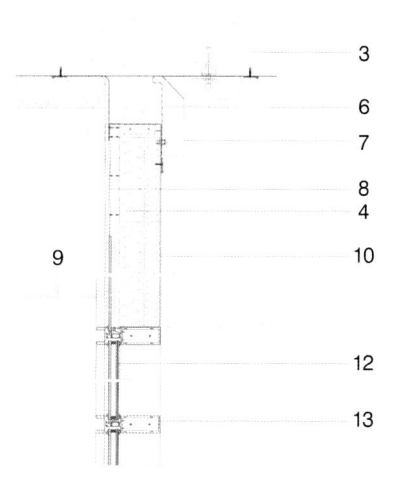

1. Outer face of unitized cladding pre-patinated copper
2. Floor finish
3. Concrete slab
4. Insulation
5. Suspended soffit, copper
6. Water proofing fixed back to backing tray of the unitized cladding system
7. Fixing bracket
8. Outer face of unitized cladding, PPC - Aluminum
9. Soffit, PPC - Aluminum
10. Backing tray of unitized cladding, galvanized steel
11. Back painted toughened single glazing
12. DGU with high performance solar and low-energy coating
13. Intermediate mullion
14. Interlocking frame of unitized cladding system
15. Fire / smoke stop between floors
16. 3 Dimensional adjustable fixing bracket connecting concrete slab with frame of unitized cladding
17. Suspended ceiling
18. Expressed capping on top of pressure cap of glazing system
19. Feature channel, PPC - aluminium
20. Base bracket of unitized cladding
21. Coping, pre-patinated copper
22. Outer face of unitized cladding pre-patinated copper
23. Cementious board
24. Continuous water proofing around upstand, fixed back to backing tray of unitized cladding system
25. Waterproofing line of inverted cold roofing system
26. Balustrade, stainless steel

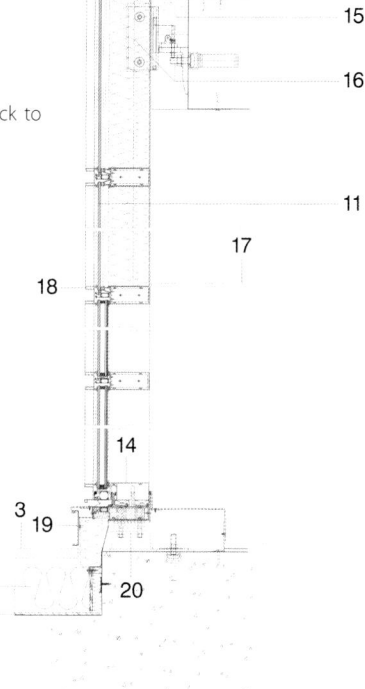

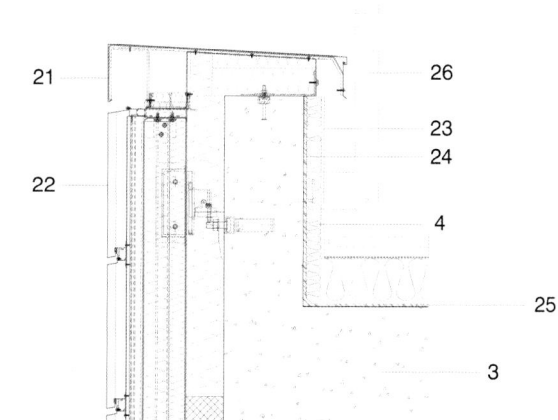